OPHTHALMOLOGY
principles and concepts

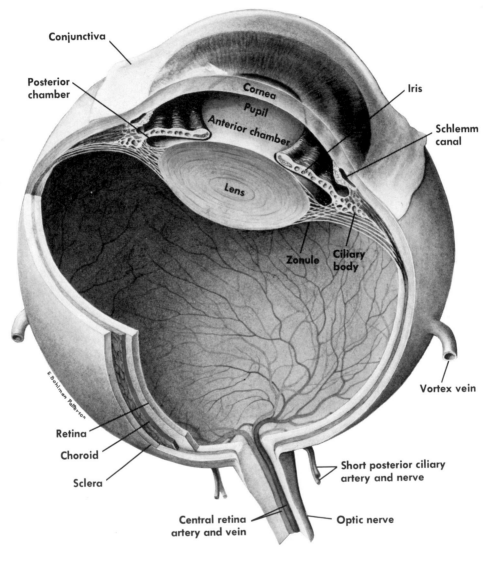

Conjunctiva

Posterior chamber

Cornea

Pupil

Anterior chamber

Iris

Schlemm canal

Lens

Zonule

Ciliary body

E. Bohlman Patterson

Vortex vein

Retina

Choroid

Sclera

Short posterior ciliary artery and nerve

Central retina artery and vein

Optic nerve

THE HUMAN EYE

OPHTHALMOLOGY

principles and concepts

FRANK W. NEWELL, M.D., M.Sc. (Ophth.)

The James N. and Anna Louise Raymond Professor,
Department of Ophthalmology,
The University of Chicago;
Profesor Extraordinario de Oftalmología,
Universidad Autónoma de Barcelona

SIXTH EDITION

with **422** *illustrations*
and **64** *color illustrations*

The C. V. Mosby Company

ST. LOUIS • TORONTO • PRINCETON   1986

MOSBY

A TRADITION OF PUBLISHING EXCELLENCE

Editor: Eugenia A. Klein
Cover design: Christine Leonard Raquepaw

Top Graphics
Project manager: Billie Forshee
Manuscript editor: Connie Leinicke
Book design: Joanne Kluba
Production: Judy Bamert, Susan Trail

SIXTH EDITION

The C.V. Mosby Company
11830 Westline Industrial Drive, St. Louis, Missouri 63146

Library of Congress Cataloging in Publication Data

Newell, Frank W.
  Ophthalmology: principles and concepts.

  Includes bibliographies and index.
  1. Ophthalmology. I. Title. [DNLM: 1. Eye Diseases. WW 100 N544o]
RE46.N57 1986   617.7   85-21366
ISBN 0-8016-3643-4

C/MV/MV 9 8 7 6 5 4 3 2 1   01/C/024

To
Marïan, Frank, Mary Susan,
Elizabeth Ann, and **David Andrew**

PREFACE

It is gratifying for me to prepare the sixth edition of *Ophthalmology: Principles and Concepts* 20 years after the first edition appeared. These years have seen exciting advances in ophthalmology: intraocular lenses, laser therapy, vitreous surgery, routine electron microscopy, computed tomography, new drugs, a new science of neurobiology, and many others. All of these have influenced clinical ophthalmology, and I have tried to make the text reflect their impact.

As in the past, I have been impressed with the scholarly volumes assigned to medical students in their classes in anatomy, physiology, pathology, pharmacology, medicine, and others. By bringing the lessons of these volumes to this textbook, I have tried to simplify the study of ophthalmology. An atlas of ophthalmic disorders has been added, together with a series of case histories of typical conditions likely to be encountered by a physician in any field.

Mrs. Karen Ku, of the audiovisual depart-ment of the University of Chicago Medical Center, prepared many illustrations. Mr. Charles Welleck, of the audiovisual department, Mr. Ernest Heath, and Mr. Joseph Barabe prepared many of the photographs. Mrs. Karin Cassel, my capable assistant of 23 years, was as always exceptional in the care with which she prepared material.

A generation of medical students have delineated their needs and their interests. Thousands of readers and contributors to the *American Journal of Ophthalmology* together with a dedicated staff have maintained my awareness of current trends in ophthalmology. The clinical photographs in the text and atlas reflect the diagnostic and therapeutic skills of many physicians past and present at the University of Chicago. My particular thanks go to the patients who have cooperated so fully in the often tedious teaching sessions and who have contributed so generously to clinical education.

Frank W. Newell

CONTENTS

PART ONE

BASIC MECHANISMS

1
ANATOMY AND EMBRYOLOGY

ANATOMY

Dissection of a fresh animal eye readily reveals the interrelationship of the intraocular tissues and the organization of the eye as a multichambered, nearly spherical structure. The surface anatomy is easily studied in a living subject by direct inspection using a small penlight for illumination and a +20 diopter lens for magnification.

THE EYE

The eye (frontispiece) rests in the front half of the cavity of the orbit upon a fascial hammock surrounded by ocular muscles, fat, and connective tissue. Only its anterior aspect is exposed, and it is protected by the bony orbital rim. Attached to the eye are four recti and two oblique muscles. These are innervated by the oculomotor (N III), trochlear (N IV, superior oblique muscle), and abducent (N VI, lateral rectus muscle) cranial nerves, which enter the orbit through the superior orbital fissure in the posterior orbit. The ophthalmic branch of the trigeminal nerve (N V) that transmits sensory fibers from the upper face and the eye also enters the cranial cavity through the superior orbital fissure. The optic nerve leaves the orbit through the optic foramen, which also transmits the ophthalmic artery and the sympathetic innervation of the eye. The exposed anterior one third of the eye consists of a central transparent portion, the cornea, and a surrounding white portion, the sclera. The sclera is covered with the bulbar conjunctiva, which is continuous with the palpebral conjunctiva lining the inner surface of the protective tissue curtains, the eyelids. The lacrimal gland is located in the upper outer portion of the bony orbit.

The anterior pole of the eye is the center of curvature of the cornea. The posterior pole marks the center of the posterior curvature of the globe, and it is located slightly temporal to the optic nerve. The geometric axis is a line connecting these two poles. The equator encircles the eye midway between the two poles (Fig. 1-1).

The anteroposterior diameter of the normal eye, measured by ultrasonic methods, is about 22 to 27 mm. The circumference is between 69 and 85 mm. In the average eye (24 mm in diameter), the equator is on the surface of the sclera 16 mm posterior to the corneoscleral limbus. The posterior pole is 32 mm behind the corneoscleral limbus. Internally the anterior termination of the sensory retina (ora serrata) is approximately 5.75 to 6.5 mm posterior to the termination of the Descemet membrane of the cornea (Schwalbe line) (Fig. 1-2).

The globe has three main layers, each of which is further divided. The outer supporting coat consists of the transparent cornea, the opaque sclera, and their junction, the corneoscleral limbus or sulcus. The middle layer, or the uvea, consists of the choroid, the ciliary body, and the iris, which contains a central opening, the pupil. The inner layer consists of the retina, which is composed of two parts, a sensory portion and the layer of retinal pigment epithelium.

The lens is a transparent structure located immediately behind the iris and supported in position by a series of fine fibers, the zonule. These are attached to the ciliary body and the capsule of the lens.

The eye encloses three chambers: (1) the vitreous cavity, (2) the posterior chamber, and (3) the anterior chamber. The *vitreous cavity*, by far the largest, is located behind the lens and zonule and is adjacent to the sensory retina. The *posterior chamber* is minute in size and is bounded by the lens and zonule behind and the iris in front. The *anterior chamber* is located between the iris and the posterior surface of the cornea and communicates with the posterior chamber through the pupil. Aqueous humor is secreted by the ciliary processes into the

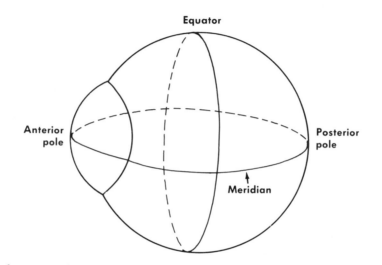

Fig. 1-1. The principal coordinates of the eye. The visual line that connects an object in space with the fovea centralis does not correspond exactly to the geometric axis, which connects the anterior to the posterior pole.

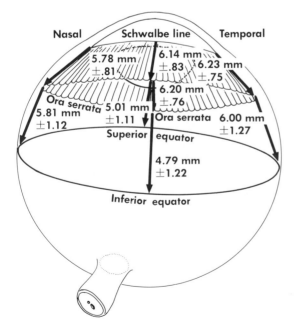

Fig. 1-2. The relationship of the ora serrata to the line of Schwalbe and to the equator of the eye. The measurements are determined in millimeters from the internal surfaces in the four principal meridians. The average measurements and the standard deviations are shown. The average internal diameter at the equator is 24.08 ± 0.94 mm. (Redrawn from Straatsma, B.R., Landers, M.B., and Kreiger, A.E.: Arch. Ophthalmol. **80:**30, 1968. Copyright 1968, American Medical Association.)

posterior chamber and passes through the pupil into the anterior chamber. The aqueous humor leaves the anterior chamber through the trabecular meshwork that opens into the canal of Schlemm, an endothelium-lined channel that encircles the anterior chamber.

Outer coat

The outer coat of the eye consists of relatively tough fibrous tissues shaped as segments of two spheres: the sclera, with a radius of curvature of about 13 mm, and the cornea, with a radius of curvature of about 7.5 mm. The white, opaque sclera constitutes the posterior five sixths of the globe, and the transparent cornea provides the anterior one sixth of the globe. The junction of the cornea and the sclera, the corneoscleral limbus, contains the trabecular meshwork and the aqueous humor drainage system, the canal of Schlemm, which is an important functional and anatomic area.

The sclera. The sclera is a dense, fibrous, collagenous structure that comprises the pos-terior five sixths of the eye. Anteriorly, it forms the "white" of the eye and is covered with a richly vascular episclera, the fascia bulbi (Tenon capsule), and the conjunctiva. The fine blood vessels of the episclera are visible anteriorly through the transparent conjunctiva. Posteriorly, the sclera is connected by loose, fine collagen fibers to the dense fascia bulbi (Tenon capsule).

The sclera has two large openings, the anterior and posterior scleral foramina, and numerous smaller openings through which nerves and blood vessels pass. The sclera is perforated 3 mm medial to the posterior pole by the posterior scleral foramen, the canal through which the optic nerve and central retinal vein leave the eye and through which the central retinal artery enters the eye. The canal is cone-shaped and measures 1.5 to 2.0 mm in diameter on the inner surface of the sclera and 3.0 to 3.5 mm on the outer surface. The scleral foramen is bridged by a sievelike structure, the lamina cribrosa (Fig. 1-3), the most posterior portion of

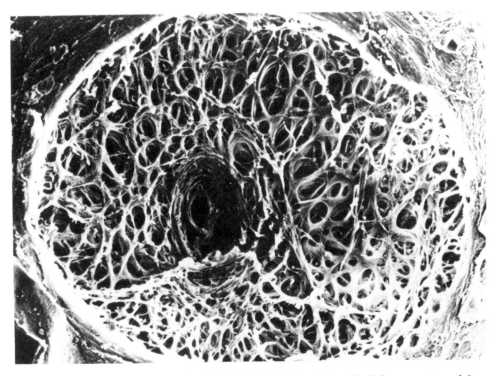

Fig. 1-3. Scanning electron micrograph of the human posterior scleral foramen viewed from the vitreous cavity. It is bridged by a sievelike structure, the lamina cribrosa. (With permission from Miller, N.R.: Walsh and Hoyt's clinical neuro-ophthalmology, ed. 4, vol. 1, Baltimore, 1982, The Williams & Wilkins Co.)

which is formed by scleral fibers. The anterior portion, derived from the choroid and Bruch membrane, is rich in elastic tissue.

The anterior sclera foramen is bridged by the transcript cornea. The anterior scleral foramen is bounded by a transitional area between the cornea and sclera. On its inner surface is the scleral spur to which the longitudinal portion of the ciliary muscle (N III) is attached. Slightly anterior to this is the canal of Schlemm.

About 4 mm posterior to the equator of the eye in the region between the recti muscles are the openings for the vortex veins that are the collecting channels for choroidal veins. In the area surrounding the optic nerve, the sclera is perforated by the long and short ciliary nerves and the long and short posterior ciliary arteries. About 4 mm posterior to the corneoscleral limbus and just anterior to the insertions of the recti muscles, the anterior ciliary arteries pierce the sclera at a site sometimes marked with a dot of uveal pigment. Occasionally a loop of a long ciliary nerve penetrates into the sclera, returns to the ciliary body, and with uveal melanin appears as a small pigmented dot 2 to 4 mm from the corneoscleral limbus.

The sclera is thickest (1.0 mm) in the region surrounding the optic nerve, where the meningeal coverings (mainly dura mater) of the nerve blend into the sclera. It is thinnest (0.3 mm) immediately posterior to the insertions of the recti muscles.

Structure. The sclera (Fig. 1-4) has three parts: (1) the episclera, (2) the scleral stroma, and (3) the lamina fusca.

The *episclera* is the outermost layer. It is a moderately dense, vascularized connective tissue that merges with the scleral stroma and

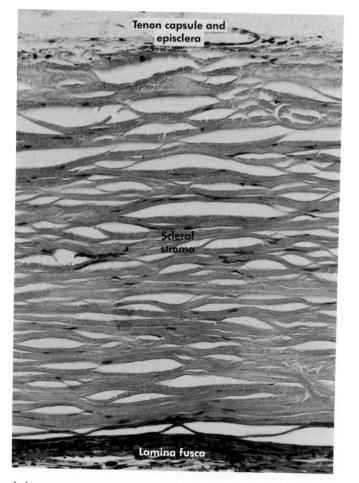

Fig. 1-4. Transverse section of sclera. (Masson trichrome stain; ×160.)

sends connective tissue bundles into the fascia bulbi (Tenon capsule). The anterior portion of the episclera has a rich blood supply that may become violently congested in inflammation. The episclera becomes progressively thinner toward the back of the eye. Both the fascia bulbi and the episclera are attenuated behind the ocular equator; this accounts for the relative avascularity of the posterior sclera.

The dense *scleral stroma* consists mainly of bundles of typical collagen fibers (Fig. 1-5) that vary in diameter from 10 μm to 16 μm and in length from 30 μm to 140 μm. The fibers are oriented parallel to the corneoscleral limbus to form an interlacing basketlike weave in that region. In the region of the insertion of the extraocular muscles, they become more meridional, apparently in response to mechanical stresses induced by traction of the ocular muscles and intraocular pressure. The sclera is white because of the variable diameter and irregular arrangement of the collagen fibers of the stroma.

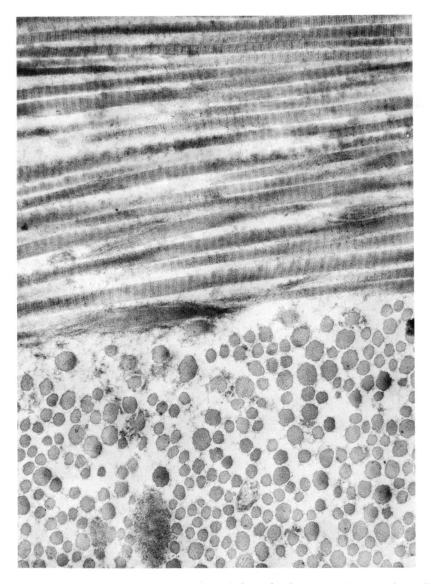

Fig. 1-5. Transmission electron micrograph of the scleral stroma showing the collagen bundles. The collagen fibrils in the lamellae are of variable diameter and much more irregularly arranged than those of the cornea. (×45,000.) (Courtesy Ramesh C. Tripathi.)

When the water content of the sclera (usually between 65% and 70%) is reduced to less than 40% or increased to more than 80%, the sclera becomes transparent.

The *lamina fusca* is the innermost layer of the sclera adjacent to the choroid, which provides many melanocytes that give it a brown color. Fine collagen fibers blend with the choroid and form delicate connections between the choroid and the sclera.

Blood supply. The scleral stroma derives its nutrition from both the episcleral and choroidal vascular network. Anterior to the insertions of the recti muscles, the anterior ciliary arteries form a dense episcleral plexus. These vessels become congested in "ciliary injection." Small branches of the long and short posterior ciliary arteries supply the scleral stroma posterior to the recti muscles.

Nerve supply. The posterior sclera is innervated by branches of the short ciliary nerves that enter the sclera close to the optic nerve. The long ciliary nerves provide sensory innervation anteriorly. Because of the generous innervation, inflammations of the sclera are extremely painful.

The cornea. The cornea is the transparent anterior one sixth of the eye. Its anterior peripheral margin is covered with conjunctiva, whereas its internal margin terminates at the trabecular meshwork. Anteriorly, it measures about 10.6 mm vertically and about 11.7 mm horizontally; the peripheral conjunctival covering makes exact measurement difficult. Internally the cornea is circular with a diameter of 11.7 mm. The central optical portion is 0.52 mm thick with nearly parallel anterior and posterior surfaces. It thickens to about 1.0 mm at the periphery. Its growth is complete in humans at about 6 years of age. The radius of curvature of the anterior surface is 7.8 mm, and the radius of curvature of the concave posterior surface is 6.2 to 6.8 mm. The cornea separates air with an index of refraction of 1.00 and aqueous humor with an index of refraction of 1.33 and is the main refracting structure of the eye. Variations in the radius of curvature in different corneal meridians cause astigmatism.

Structure. The cornea (Fig. 1-6) has three layers: (1) the epithelium and its basement membrane, (2) the substantia propria (stroma) and its anterior condensation, Bowman zone,

and (3) the mesothelium (endothelium) and its basement membrane (Descemet membrane), which separates the endothelium from the stroma (Table 1-1).

The *epithelium* is 50 μm to 90 μm thick and covers the stroma anteriorly. It is continuous with the epithelium of the conjunctiva. The epithelium is stratified, five to six cell layers thick. It has an outermost layer two to three cell layers thick, a midzone layer formed by two or three layers of polyhedral cells (wing cells), and a single layer of tall, columnar, basal, germinal cells that rest upon a thin base-

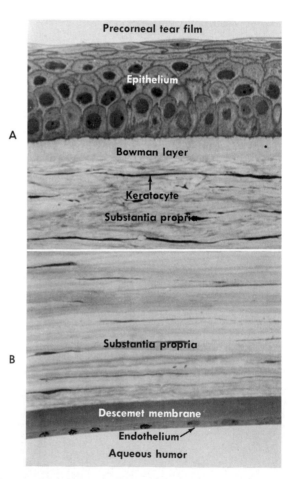

Fig. 1-6. Cross section of the axial area of the cornea. The substantia propria constitutes 90% of the thickness. **A,** The basement membrane of the epithelium is firmly adherent to the Bowman zone, the anterior condensation of the substantia propria. **B,** The lamellae of the posterior substantia propria are much more regularly arranged than those of the anterior substantia propria. (×500.) (Courtesy Ramesh C. Tripathi.)

ment membrane. The epithelial cells form in the deepest layer, become progressively flatter, and are shed from the superficial layer 7 days later. The superficial squamous cells (Fig. 1-7) have many microvilli. These cells are flat, have horizontal nuclei, and are joined to each other with desmosomes that prevent aqueous solutions (such as tears) from penetrating the cornea. As superficial cells age, they lose their interdigitation and disintegrate or are swept away by the eyelids in blinking. Wing cells in the midzone are polyhedral with a convex anterior surface, parallel with the surface of the cornea, and a concave posterior surface. Those immediately adjacent to the columnar epithelium have round nuclei that become successively flatter as the cells approach the surface. The cells are joined together from base to apex by desmosomes (maculae adherentes). The deepest basal cells are tall and columnar in shape. They have a flattened base that rests on the basement membrane to which it is attached by hemidesmosomes. Their interdigitating lateral cell borders are joined by desmosomes. The cells often show mitosis. The basement membrane is PAS-positive and is firmly attached to the underlying anterior condensation of the substantia propria (Bowman zone) by irregular filaments. After injury, this attachment may take up to 6 weeks to reestablish itself. The basement membrane forms a barrier that

separates superficial corneal disorders from the underlying substantia propria.

The *substantia propria* (Fig. 1-8), or stroma, constitutes 90% of the corneal thickness. Its anterior portion, the Bowman zone (Bowman membrane or layer to the light microscopist), is made up of randomly oriented collagen fibers that form an acellular region resistant to deformation, trauma, and the passage of foreign bodies or infecting organisms. Once damaged, its typical architecture is not restored and causes scarring or irregularity in corneal thickness that results in irregular astigmatism. The stroma is composed of lamellae of collagen fibrils of uniform diameter and regular spacing that extend the entire width of the cornea. They have a periodicity typical of embryonic collagen. In the posterior cornea, the lamellae are of almost equal thickness; they become more irregular in the anterior portion. All fibers within a lamella are parallel but at a right angle to fibers in the adjacent lamellae. They are enmeshed in glycosoaminoglycans. Scattered throughout are fixed, long, and flat cells known as keratocytes or corneal corpuscles that function as fibroblasts do in other tissues. There are a few wandering cells (leukocytes and macrophages).

The posterior surface of the stroma is lined with a loosely attached PAS-positive glassy membrane, the Descemet membrane, the basement membrane of endothelial cells. Descemet's membrane is composed of collagen fibers, different from those of the corneal stroma, arranged in a hexagonal pattern. After injury the membrane regenerates readily (but not its endothelial cells in humans) and may form glass membranes that extend into the anterior chamber. The abrupt peripheral termination of Descemet's membrane marks the peripheral margin of the cornea, the anterior border ring of the trabecular meshwork (the line of Schwalbe).

The *endothelium* of the cornea is a single layer of mesothelium (Fig. 1-9) with centrally located large oval nuclei. These cells are rich in intracellular organelles. Their apices are in direct contact with the aqueous humor and have occasional microvilli. The cells are tightly bound together with desmosomes (maculae adherentes); near the apical region a terminal bar is constantly present. The endothelium is re-

Table 1-1. Layers of cornea and sclera

I. Precorneal tear film
   A. Oil layer (from meibomian glands)
   B. Aqueous layer (from lacrimal glands)
   C. Mucoid layer (from goblet cells)
II. Cornea
   A. Epithelium
      1. Surface cell layer
      2. Wing cell layer
      3. Basal cell layer (columnar cells)
      4. Basement membrane
   B. Stroma
      1. Anterior condensation (Bowman zone)
      2. Lamellar stroma
   C. Mesothelium (endothelium)
      1. Descemet membrane (basement membrane)
         separates endothelium from stroma
III. Sclera
   A. Episclera
   B. Scleral stroma
   C. Lamina fusca

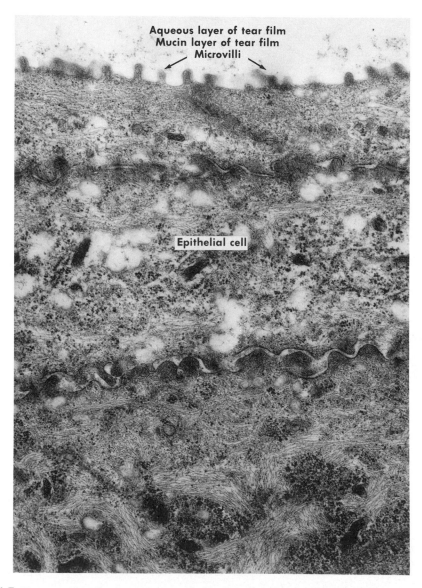

Fig. 1-7. Transmission electron micrograph of corneal epithelium with the surface cells *(top)* showing microvilli. The surface barrier of the epithelium is formed by the integrity of the most anterior squamous cells that are bound together by terminal bars. (×37,000.) (Courtesy Ramesh C. Tripathi.)

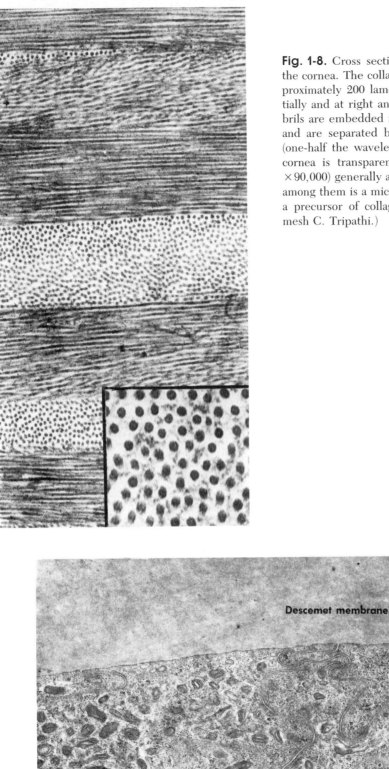

Fig. 1-8. Cross section of the substantia propria of the cornea. The collagen fibers are in bundles of approximately 200 lamellae that are arranged tangentially and at right angles to each other. Collagen fibrils are embedded in a mucopolysaccharide matrix and are separated by a distance of about 200 nm (one-half the wavelength of blue light, so that the cornea is transparent). The collagen fibrils (*inset*, ×90,000) generally are of uniform size; interspersed among them is a microfibrillar structure that may be a precursor of collagen. (×32,500.) (Courtesy Ramesh C. Tripathi.)

Fig. 1-9. Corneal mesothelium (endothelium.) The cells are rich in organelles; adjacent cell borders are markedly convoluted but parallel and are attached by terminal bars near the anterior chamber aspect. (×24,000.) (Courtesy Ramesh C. Tripathi.)

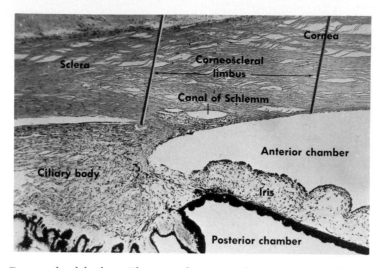

Fig. 1-10. Corneoscleral limbus. The central margin of the corneoscleral limbus is a line drawn between the termination of the Bowman zone and the point where the Descemet membrane becomes discontinuous (line of Schwalbe). The posterior margin is a line drawn parallel to the central margin and passing through the root of the iris. (Hematoxylin and eosin stain; ×105.)

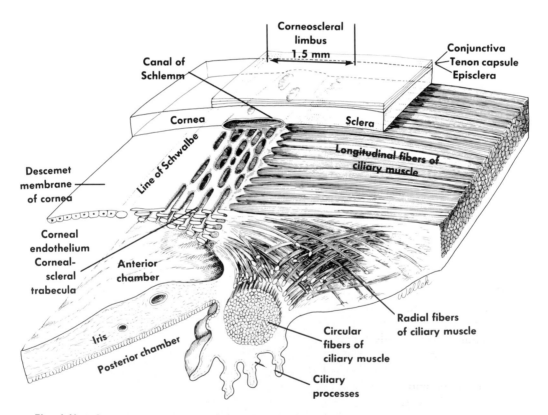

Fig. 1-11. Schematic construction of the ciliary body and angle recess in humans. Anteriorly the area is covered by the cornea and posteriorly by the sclera, which contains the canal of Schlemm. The termination of the corneal endothelium is marked by the line of Schwalbe. The ciliary muscle consists of longitudinal fibers, which are mainly parallel to the sclera; radial fibers, which are intermediate; and a circular muscle, which is most internal. The corneoscleral trabecula provides a filtering area between the anterior chamber angle and the canal of Schlemm. (Redrawn from Rohen, J.W.: Das Auge und seine Hilfsorgane. In Von Mollendorf, W., and Bargmann, W., editors: Handbuch der mikroskopischen Anatomie des Menschen, Berlin, 1964, Springer-Verlag.)

sponsible for the deturgescence (dehydration) of the corneal stroma. Injury to the endothelium (or epithelium) results in edema of the corneal stroma. The corneal endothelium does not regenerate in adult humans.

At the corneal periphery, the Bowman zone and the Descemet membrane stop abruptly. A line connecting these terminations constitutes the anterior margin of the corneoscleral limbus. (Fig. 1-10.)

Nerve supply. The corneal nerves are branches of the ophthalmic division of the trigeminal nerve and are solely sensory. Within the cornea the nerves are nonmyelinated, but they gain a myelin sheath at the corneoscleral limbus. Most are concentrated in the anterior stroma beneath the Bowman zone and send branches forward into the epithelium with either beadlike thickening or bare fibers. The axons pass in the long ciliary nerves through the ciliary ganglion to the semilunar ganglion. The Descemet membrane and the endothelium are not innervated.

Blood supply. The central cornea is avascular, but the corneoscleral limbus is generously supplied by the anterior conjunctival branches of the anterior ciliary arteries. These vessels course circumferentially around the corneoscleral limbus, giving off small radial branches that end either in the deep or superficial corneal plexus with recurrent branches that anastomose with posterior conjunctival arteries.

Corneoscleral limbus. The corneoscleral limbus (junction) (Fig. 1-11) is a transitional zone 1 to 2 mm wide that contains the trabecular meshwork through which aqueous humor leaves the eye. It is covered by the conjunctiva. At the corneoscleral limbus the corneal epithelium loses its regular structure and becomes continuous with the conjunctival epithelium that contains goblet cells and lymphatic channels. The Bowman zone of the stroma ends abruptly in a loose arrangement of collagen fibers, filaments, and amorphous material. The regularity of the corneal lamellae is lost and the collagen fibrils vary in diameter. Some are characteristic of the central cornea, and others are characteristic of the sclera. The Descemet membrane terminates and splits into narrow bands that form the anterior chamber surface of the trabecular meshwork. The corneal endothelium loses its continuity and continues as the endothelium that covers each of the bands of the trabecular meshwork.

The anterior margin of the corneoscleral limbus is an imaginary line drawn between the terminations of the Bowman zone and the Descemet membrane. The posterior margin is a line drawn parallel to the anterior margin that passes through the root of the iris. Enmeshed in the corneoscleral limbus is the trabecular meshwork with its canal of Schlemm, which forms the drainage system of the anterior chamber. Clinically, the area is viewed with a goniolens. (See Chapter 20.)

Trabecular meshwork. Encircling the circumference of the anterior chamber is the trabecular meshwork through which anterior aqueous humor filters en route to the canal of Schlemm (Fig. 1-12). It is composed of the uveal meshwork and the corneoscleral meshwork. The uveal meshwork faces the anterior chamber and extends from the scleral spur, the anterior face of the ciliary body and iris root, to the termination of the Descemet membrane (the line of Schwalbe). The corneoscleral meshwork is adjacent to the canal of Schlemm and extends from the line of Schwalbe to the scleral spur. The meshwork consists of a number of superimposed fibrocellular cords (L. *trabecula*, beam) that enclose oval, circular, or rhomboidal spaces. Near the scleral spur the meshwork contains approximately 12 layers of cords, whereas there are only two or three near the line of Schwalbe. Each cord contains a collagen core, surrounded by a thin matrix containing fibrils covered by endothelium. Fibers of the longitudinal portion of the ciliary muscle terminate in the region adjacent to the canal of Schlemm.

The trabecular meshwork is innervated by a plexus of delicate axons that terminate without specialized endings within the endothelium of the canal of Schlemm. The nerves originate from both divisions of the autonomic nervous system and from the trigeminal nerve.

Canal of Schlemm. The canal of Schlemm is an oval channel that encircles the entire circumference of the anterior chamber. It is lined with a single layer of mesothelial cells (endothelium) that contain giant vacuoles. On its inner surface, the canal of Schlemm communicates with the anterior chamber through the trabecular meshwork. Its outer wall is buried in the stroma of the corneoscleral limbus. The canal of Schlemm connects with the venous system through a series of 25 to 35 collector channels that anastomose to form a deep scleral plexus. This scleral plexus drains aqueous humor from the canal of Schlemm into anterior ciliary veins and episcleral veins. Several of the collector channels bypass this plexus and continue through the sclera. They may be seen subconjunctivally as minute vessels, the aqueous veins, which contain clear aqueous humor. They terminate in conjunctival veins within a few millimeters of the corneoscleral limbus.

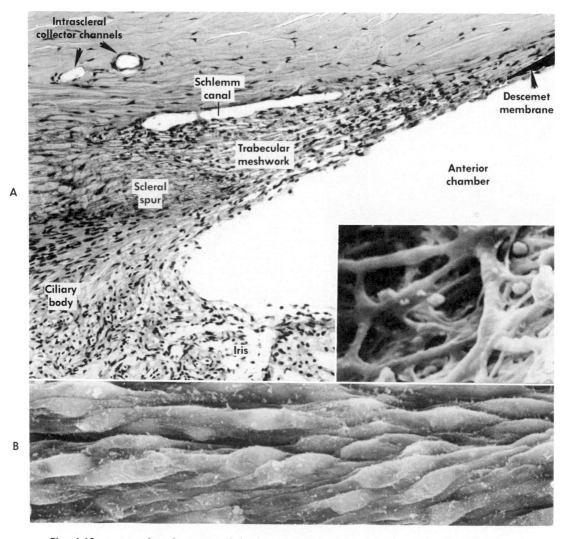

Fig. 1-12. A, Meridional section of the human trabecular meshwork. The aqueous drainage pathway consists of the trabecular meshwork, Sclemm canal, and intrascleral collector channels. The trabecular meshwork, located in the inner corneoscleral limbus, extends from the scleral spur, anterior face of the ciliary body, and iris root to the deeper corneal lamellae and peripheral termination of the Descemet membrane. (×138.) The inset shows the rounded trabeculae from the anterior chamber aspect. **B,** Scanning electron micrograph of the endothelial lining of the trabecular wall of the canal of Schlemm viewed from the anterior chamber aspect. Note the crypts between the cells, their spindle shape, and the central bulges that correspond to the location of nuclear and microvascular structures. The long axes of the cells usually parallel the canal circumference. (With permission from Tripathi, R.C.: Exp. Eye Res. **25:**65, 1977. Copyright by Academic Press Inc. [London] Ltd.)

Middle coat

The middle, or uveal, coat of the eye (L. *uva*, grape) consists of the choroid, the ciliary body, and the iris. The choroid is a vascular layer that provides the blood supply to the retinal pigment epithelium and the outer half of the sensory retina adjacent to it. The ciliary body secretes aqueous humor and contains the smooth muscle responsible for changing the shape of the lens in accommodation. The iris surrounds the pupil, a central opening that controls the amount of light entering the eye.

The choroid. The choroid (Fig. 1-13) is the vascular sheet that provides the blood supply for the retinal pigment epithelium and the outer one-half of the sensory retina adjacent to it. It is composed of an inner layer of fenestrated, large-diameter capillaries (21 μm), the choriocapillaris, and successively larger collecting veins approximately arranged in layers. The choroid extends from the optic nerve posteriorly to the ciliary body anteriorly. It is thickest (0.25 mm) at the posterior pole and gradually thins anteriorly (0.10 mm). It is attached firmly to the sclera in the region of the optic nerve where the posterior ciliary arteries enter the eye and at the points of exit of the vortex veins.

Structure. The three layers of blood vessels of the choroid have supporting structures on either side: the suprachoroid (lamina fusca) on the outer side and the basal lamina (Bruch membrane) on the inner side (Table 1-2).

The outermost layer, the *suprachoroid (lamina fusca)*, is made up of lamellae composed of elastic and collagenous fibers to form a syncytium that is dense posteriorly and becomes looser anteriorly. Melanocytes (fibroblasts that contain pigment) are abundant in this layer and decrease in number in the vascular layers. Found in this layer are smooth muscle fibers, fibroblasts, endothelial cells, long and short posterior ciliary arteries, and nerves. The short posterior ciliary arteries have but a short course in the suprachoroid and extend directly to the choriocapillaris layer.

The blood vessel layer has three components: (1) the outer (nearest the sclera) vessel layer (of Haller), which consists of large veins that lead to the vortex veins and have no valves; (2) the middle vessel layer (of Sattler), which consists of medium-sized veins and some arterioles and which contains a loose, collagenous stroma with numerous elastic fibers, fibroblasts, and melanocytes; and (3) the choriocap-

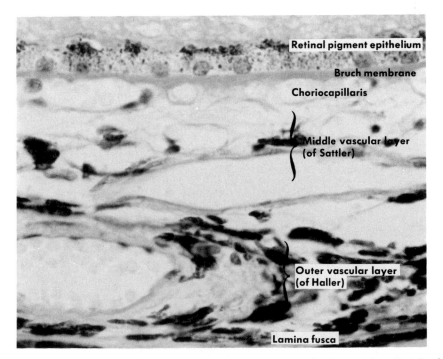

Fig. 1-13. Transverse section of the choroid. The outer vascular layer (of Haller) leads to vortex veins; the middle vascular layer (of Sattler) drains the choriocapillaris. (Hematoxylin and eosin stain; ×625.)

Table 1-2. Layers of uvea and Bruch membrane

I. Uvea
  A. Choroid
    1. Lamina fusca
    2. Layer of large veins (of Haller)
    3. Layer of smaller veins (of Sattler)
    4. Choriocapillaris (blood supply of the outer retina)
  B. Ciliary body
    1. Uveal portion
      a. Lamina fusca
      b. Vessel layer
      c. Ciliary muscle
        (1) Longitudinal
        (2) Radial
        (3) Circular
    2. Epithelial portion
      a. Pigmented epithelium
      b. Nonpigmented epithelium
  C. Iris
    1. Anterior border layer (fibroblasts and melanocytes, absent in pupillary zone)
    2. Stroma (connective tissue, blood vessels, sphincter pupillae muscle [N III])
    3. Epithelium
      a. Anterior (myoepithelium: dilatator pupillae muscle [sympathetics])
      b. Posterior pigmented layer
II. Bruch membrane (lamina basilis choroideae) (lamina vitrea [obsolete])
  A. Basement membrane of choriocapillaris endothelium
  B. Outer collagen layer
  C. Elastic layer
  D. Inner cuticular layer
  E. Basement membrane of pigment epithelium

illaris, which consists of large fenestrated capillaries that form a dense, flat network extending from the optic disk to the ora serrata. The choriocapillaris (Fig. 1-14) has a distinct lobular structure with a feeding arteriole in the center and draining venules at the lobular periphery.

The *lamina basalis choroideae (Bruch membrane)* (Fig. 1-15) is about 7 μm thick and separates the choriocapillaris from the retinal pigment epithelium. It is composed of layers contributed by both the choriocapillaris and the retinal pigment epithelium. The outer layer, nearest the choroid, is composed of the basement membrane of the endothelial cells of the choriocapillaris. Adjacent to this is a fine layer of collagen fibers. Centrally, a layer of elastic tissue fibers extends outward to form

the supporting structure of the choriocapillaris. The inner (cuticular) layer originates from the retinal pigment epithelium and is composed of collagen fibers surrounded by glycosaminoglycans. Resting upon this layer is the thin basement membrane of the retinal pigment epithelium. The Bruch membrane stops abruptly at the optic nerve as does the retinal pigment epithelium.

Blood supply. The blood supply of the choroid is derived from the short posterior ciliary arteries, the two long posterior ciliary arteries, and the seven anterior ciliary arteries (Fig. 1-16). The short posterior ciliary arteries originate as two or three branches of the ophthalmic artery. These branches subdivide into 10 to 20 branches that perforate the sclera around the circumference of the optic nerve. The majority pass at once into the choroid and communicate directly with the choriocapillaris layer. The two long posterior ciliary arteries perforate the sclera just medial and lateral to the optic nerve. They extend forward in the suprachoroidal space on the medial and lateral sides of the globe to the ciliary body. There each divides into two branches that extend circumferentially to form the major arterial circle of the iris (see Fig. 1-23) that is located in the ciliary body. Branches extend anteriorly to the iris. Recurrent choroidal branches extend posteriorly to terminate in the choriocapillaris.

The anterior ciliary arteries are the terminal branches of the two muscular arteries of each rectus muscle (except the lateral rectus muscle, which has but one muscular artery). The anterior ciliary arteries bifurcate into vessels that penetrate the sclera and nonpenetrating vessels that extend toward the cornea. The penetrating vessels provide the blood supply to the ciliary body and send recurrent branches to the anterior extremity of the choriocapillaris and to the major arterial circle of the iris. The nonpenetrating vessels extend forward in the episclera as anterior conjunctival arteries, anastomose with posterior conjunctival arteries, and terminate in the superficial (conjunctival) and deep (episcleral) pericorneal plexus (see conjunctival blood supply and Fig. 1-22).

Venous blood from the choroid, ciliary body, and iris is collected by a series of veins of increasingly larger diameter. These lead to four or more large vortex veins located behind the

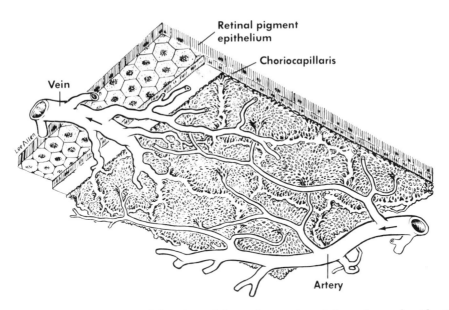

Fig. 1-14. Lobular structure of the choroidal circulation viewed from the underside. The short posterior ciliary arteries divide soon after their entry into the eye and send branches to the center of each lobule, which drains into peripheral veins. (Courtesy Lee Allen.)

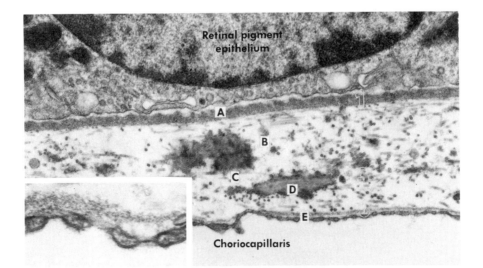

Fig. 1-15. Electron micrograph of the Bruch membrane, which separates the choriocapillaris from the retinal pigment epithelium. *A*, Basement membrane of the retinal pigment epithelium; *B*, inner collagen layer; *C*, elastic layer; *D*, outer collagen layer; *E*, basement membrane of the choriocapillaris. (×21,000.) *Inset*, The choriocapillaris showing its fenestrations bridged by membranous diaphragms. (×77,000.) (Courtesy Ramesh C. Tripathi.)

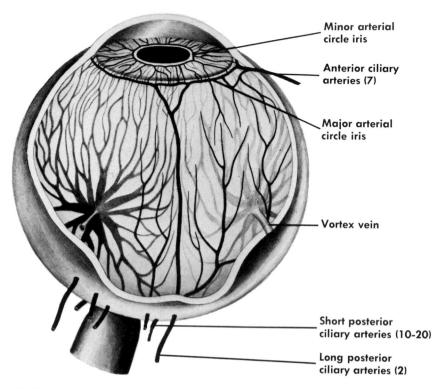

Minor arterial
circle iris

Anterior ciliary
arteries (7)

Major arterial
circle iris

Vortex vein

Short posterior
ciliary arteries (10-20)

Long posterior
ciliary arteries (2)

Fig. 1-16. Blood supply of the uveal tract. The two long posterior arteries mainly supply the iris. The anterior ciliary arteries supply the ciliary body, whereas the short posterior ciliary arteries supply the choroid. Note that there are no corresponding veins; rather the blood is collected into four or more vortex veins that empty into the superior and inferior ophthalmic veins, which drain into the cavernous sinus.

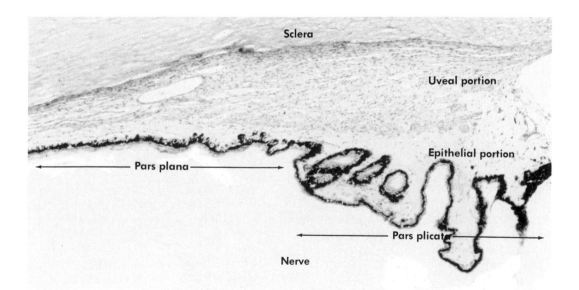

Sclera

Uveal portion

Epithelial portion

Pars plana

Pars plicata

Nerve

Fig. 1-17. Cross section of the ciliary body that encircles the eye. The pars plicata portion is about 2 mm in width; the pars plana about 4 mm. Intraocular surgeons often use an incision through the sclera and the adjacent pars plana. (Hematoxylin and eosin stain; ×60.)

equator of the globe. The vortex veins empty into the superior and inferior ophthalmic veins, each of which drains into the cavernous sinus.

Nerve supply. The choroid is innervated mainly by sympathetic nerves that pass through the ciliary ganglion without synapse and are distributed through the short ciliary nerves. As they enter the suprachoroid, they lose their myelin sheath and branch repeatedly to form a plexus. There are many adrenergic vesicles, and nerve endings contact pigment cells and smooth muscle in the walls of arterioles.

The ciliary body. The ciliary body (Fig. 1-17) is a ring of tissue about 6 mm wide that extends from the scleral spur to the ora serrata of the retina.

Structure. It is divided into uveal and epithelial portions. The uveal portion is adjacent to the sclera and includes the suprachoroid (lamina fusca), the ciliary muscles, the blood vessel layer, and the lamina basalis choroideae (lamina vitrea). The epithelial portion is adjacent to the posterior chamber and includes the pars plana (orbiculus ciliaris) and the pars plicata (corona ciliaris) or ciliary processes.

Uveal portion. The ciliary muscle (Fig. 1-18) is the most prominent structure in the uveal portion of the ciliary body. It is composed of three groups of smooth muscle: (1) the longitudinal fibers (Brücke muscle), which are the outermost, parallel the surface of the overlying sclera, and constitute the main bulk of the muscle; (2) the radial fibers that originate from the anterior portion of the longitudinal fibers and run obliquely to become continuous with circular fibers; and (3) the circular fibers (Müller muscle) that are the innermost portion of the ciliary muscle and parallel the lens equator.

Contraction of the circular fibers relaxes the lens zonule, which allows a greater curvature of the lens (accommodation). Parasympathetic (cholinergic) motor innervation originates in the Ediger-Westphal nucleus of the oculomotor (N III) nerve. Efferent visceral motor fibers pass from the inferior division of N III to synapse in the ciliary ganglion. Postganglionic fibers in 6 to 20 short ciliary nerves innervate the ciliary muscle and sphincter pupillae muscle. Contraction of the longitudinal portion of the ciliary muscle may retract the scleral spur and enlarge the canal of Schlemm.

The scleral surface of the ciliary body is the suprachoroid (lamina fusca). The vessel layer is composed mainly of the major arterial circle of

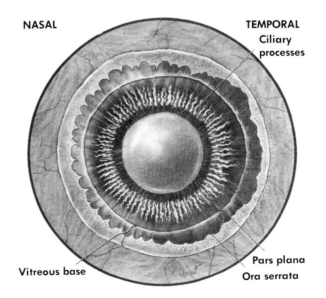

NASAL

TEMPORAL
Ciliary processes

Vitreous base

Pars plana
Ora serrata

Fig. 1-18. View from behind the epithelial portion of the ciliary body. The indentations of the ora serrata are irregular. The vitreous humor has firm attachments (vitreous base) to the periphery of the sensory retina and the posterior pars plana (orbicularis ciliaris). (With permission from Michels, R.G.: Vitreous surgery, St. Louis, 1981, The C.V. Mosby Co.)

the iris, its tributaries, and veins. There is no choriocapillaris. At the anterior termination of the choroid, Bruch membrane divides. The elastic layer derived from choroid disappears, but the inner cuticular layer that originates from the retinal pigment epithelium continues forward to the iris root as the basement membrane of the pigmented epithelium of the ciliary body.

Epithelial portion. The epithelial portion of the ciliary body (Fig. 1-19) is divided into the pars plana (orbiculus ciliaris) and the pars plicata (corona ciliaris). The pars plana is about 4 mm wide and extends anteriorly from the ora serrata of the retina. The pars plicata forms the most anterior 2 mm of the ciliary body. It is formed of 60 to 70 folds, the ciliary processes, each of which is about 0.8 mm high and 1.0 mm wide. Each ciliary process consists of a finger of tissue covered with an outer layer of nonpigmented epithelium that covers a layer of pigmented epithelium surrounding a central vascular core (see Fig. 1-19).

The nonpigmented epithelium constitutes the anterior continuation of the sensory retina. Its basement membrane is continuous with the internal limiting membrane of the retina and is located on the posterior chamber side of the cell. The basement membrane of the pigmented epithelium is on the side of the cell nearest the sclera. Aqueous humor and hyaluronic acid are secreted through the apices of the nonpigmented epithelial cells of the ciliary processes. These cells have prominent Golgi complexes comparable to those of other secreting glandular cells. The apices of the cells of the pigmented epithelium and nonpigmented epithelium are in apposition, and the posterior aqueous humor secreted must pass between the cells of the nonpigmented epithelium to reach the posterior chamber.

The posterior margin of the pars plana portion of the ciliary body has a scalloped edge that corresponds to the retinal ora serrata. Each retinal tooth corresponds to a valley of the ciliary body. In this region the sensory retina abruptly changes into a single layer of elongated nonpigmented epithelium of the ciliary body. The retinal pigment epithelium continues forward on the pigmented epithelium of the ciliary body. Surgical instruments may be introduced into the vitreous cavity and into the crystalline lens through the pars plana.

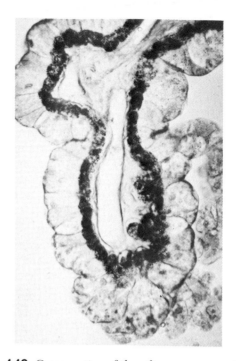

Fig. 1-19. Cross section of the ciliary processes. The nonpigmented epithelium is on the surface; its base faces the posterior chamber, and the cell apex faces the pigmented epithelium. The nonpigmented epithelium is a forward extension of the sensory retina, whereas the pigmented epithelium is continuous with the retinal pigment epithelium. (Periodic acid–Schiff stain; ×63.)

Blood supply. The blood supply of the ciliary body is mainly from the major arterial circle of the iris formed by the two long ciliary arteries and the penetrating branches of the seven anterior ciliary arteries.

Nerve supply. The motor nerve supply to the ciliary muscle is from the oculomotor nerve by postganglionic parasympathetic fibers that synapse in the ciliary ganglion and are distributed by the short ciliary nerves. These nerves also carry the sympathetic nerve supply of the uveal blood vessels.

The iris and pupil. The iris is a diaphragm that lies in front of the lens and ciliary body and separates the anterior chamber from the posterior chamber. It rests upon the lens, and without this support the iris is tremulous (iridodonesis). The iris inserts into the scleral spur through the anterior chamber face of the ciliary body. Located slightly to its nasal side is a circular aperture, the pupil, which controls the amount of light entering the eye.

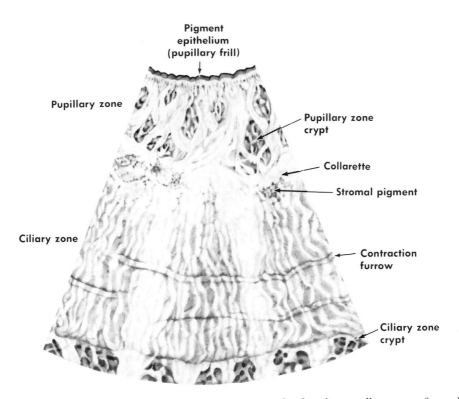

Pigment
epithelium
(pupillary frill)

Pupillary zone

Pupillary zone
crypt

Collarette

Stromal pigment

Ciliary zone

Contraction
furrow

Ciliary zone
crypt

Fig. 1-20. Surface pattern of the iris. The collarette divides the pupillary zone from the ciliary zone and marks the position of the minor vascular circle of the iris, from which the pupillary membrane originated in fetal life.

The anterior iris surface (Fig. 1-20) is divided into a central pupillary zone, from which the anterior border layer is absent, and a peripheral ciliary zone. These are divided by a circular ridge, the collarette, that marks the site of the minor vascular circle of the iris from which the pupillary membrane originated in embryonic life. Atrophy of the pupillary membrane begins in the seventh gestational month and is usually completed by 8½ months, sometimes leaving behind a few delicate strands that extend from the collarette to the anterior lens capsule.

The pupillary zone of the iris is relatively flat with its width varying with the amount of atrophy of the anterior border layer and the degree of pupillary dilation. The ciliary zone is marked by more radial interlacing ridges, giving a gossamerlike appearance. In blue irises concentric contraction furrows may be seen. The color of the iris depends on the amount of melanin in the anterior border layer. If slight, reflection from the pigment of the pigmented epithelium causes scattering and thus a blue color. If there is a moderate amount of melanin, the iris is hazel; if there is a large amount, the iris is brown.

Structure. The iris consists of two layers: (1) stroma, located anteriorly and originating from mesoderm and (2) pigmented epithelium, located posteriorly and originating from neural ectoderm (Fig. 1-21).

The stroma may be divided into an anterior border layer and a deeper stroma proper. The anterior border layer of the iris is a loose collagen tissue in which pigmented or nonpigmented cells are densely packed. The layer develops maximally about the seventh month of fetal life. Thereafter generalized atrophy occurs in the pupillary zone. Irregular atrophy in the ciliary zones forms iris crypts. In brown irises the surface is smooth and heavily pigmented and in blue or hazel irises it is irregular with crypts. The anterior border layer ends abruptly at the iris root, but spokelike processes may continue as iris processes to the line of Schwalbe.

The stroma proper has a similar appearance irrespective of the color of the iris. It is visible

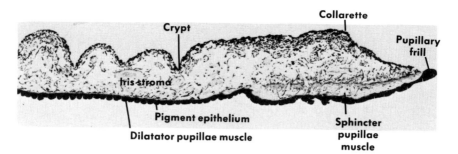

Fig. 1-21. Transverse section of the iris. The stroma is derived from mesoderm, whereas the pigment epithelium constitutes a fusion of the two layers of the primitive optic vesicle and is a forward extension of both the sensory retina and retinal pigment epithelium. The pupillary zone extends from the pupillary frill to the collarette. The ciliary zone of the iris extends from the collarette to the peripheral termination of the iris. (Hematoxylin and eosin stain; ×43.)

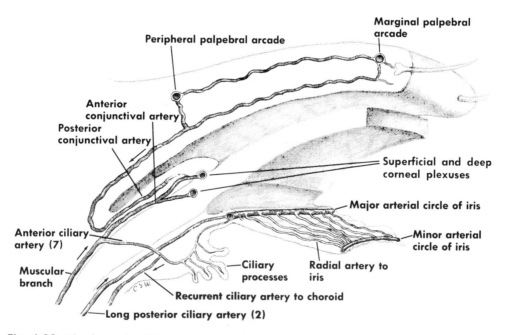

Fig. 1-22. Blood supply of the anterior ocular segment. Two anterior ciliary arteries arise from the muscular branches of each rectus muscle except for the lateral rectus muscle, which contributes only one. Two long posterior ciliary arteries enter the globe on the nasal and temporal sides of the optic nerve and extend forward in the suprachoroidal space to the ciliary body. The vascular arcades of the eyelid are derived from the lateral palpebral branches of the lacrimal artery and the medial palpebral branches of the dorsonasal artery. They have generous anastomoses with branches of the external carotid artery distributed to the face.

PLATE 1

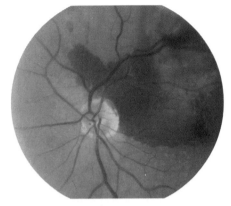

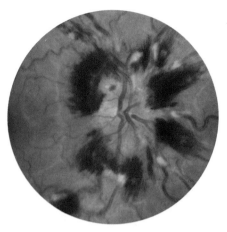

Preretinal hemorrhages.

Flame-shaped hemorrhages and cotton-wool patches in lupus erythematosus.

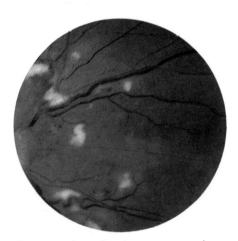

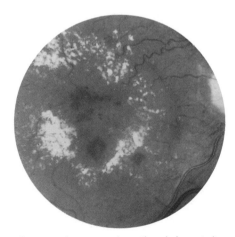

Cotton-wool patches in severe vascular hypertension.

Chronic edema residues (hard deposits) surrounding an area of retinal capillary leakage.

PLATE 2

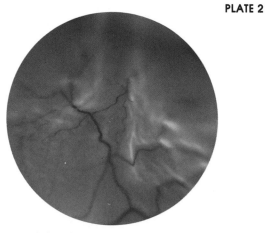

Retinal detachment.

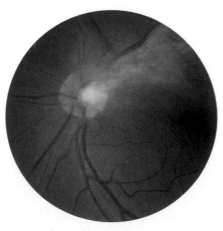

Carcinoma of the breast metastatic to the choroid.

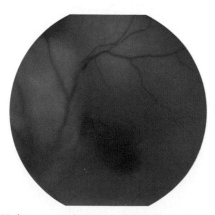

Malignant melanoma of the choroid.

Epiretinal membrane superior to the disk.

PLATE 3

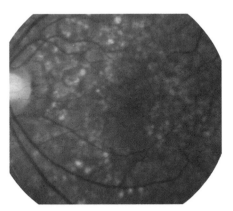

Retinal drusen.

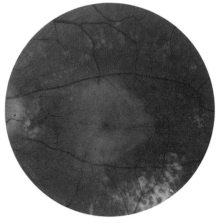

Retinal drusen.

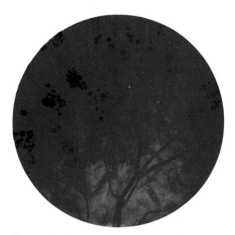

Grouped pigmentation of the retina.

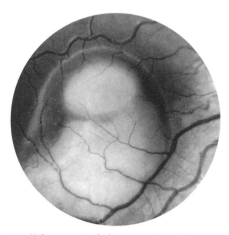

Vitelliform retinal degeneration (Best disease).

PLATE 4

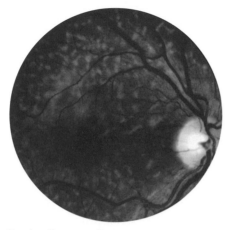

Fundus flavimaculatus.

Retinitis pigmentosa.

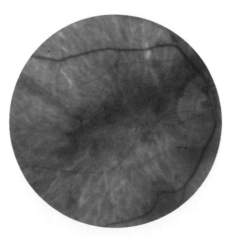

Choroidal atrophy.

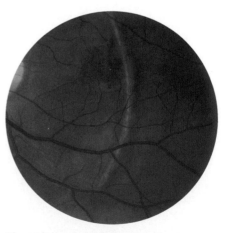

Choroidal rupture following blunt trauma to the eye.

PLATE 5

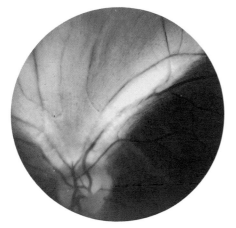

Medullated nerve fibers of the retina.

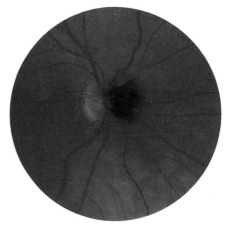

Melanocytoma of the optic disk.

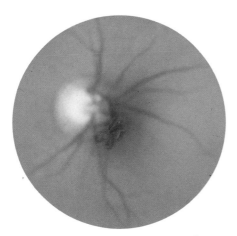

Patent hyaloid vascular system at the disk.

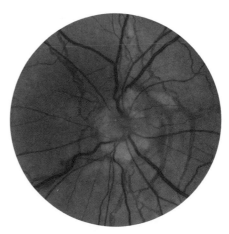

Drusen of the optic nerve. There are also angioid streaks and retinal hemorrhage.

PLATE 6

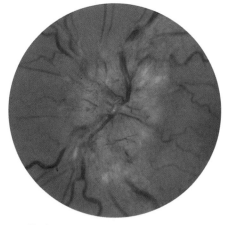

Papilledema.

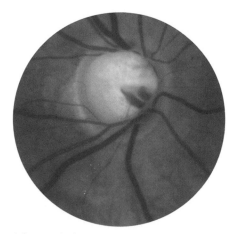

Advanced glaucomatous optic atrophy with excavation of the optic cup and nasal displacement of the blood vessels.

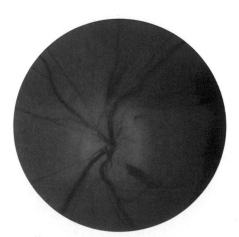

Papillitis with vision reduced to 20/200.

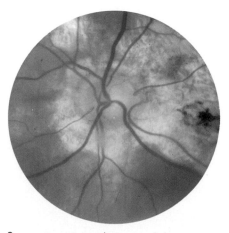

Severe myopia with conus of the optic nerve and severe chorioretinal atrophy.

PLATE 7

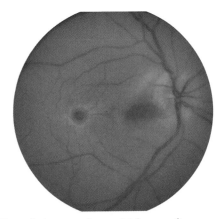

Foveal cherry-red spot 24 hours after
central retinal artery occlusion in
patient with subacute bacterial
endocarditis.

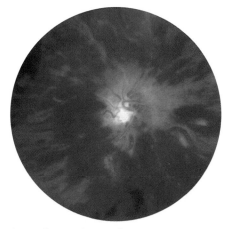

Central retinal vein closure.

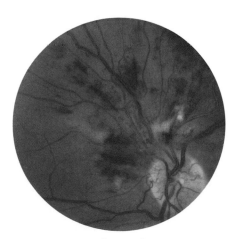

Superior temporal vein closure.

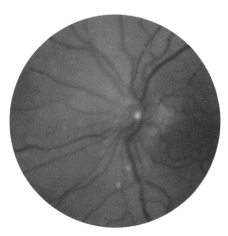

Central retinal artery embolus in
subacute bacterial endocarditis.

PLATE 8

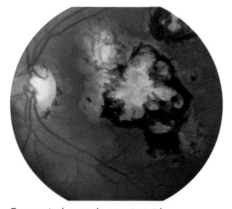

Congenital toxoplasmosis with papillomacular atrophy of the optic nerve.

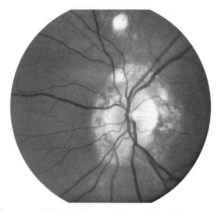

Presumed histoplasmosis peripapillary (adjacent optic disk) chorioretinitis and peripheral "histo" spot.

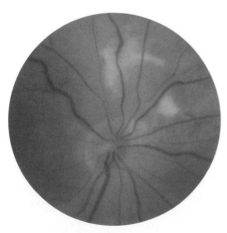

Placoid epitheliopathy.

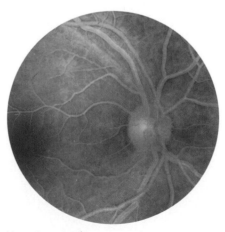

Lipemia retinalis.

PLATE 9

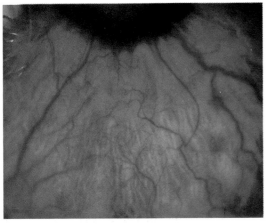

Rubeosis of the iris in diabetes.

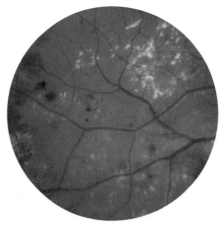

Diabetes: background retinopathy with chronic edema residues (hard exudates or hard deposits) and hemorrhages.

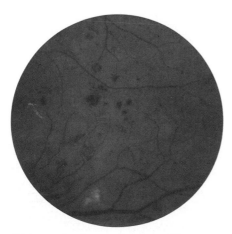

Diabetes: background retinopathy, predominantly with deep, round hemorrhages (blot hemorrhages).

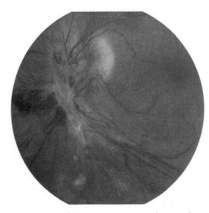

Diabetes: proliferative retinopathy with neovascularization of the optic disk.

PLATE 10

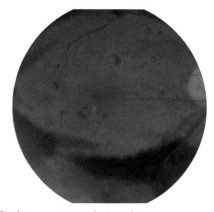

Diabetes: vitreous hemorrhage.

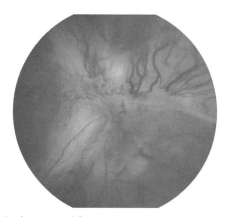

Diabetes: proliferative retinopathy with retinal detachment.

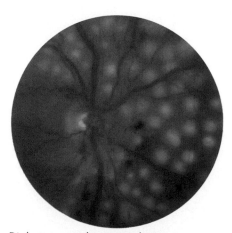

Diabetes: panphotocoagulation immediately after laser therapy.

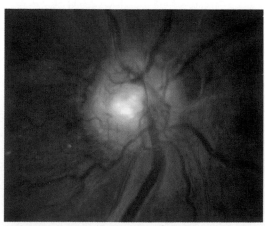

Diabetes: neovascularization of optic disk.

PLATE 11

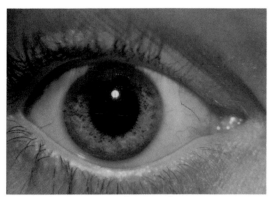

Kayser-Fleisher ring in hepaticolent
degeneration.

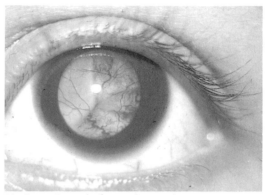

"Cat's-eye" pupil of an advanced
retinoblastoma.

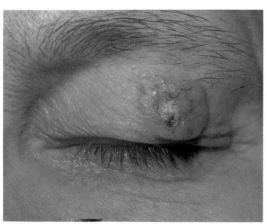

Basal cell carcinoma of the upper eyelid.

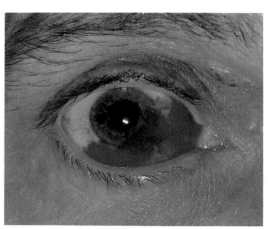

Subconjunctival hemorrhage.

PLATE 12

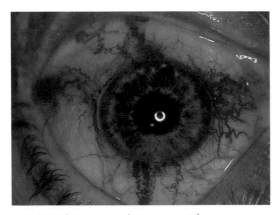

Caput medusae secondary to carotid artery fistula into the cavernous sinus.

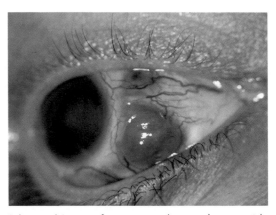

Scleromalacia perforans secondary to rheumatoid arthritis.

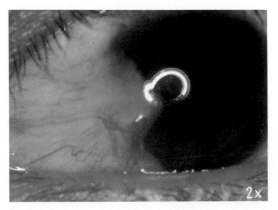

Pterygium.

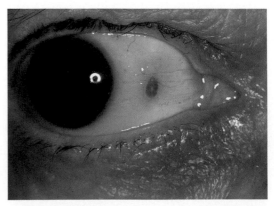

Senile hyaline plaque.

PLATE 13

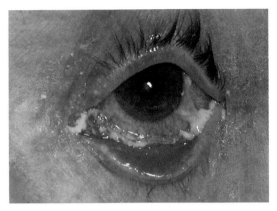

Acute conjunctivitis.

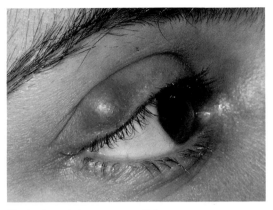

Chalazion, right upper eyelid.

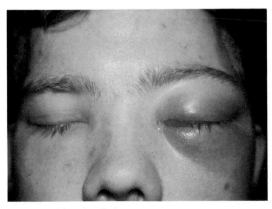

Anterior orbital cellulitis.

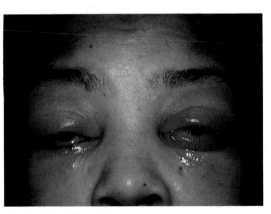

Conjunctival chemosis.

PLATE 14

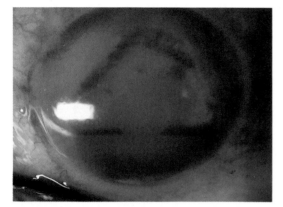

Blood in the anterior chamber (hyphema).

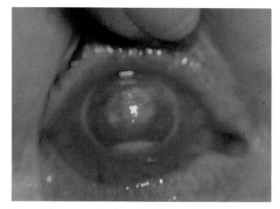

Pus in the anterior chamber (hypopyon). A corneal ulcer has been stained with sterile fluorescein.

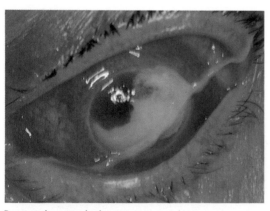

Bacterial corneal ulcer.

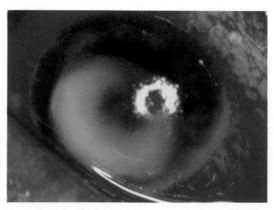

Fungus corneal ulcer.

PLATE 15

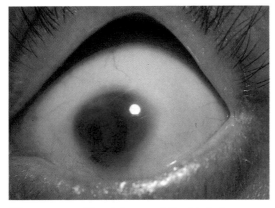

Microcornea with coloboma of the iris below. There is also corneal clouding and a coloboma of the choroid.

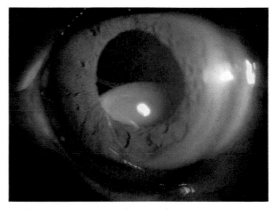

Dislocated lens in Marfan syndrome.

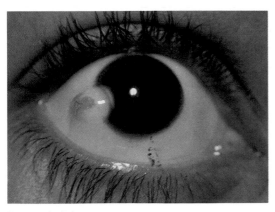

Dermoid of the cornea.

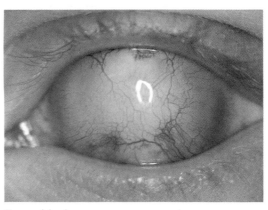

Corneal leukoma.

PLATE 16

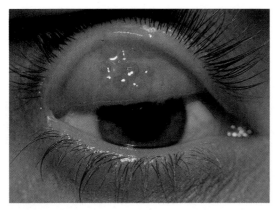

Follicles of the upper eyelid in vernal conjunctivitis.

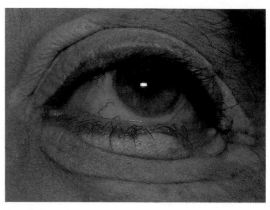

Xanthelasma.

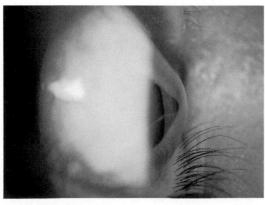

Profile of keratoconus.

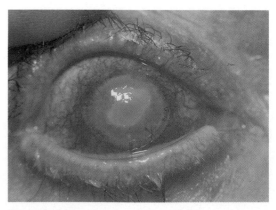

Corneal ulcer stained with fluorescein.

in the pupillary zone and in the depth of iris crypts. It consists of bundles of collagen fibrils arranged in columns around blood vessels and nerves, pigment and nonpigmented cells, all enmeshed in a hyaluronidase-sensitive glycosaminoglycans. The stroma proper contains more elastic tissue and fewer pigment cells than the anterior border layer. Its capillaries are nonfenestrated with a structure similar to that of other nonfenestrated capillaries.

The *iris pigmented epithelium* consists of two layers of cells that constitute a fusion of the two layers of the primitive optic vesicle. They are densely packed with melanin. The anterior layer of pigment cells intermingles with the dilatator pupillae muscle and is absent in the region of the sphincter pupillae muscle. The posterior layer of epithelium is covered on its lenticular surface with a basement membrane continuous with that of the retina and the ciliary body. Often the pupillary margin has a pigment frill continuous with the ectodermal pigmented epithelium that constitutes the anterior extremity of the optic cup.

The sphincter pupillae muscle is located in the pupillary zone of the posterior stroma. It is a smooth muscle about 1 mm wide that forms a sphincter surrounding the pupillary margin. The dilatator pupillae muscle is a thin sheet of smooth muscle (myoepithelium) located between the stroma and the posterior layer of the pigmented epithelium. It extends from the iris root at the ciliary body as far as the sphincter pupillae muscle. Both muscles are derived from neural ectoderm from the outer layer of the optic cup.

Blood supply. The blood supply of the iris is provided by radial vessels in the stromal layer that extend from the major arterial circle of the iris (circulus arteriosus iridis major) located in the ciliary body (Fig. 1-22). This is formed by the two long posterior ciliary arteries and the seven anterior ciliary arteries. The iris blood vessels pass radially in a corkscrew pattern toward the pupillary margin, causing the meridional striations of the ciliary portion of the iris. At the collarette they anastomose to form the incomplete minor vascular circle of the iris. The vessels have thick collagen adventitia and a thin muscularis layer. The endothelial cells of the veins have a perivascular sheath. They drain into the vortex veins. The endothelial cells of the capillaries are typically nonfenestrated with junctional complexes (zonulae occludentes) that prevent the passage of large molecules. This vascular endothelium, together with the tight junctions of the pigment epithelium of the ciliary body processes, forms the blood-aqueous barrier. The ciliary body vessels, like those of the choroid, are fenestrated.

Nerve supply. The iris is richly supplied with nerves from the short ciliary (cholinergic) and long ciliary (sensory, adrenergic) nerves. The nerves are partially medullated and have a thick neurilemma. The motor innervation of the dilatator pupillae muscle emerges from adrenergic nerves accompanying the long ciliary nerves. Additionally, the long ciliary nerves transmit sensory fibers from the iris. The sphincter pupillae muscle is innervated by cholinergic fibers from the Edinger-Westphal nucleus of the oculomotor nerve that synapse in the ciliary ganglion and are distributed with short ciliary nerves. The adrenergic nerve supply of iris arteries is carried by the short ciliary nerves.

Inner coat

The retina. The retina develops from invagination of the optic vesicle (see discussion on embryology) to form an outer layer, the retinal pigment epithelium, and an inner layer, the sensory retina. The inner layer is stratified into many layers, but the pigment epithelium is only one layer thick. The layers of the retina nearest the choroid are designated as the outer layers, and those nearest the vitreous humor as the inner layers. The retina extends from the optic nerve posteriorly to its scalloped margin (the ora serrata) anteriorly, where it continues as the epithelium of the ciliary body (Table 1-3).

Retinal pigment epithelium. The retinal pigment epithelium (Fig. 1-23) is a single layer of cells that extends to the optic nerve margin posteriorly and to the ora serrata anteriorly, where it fuses with the anterior continuation of the sensory retina and continues forward as the pigmented ciliary epithelium. The cells of the retinal pigment epithelium contain varying amounts of melanin, which, on ophthalmoscopic examination, give a granular appearance to the fundus (the pigment is of neural ectoderm origin and not of neural crest origin). In the

Table 1-3. Layers of the retina

I. Retinal pigment epithelium (outer layer of optic vesicle)
  A. Base (plasma membrane, mitochondria)
  B. Body (nucleus, endoplasmic reticulum, lipofuscin)
  C. Apex (pigment, ingested outer segment [phagosomes])
    1. Microvilli
    2. Lateral terminal bars (zonula adherens and zonula occludens)
II. Sensory retina (inner layer of optic vesicle)
  A. Photoreceptor cells (nuclei form the outer nuclear layer)
    1. Outer segment (rods and cones)
    2. Cilium
    3. Inner segment
      a. Ellipsoid
      b. Myoid
      c. Outer fiber (surrounded by terminal bars of Müller cells)
      d. Cell body (nucleus), the outer nuclear layer
      e. Inner fiber
      f. Synaptic vesicle
  B. Modulator cells (the nuclei form the inner nuclear layer)
    1. Bipolar*†
      a. Midget
      b. Flat midget
      c. Diffuse
      d. Interplexiform
    2. Horizontal*
    3. Amacrine†
  C. Transmitter cells
    1. Ganglion†
      a. Nerve fiber layer (axons of ganglion cells)
  D. Skeletal support
    1. Müller cells (nuclei within inner nuclear layer)
    2. Internal limiting membrane (retinal basement membrane)
    3. Accessory glia
      a. Small astrocytes
      b. Oligodendrocytic-like cells

*The axons of photoreceptor cells and horizontal cells and the dendrites of bipolar cells and horizontal cells form the outer plexiform layer of the retina (outer molecular layer).
†The axons of bipolar cells and processes of amacrine cells and the dendrites of ganglion cells form the inner plexiform layer (inner molecular layer).

region underlying the central sensory retina, the cells are slender and tall, but they are more cuboidal and irregular in the periphery. Their basement membrane is firmly attached to the cuticular portion of the Bruch membrane. The villous projections of the apices surround the outer segments of rods and cones in an interphotoreceptor matrix without specialized attachments.

Pigment epithelial cells are generally hexagonal; in flat section individual cells may have four to eight sides. The cells fit together like cobblestones in a regular arrangement. In cross-section, the pigment epithelial cells are divided into thirds, consisting of a base, a body, and an apex.

The base is adjacent to the cuticular portion of the Bruch membrane. It contains prominent infoldings of the basal plasma membrane, many mitochondria, and little or no pigment. The cell nucleus and assorted organelles and lipofuscin occupy the body. The apex is topped with microvilli that enmesh the outer segments of rods and cones embedded in glycosaminoglycans. The apical cytoplasm contains ovoid pigment granules and partially digested outer segment disks (phagosomes). The lateral surfaces of adjacent cells at the apices (but not the microvilli) are bound together by terminal bars that are composed of a basilar portion (zonula adherens) and an apical portion (zonula occludens). There is no intercellular space at the level of these junctions, and together with the nonfenestrated retinal blood vessels they constitute the blood-retina barrier. After 30 years of age, lipofuscin is prominent in the pigment epithelium underlying the central retina. In fluorescein angiography, lipofuscin and the melanin in the retinal pigment epithelium obscure fluorescence from the underlying choroid.

Sensory retina. The sensory retina (pars optica retinae) develops from the inner wall of the secondary optic vesicle. It consists of a layer of photoreceptor cells whose axons synapse with cells that modulate their response (Fig. 1-24). These modulator cells in turn synapse with

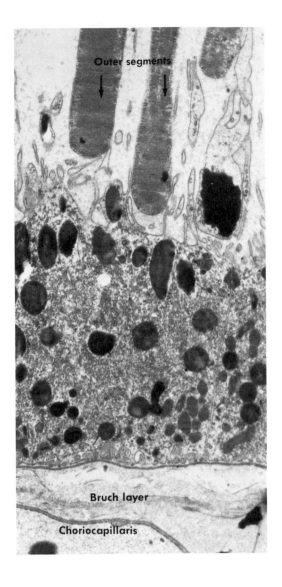

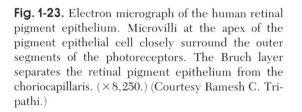

Fig. 1-23. Electron micrograph of the human retinal pigment epithelium. Microvilli at the apex of the pigment epithelial cell closely surround the outer segments of the photoreceptors. The Bruch layer separates the retinal pigment epithelium from the choriocapillaris. (×8,250.) (Courtesy Ramesh C. Tripathi.)

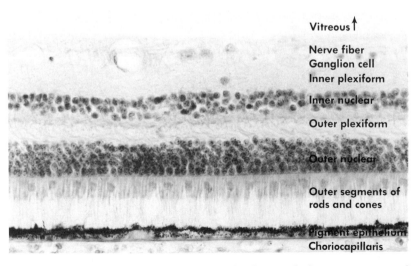

Fig. 1-24. Cross section of the human retina. The larger, darker structures in the outer segments of the rod and cone layer are cones. (Hematoxylin and eosin stain; ×625.)

cells that transmit spike discharges to the brain. The rods and cones, the light-sensitive cells of the retina, correspond to the sensory endings elsewhere in the nervous system. The glial system of Müller cells provides mechanical support of the retina.

Photoreceptor cell. The photoreceptor cell (Fig. 1-25) may be divided into the following: (1) an outer segment, which is embedded in the microvilli of the retinal pigment epithelium cells; (2) a cilium, a tubular structure that connects the outer and inner segments; (3) an inner segment composed of an ellipsoid and a myoid; (4) the outer rod (or cone) fiber connecting the inner segment to the cell body; (5) the cell body that contains the nucleus; and (6) the inner rod (or cone) fiber that terminates in a specialized synaptic ending.

The *outer segment* consists of a dense vertical stack of 700 flattened sacs or disks. The outer segment is surrounded by a plasma membrane that is continuous with the disks of cones but separate from rod disks. The space within each sac is occupied by the visual pigments. Most (111 to 130 million) outer segments in humans consist of cylindrical disks (rods) containing the photopigment rhodopsin. Other outer segments (6.3 to 6.8 million) have a conical shape (cones) with the apex pointing outward and containing three different photopigments responsible for color vision. The outer tip of the rod is surrounded by the microvilli of the retinal pigment epithelium and the extracellular space containing glycosaminoglycans. Outside of the fovea centralis, the tapered portion of the cone does not reach the retinal pigment epithelium, and the microvilli of the retinal pigment epithelium are lengthened to reach the cone outer segment. In the foveal region, cones are more slender and resemble the cylindrical structure of rods.

The outer segment is connected to the inner segment by the *cilium.* The connecting cilium contains nine pairs of microtubules but lacks the central pair seen in mobile cilia. This structure transmits cellular components from the inner segment and cell nucleus to the disks and their plasma membrane.

The *inner segment* is divided into a refractile outer ellipsoid and a nonrefractile, basophilic inner myoid. The ellipsoid contains mitochondria grouped around the base of the cilium.

The myoid portion (contractile in some amphibia) of the inner segment contains free and membrane-bound ribosomes, Golgi complexes, and a variety of vesicles and vacuoles. The division into ellipsoid and myoid portions is more distinct in rods than in cones.

The inner segment is connected to the cell body, which contains the nucleus, by an *outer fiber* (rod or cone). This fiber may be long or short depending on the distance between the myoid and the cell body. Most of the outer fibers of cones are shorter than those of rods.

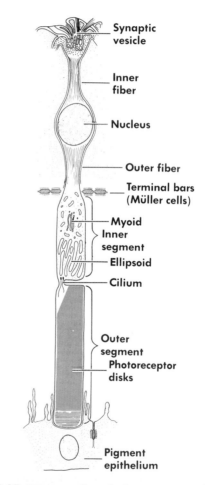

Synaptic vesicle

Inner fiber

Nucleus

Outer fiber

Terminal bars (Müller cells)

Myoid

Ellipsoid — Inner segment

Cilium

Outer segment Photoreceptor disks

Pigment epithelium

Fig. 1-25. Diagram of a rod photoreceptor cell. Photoreceptor disks of the outer segment form in the inner segment and migrate in the outer segment to the pigment epithelium where they are phagocytized. The visual cell does not undergo mitosis but constantly forms new photoreceptors. The terminal bars of the outer process of Müller cells orient the outer segments vertically for maximal visual efficiency.

The outer fiber is surrounded by the terminal bars (zonula adherens) of Müller cells. In light microscopy this is the external limiting membrane. These bars provide vertical orientation for the photoreceptors.

The *cell body*, located in the outer nuclear layer, consists almost entirely of nucleus.

An *inner fiber* (rod or cone) passes in the outer plexiform layer and terminates in a synaptic expansion, the rod spherule, or in a cone pedicle, the cone-foot. These synapse in the outer plexiform layer with cells whose nuclei are in the inner nuclear layer. There are several different types of synaptic endings, and it is possible that at this level there are both inhibition and integration of the nervous impulse. At this level chemical intermediates are secreted that are involved in the synaptic transmission of impulses.

Mature visual cells do not replicate, and their DNA is stable. In contrast, ribosomal RNA, transfer RNA, and messenger RNA are constantly renewed by the cell nucleus and passed to

the myoid. The organelles of the myoid synthesize the visual pigments, the phospholipids and proteins of the outer segments, and the interphotoreceptor matrix. Proteins reach the outer segment through the connecting cilium (Fig. 1-26). The rod's oldest disks, which are surrounded by the retinal pigment microvilli, are detached in small groups from the tip of the cell; they are phagocytized and destroyed by the pigment epithelium. Sodium channels in the ellipsoid portion of the cell are active in visual transduction (Chapter 2).

Modulator cells. The signal initiated by stimulation of the outer segments is modulated and transmitted by three different cell types: (1) bipolar cells, (2) horizontal cells, and (3) amacrine cells. Their nuclei are located in the inner nuclear layer.

In primates there are four types of bipolar cells: (1) midget, (2) flat midget, (3) diffuse, and (4) interplexiform bipolar cells. Their dendrites attach to photoreceptor synaptic vesicles with desmosomes. Synapse with horizontal cells is

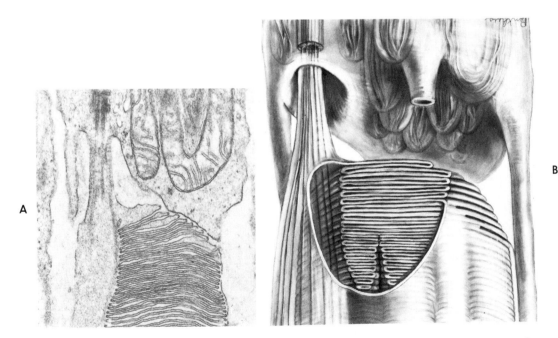

Fig. 1-26. A, Electron micrograph showing the junction of the outer and inner segments of the retinal rod of the rhesus monkey. The membranous disks form by inward folding of the outer cell membrane adjacent to the inner segment. As the disks mature they are displaced away from the base by newer disks and lose their attachment to the outer membrane and to each other. **B,** Drawing of this region reconstructed from electron micrographs to illustrate the process of disk formation. (From Young, R.W.: Invest. Ophthalmol. **15:**700, 1976.)

by desmosomes and gap junctions. A basketlike configuration of the dendrites at the border of the inner and middle thirds of the outer plexiform layer forms a dense structure that divides the retina into an outer portion, which, in humans, is dependent on choroidal circulation, and an inner portion, which is nurtured by the branches of the central retinal artery.

All cones synapse with at least one midget bipolar cell and commonly with other bipolar cells, but midget bipolar cells generally synapse with a single cone. Formerly, the midget bipolar cells were thought to synapse with a single foveal cone and a single ganglion cell. Physiologically, this one-to-one representation of cones in the fovea centralis is an oversimplification. Bipolar cells synapse with more than one foveal photoreceptor and ganglion cell but synapse with fewer of these cells than elsewhere in the retina.

Bipolar axons have branches that terminate in synaptic vesicles comparable to those of photoreceptors. In the inner plexiform layer, they synapse with the dendrites of ganglion cells and the processes of amacrine cells.

The nuclei of *horizontal cells* are located in the outer portion of the inner nuclear layer, and both their axons and dendrites are located in the outer plexiform layer. Horizontal cell dendrites synapse with several closely adjoining photoreceptors, and their axons synapse with several photoreceptors in a distant part of the retina. Other axons synapse with bipolar cells. Possibly, they act as condensers, as in an electric circuit, and collect impulses from a group of photoreceptors and, with discharge, trigger a visual impulse.

Amacrine cells are oriented in the wrong direction in terms of the transmission of the light impulse. The amacrine cell processes synapse with ganglion cells and bipolar cells. Their cell bodies lie at the inner portion of the inner nuclear layer, and their processes are directed inward toward the ganglion cell layer. Some contain large vesicles in their nuclei and cell processes that may contain dopamine. They may inhibit the integration of the visual impulse.

Transmitter cells. Ganglion cells transmit spike discharges through their axons to the midbrain. Their nuclei are located in the innermost cellular layer of the retina. In the region surrounding the fovea centralis, the ganglion cell layer is five to seven layers thick. In the retinal periphery, the ganglion cell layer is but a single cell thick. Transmitter cells may be classified anatomically on the basis of their dendrites: nonstratified, multistratified, diffuse, small, or large. Ganglion cell dendrites synapse with the axons of bipolar cells and the axons of amacrine cells in the inner plexiform layer. Physiologically, they may be divided into those subserving vision and those transmitting afferent pupillary impulses to the pretectal nuclei or the midbrain.

The axons of ganglion cells form the nerve fiber layer. The layer is sometimes visible in red-free light and may often be seen ophthalmoscopically in black individuals. The nerve fibers originating from ganglion cells of the fovea centralis extend directly medially to the optic nerve. Other axons form the temporal retina arch above and below these fibers but do not cross the horizontal raphe of the retina, which extends temporally from the fovea centralis to the ora serrata. The fibers to the nasal side of the optic disk have an approximately straight radial course. The distribution is important in the configuration of field defects in glaucoma. The major branches of the central retinal artery and vein are located in the nerve fiber layer.

The supporting astroglia. Müller cells are large astrocytes that mechanically support the retina partially aided by smaller glia and fibrous and protoplasmic astrocytes in the inner plexiform, ganglion cell, and nerve fiber layers of the retina. The nuclei of Müller cells are located in the middle portion of the inner nuclear layer of the retina. Terminal bars (zonula adherens) of the outer processes attach to the outer fibers of the photoreceptors and orient the outer segments for maximum efficiency. Inner processes extend toward the nerve fiber layer where their footplates separate this layer from the internal limiting lamina. Many filaments of the inner processes pass between axons of the nerve fiber layer. Müller cells furnish the enzymes for glycolysis. They accumulate retinal potassium and pass it to the vitreous (in some species).

Regions of the retina. The sensory retina is divided histologically as follows: (1) the ora serrata, the scalloped anterior termination of the

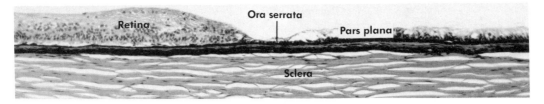

Fig. 1-27. The laminated sensory retina terminates in a serrated border at the ora serrata and continues forward as the epithelium of the pars plana portion of the ciliary body. The retinal pigment epithelium continues as the pigment epithelium of the ciliary body. (Hematoxylin and eosin stain; ×43.)

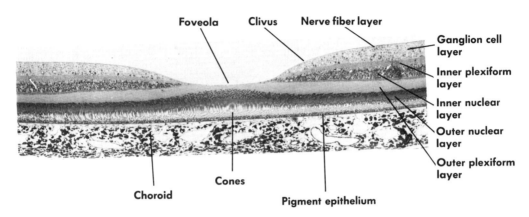

Fig. 1-28. Human fovea centralis. The fovea centralis is a depression with sloping walls, the clivus. The floor of the fovea centralis, the foveola, is flat. The fibers of the outer plexiform layer are tangential to the surface of the retina. The inner layers of the retina are absent, so that light falls directly upon the cones. The floor of the fovea centralis corresponds closely to the capillary-free region of the retina, and this area is nurtured solely by the choriocapillaris. (×105.) (Courtesy Ramesh C. Tripathi.)

sensory retina; (2) the central retina, with the fovea centralis and adjacent retina; and (3) the extracentral, or peripheral, retina, which includes the other portions of the retina.

Ora serrata. The ora serrata is the anterior termination of the retina; it consists of a dentate fringe adjacent to the pars plana (Fig. 1-27). It is located about 6 mm from the corneoscleral limbus. In this area, the sensory retina abruptly loses its laminated structure, and the two layers of the primitive optic vesicle fuse and continue forward as the ciliary epithelium.

Central retina (macula lutea). This region is about 4.5 mm in diameter. (The optic disk is 1.5 mm in diameter and is the unit customarily used in the measurement of retinal lesions.) The central retina extends from the fovea centralis nasally almost to the optic disk, about the same distance temporally, and a similar distance above and below the fovea centralis. In this region, the ganglion cell layer has more than one layer of nuclei. The retinal layers of the central retina from the outer nuclear layer inward have a yellow carotenoid pigment, xanthophyll, and this region is called the macula lutea (yellow spot). Clinically, the region is often called the macula.

The fovea centralis (Fig. 1-28) is a depressed area located in the central retina about 3 mm temporal to the optic disk and 0.8 mm below the horizontal meridian. It measures 1.5 mm in diameter. The sides of the depression form the clivus; its center is the foveola (Fig. 1-29) and measures about 0.4 mm in diameter. The photoreceptors in the fovea centralis are exclu-

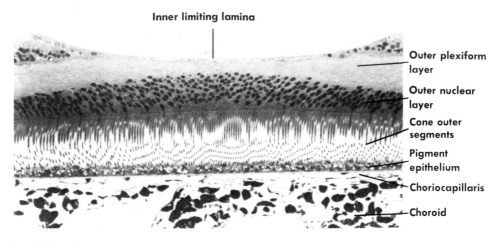

Inner limiting lamina

Outer plexiform layer

Outer nuclear layer

Cone outer segments

Pigment epithelium

Choriocapillaris

Choroid

Fig. 1-29. The human foveola. The outer segments of cones of the foveola are densely packed, thin, long, and attenuted. The inner layers of the retina are absent and only the outer nuclear layers and the outer plexiform layer are present. (×350.) (Courtesy Ramesh C. Tripathi.)

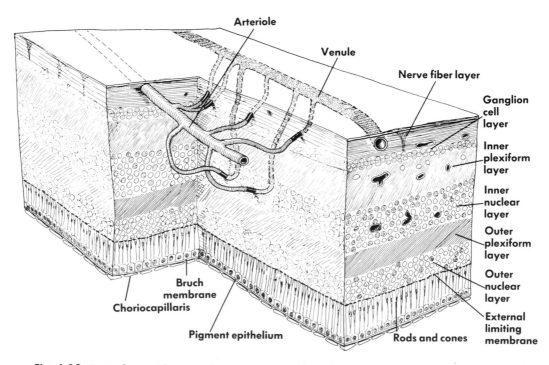

Arteriole

Venule

Nerve fiber layer

Ganglion cell layer

Inner plexiform layer

Inner nuclear layer

Outer plexiform layer

Outer nuclear layer

External limiting membrane

Rods and cones

Pigment epithelium

Choriocapillaris

Bruch membrane

Fig. 1-30. Retinal arterioles provide two major capillary layers in the retina: one in the nerve fiber layer and one in the inner nuclear layer. In general, diseases affecting primarily the arteries, such as vascular hypertension, involve the capillary network in the nerve fiber layer, whereas predominantly venous diseases, such as diabetes mellitus, involve the layer of capillaries in the inner nuclear layer. The photoreceptors together with their cell bodies in the outer nuclear layer and the outer one third of the outer plexiform layer are nurtured by the choriocapillaris of the choroid. Both systems are necessary to the function of the retina.

sively cones. The outer segments of cones in the foveola are densely packed, thin, long, and attenuated. The foveola is nurtured solely by the choriocapillaris of the choroid and does not contain the capillaries of the sensory retina located in the inner layers of the retina. The inner cell layers are displaced peripherally, and only the layer of cones, their nuclei in the outer nuclear layer, and their connections in the outer plexiform layer are present. The fibers in the outer plexiform layer extend radially to the inner nuclear layer. The region is nurtured solely by the choriocapillaris.

Peripheral retina. In the peripheral retina the photoreceptors are mainly rods, and the cones present are thicker than those in the central retina. The outer plexiform layer is vertically arranged, and the inner nuclear layer has a regular orientation. The ganglion cells are larger than those in the central retina, and their cell bodies are arranged in a single layer.

Retinal layers. The sensory retina is divided into three layers of nuclei and three layers of fibers. Conventionally, the layers closest to the sclera are the outer layers, and the layers closest to the vitreous are the inner layers.

The three nuclear layers are (1) the outer nuclear layer, which contains the nuclei of photoreceptors (rods and cones); (2) the inner nuclear layer, which contains the nuclei of bipolar, horizontal, amacrine, and Müller cells; and (3) the ganglion cell layer, which contains the nuclei of ganglion cells. The three nerve layers are (1) the outer plexiform layer where there is synapsis between rods and cones and the dendrites of bipolar cells and horizontal cells; (2) the inner plexiform layer where there is synapsis between bipolar cells, amacrine cells, and ganglion cells; and (3) the nerve fiber layer composed of axons of ganglion cells.

Functionally, the retina is divided into temporal and nasal portions by a line drawn vertically through the center of the fovea. Light impulses originating from cells temporal to this line pass to the lateral geniculate body on the same side. Light impulses originating from cells nasal to this line cross in the optic chiasm to the opposite side of the brain.

Ophthalmoscopically, the clinician uses the optic nerve as a hub to divide the retina into superior and inferior temporal portions, superior and inferior nasal portions, and a central area. The different quadrants are further divided into the regions posterior and anterior to the equator.

Blood supply. The retina is nurtured from two sources: (1) the outer portion is nurtured mainly by the choriocapillaris of the choroid, and (2) the inner portion is nurtured mainly by branches of the central retinal artery. The border is the basketlike configuration of bipolar cell dendrites at the junction of the outer and middle thirds of the outer plexiform layer. This does not provide a double blood supply—both circulations must be intact to maintain retinal function.

The central retinal artery, the first branch of the ophthalmic artery, enters the inferior medial side of the optic nerve about 12 mm posterior to the globe. It extends forward to the optic disk, where it bifurcates into superior and inferior papillary branches. As the vessel passes through the lamina cribrosa, its wall is reduced to about half its previous thickness, the internal elastic lamella is lost, and the medial muscle coat becomes incomplete. Thus its branches within the eye are arterioles.

The superior and inferior papillary branches of the central retinal artery bifurcate within the optic nerve or on the surface of the optic disk to form nasal and temporal branches. The nasal branches follow a relatively direct course to the periphery. The temporal vessels arch above and below the fovea centralis and pass to the periphery.

Capillaries. The capillaries are distributed in a superficial network at the level of the nerve fiber layer and in an intraretinal network at the level of the inner nuclear layer (Fig. 1-30). The intraretinal capillaries receive blood from the capillaries in the nerve fiber layer. Arterial abnormalities (such as vascular hypertension) tend to involve the capillaries in the nerve fiber plexus, whereas venous abnormalities (such as diabetes mellitus) tend to involve those located in the inner nuclear layer. The arterioles have a capillary-free zone surrounding them.

The endothelial cells that line retinal capillaries are regularly arranged with their nuclei parallel to the direction of the vessel. The vessel wall contains pericytes (mural cells) that are separated from the endothelium by its basement membrane. The endothelial cells are joined by terminal bars and constitute, together with the tight junctions of retinal pigment epithelium, the blood-retinal barrier.

Veins. The veins in the retina essentially follow the distribution of the arteries. They consist of an endothelial coat supported by a small amount of connective tissue. At points in the retina where arteries cross veins, the vessels are bound together with a common adventitial sheath. The central retinal vein emerges from the optic nerve at about the same point where the central retinal artery enters 12 mm behind the globe. As the central retinal vein passes through the meninges surrounding the optic nerve, it is considered vulnerable to increases in intracranial pressure, a factor important in the production of papilledema.

Chambers of the eye

The eye contains three chambers: the anterior chamber, the posterior chamber, and the vitreous cavity.

Anterior chamber. The anterior chamber (frontispiece) is bounded anteriorly by the cornea, posteriorly by the front surface of the iris and lens, and peripherally by the anterior chamber angle. The anterior chamber is deepest in its central portion (3 mm) and shallowest at the peripheral insertion of the iris. In humans, its volume is approximately 0.20 ml.

Posterior chamber. The posterior chamber (frontispiece) is bounded anteriorly by the iris, peripherally by the ciliary processes, and posteriorly by the anterior lens capsule and its zonule. Its volume in adults is about 0.06 ml. Aqueous humor is secreted by the nonpigmented epithelium of the ciliary processes into the posterior chamber and flows through the pupil into the anterior chamber.

Vitreous cavity. The vitreous cavity is the largest cavity of the eye. It is bounded anteriorly by the lens, zonule, and ciliary body and posteriorly by the retina and optic nerve. It has a volume of 4.5 ml.

The vitreous humor

The vitreous humor is a transparent gel structure composed of a random network of uniformly thin collagen fibrils suspended in a highly dilute solution of salts, protein, and hyaluronic acid. Its main component is water (98.5% to 99.7%). In young adults it is about

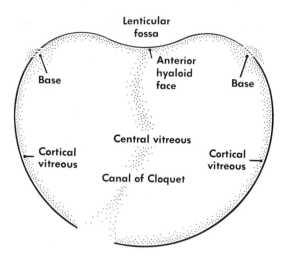

Fig. 1-31. The vitreous body that fills the vitreous chamber. The vitreous is strongly attached to the peripheral retina and the pars plana at its base and attached to the periphery of the optic nerve. It is divided into peripheral cortical vitreous and central vitreous.

80% gel and 20% liquid vitreous humor that contains hyaluronic acid but no fibrils. With aging, the volume of liquid vitreous increases to about 50%.

The vitreous is shaped like a sphere with a segment removed anteriorly to provide a saucer-shaped depression for the lens (lenticular fossa). In the region of the depression, the vitreous humor is condensed and described clinically as the anterior hyaloid face (Fig. 1-31). The vitreous humor adheres firmly to the peripheral retina and to the ciliary epithelium in the region of the pars plana (vitreous base) and to the margin of the optic disk. Sometimes it is strongly attached to retinal blood vessels. The anterior hyaloid may be loosely attached to the posterior capsule of the lens (Weigert hyaloideocapsular ligament).

In the healthy young eye, the vitreous humor is in contact with the entire retina and is attached to the internal limiting lamina of the retina by scattered collagenous filaments. These attachments may cause retinal tears by traction if the vitreous humor degenerates and collapses.

The vitreous humor may be divided into two portions: a cortical portion, which circumscribes the entire vitreous body adjacent to the

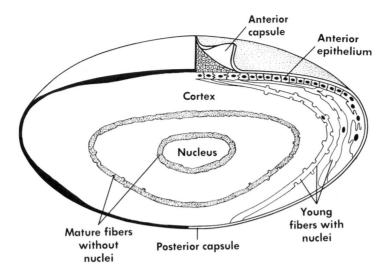

Fig. 1-32. Cross section of the lens. Young lens fibers form at the equator and migrate centrally. They contain nuclei and attach to their basement membrane, the posterior capsule. They occupy only a thin peripheral portion of the lens. The anterior epithelial cells attach to their basement membrane, the anterior capsule. Anterior epithelial cells do not have lens fibers. The majority of lens fibers in both the deeper cortex and nucleus do not have nuclei and do not attach to the lens capsule. Lens fibers join each other by gap junctions and ball-and-socket attachments.

lens and retina, and a central portion. The vitreous base is a 2 mm band of vitreous that straddles both the ora serrata and pars plana to which it is attached by many fibrils. At the periphery of the optic disk, fibrils extend between the vitreous and the footplates of Müller cells. Embryologically, the vitreous is divided into primary (mesenchymal, canal of Cloquet), secondary (most of the adult vitreous), and tertiary (the lens zonule) parts.

The central vitreous has a less dense structure with fewer fibrils than the vitreous of the cortex. The vitreous cortex contains a few cells called "hyalocytes," which are believed to be phagocytes, connective tissue cells of the macrophage type.

Lens and zonule

The crystalline lens. The crystalline lens (Fig. 1-32) is a grossly transparent, biconvex structure, located directly behind the iris and pupil and anterior to a shallow depression in the vitreous face, the lenticular fossa. It is held in position by its suspensory ligament, the zonule. It is approximately 10 mm in diameter and 4 mm thick. The center of curvature of the anterior surface is the anterior pole; the posterior

pole is the corresponding point on the posterior surface. The anterior surface has a radius of curvature of 10 mm. The posterior pole has a radius of curvature of 6.0 mm. The equator is separated from the free edge of the processes of the ciliary body by a distance of 0.5 mm. The zonular fibers insert into the anterior and posterior lens capsule near the equator and extend further over the anterior than the posterior surface.

The lens forms new fibers throughout life. In humans old fibers are compressed centrally to form an increasingly larger inelastic lens nucleus. Although the lens appears brilliantly transparent when viewed grossly, biomicroscopy discloses minute opacities and concentric areas with different indices of refraction.

The lens is composed of (1) a lens capsule that envelops the entire lens, (2) an anterior lens epithelium located immediately beneath the anterior lens capsule, and (3) a lens substance consisting of the cortex (newly formed soft lens fibers with nuclei) and the nucleus (a dense central area of fibers that have lost their nuclei).

The lens capsule is a smooth, homogenous, acellular structure. It is thickest on the anterior and posterior surfaces just central to the insertion of the zonular fibers. The anterior capsule is the basement membrane of the anterior lens epithelium and is the thickest basement membrane in the body. The posterior capsule is the basement membrane of lens cells that have their nuclei in the nuclear bow. The anterior lens epithelial cells consist of a single row of cuboidal cells of irregular shape with numerous interdigitations.

The lens substance consists of elongated lens cells (fibers). The less mature fibers have nuclei at the lens equator in the nuclear bow. Their posterior processes extend to their basement membrane, the posterior capsule. Mature lens fibers have lost their nuclei and are no longer in contact with the posterior capsule. These form most of the lens substance of the lens. They are packed into an increasingly dense, central nucleus. The nuclei of young cells migrate inward from the lens equator toward the center of the lens to form a nuclear bow zone. In fetal life, the apices of lens processes join at

the anterior central area and maintain junctions with cells extending from corresponding cells of the opposite side to form the upright, anterior Y-suture of the lens. When cells lose their nuclei, the posterior fibers are detached from the posterior capsule and are pushed deeper into the central zone to form the inverted Y-shaped posterior suture. After the fetal nucleus forms, the developing lens fibers form more complicated junctions than the Y-sutures. Lens fibers are curved, narrow, membranous cylinders that have numerous ridges and socket invaginations to receive knobs, especially in their lateral edges. Their apical ends are flat with lobulated edges.

The zonule. The lens zonule (zonule of Zinn, or suspensory ligament of the lens, Fig. 1-33) supports the lens in position and connects the lens to the ciliary muscle. It is composed of a series of fine fibrils modified of collagenous tissue on the outer surface of the lens capsule. The zonules attach to the lamellar portion of the lens capsule on either side of the equator

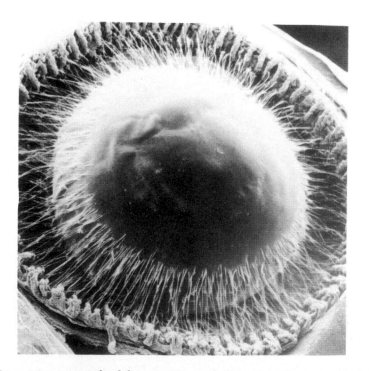

Fig. 1-33. Scanning micrograph of the anterior zonular insertion after removal of the cornea and iris. The anterior heads of the ciliary processes are free of zonules, and the angle between the anterior and the posterior zonules is evident. The lens is 25% smaller than normal owing to processing shrinkage. ($\times$25.) (By permission of Streeten, B.W.: Zonular apparatus. In Duane, T.D., and Jaeger, E.A., editors: Biomedical foundations of ophthalmology, vol. 1, Philadelphia, 1983, Harper & Row, Publishers.)

and to the basement membrane of the ciliary epithelium in the valleys between the ciliary processes. The ciliary attachment is long, and fibers may extend to the pars plana of the ciliary body. Other fibers attach to the anterior vitreous face. The lens insertion extends about 2 mm in front and 1 mm behind the lens equator.

THE ORBIT

The eyes rest in the anterior portion of two bony cavities, the orbits (Fig. 1-34), located on either side of the nose. Although each orbit appears to be positioned directly forward, only the medial walls are parallel, and the lateral walls diverge at an angle of about 45°. The posterior openings of each orbit, the optic foramen and the superior orbital fissure, are located me-

dial to the eye, so that the optic nerve, blood vessels, and ocular muscles must pass laterally, a factor in ocular rotations.

The anterior two thirds of the orbit are roughly the shape of a truncated quadrilateral pyramid with a base of about 35 to 40 mm. The posterior third narrows to the shape of a triangular pyramid. The adult orbit is usually considered to be approximately 40 mm in height, width, and depth, and its volume is about 29 ml.

Structure

The anterior margin of the orbit is thickened and provides protection for the eye. The zygomatic bone and the zygomatic process of the frontal bone form the sturdy lateral margin. The superior margin is formed entirely by the

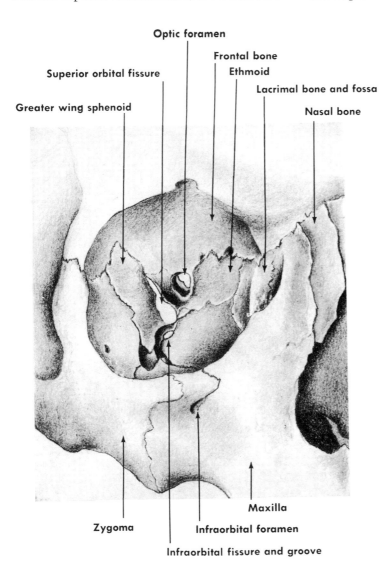

Fig. 1-34. The bony orbit.

frontal bone. The medial angular process of the frontal bone and the frontal process of the maxilla form the medial margin, which is poorly defined because of the fossa for the lacrimal sac. The inferior margin is formed by the zygoma and the body of the maxilla. Each wall of the orbit, except the medial, is approximately triangular with the base directed forward.

Two bones form the lateral wall: the zygoma anteriorly and the greater wing of the sphenoid posteriorly. The zygomatic portion of the lateral wall is composed of dense bone that separates the orbit from the fossa of the temporalis muscle. The lateral orbital tubercle is situated on the anterior margin of the lateral wall. To it is attached the aponeurosis of the levator palpebrae superioris muscle, the suspensory ligament of the globe (ligament of Lockwood), the check ligament of the lateral rectus muscle, and the lateral palpebral ligament. The greater wing of the sphenoid bone forms the posterior two thirds of the lateral wall. This posterior portion is extremely thin, and it separates the orbit from the temporal lobe of the brain.

The roof of the orbit is mainly formed by the orbital plate of the frontal bone. The lesser wing of the sphenoid bone contributes slightly to the apex. Laterally, the orbital roof is adjacent to the zygoma anteriorly and to the greater wing of the sphenoid posteriorly. The fossa for the lacrimal gland is located in its anterior lateral portion. Medially, the roof is adjacent to the lacrimal bone anteriorly and the ethmoid bone posteriorly. Medially, near the anterior margin, is the trochlea, a fibrous tissue that forms a pulley for the tendon of the superior oblique muscle. Immediately above the orbital roof is the frontal sinus anteriorly and the frontal lobe of the brain posteriorly.

The orbital floor does not extend to the apex. The floor is formed mainly by the orbital plate of the maxilla. The orbital surface of the zygoma extends laterally, and the orbital process of the palatine bone extends medially. Posteriorly, the infraorbital sulcus (Fig. 1-35) extends across the floor of the orbit from the infraorbital fissure. It contains the infraorbital artery and maxillary nerve. At about its midpoint, the sulcus becomes a canal that opens into the in-

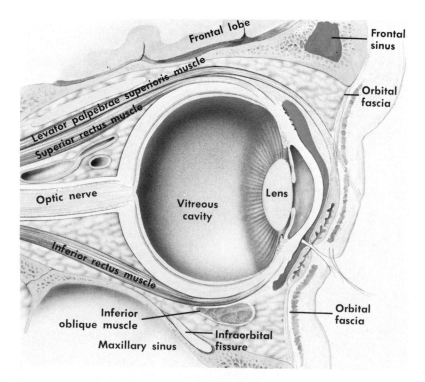

Fig. 1-35. Sagittal section of the orbit. The infraorbital fissure is the weakest area of the orbit and may incarcerate the inferior rectus muscle in fractures (blow-out) of the floor of the orbit.

fraorbital foramen through which the artery and nerve emerge on the face.

The medial wall is quadrilateral. It is formed mainly by the orbital plate of the ethmoid bone, but it has sutures anteriorly with the lacrimal bone and posteriorly with the body of the sphenoid bone. The lamina papyracea of the ethmoid bone is extremely thin, and the sinus may rupture into the orbit when inflamed or when fractured and allow air to enter the orbit. In the anterior portion of the orbit, the fossa of the lacrimal sac is located between the anterior lacrimal crest of the frontal process of the maxilla and the posterior lacrimal crest of the lac-

rimal bone. The lacrimal sac occupies this fossa and extends downward through the nasal lacrimal duct into the nose. The two leaves of the medial canthal ligament insert into the anterior and posterior lacrimal crests. The posterior portion of the medial wall of the orbit formed by the body of the sphenoid bone contains the optic foramen.

Optic foramen and orbital fissures

The optic foramen is located at the posterior medial portion of the orbit in the body of the sphenoid bone. The optic canal measures 4 to 10 mm in length. Through it passes the optic

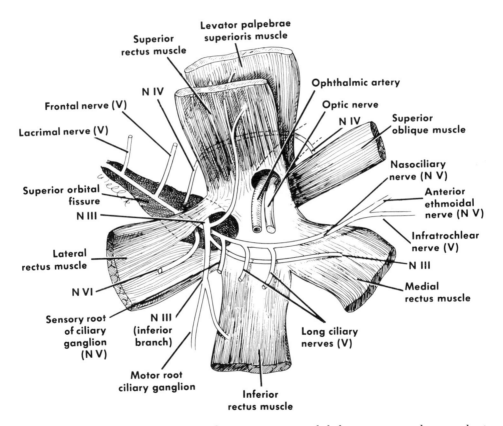

Fig. 1-36. Apex of the right orbit. The optic nerve, ophthalmic artery, and sympathetic nerves are transmitted through the optic foramen. The optic foramen and the medial portion of the superior orbital fissure are encircled by the annulus of Zinn. The lacrimal and frontal branches of the ophthalmic division of the fifth nerve and the trochlear nerve (N IV) enter the orbit in the lateral portion of the superior orbital fissure outside of the annulus. The other branches of the ophthalmic division of the fifth nerve and the oculomotor (N III) and abducent (N VI) nerves enter the orbit more medially within the annulus. The maxillary, or second, division of the trigeminal nerve enters the orbit through the inferior orbital fissure and emerges on the face at the intraorbital foramen. The lateral rectus muscle is divided into upper and lower origin by the annulus of Zinn as it bridges the superior orbital foramen. The superior oblique muscle is exceptional in receiving its motor nerve, the trochlear (N IV), on its orbital surface. All the other muscles are innervated on the side closest to the globe.

nerve, the ophthalmic artery, and sympathetic nerves from the carotid plexus. Just lateral to the optic foramen is a superior orbital fissure that separates the greater and lesser wings of the sphenoid bone. The fissure is divided into lateral and medial portions by the fibrous annulus of Zinn, from which the ocular muscles originate. Passing through the superior orbital fissure within the annulus of Zinn are the oculomotor nerve (N III), abducent nerve (VI), and all branches of the ophthalmic division of the trigeminal nerve (N V) except the lacrimal and frontal branches. These latter nerves and the trochlear nerve (N IV) emerge from the lateral portion of the superior orbital fissure outside the annulus of Zinn and the muscle cone (Fig. 1-36).

The inferior orbital fissure (sphenomaxillary) is formed at the junction of the orbital plate of the greater wing of the sphenoid bone and the lateral margin of the orbital process of the maxillary bone. It transmits the second branch (maxillary) of the trigeminal nerve and provides anastomosis between the inferior ophthalmic vein and the pterygoid plexus. The fissure is covered by smooth muscle of Müller, which has a doubtful function in humans and is the analogue of the retractor bulbi muscle of lower animals.

The dura mater layer of the meninges that surrounds the optic nerve in the optic foramen divides into two layers at the orbital apex. One portion lines the orbit as the periosteum; the other continues forward as the dural sheath of the optic nerve. The annulus of Zinn inserts medially into the cleft formed by this splitting; laterally, it is attached at the spina recti lateralis at the tip of the greater wing of the sphenoid. Each of the recti muscles originates at the annulus of Zinn. The lateral rectus muscle is divided into an upper and lower head by the superior orbital fissure.

Orbital fascia

The orbital contents are bound together and supported by connective tissues that divide the orbit into spaces of clinical importance in limiting the spread of hemorrhage and inflammation. The main orbital fasciae are (1) the periorbita (periosteum of the orbit), (2) the orbital septum (palpebral fascia), (3) the bulbar fascia (Tenon capsule), and (4) the muscular fascia.

The *periorbita (periosteum of the orbit)* is the periosteal lining of the orbit. It is derived from the dura mater, which splits at the optic foramen into two layers, one constituting the periosteum and the other continuing as the dural sheath of the optic nerve.

The *orbital septum (palpebral fascia)* stretches from the bony margins of the orbit to the eyelid in close relationship with the posterior surface of the palpebral portion of the orbicularis oculi muscle. It divides the orbit into anterior and posterior portions. The septum prevents orbital fat from entering the eyelids and limits the spread of inflammation.

The *bulbar fascia (Tenon capsule)* separates the globe from orbital fat and provides the socket in which the eye moves. It extends anteriorly to the insertion of the conjunctiva at the corneoscleral limbus. Its lower portion is thickened to form a sling (the ligament of Lockwood), upon which the globe rests. Posteriorly, the fascia is thin and perforated by the structures passing to or from the globe.

The *muscular fascia* surrounds the ocular muscles, particularly their anterior portions, like the sleeve of a coat surrounds an arm. The portion that covers the medial and lateral recti muscles sends expansions to the orbital margins as check ligaments. Other fibers extend to the conjunctiva and hold it taut in ocular rotation.

EXTRINSIC MUSCLES

The extrinsic muscles of the eye (Fig. 1-37) are the four recti and the two oblique muscles. (The ciliary muscles and the sphincter pupillae and dilatator pupillae muscles are the intrinsic muscles.)

Origin

The four recti muscles originate at the apex of the orbit from the ligament of Zinn (annulus tendineus communis), which encircles the optic foramen and the medial portion of the superior orbital fissure (see Fig. 1-36). The superior oblique muscle originates at the apex of the orbit from the periosteum of the lesser wing of the sphenoid bone medial to and above the optic foramen. The inferior oblique muscle originates on the floor of the orbit from the periosteum covering the anteromedial portion of the maxilla. The four recti muscles insert

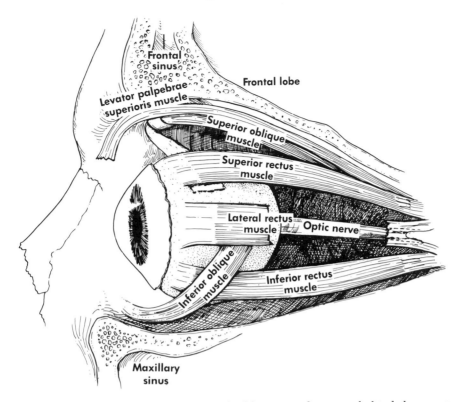

Fig. 1-37. Extrinsic muscles of the eye. Both oblique muscles insert behind the equator of the globe. The inferior oblique muscle passes inferior to the body of the inferior rectus muscle but beneath the lateral rectus muscle. The numbers indicate the distance of the insertion from the corneoscleral limbus and the length of the muscle tendon.

into the sclera anterior to the equator of the globe. The two oblique muscles insert into the sclera posterior to the equator.

The extraocular muscles are the most highly differentiated of all striated muscles. They contain slow fibers capable of a graded contracture on their exterior surface and fast fibers responsible for rapid movements in the central mass of the muscle. The slow fibers correspond to red muscle fibers, which contain a high content of mitochondria and oxidative enzymes. They are innervated by grapelike motor nerve terminals. The fast fibers correspond to white muscle fibers and contain greater amounts of glycogen and glycolytic enzymes and less oxidative enzymes than do the slow fibers. They have plaquelike motor nerve endings.

Recti muscles

The recti muscles are (1) the medial rectus muscle, (2) the lateral rectus muscle, (3) the superior rectus muscle, and (4) the inferior rectus muscle. They originate from the ligament of Zinn and pass forward in the orbit, gradually diverging to form the ocular muscle cone. Each muscle is about 40 mm long and about 10 to 11.5 mm wide at its point of insertion into the sclera. By means of a tendon, the muscles insert into the sclera between 5.3 and 7.9 mm from the corneoscleral limbus (Fig. 1-38).

The *medial rectus muscle* originates from the medial portion of the ligament of Zinn in close contact with the optic nerve. It is innervated by the inferior division of the oculomotor nerve (N III), which enters on the bulbar side. It functions in adduction (medial rotation) of the globe.

The *lateral rectus muscle* originates from two heads from the upper and lower portions of the ligament of Zinn, where the ligament bridges the superior orbital fissure. It passes forward, over the insertion of the inferior oblique muscle, to insert into the sclera. It is innervated by the abducent nerve (N VI), which enters on its bulbar surface at about the middle. It functions in abduction (lateral rotation) of the eye.

The *superior rectus muscle* originates from the superior portion of the ligament of Zinn in close contact with the meningeal sheaths surrounding the optic nerve.* The muscle passes forward and laterally from the apex, forming an angle of 23° with the sagittal diameter of the globe. Superiorly, it is adjacent to the levator palpebrae superioris muscle throughout its course. The superior rectus muscle is innervated by the superior division of the oculomotor nerve, which enters its bulbar surface at the junction of the anterior one third with the posterior two thirds. The muscle functions mainly as an elevator, with elevation becoming more efficient as the eye abducts and becoming entirely absent as the eye adducts. When the eye is turned medially, the muscle aids in adduction. The muscle intorts (rotates inward) the superior meridian of the cornea.

The *inferior rectus muscle* originates from

---

*Rotation of the eye causes pain in retrobulbar neuritis because of the close association of the superior and medial recti muscles with the optic nerve.

the inferior portion of the ligament of Zinn and passes forward and laterally, forming an angle of 23° (as does the superior rectus muscle) with the sagittal diameter of the globe. It is innervated by a branch of the inferior division of the oculomotor nerve, which enters on its superior edge at the junction of the anterior one third with the posterior two thirds. The muscle functions mainly as a depressor, with depression becoming more efficient as the eye abducts and becoming entirely absent as the eye adducts. In medial rotation, the muscle aids in adduction. The muscle extorts (rotates outward) the superior meridian of the cornea. Through fibrous tarsal and subconjunctival attachments, it also acts as a retractor of the lower eyelid.

Oblique muscles

There are two oblique muscles, the superior oblique and the inferior oblique.

The *superior oblique muscle* originates from the periosteal covering of the lesser wing of the sphenoid bone above and medial to the optic foramen. It consists of two parts: a direct muscular portion that extends from its origin to the trochlea and a reflected portion, composed en-

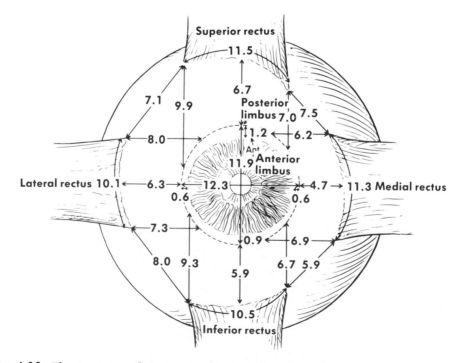

Fig. 1-38. The insertion of rectus muscles into the sclera. (From Apt, L.: Trans. Am. Ophthalmol. Soc. **78:**365, 1980.)

tirely of tendon, that extends from the trochlea, passing beneath the superior rectus muscle, to its insertion to the globe.

The direct portion passes forward in the angle between the roof and the medial wall of the orbit to the trochlea. The trochlea is a synovial-lined fibrocartilage sling attached to the trochlear spine of the medial aspect of the frontal bone a few millimeters behind the superior orbital margin. The tendon of the superior oblique muscle begins about 10 mm behind the trochlea. From the trochlea the tendon passes downward, laterally, and posteriorly beneath the superior rectus muscle to be inserted on the upper outer quadrant of the eye behind the equator. The tendon is a fibrous cord, about 1 × 2 mm in size, that becomes flatter and wider as it approaches the medial margin of the superior rectus muscle. The main function of the muscle is intorsion (inward rotation) of the 12 o'clock meridian of the cornea; this action is absent when the eye is adducted. In adduction the muscle depresses the eye, and in the straight ahead position the muscle aids in abduction.

The *inferior oblique muscle* originates at the periosteum covering the orbital plate of the maxilla a few millimeters behind the orbital margin and near the orifice of the nasolacrimal duct. It passes laterally and posteriorly between the inferior rectus muscle and the floor of the orbit in a tunnel in the fascia that envelops the inferior rectus muscle. It then curves upward around the globe to insert into the posterior sclera on the inferior lateral surface of the globe. It has no tendon. The muscle is innervated by the inferior division of the oculomotor nerve (N III), which enters the bulbar surface just after the muscle has passed to the lateral side of the inferior rectus muscle. The main function of the inferior oblique muscle is elevation, which increases as the eye is adducted and is absent in abduction. In lateral rotation the muscle aids in abduction. The muscle extorts (rotates outward) the 12 o'clock meridian of the cornea.

EYELIDS

The eyelids (Fig. 1-39) are thin curtains of skin, muscle, fibrous tissue, and mucous membrane that protect the eye from external irritation, interrupt and limit the amount of light entering the eye, and distribute tears over the surface of the globe. The upper eyelid is limited above by the eyebrow; the lower eyelid merges with the cheek. Each eyelid is divided by a horizontal furrow (sulcus) into an orbital and a tarsal portion. The upper furrow is

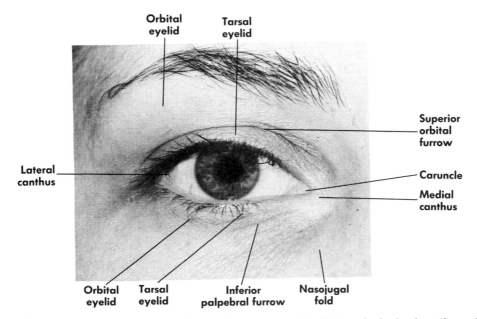

Fig. 1-39. Eyelids and palpebral sulcus. The superior and inferior palpebral sulcus (furrow) divide the eyelids into tarsal and orbital portions.

formed by skin insertions of the levator palpe-brae superioris muscle. The lower furrow is poorly defined and is formed by a few cutaneous connections from the orbicularis oculi muscle. The corneoscleral limbus is covered above and below by the eyelids.

When open, the eyelids form an elliptic opening, the palpebral fissure, which measures about 12 by 30 mm. Laterally the fissure forms a 60° angle; medially it is rounded. In blacks and whites the lateral margin (canthus) is about 2 mm higher than the medial; in orientals it may be 5 mm higher. In blacks and whites the fissure is widest at the junction of the inner one third with the outer two thirds. In orientals the fissure is widest at the junction of the inner one half with the outer one half. In orientals the medial canthus is obscured by a characteristic vertical skin fold (epicanthus), which, when present in whites, may cause the eyes to appear to be turned in (pseudostrabismus).

Each eyelid margin is 2 mm thick and 30 mm long. At a point 5 mm from the medial angle is a small eminence, the papilla lacrimalis, which contains the minute central opening of the lacrimal canaliculus, the punctum (Fig. 1-40). The medial one sixth of the eyelid, or the lacrimal portion, has no cilia or gland openings, and the eyelid margins are rounded. The lateral five sixths of the eyelid margin, the ciliary portion, has squared edges.

The intramarginal sulcus, or gray line, of the margin of the eyelid divides the eyelid into an anterior leaf containing muscle and skin and a posterior leaf containing tarsus and conjunctiva. The eyelashes originate anterior to the gray line, and the orifices of the tarsal glands are posterior to it. The junction of the conjunctiva and the stratified epithelium of the skin is at the level of the orifices of the tarsal glands.

The eyelashes on the upper eyelid margin curve upward and are more numerous than those on the lower eyelid margin, which curve downward. Opening into the follicle of each cilium are the ducts of the sebaceous glands of Zeis. Large sweat glands (of Moll) open into these follicles or directly onto the eyelid margin between the cilia.

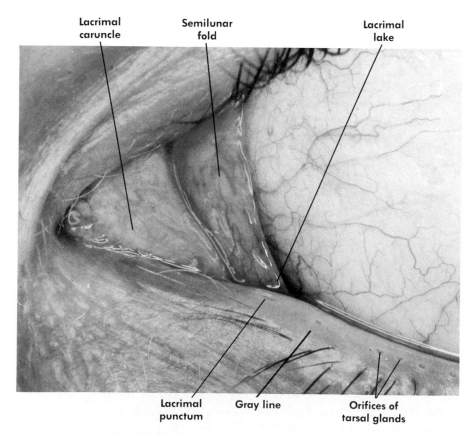

Fig. 1-40. Lacrimal portion of the eyelid margin.

Structure. The eyelids contain the following parts (Fig. 1-41):

Skin
Muscles
  Orbicularis oculi (N VII)
    Orbital portion
    Palpebral portion
      Preseptal portion
      Pretarsal portion

Eyelid retractors
  Levator palpebrae superioris (N III)
  Superior tarsal muscle (sympathetic)
  Inferior rectus muscle (N III)
  Inferior tarsal muscle (sympathetic)
Fibrous tissue
  Septum orbitale
  Tarsal plates
Conjunctiva

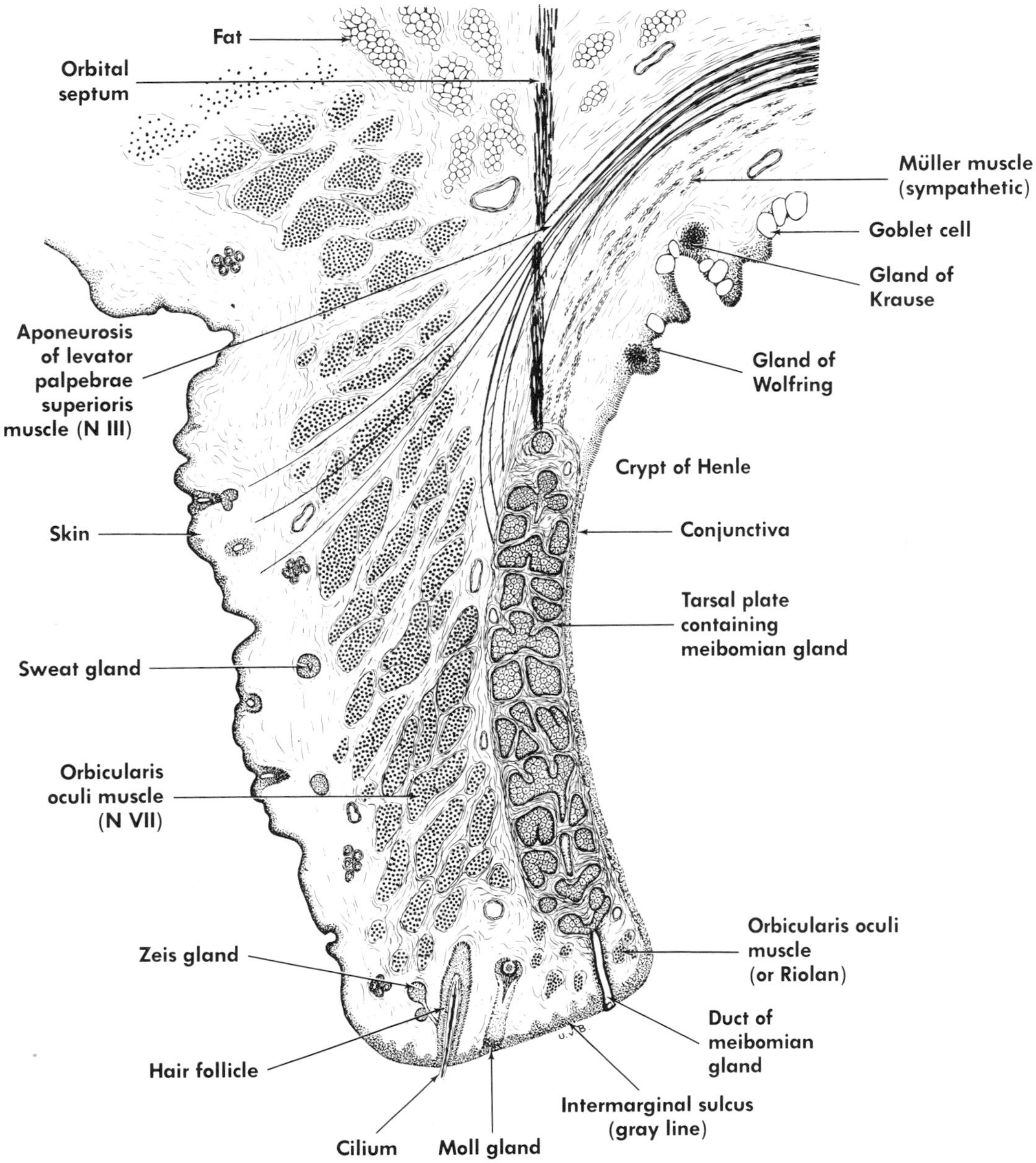

Fig. 1-41. Eyelid in cross section. The orbital septum separates the intraorbital contents from the eyelid. The intermarginal sulcus provides a line of surgical dissection separating the anterior structures of the eyelid from the tarsus and tarsal conjunctiva.

The skin of the eyelids is the thinnest in the body. It contains no fat in the subcutaneous areolar area and is thrown into numerous folds. The skin may be markedly distended by blood or fluid and, because of its thinness, underlying blood vessels may appear as dark blue channels.

The orbicularis oculi muscle (N VII), the sphincter of the eyelids, is a thin oval sheet of striated muscle composed of concentric fibers surrounding the palpebral fissure. It is divided into a peripheral orbital portion involved in forcible closure of the eyelids and a central palpebral portion that functions in involuntary blinking. The orbital part of the muscle originates from the medial margin of the orbit and the anterior surface of the medial palpebral (canthal) ligament. It inserts into the periorbita of the superior and inferior orbital margin and into the lateral palpebral (canthal) ligament. The palpebral part of the orbicularis oculi muscle is divided into a preseptal portion overlying the orbital septum and a pretarsal part overlying the upper and lower tarsal plates. The upper and lower preseptal portions have deep heads that originate in the region of the posterior lacrimal crest and a superficial origin from the medial palpebral ligament. The preseptal portions of the orbicularis oculi muscles pass laterally anterior to the orbital septum and join to form the lateral palpebral raphe that inserts into the fascia investing the orbital muscle in the zygomatic region. The upper and lower pretarsal muscles originate from the posterior lacrimal crest and from the medial canthal ligament that inserts into the anterior lacrimal crest. They sweep laterally to insert into the lateral canthal ligament that inserts into the lateral orbital tubercle. The fibers at the medial canthus support the lacrimal puncta and with each blink create suction in the lacrimal sac.

The orbital septum separates the eyelids from the contents of the orbit. In the upper eyelid it fuses with the levator aponeurosis, slightly above the upper level of the tarsus. It attaches laterally to the lateral canthal ligament and to the periorbita overlying the orbital tubercle. Nasally the orbital septum attaches to the region of the posterior lacrimal crest. In the lower eyelid the orbital septum attaches to the lateral reticulum along the entire width of the lower border of the tarsus and to the posterior lacrimal crest.

The levator palpebrae superioris muscle (N III) is closely related to the superior rectus muscle in its origin and course. It originates from the periosteal covering of the lesser wing of the sphenoid bone, and its origin blends with that of the superior rectus muscle below and the superior oblique muscle medially. It runs forward beneath the roof of the orbit to a point about 1 cm behind the septum orbitale, where it expands into an aponeurosis, which passes through the orbital septum. The aponeurosis inserts into the skin of the eyelid to form the superior palpebral furrow, into the anterior surface of the tarsal plate, and into the medial and lateral palpebral ligaments. The nerve supply is from the superior division of the oculomotor nerve (N III), which passes through the underlying superior rectus muscle to reach the inferior surface of the levator muscle.

The capsulopalpebral fascia in the lower eyelid is equivalent to the levator aponeurosis in the levator palpebrae superioris muscle aponeurosis in the upper eyelid. It extends between the fascia components and the inferior transverse ligament (Lockwood), and the inferior border of the lower tarsus and passes under the inferior oblique muscle. The connection between the suspensory ligament and the tarsus makes this fascia the principal retractor of the lower eyelid.

The inferior tarsal muscle originates from the sheath of the inferior rectus muscle where it surrounds the inferior oblique muscle. It courses upward, forward, and inserts into the bulbar conjunctiva and to the expansion of the fascia of the inferior rectus muscle that inserts into the tarsus. Its fibers are continuous over the lateral orbital rim.

The superior and inferior palpebral smooth muscles of Müller (sympathetics) are small sheets of smooth muscle located immediately beneath the orbital portion of the palpebral conjunctiva. The superior palpebral muscle originates from the undersurface of the levator palpebrae superioris muscle.

The fibrous tissue of the eyelids consists of a peripheral layer, the palpebral fascia or septum orbitale, and a thickened central portion, the tarsal plates.

The tarsal plates consist of firm connective tissue (not cartilage) that gives form and density to the free margin of the eyelids. Each tarsal plate is about 1 mm thick and 25 to 30 mm long. They extend from the lacrimal puncta medially to the lateral canthus. The upper tarsus measures about 11 mm vertically, and the lower tarsus about 5 mm.

The free edge of the tarsal plate extends the length of the ciliary portion of the eyelid margin. The posterior surface of the tarsus is firmly attached to the tarsal conjunctiva and conforms to the curvature of the globe. The anterior surface of the tarsus is separated from the orbicularis oculi muscle by loose areolar tissue, so that the muscle moves freely over its surface. The attached margin of the tarsus gradually merges into the orbital septum. Medially and laterally, the tarsal plates attach to palpebral ligaments.

Each tarsus contains sebaceous (meibomian) glands, the ducts of which open onto the eyelid margin. These glands are arranged in a single row in the tarsal plate, and each consists of 10 to 15 acini placed irregularly around a central canal that opens onto the eyelid margin. The sebaceous secretion prevents the overflow of tears, makes possible an airtight closure of the eyelids, provides the external layer of the precorneal tear film, and prevents the rapid evaporation of tears.

Blood supply. The blood supply to the eyelid is derived from marginal and peripheral vascular arcades. These are formed by the lateral palpebral branches of the lacrimal artery and the medial palpebral branches of the dorsonasal artery, both of which are derived from the internal carotid artery through the ophthalmic artery. There is a wide anastomotic circulation provided by branches of the external carotid artery through the facial, superficial temporal, and infraorbital arteries.

Nerve supply. The ophthalmic (first) division of the trigeminal nerve (N V) provides the sensory innervation to the upper eyelid and to a small lateral portion of the lower eyelid. Innervation of the remaining portion of the lower eyelid is by the maxillary (second) division of the trigeminal nerve through the infraorbital nerve. The facial nerve (N VII) innervates the orbicularis oculi muscle, and the oculomotor nerve (N III) supplies the levator palpebrae superioris muscle. Postganglionic sympathetic fibers from the superior cervical ganglion innervate the palpebral muscles of Müller.

Lymphatic supply. The eyelids are drained by two groups (Fig. 1-42) of lymphatic vessels: (1) a medial group drains the medial two thirds of the lower eyelid and the medial one third of

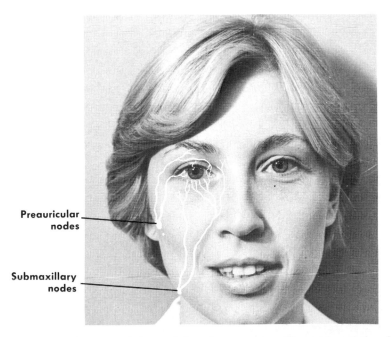

Preauricular nodes

Submaxillary nodes

Fig. 1-42. Lymphatic drainage of the eyelids and conjunctiva. The orbit and the globe and its contents have no lymphatics.

the upper eyelid into the submaxillary lymph nodes, and (2) a lateral group drains the remaining portion of the eyelids into the preauricular nodes.

THE CONJUNCTIVA

The conjunctiva is a thin, transparent mucous membrane (Fig. 1-43) that lines the inner surface of the eyelids and covers the anterior portion of the sclera. Its epithelium is continuous with that of the cornea and with the lacrimal drainage system through the puncta. The conjunctiva is divided into three areas: (1) the palpebral conjunctiva, (2) the conjunctiva of the superior and inferior fornices, and (3) the bulbar conjunctiva.

The *palpebral conjunctiva* is divided into marginal tarsal and orbital portions. The tarsal portion is closely adherent to the tarsal plate, from which it can be removed only with difficulty. The orbital portion is thrown into folds.

The *conjunctiva of the superior and inferior fornices* forms transitional areas between the palpebral and bulbar conjunctivae. It is but loosely attached to the underlying tissue and may become markedly swollen.

The *bulbar conjunctiva* is closely adherent to the sclera, which can be seen as the "white" of the eye through the transparent conjunctival tissue.

At the medial angle of each eye are two specialized structures formed in part by the conjunctiva: the semilunar fold and the lacrimal caruncle. The semilunar fold (plica semilunaris) consists of a delicate vertical crescent of conjunctiva, the free edge of which is concave and

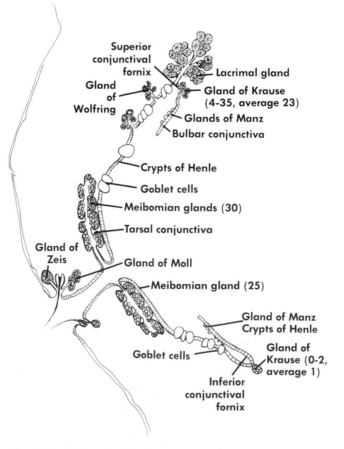

Fig. 1-43. Sagittal section of the eyelids to show the glandular structures of the conjunctiva. Mucin, the wetting agent of the precorneal tear film, is mainly secreted by goblet cells with minor amounts secreted by the glands of Wolfring and Manz. The lacrimal gland and the glands of Krause secrete the aqueous portion of tears. The meibomian glands secrete the oily exterior layer of the tear film.

concentric with the corneal margin. It is separated from the bulbar conjunctiva by the cul-de-sac 2 mm deep. The lacrimal caruncle is a minute piece of modified skin located in the lacus lacrimalis medial to the semilunar fold. It is covered by stratified epithelium that is not keratinized. It consists of large sebaceous glands similar to meibomian glands and has fine hairs with sebaceous glands similar to the glands of Zeis. The caruncle is conspicuous when the eye is rotated laterally.

Structure. Like other mucous membranes, the conjunctiva is composed of two layers: (1) stratified columnar epithelium, and (2) lamina propria composed of an adenoid and a fibrous layer.

The *stratified epithelium* varies in thickness from two cell layers in its upper tarsal portion to five to seven layers at the corneoscleral junction. It is never keratinized in healthy individuals. After 3 months of age, the development of the adenoid tissue makes the conjunctival surface moderately irregular.

The *lamina propria* is composed of connective tissue containing blood vessels, nerves, conjunctival glands, polymorphonuclear leukocytes, mast cells, and macrophages. The bulbar and fornix conjunctiva and the orbital portion of the palpebral conjunctiva contain adenoid tissue with many lymphocytes enmeshed in a fine reticular network. True lymphatic follicles are not present except in childhood and in follicular conjunctivitis. The fibrous layer of the conjunctiva is continuous with the inner margins of the tarsal plates and contains the smooth palpebral muscles of Müller (sympathetic nervous system).

Glands. The conjunctival epithelium contains numerous glands (see Fig. 1-43) responsible for maintaining moisture and secreting the constituents of the precorneal tear film. Unlike the corneal epithelium, the conjunctival epithelium contains numerous unicellular mucous glands (goblet cells) that secrete mucin, the wetting agent of the precorneal tear film responsible for wetting the corneal epithelium. The glands are most numerous in the conjunctival fornices, occur less frequently in the bulbar conjunctiva, and are absent at the eyelid margins and corneoscleral margin.

The accessory lacrimal glands of Krause are located deep in the substantia propria, particularly in the fornices. They have the histologic structure and secretion of the lacrimal gland proper. Most are located in the temporal one third of the conjunctiva. The glands of Wolfring and Manz are less common and secrete a mucinous substance similar to goblet cells. The conjunctiva has a papillary arrangement, the crypts of Henle, above and below the tarsal plates.

Blood supply. The blood supply of the palpebral conjunctiva comes from the peripheral and marginal arterial arcades of the eyelid. The marginal arcade nourishes the margins of the eyelids and part of the tarsal area of the palpebral conjunctiva. The bulbar and fornix conjunctiva is nourished by the peripheral arcade.

The posterior conjunctival branches of the peripheral arterial arcade provide the blood supply of the peripheral bulbar conjunctiva. These vessels are superficial, nearly invisible, and extend to within 4 mm of the corneoscleral limbus. In the area adjacent to the corneoscleral limbus, the anterior conjunctival branches of the seven anterior ciliary arteries divide to form a superficial (conjunctival) and a deep (episcleral) pericorneal plexus. The anterior and posterior conjunctival vessels anastomose (see Fig. 1-22).

The posterior conjunctival vessels are dilated in inflammations of the bulbar conjunctiva. Because of their superficial position, they appear bright red and move with the conjunctiva. They are most evident in the fornices and fade toward the corneoscleral limbus. Because they are superficial, they may be constricted with the instillation of 1:1,000 epinephrine.

The superficial (conjunctival) pericorneal plexus, which is derived from the anterior ciliary arteries, is injected in inflammations of the cornea. The deep (episcleral) pericorneal plexus is injected in inflammations of the iris and the ciliary body and in closed-angle glaucoma. Because of their deep position, these vessels appear dull red to purple and do not move with the conjunctiva. They are not constricted by topical epinephrine. These vessels are most evident near the corneoscleral limbus and fade toward the fornices. Because of the generous anastomoses between the anterior and posterior conjunctival arteries, severe inflammations always cause injection of both ciliary and conjunctival vessels.

Nerve supply. The bulbar conjunctiva is innervated by ciliary nerves and by sympathetic nerves accompanying blood vessels. Sensory innervation of the superior palpebral conjunctiva is by the frontal nerve medially and lacrimal nerve laterally. Sensory innervation of the inferior palpebral conjunctiva is by the lateral palpebral branch of the lacrimal nerve laterally (ophthalmic division, N V) and the infraorbital nerve (maxillary division, N V) medially.

Lymphatic supply. The lymphatics of the conjunctiva parallel those of the eyelid.

LACRIMAL APPARATUS

The lacrimal apparatus consists of a secretory and a collecting portion. The secretory portion is composed of the lacrimal gland and the accessory lacrimal glands of Krause and Wolfring. The collecting portion consists of the canaliculi with their orifices (the puncta), the lacrimal sac, and the lacrimal duct, which has its opening in the inferior nasal meatus.

Secretory portion

Lacrimal gland. The lacrimal gland is located in the anterior lateral portion of the roof of the orbit in the lacrimal fossa. It is divided into a large orbital portion and a small palpebral portion by the lateral part of the aponeurosis of the levator palpebrae superioris muscle. The lacrimal gland is of the tubuloalveolar type and has numerous acini composed of a double layer of cells surrounding a central canal. The canals open into the larger ducts that in turn open into excretory ducts. Three to five ducts drain the orbital portion of the gland, and five to seven ducts drain the palpebral portion. The ducts of the orbital portion pass through the palpebral lobe, and each of the ducts opens separately onto the superior temporal fornix.

Secretory innervation to the lacrimal gland begins in the lacrimal (salivatory) nucleus of the facial nerve (N VII) in the floor of the fourth ventricle and runs through the facial nerve to the geniculate ganglion. The nerve does not synapse here but leaves the facial pathway via the greater superficial petrosal nerve to synapse in the sphenopalatine (Meckel) ganglion. From here, postganglionic fibers are distributed to the lacrimal gland, passing either directly or with the zygomatic branch of the maxillary branch of the trigeminal nerve (N V).

Postganglionic sympathetic fibers from the superior cervical ganglion pass by way of the deep petrosal nerve to the sphenopalatine ganglion, where they are distributed with fibers destined for the lacrimal gland. The sympathetic innervation is mainly to blood vessels of the gland and has no direct effect on secretion. The lacrimal gland is drained by the lymphatic vessels ending in the preauricular lymph nodes.

Collecting portion

The collecting portion of the lacrimal apparatus (Fig. 1-44) is composed of the puncta, the canaliculi, the lacrimal sac, and the nasolacrimal duct.

Puncta. The puncta are slightly elevated openings that are round or slightly oval, about 3 mm in size, and located on the upper and lower eyelid margins about 6 mm from the medial canthus. The openings are surrounded by relatively dense, avascular connective tissue.

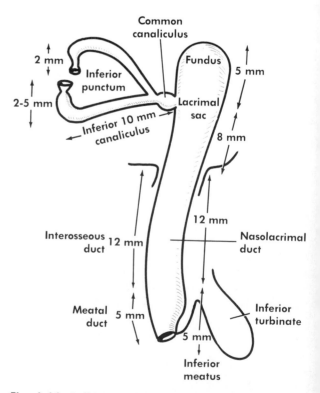

Fig. 1-44. Collecting portion of the lacrimal apparatus. Tears enter the canaliculi through the puncta and then pass through the lacrimal sac and nasal lacrimal duct to the inferior nasal meatus.

Canaliculi. The upper and lower canaliculi each consist of a vertical portion 2.0 to 3.5 mm in length and a horizontal portion directed medially for about 8 mm where the two join to form the common canaliculus. Each canaliculus is about 0.5 mm in diameter, lined by stratified squamous epithelium, and surrounded by elastic tissue. The puncta openings of the lacrimal canaliculi are inverted into the lacrimal lake when the eyelids are closed. The surrounding orbicularis oculi muscle prevents their collapse.

Lacrimal sac. The lacrimal sac is located in the medial portion of the orbit in the lacrimal fossa. The medial palpebral ligament lies anterior to it. The ligament attaches to the anterior lacrimal crest and a portion is reflected to the posterior lacrimal crest. The fundus of the sac rises 3 to 5 mm above the palpebral ligament, and immediately posterior to the ligament, the sac receives the canaliculi. Inferiorly, the sac is continuous with the nasolacrimal duct.

Nasolacrimal duct. The nasolacrimal duct is a downward extension of the sac and opens into the inferior nasal meatus. The duct is surrounded by the bone of the nasolacrimal canal, and it opens in the inferior nasal meatus at the anterior portion of the lateral wall. The duct may pass for several millimeters in the nasal mucous membrane before the opening. A variety of constrictions and folds in the sac and the nasolacrimal duct are described as "valves."

BLOOD SUPPLY
Arteries

The eye and the orbital contents receive their main blood supply from the ophthalmic artery. The eyelids and conjunctiva have a generous anastomotic supply from the branches of both the external carotid and the ophthalmic arteries. There are numerous variations in the pattern of vasculature.

Ophthalmic artery. The ophthalmic artery is the first intracranial branch of the internal carotid artery and begins just as the artery exits from the cavernous sinus. The ophthalmic artery enters the orbit through the optic foramen below and lateral to the optic nerve, turns for-

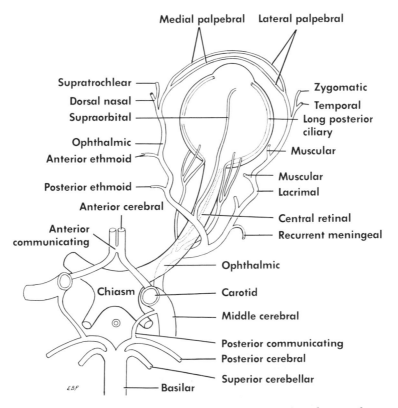

Fig. 1-45. Arteries that supply blood to the orbit and the ocular adnexa. There are many variations.

ward and upward, and passes over the optic nerve to its medial side. It ascends to the medial wall of the orbit, passes forward with the nasociliary nerve between the medial rectus and the superior oblique muscles, and terminates by dividing into dorsonasal and supratrochlear branches (Fig. 1-45).

The majority of branches of the ophthalmic artery are given off while the vessel is lateral to the optic nerve. These branches include the following arteries.

1. The central retinal artery sends nutrient vessels to the optic nerve. It then divides into superior and inferior optic disk branches (papillary), which in turn divide into nasal and temporal branches providing blood to the inner layers of the retina.

2. The medial and lateral ciliary arteries enter the globe on either side of the optic nerve and pass forward in the suprachoroidal space as the long ciliary arteries to the ciliary body. Here they anastomose with the anterior ciliary arteries to form the circulus arteriosus iridis major. Before penetrating the globe, they give off 6 to 20 posterior ciliary arteries that enter the globe to be distributed to the choroid and optic disk (see blood supply, optic nerve).

3. The lacrimal artery and its branches provide much of the blood supply to orbital structures other than the eye itself. Its recurrent meningeal branch passes into the cranial cavity through the superior orbital fissure. It anastomoses with the middle meningeal branch of the maxillary artery, which is the terminal branch of the external carotid artery. There is usually a superior and inferior muscular branch together with a branch to the lateral rectus muscle. The superior branch is distributed to the superior rectus, superior oblique, and levator palpebrae superioris muscles. The inferior branch is distributed to the inferior oblique, the medial, and the inferior recti muscles.

The muscular branches to the recti muscles provide the anterior ciliary arteries. Each rectus muscle has two muscular arteries except the lateral muscle, which has one. The anterior ciliary vesicles extend to the corneoscleral limbus as the anterior conjunctival arteries and form the pericorneal arcade. The anterior conjunctival arteries anastomose with the posterior conjunctival arteries derived from the palpebral arcade. About 4 mm from the corneo-

scleral limbus, branches of the anterior ciliary arteries penetrate the sclera to contribute, together with long posterior ciliary arteries, to the circulus arteriosus iridis major and to provide blood vessels to the ciliary processes.

The lacrimal artery terminates in temporal and zygomatic branches that anastomose with the anterior deep temporal and transverse facial arteries. These form lateral palpebral branches that anastomose with medial palpebral arterial arcades of the eyelid. Branches of the peripheral arterial arcade are distributed to the conjunctiva as the posterior conjunctival arteries.

4. The supraorbital artery originates from the ophthalmic artery where it is superior to the optic nerve. It extends anteriorly to anastomose with the superficial temporal and superficial trochlear arteries in the scalp.

5. As the ophthalmic artery courses medial to the optic nerve it gives off the anterior and posterior ethmoidal arteries. The anterior ethmoidal artery provides a recurrent meningeal artery. Superior and inferior palpebral branches anastomose through the tarsal and peripheral palpebral arcades with the corresponding branches of the lacrimal artery. The ophthalmic artery terminates in two branches: (1) the dorsonasal artery, which is distributed to the skin of the nose and anastomoses with the angular artery, the terminal branch of the facial artery; and (2) the supratrochlear artery that supplies the forehead and scalp.

External carotid artery. The blood supply to the eye and eyelids from branches of the external carotid artery originates from (1) the external maxillary (facial) artery, (2) the superficial temporal artery, and (3) the internal maxillary artery.

The *external maxillary (facial) artery* has a number of branches to the face. Its terminal branch is the angular artery, which anastomoses at the medial canthus with the dorsonasal branch of the ophthalmic artery to provide blood for the inferior arterial arcades of the eyelids. It also anastomoses with the infraorbital artery, a branch of the maxillary artery.

The *superficial temporal artery* is the smaller terminal branch of the external carotid artery. The transverse facial artery, the largest branch of the superficial temporal artery, anastomoses with the infraorbital and angular arteries. The zygomatico-orbital artery anastomoses with the lacrimal artery and its palpebral branches to participate in the arterial arcade of the eyelids. The frontal artery anastomoses with the supraorbital and frontal branches of the ophthalmic artery and with the corresponding artery from the opposite side.

The *internal maxillary artery* is the larger of the terminal branches of the external carotid artery. Its largest branch is the middle meningeal artery, which supplies the bone and dura mater at the base of the skull. The internal maxillary artery sends an orbital branch through the superior orbital fissure and anastomoses with a recurrent branch of the ophthalmic artery. The infraorbital artery originates in the pterygopalatine (sphenomaxillary) fossa; it enters the orbit through the infraorbital fissure, runs in the infraorbital sulcus and canal in the orbital plate of the maxilla, and passes forward to emerge on the face from the infraorbital foramen. The infraorbital branch anastomoses with the angular branch of the external maxillary (facial) artery, the transverse facial branch of the superficial temporal artery,

and the lacrimal and dorsonasal branches of the ophthalmic artery.

Veins

Venous drainage of the orbit is mainly through the superior and inferior orbital veins. These are markedly tortuous, have no valves and pass through the superior orbital fissure to empty into the cavernous sinus. The superior orbital vein communicates with the angular vein, which is continuous with the facial vein. The inferior ophthalmic vein communicates with the pterygoid plexus through the inferior orbital fissure. The inferior ophthalmic vein may communicate either directly with the cavernous sinus or may empty into the superior ophthalmic vein. The two or more superior vortex veins empty into the superior orbital vein, and the four or more inferior vortex veins join the inferior orbital vein. The central retinal vein usually exits from the optic nerve close to the entrance of the artery. It enters the cavernous sinus separately or empties into the superior ophthalmic vein.

The carvenous sinus (Fig. 1-46) is an irregu-

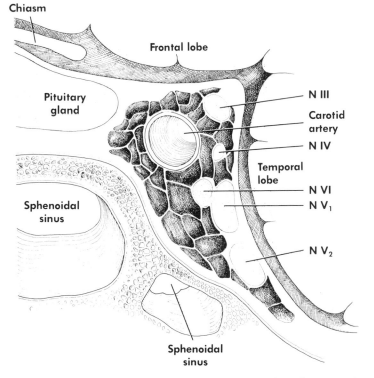

Fig. 1-46. Coronal section of the cavernous sinus posterior to the orbit. It is almost continuous with the superior orbital vein.

lar-shaped, endothelium-lined venous space situated between the meningeal and periosteal layers of the dura mater on either side of the body of the sphenoid bone. It extends from the medial end of the superior orbital fissure to the apex of the petrous bone behind. Anteriorly it receives the superior orbital vein, with which it is almost continuous. Medially, it communicates with the opposite sinus, and posteriorly, with the superior and inferior petrosal sinuses. The internal carotid artery passes through the cavernous sinus on its medial wall; the abducent nerve (N VI) is just lateral to the artery. The oculomotor nerve (N III) and trochlear nerve (N IV) are in its lateral wall on its superior aspect, whereas the ophthalmic and maxillary branches of the trigeminal nerve (N V) are located lateral to and below the artery. One or a combination of these nerves may be affected by diseases of the cavernous sinus, such as inflammation or internal carotid artery fistula or aneurysm.

NERVES OF THE EYE

The visual, motor, and mixed motor and sensory nerves of the eye include the following:

Visual system
    Optic nerve
    Optic chiasm
    Optic tract
    Lateral geniculate body
    Optic radiation
    Visual cortex
Motor nerves
    Oculomotor (N III)
    Superior division to superior recti and levator palpebrae superioris muscles
    Inferior division to medial and inferior recti and inferior oblique muscles and motor (short) root to ciliary ganglion (ciliary muscle and sphincter pupillae muscle)
    Trochlear (N IV) to superior oblique muscle
    Abducent (N VI) to lateral rectus muscle
Mixed motor and sensory nerves
    Trigeminal (N V)
      Motor to muscles of mastication
      Sensory from face and eye
      Proprioceptive from muscles of mastication (mesencephalic nucleus and perhaps ocular muscles)
    Facial (N VII)
      Motor to face
      Secretory to submaxillary, sublingual, and lacrimal glands
      Taste from anterior two thirds of tongue

Autonomic nervous system
    Parasympathetic
    Sympathetic

THE VISUAL PATHWAYS

Visual stimuli originating in the retina pass to the brain in the optic nerve. Fibers originating from the retina nasal to a vertical line through the foveola decussate in the optic chiasm and join axons from the contralateral temporal retina in the optic tract. They synapse in the lateral geniculate body, and axons from the lateral geniculate body pass in the optic radiation to the visual cortex in the occipital lobe (Fig. 1-47).

Visual nerve

The optic nerve. The optic nerve is a portion of a white fiber tract of the central nervous system that consists of axons of retinal ganglion cells. It extends from the optic disk at a level with the retina within the eye to the optic chiasm, where, in normal humans, half of the fibers decussate to the opposite side of the brain in the optic chiasm. Thereafter, crossed nasal fiber and uncrossed temporal fibers constitute the optic tract.

The optic nerve is divided into four portions: (1) intraocular, 1 mm; (2) orbital, 30 mm; (3) intracanalicular, 4 to 10 mm; and (4) intracranial, 10 mm.

The *intraocular portion* of the optic nerve includes the optic disk and the portion of the optic nerve within the posterior scleral foramen. The optic disk (Fig. 1-48) is located about 3 mm nasal to and about 0.8 mm above the foveola. It is composed of axons of ganglion cells. The choroid and all layers of the retina, except the nerve fiber layer, terminate at the optic disk margin. Because the photosensitive rods and cones are absent, this area is blind (the blind spot of Mariotte in visual field testing).

The optic nerve exits from the eye through the posterior scleral foramen bridged with the lamina cribrosa that is formed by fibrous tissue from the sclera, elastic tissue of the choroid and Bruch membrane, and astroglia derived from the septal system of the nerve. Posterior to the optic disk the nerve fibers are myelinated, whereas anterior to the optic disk they are normally not myelinated. The portion of the optic nerve visible within the eye is about

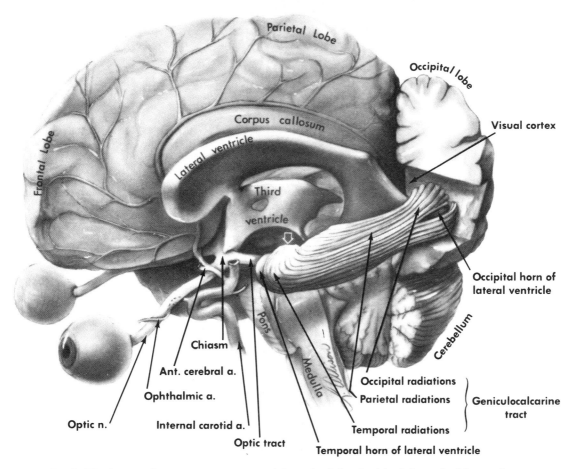

Fig. 1-47. The visual-sensory system viewed from the left side. The left cerebral hemisphere has been removed except for a portion for the occipital lobe and the ventricular system. The arrow beneath the third ventricle points to the lateral geniculate body. The cerebral falx and the cerebellar tentorium are not shown. (By permission from Glaser, J.S.: Neuro-ophthalmology, Hagerstown, Md., 1978, Harper & Row, Publishers.)

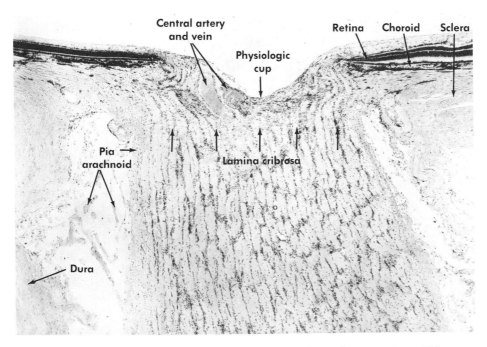

Fig. 1-48. Optic disk and optic nerve. (Hematoxylin and eosin stain; ×43.)

1.5 mm in diameter. (The optic disk is not elevated above the surrounding retina and the term "optic papilla" is a misnomer. Nonetheless the central retinal artery divides into papillary branches. The fundus surrounding the disk is called peripapillary, and edema of the disk is papilledema.)

The *orbital portion* of the optic nerve has an S-shaped curve to permit movements of the eye. It is sheathed with a dense outer dura mater, a middle arachnoid mater, and an innermost pia mater. These extend from the optic foramen to the globe, where the dura mater and arachnoid sheaths blend into the sclera. Near the globe the long and short ciliary arteries and nerves are arranged about its circumference. The central retinal artery and vein penetrate the optic nerve 12 mm behind the globe. At the apex of the orbit, the optic nerve is surrounded by the tendinous origin of the recti muscles, the ligament of Zinn.

In its *intracanalicular portion*, the optic nerve passes through the optic foramen together with the ophthalmic artery and the sympathetic nerves accompany this artery. At the anterior margin of the optic foramen the dura mater covering the nerve divides so that one portion continues as the periosteum of the orbit and the other continues as the dural sheath of the optic nerve. Within the optic canal, the dura mater is adherent to bone, arachnoid, and pia mater so that the nerve is firmly fixed.

The *intracranial portion* of the optic nerve passes medially to form the chiasm.

Structure. The optic nerve contains between 1.1 and 1.3 million afferent axons of ganglion cells subserving vision, pupillary reflex, and ocular movements. Axons from ganglion cells of the fovea centralis may provide up to 90% of the axons of the optic nerve.

The nerve is composed of bundles of nerve fibers separated by septa that are continuous with the pia mater and carry minute blood vessels to the nerve (Fig. 1-49). As in the brain, nerve fibers are supported by astroglia and oligodendroglia derived from the neural ectoderm and by mesenchymal microglia that have a phagocytic function. Myelinization of the optic nerve begins at the chiasm at about the twenty-fourth week of fetal life and, at birth, has reached a point just behind the lamina cribrosa. Oligodendrocytes are associated with

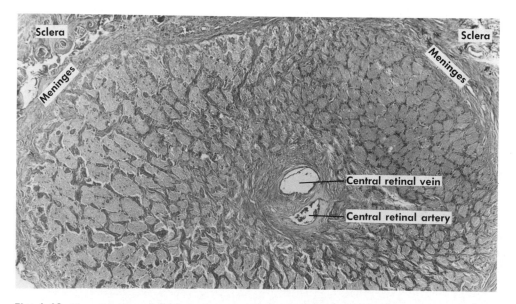

Fig. 1-49. Cross-section of the human optic nerve just posterior to the globe. The contribution of the dura mater to the sclera is shown above. The central artery and vein share a common adventitial sheath, as they do at points of crossings within the eye. In the nerve the myelinated nerve fibers are divided into septa by delicate, collagenous fibers from the pia. The nerve fiber bundles are separated from the septal system by a layer of astrocytes. (×70.) (Courtesy Ramesh C. Tripathi.)

the synthesis and metabolism of myelin; these cells are more numerous behind the lamina cribrosa. Astrocytes provide a skeletal framework on the intraocular surface of the optic nerve and are important in providing mechanical support as nerve fibers make the right angle turn from the retina.

Blood supply. The blood supply of the optic nerve is derived from several sources. The intraocular portion is supplied by the short posterior ciliary arteries that, as they penetrate the sclera, give off branches to form the anastomotic partial circle of Haller-Zinn. The central retinal artery does not furnish branches to the optic nerve in this region. Much attention has been focused on the blood supply to this area because of involvement of the optic disk in glaucoma.

The intraorbital portion of the nerve has a peripheral and possibly an axial blood supply. The peripheral vessels originate from those of the pia mater and are derived from the neighboring blood vessels. The axial vessels are derived from the central retinal artery, a branch of the ophthalmic artery. The axial vascular system nurtures the central retinal fibers.

The intracanalicular and intracranial portions of the optic nerve are nurtured by the pial fibrovascular meshwork from branches of the internal carotid artery.

Optic chiasm. The optic chiasm is about 13 mm wide. It is attached by the pia mater and the arachnoid to the dorsal surface of the diencephalon, and it forms a portion of the floor of the third ventricle. Its posterior surface is in close contact with the tuber cinereum from which extends the infundibulum or stalk of the pituitary gland (hypophysis cerebri). The chiasm is superior to the tuberculum sellae turcicae and the diaphragma sellae and is usually posterior to the optic groove of the sphenoid bone. It is closely related to the internal carotid arteries laterally and to the anterior cerebral arteries and anterior communicating artery anteriorly.

Optic tract. The optic tract extends from the chiasm to the lateral geniculate body. It is composed of axons from ganglion cells of the nasal retina of the opposite side and the temporal retina on the same side. These axons sweep laterally, encircle the hypothalamus posteriorly (in the ventral wall of the third ventricle), and

wind around the ventrolateral aspect of the pes pedunculi (the ventral portion of the midbrain). The majority of axons terminate in the lateral geniculate body. A smaller number continue in the superior quadrigeminal brachium to the superior colliculi (reflex ocular movements) and to the pretectal area (pupillary reflexes). Other fibers enter the hypothalamus and terminate in the supraoptic nucleus and the medial nuclei of the tuber cinereum. The significance and extent of this distribution in humans is not known. The superior colliculi are sensitive to moving visual stimuli and may direct the eyes and the head toward a visual stimulus.

Lateral geniculate body. The axons of retinal ganglion cells that carry visual impulses synapse in the lateral geniculate body (Fig. 1-50). This is located in the diencephalon lateral to the medial geniculate body and consists of a dorsal and inconspicuous (in humans) ventral nucleus. In primates the dorsal nucleus is composed of six cellular layers, numbered 1 to 6, beginning at the hilus and continuing toward the dorsal portion of the nucleus. Cells in the ventral layers 1 and 2 (magnocellular laminae) are larger and more uniform in size and shape than cells in the remaining four layers (parvocellular laminae). Axons from the temporal ret-

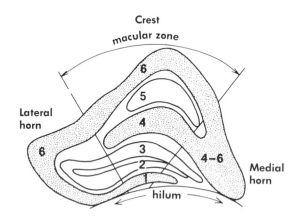

Fig. 1-50. Schema of a coronal section through the lateral geniculate body viewed from its posterior aspect. Uncrossed axons from the terminal retina synapse in layers 2, 3, and 5. Crossed axons from the contralateral nasal retina synapse in layers 1, 4, and 6. (By permission from Miller, N.: Walsh and Hoyt's clinical neuro-ophthalmology, ed. 4, vol. 1, Baltimore, 1982, The Williams & Wilkins Co.)

ina (uncrossed) on the same side synapse in layers 2, 3, and 5. Axons from the nasal one half of the retina of the opposite eye decussate in the chiasm and terminate in layers 1, 4, and 6. The axons from the lower one half of the retina synapse in the lateral portion of the lateral geniculate body; those from the upper one half in the medial portion. Foveal axons are located posteriorly. Central visual fibers are represented in all six layers, whereas peripheral axons are represented in the two magnocellular layers and in two parvocellular layers.

In addition to visual fibers, the lateral geniculate body receives input from the visual cortex, oculomotor centers in the brain stem, and from the brain stem reticular formation. The lateral geniculate body modulates the strength and the pattern of the retinal input and may play a fundamental role in color vision and stereoscopic vision.

Optic radiation. The optic radiation (geniculocalcarine tract) extends from the lateral geniculate body to the superior and inferior lips of the calcarine fissure (area striata; area 17) of the occipital lobe (Fig. 1-51). Axons from cells located in the lateral aspect of the lateral geniculate body representing the inferior retinal quadrants (superior visual field quadrants) pass anteriorly around the tip of the temporal horn of the lateral ventricle to form the temporal loop of Flechsig-Archmabault-Meyer (see Fig. 1-51). Damage to the axons in this loop produces superior homonymous quadrantic field defects. The axons of the temporal loop continue posterior to terminate in the ventral (inferior) lip of the calcarine fissure. Axons from

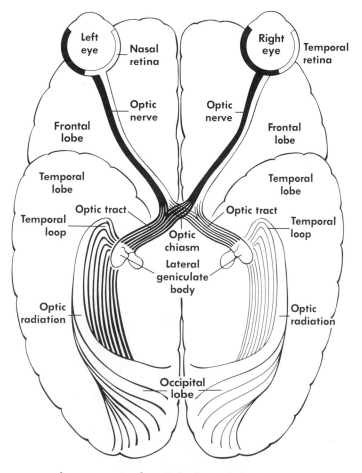

Fig. 1-51. The optic pathways projected onto the base of the brain. All of the nasal fibers of the right and left eye decussate (cross) at the optic chiasm.

cells located in the medial portion of the lateral geniculate body, representing the superior retinal quadrants (inferior visual field quadrants), pass nearly directly posterior through the parietal lobe to terminate in the dorsal (superior) lip of the calcarine fissure.

Visual cortex. The axons of cells located in the lateral geniculate body terminate along the superior and inferior lips of the calcarine fissure. This area is often called the striate cortex (area 17 of Brodmann) because of the prominent band of geniculocalcarine fibers (striae of Gennari). The upper one half of each retina is represented on the dorsal (superior) part of each occipital cortex, and the lower one half covers the ventral (inferior) part. Fibers representing the central retina terminate at the tip of the posterior pole, and more peripheral portions of the retina are represented more anteriorly (Fig. 1-52). The visual cortex is composed of six cell layers typical of cortex; most axons from the lateral geniculate body terminate in layer IV (lamina granularis interna of Brodmann) that is divided (in monkeys) into three major layers.

Optic pathways. The retina, as discussed previously, is divided into a central portion (mainly cones), used in form vision and color vision, and a peripheral portion (mainly rods), used in dark adaptation and in the detection of movement. In the distribution of nerve impulses in the visual pathways, the retina is divided into four quadrants by horizontal and vertical lines that intersect at the fovea centralis. (Note that the fovea centralis and not the optic nerve is the point of division.) Thus each retina is divided into superior, inferior, temporal, and nasal portions, which in turn may be divided into peripheral and central portions.

All axons coming from the nasal half of each retina decussate to the opposite side at the chiasm and join uncrossed temporal fibers to form the optic tract. Visual axons synapse in the lateral geniculate body and then pass to the optic radiation as the geniculocalcarine tract (Fig. 1-53).

Localization in the visual pathways. The visual field is composed of the total perception resulting from retinal stimulation at one moment. It is oriented according to the origin of the visual stimulus and is thus opposite the portion of the retina stimulated. Objects located in the temporal field stimulate the nasal retina, objects located below stimulate the retina above, and so on.

As axons enter the optic nerve, central retinal axons occupy the lateral portion nearest the fovea. Thereafter the various sectors have the same distribution in the optic nerve as in the retina. The central axons are surrounded by the peripheral axons; axons from the inferior retina are below, and those from the superior retina are above. (Axons from the central retina may provide as many as 90% of the afferent axons in the optic nerve.)

Axons of ganglion cells from the nasal portion of both the central and peripheral retina decussate in the optic chiasm. Axons from the inferior nasal retinas are located in the anterior and inferior surfaces of the chiasm (closest to the pituitary gland). Axons from the inferior nasal retinas, after decussating, loop forward slightly in the opposite optic nerve before passing into the optic tract. The anterior loop in the contralateral optic nerve is responsible for the occasional involvement of the visual field of both eyes in lesions affecting the optic nerve just anterior to the chiasm. The position of inferior nasal axons in the inferior portion of the chiasm makes them vulnerable in pituitary enlarge-

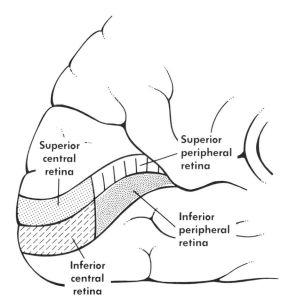

Fig. 1-52. Striate area of left occipital lobe with calcarine fissure widely opened. The central retina is represented posteriorly in the brain and is relatively large; the peripheral retina is represented anteriorly and is relatively small.

ment, so that the initial visual field defect in pituitary tumors is loss of the superior temporal visual field.

The superior nasal axons cross in the superior portion of the chiasm in its posterior aspect. They first pass posteriorly in the optic tract on the same side and then loop forward to decussate.

The distribution of axons in the anterior portion of the optic tract is similar to that in the optic nerve, except that the nasal axons are those that have crossed from the opposite side. The axons are rapidly redistributed so that those from corresponding parts of each retina become associated. Thus axons from the inferior nasal retina become related to inferior

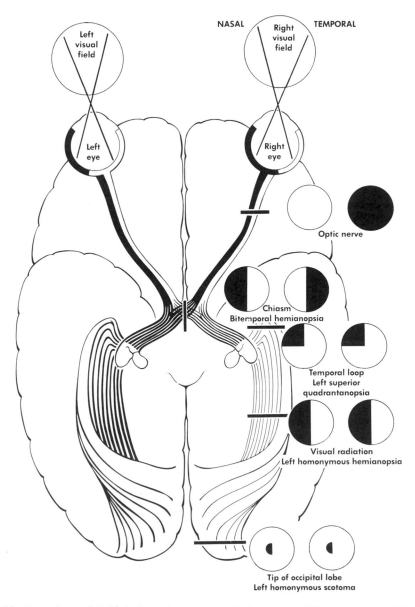

Fig. 1-53. Typical visual field defects that occur with damage to different regions of the optic pathways. The visual fields are diagrammed to reflect the source of the light that stimulates the retina. Light from the temporal side stimulates the nasal portion of the retina; light from above stimulates the lower portion, and so on. Thus the visual field defect caused by a lesion affecting fibers arising from the nasal half of the retina is diagrammed as a temporal field defect. (The visual pathways are projected onto the base of the brain.)

temporal retinal axons and superior nasal retinal axons become related to uncrossed superior temporal retinal axons. Transmission defects in the optic tracts produce homonymous (same side, both eyes) visual field defects, because axons from corresponding parts of each retina are involved in a single lesion (hemianopsia is half-blindness; the reference is to the blind portion of the field).

In the lateral geniculate body, uncrossed (temporal) retinal axons synapse in layers 2, 3, and 5; crossed (nasal) retinal axons synapse in layers 1, 4, and 6.

The axons emerging from the cells of the lateral geniculate body have exact correspondence in each eye so that a lesion in them causes exactly similar visual field defects in each eye (homonymous congruous defects). Lesions in axons carrying stimuli from the inferior retinas as they pass around the temporal horn of the lateral ventricle cause a superior homonymous quadrantanopsia (often a sign of a vascular lesion). Lesions in the superior axons passing more directly to the cortical striate area cause an inferior quadrantanopsia.

Fibers that represent corresponding portions of the fovea centralis of each eye and the immediately surrounding areas occupy a relatively large area in the striate area of the visual cortex of the occipital lobe (Brodmann area 17). More peripheral portions of the retina are represented anteriorly. The superior areas of the retinas (inferior visual fields) are represented on the upper lip of the calcarine fissure; inferior binocular areas (superior visual fields) are on the lower lip. All nasal axons from the fovea decussate completely. The "sparing of the macula," in which destruction of the occipital lobe on one side seems not to affect all of the central retinal fibers, may be the result of incomplete destruction inasmuch as many arteries supply the area. Alternatively, "central retinal sparing" may be caused by minute changes in visual fixation.

Motor nerves

Oculomotor (third cranial nerve). The oculomotor nerve supplies the inferior oblique muscle, the superior, medial, and inferior recti muscles, and the levator palpebrae superioris muscle. Its visceral efferent fibers innervate the ciliary muscle and the sphincter pupillae muscle after synapse in the ciliary ganglion.

Nucleus. The oculomotor nuclear complex (Fig. 1-54) is a small (5 mm) collection of cells arranged medial to the diverging medial lateral

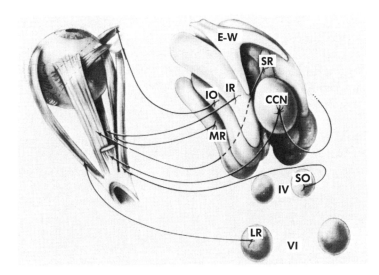

Fig. 1-54. Organization of the oculomotor nucleus viewed from above, left posterior. *E-W,* Edinger-Westphal parasympathetic subnucleus; *IR,* inferior rectus muscle nucleus; *IO,* inferior oblique muscle nucleus; *MR,* medial rectus muscle nucleus. The efferent fibers of superior rectus, *SR,* and superior oblique, *SO,* motor pool innervate muscles on the opposite side. *CCN,* caudal nucleus, is distributed to the levator palpebrae superioris on both sides. *LR,* abducent nucleus for lateral rectus muscle. (From Glaser, J.S.: Neuro-ophthalmology, New York, 1978, Harper & Row, Publishers.)

fasciculi and beneath the aqueduct of Sylvius at the level of the superior colliculus. The trochlear nerve nucleus is continuous caudally. An unpaired mass of cells located caudally and centrally sends efferent fibers to the levator palpebrae superioris muscles. The motor cell pool of the superior rectus muscle sends efferent fibers to the contralateral superior rectus muscle. Paired lateral nuclei send efferent fibers to the ipsilateral medial and inferior recti muscles and the inferior oblique muscle. A pair of nuclei (of Edinger-Westphal) located rostrally and ventrally sends preganglionic parasympathetic fibers to the ciliary ganglion where they synapse and are then distributed to the ciliary muscle (accommodation) and the sphincter pupillae muscle (constriction).

The medial (posterior) longitudinal fasciculus connects motor cells of the oculomotor complex to each other and to the nuclei of the trochlear and abducent cranial nerves, the supranuclear centers for gaze, the cerebellum, and the sensory nuclei of the trigeminal nerves. This important fiber tract transmits stimuli that coordinate conjugate movements of the eyes (eyes right, eyes left, eyes up, or eyes down). Axons from the abducent nuclei decussate to the opposite medial fasciculus bundle and are distributed mainly to the medial rectus muscle nucleus. Thus on the signal "eyes left," the left lateral rectus muscle contracts as does the right medial rectus muscle. (A lesion in an abducent nucleus thus causes a failure to move both eyes to the right or left. A lesion in an abducent nerve affects only the lateral rectus muscle of that side.) Anterior lesions of the medial longitudinal fasciculus produce an internuclear ophthalmoplegia in which convergence is normal but, on attempts to turn the eyes laterally, the adducting eye does not pass beyond the midline and there is a coarse nystagmus of the abducting eye.

Intracerebral course. From the third cranial nerve nuclei, efferent fibers run through the tegmentum, red nucleus, and substantia nigra and leave the midbrain in the interpeduncular fossa between the cerebral peduncles.

Intracranial course. In their intracranial course, the oculomotor nerves are closely associated with the posterior cerebral arteries above and the superior cerebellar arteries below. From the midbrain, they pass down forward, outward, and downward to pierce the dura mater and enter the roof and lateral wall of the cavernous sinus about midway between the anterior and posterior clinoid processes. In the cavernous sinus, each nerve is close to the trochlear and ophthalmic division of the trigeminal nerve.

Orbital distribution. Each oculomotor nerve leaves the cavernous sinus near the lesser wing of the sphenoid bone and enters the orbit through the superior orbital fissure. Here it divides into a small superior and larger inferior division. The superior division is distributed to the superior rectus muscle on its bulbar surface and passes through this muscle to terminate in the levator palpebrae superioris muscle. The inferior division is distributed to the medial and inferior recti muscles. Its terminal portion ends in the posterior border of the inferior oblique muscles. The terminal portion ends in the posterior border of the inferior oblique muscles. This terminal branch to the inferior oblique muscle sends the short, or motor, root branch to the ciliary ganglion.

Ciliary ganglion. The ciliary ganglion is located between the lateral rectus muscle and the optic nerve near the apex of the orbit. It has three roots: parasympathetic, sympathetic, and sensory.

Parasympathetic root (N III)
    Ciliary muscle
    Sphincter pupillae muscle
Sympathetic root
    Uveal blood vessels
Sensory root (N V)
    Globe

The *parasympathetic root* consists of visceral motor fibers (Edinger-Westphal nucleus) given off by the terminal branch of the inferior division of the oculomotor nerve, which ends in the inferior oblique muscle. After synapse in the ciliary ganglion, emerging fibers are distributed as postganglionic cholinergic fibers to the ciliary muscle (accommodation) and the sphincter pupillae muscle (pupillary constriction).

The *sympathetic root* consists of fibers derived from the cavernous sinus and internal carotid artery plexuses. The sympathetic nerves are postganglionic fibers that synapse in the superior cervical ganglion and thus pass through the ciliary ganglion without synapse. These fibers mainly provide vasoconstrictor fibers to choroidal blood vessels.

The *sensory root* is derived from the nasociliary branch of the ophthalmic division of the trigeminal nerve; these fibers do not synapse. The sensory root also contains sympathetic fibers that may entirely replace the separate sympathetic root.

The branches of the ciliary ganglion are 6 to 20 short ciliary nerves that branch and pierce the sclera around the optic nerve. They are distributed to the uveal tract and to the ciliary and sphincter pupillae muscles.

Trochlear (fourth cranial) nerve. The trochlear (fourth cranial) nerve innervates the superior oblique muscle only. Its fibers decussate in the anterior medullary vellum, and it is the only cranial nerve to emerge from the dorsal surface of the brain.

Nucleus. The nuclei of the trochlear nerves are a small group of cells located at the posterior end of the lateral (paired) portions of the oculomotor nerve. They are located beneath the cerebral aqueduct of Sylvius, near its connection with the fourth ventricle, at about the level of the inferior colliculus. The cells are connected by the medial longitudinal fasciculus to the oculomotor nucleus (but not the abducent nucleus), the vestibular nuclei, and the trigeminal sensory nucleus.

Course in the brainstem. The trochlear is the sole cranial nerve to decussate dorsally. The axons pass laterally and then curve around the aqueduct of Sylvius, progressing caudally and passing over the aqueduct, at which point they leave the brainstem.

Intracranial course. After emerging from the brainstem on its dorsal surface, the trochlear nerve passes as a slender filament around the cerebral peduncle to reach the ventral surface of the brain just posterior to the oculomotor nerve. It enters the dura mater posterior to the entrance of the oculomotor nerve at about the level of the posterior clinoid process. It is located in the lateral wall of the cavernous sinus somewhat below the oculomotor nerve. The trochlear nerve emerges from the cavernous sinus and enters the lateral portion of the superior orbital fissure outside the ligament of Zinn. In the orbit it passes anteriorly and medially, crossing above the oculomotor nerve,

the levator palpebrae superioris muscle, and the superior rectus muscle. It enters the superior oblique muscle on its orbital surface. This is the only ocular muscle that does not receive its innervation on its bulbar aspect.

Abducent (sixth cranial) nerve. The abducent (sixth cranial) nerve has the longest intracranial course of any of the motor nerves of the eye. It makes a sharp turn over the petrous ridge, which makes it vulnerable to trauma and increased intracranial pressure.

Nuclei. The nuclei of the abducent nerve (VI) are located in the gray matter of the floor of the fourth ventricle lateral to the medial longitudinal fasciculus. The genu of the facial nerve curves over the dorsal and lateral surfaces of each abducent nucleus. These structures produce an eminence on the floor of the fourth ventricle referred to as the facial colliculus.

The abducent nerve is unique since destroying a nucleus impairs not only abduction of the lateral rectus muscle on the same side but also impairs adduction of the medial rectus muscle on the opposite side. Destruction of an abducent nerve root impairs only the lateral rectus muscle on the same side. This occurs because each nucleus contains neurons whose axons cross the midline and ascend in the medial longitudinal fasciculus to the medial rectus muscle motor in the oculomotor nuclear complex.

Course in the brainstem. The axons of an abducent nucleus pass forward and downward through the pons of the medial side of the superior olivary nucleus and on the lateral side of the pyramidal tract. They emerge on the ventral surface of the brainstem in a deep groove between the pons anteriorly and the medulla posteriorly.

Intracranial course. The axons of the sixth cranial nerves pass anteriorly on the surface of the pons, to which they are bound by the anterior inferior cerebellar artery, the first branch of the basilar artery. Each nerve then pierces the dura mater and passes vertically over the posterior part of the petrous portion of the temporal bone to enter the cavernous sinus. Just before entering this sinus, each nerve passes under the petrosphenoid ligament. In the cavernous sinus it is located just below the carotid artery and is the most inferiorly located of the motor nerves to the eye. Each nerve enters the orbit through the superior orbital fissure between the two heads of the lateral rectus muscle. It passes forward and laterally in the orbit to innervate the lateral rectus muscle from its bulbar surface.

Mixed nerves

Facial (seventh cranial) nerve. The facial nerve supplies derivatives of the second branchial arch. It is mainly motor to the muscles of the face and scalp, but it has a small sensory component carrying sensations of taste from the anterior two thirds of the tongue. Additionally, it provides motor fibers to the submaxillary and sublingual salivary glands and the lacrimal glands.

Nuclei. The motor nuclei of the facial nerve are located in the pons medial to the spinal trigeminal tract and lateral to the fibers of the abducent nerve. The gustatory (taste) nuclei receive fibers from cranial nerves VII, IX, and X. The cell bodies are located in the geniculate ganglia, and the axons extend centrally to the gustatory nuclei in the medulla. Fibers that stimulate salivary and lacrimal secretions originate in the salivary nuclei.

Course in the brainstem. The motor axons pass medially and posteriorly to the floor of the fourth ventricle to form a compact genu around each abducent nucleus. The axons pass laterally to emerge from the ventral surface of the brainstem at the inferior border of the pons, considerably lateral to the abducent nerve.

Intracranial course. On emerging from the brainstem, the motor fibers of each facial nerve pass in the posterior cranial fossa anterior and lateral to the internal auditory meatus, which they enter in company with the acoustic and vestibular nerves and the intermediate nerve of Wrisberg. The facial nerve makes a sharp backward bend in the temporal bone to enter the dorsal aspect of the middle ear. It emerges from the temporal bone at its lower portion through the stylomastoid foramen.

The nerve then immediately turns anteriorly around the base of the styloid process to enter the parotid gland, where it divides into its terminal divisions, the upper temporofacial and the lower cervicofacial. The temporofacial division given off temporal and zygomatic branches supplying the orbicularis oculi, the frontalis, the corrugator supercilii, and the anterior and superior auricularis muscles. The cervicofacial division supplies the lower face. These upper and lower branches of the facial nerve have separate areas of origin in each facial nucleus. The upper branches have cortical connections with each hemisphere, but the lower branch has connections only with the opposite motor cortex. Thus, in a unilateral supranuclear lesion, structures innervated by the upper portion of the facial nerve are not affected, but those innervated by the lower portion (opposite side) are affected. The structures are similarly affected in infranuclear lesions.

The taste fibers have a complicated course. Those from the anterior tongue join the chorda tympani nerve, which runs across the middle ear cavity to join the facial nerve. Then the fibers pass with the facial nerve to a point where the internal acoustic meatus joins the facial canal. It is here that the geniculate ganglion is located. Other taste fibers are located in the petrous ganglion (glossopharyngeal nerve) and in the nodose ganglion (vagus nerve).

Motor fibers to the salivary and lacrimal glands are contained in the intermediate nerve of Wrisberg, which passes with the facial nerve into the internal auditory meatus. As the facial nerve turns to enter the facial canal, most of the visceral efferent fibers leave at the apex of the angle as the greater superficial petrosal nerve, which runs forward through the petrous bone to reach the intracranial cavity. The greater superficial petrosal nerve then runs under the semilunar ganglion to emerge from the cranial cavity through the foramen lacerum—it passes through the pterygoid canal to join the sphenopalatine ganglion. Motor fibers to the lacrimal gland join the maxillary branch of the trigeminal nerve, which joins the zygomatic branch to enter the lacrimal gland.

Fibers to the maxillary gland pass with the chorda tympani nerve to emerge from the skull by a fissure between the tympanic and petrous portions of the temporal bone. Fibers join the lingual branch of the mandibular nerve and then synapse with submaxillary ganglia; postganglionic fibers are distributed almost immediately to the maxillary and sublingual glands. The parotid gland receives its innervation from the lesser petrosal nerve.

Trigeminal (fifth cranial) nerve. The trigeminal nerve has a complicated structure. It is not only the sensory nerve of the face and head, but it also sends motor fibers to the muscles of mastication. It has extensive central connections with reflex arcs associated with cranial nerves III to XII.

Motor root
Muscles of mastication
Tensor tympani muscle
Tensor veli palatine muscle
Sensory root
Ophthalmic branch(V$_1$)
Maxillary branch (V$_2$)
Mandibular branch (V$_3$)
Mesencephalic root
Proprioceptive from muscles of mastication

Motor nucleus and root. The masticator is the motor portion of the trigeminal nerve. Its nucleus is located cephalad to the facial nerve nucleus near the floor of the cerebral aqueduct of Sylvius. The fibers are distributed with the mandibular nerve and innervate the muscles that move the mandible and the muscles of mastication: the masseter, the temporalis, the internal pterygoid, the mylohyoid, the anterior belly of the digastric, and the external pterygoid. In addition, motor fibers supply the tensor tympani muscle, which tenses the eardrum, and the tensor veli palatine muscle, which stretches out the soft palate.

The mesencephalic root of each trigeminal nerve is situated between the main sensory and the motor nuclei. Fibers of this root are distributed with each of the main divisions of the trigeminal nerve. In the act of biting, impulses pass to the mesencephalic root.

Sensory nuclei. The principal sensory nucleus of each trigeminal nerve is located near the point of entry of the sensory root into the pons; it lies near the lateral surface of the pons close to the margin of the inferior cerebral peduncle. Functionally, it appears related to tactile impulses.

The nucleus of each spiral trigeminal tract extends down to the second cervical segment of the spinal cord and becomes continuous with the substantia gelatinosa of the dorsal horn. It is functionally associated with the sensation of pain and temperature.

The sensory root is composed of fibers that originate in the semilunar (gasserian) ganglion together with a few fibers from the ciliary ganglion and possibly from other ganglia. The sensory root extends from the posterior border of the semilunar ganglion to the pons. As it leaves this ganglion, it pierces the dura mater under the attached border of the tentorium, which contains the superior petrosal sinus at this point. It lies on the trochlear nerve and then crosses over the facial and auditory foreamen. It is then related to a groove in the medial aspect of the petrous portion of the temporal bone lateral to the abducent nerve.

The sensory root of the trigeminal nerve enters the brain on the lateral surface of the pons about midway between its anterior and posterior margins. Inside the pons it divides into ascending and descending tracts. The thick ascending fibers terminate almost immediately in the principal sensory nucleus. The thin descending fibers are adjacent to the nucleus of the spinal trigeminal tract.

Semilunar ganglion. The semilunar ganglion is a crescent-shaped mass of cells lying in the Meckel cave, which is a cleft located between layers of dura mater in the middle fossa of the skull on a depression on the anterosuperior surface of the petrous bone. At its anterior concave aspect, the semilunar ganglion receives three branches: the ophthalmic division (V$_1$), the maxillary division (V$_2$), and the mandibular division (V$_3$). The *ophthalmic division* (V$_1$) may be outlined as follows:

Frontal nerve
Lacrimal nerve
Nasociliary nerve
Long (sensory) root of ciliary ganglion
Long ciliary nerves
Posterior ethmoidal nerves
Infratrochlear nerves: superior and inferior palpebral nerves
Anterior ethmoidal nevers
Interior nasal nerves: medial and lateral nasal nerves
External nasal nerves

The ophthalmic division, the smallest branch of the semilunar ganglion, is located in the lateral wall of the cavernous sinus (see Fig. 1-45). Just posterior to the superior orbital (sphenoidal) fissure, it receives the frontal, lacrimal, and nasociliary nerves. The frontal and lacrimal nerves leave the orbit above the ligament of Zinn, whereas the nosociliary branch leaves through the annulus of the ligament.

The *frontal nerve* is located in the roof of the orbit between the levator palpebrae superioris muscle and the periosteum. The supraorbital and supratrochlear are its major branches. The supraorbital nerve enters the orbit through the supraorbital notch. Its major branches, the medial and lateral frontal nerves, receive sensory impulses from the forehead, scalp, and upper eyelid. The supratrochlear nerve contains sensory nerves from the medial scalp, eyelid, and conjunctiva that enters the orbit near the trochlea.

The *lacrimal nerve* follows the upper border of the lateral rectus muscle accompanied by the lacrimal artery. Its superior branch originates as the lateral palpebral nerve, receiving sensory impulse from the skin and conjunctiva of the upper and lower eyelids. The inferior branch receives a twig from the zygomaticotemporal branch of the maxillary division (V_2) of the trigeminal nerve, which may be secretory to the lacrimal gland.

The *nasociliary nerve* has much the same course as the ophthalmic artery and provides the only sensory innervation of the globe. It receives the long (sensory) root of the ciliary ganglion at the superior orbital fissure.

Two long ciliary nerves form the nasociliary nerve as it crosses above the optic nerve. They emerge from the sclera with the short ciliary nerves and accompany the long posterior ciliary arteries. The fibers are mainly sensory, but also carry sympathetic fibers to the dilatator pupillae muscle. The infratrochlear and the anterior ethmoidal are the other branches of the nasociliary nerve.

Autonomic nervous system

The autonomic nervous system is a subdivision of the motor portion of the nervous system that carries inpulses to smooth muscles, cardiac muscle, and glands. In contrast to skeletal muscle, in which a single neuron extends from the central nervous system to the muscle fiber, the autonomic nervous system is composed of a

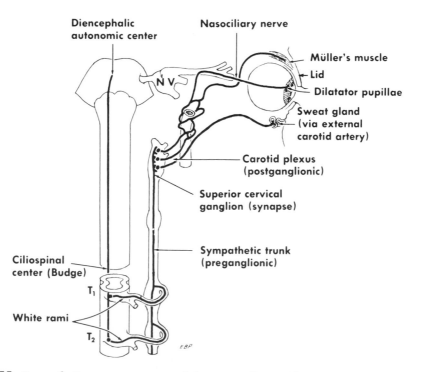

Fig. 1-55. Sympathetic nervous system of the eye. Efferent fibers synapse in the superior cervical ganglion. Postganglionic fibers then pass to the sweat glands of the face and eyelids along the external carotid artery. Other branches extend intracranially with the internal carotid artery and pass with the ophthalmic artery into the orbit. Vasomotor fibers are distributed by the short ciliary nerves to blood vessels in the choroid. Fibers to the dilatator pupillae muscle do not pass through the ciliary ganglion and are carried to the globe by the long ciliary branches of the nasociliary nerve (N V).

two-neuron chain. The first, or preganglionic neuron, has its cell body in the central nervous system and synapses in a ganglion with postganglionic neurons. The second, or postganglionic neuron, has its cell body in an autonomic ganglion and terminates in smooth muscle, cardiac muscle, or glands.

The autonomic nervous system is composed of two parts: (1) visceral efferent fibers in cranial nerves III, VII, IX, X, and XI and sacral nerves II, III, and IV, which comprise the parasympathetic portion (craniosacral division); and (2) visceral efferent fibers of thoracic and lumbar nerves, which comprise the sympathetic system (thoracolumbar division).

Parasympathetic nervous system. The visceral efferent branch of the oculomotor nerve arises from cell bodies located in the Edinger-Westphal nuclei. Together with the inferior division of the oculomotor nerve, the axons pass with the branch to the inferior oblique muscle and form the preganglionic motor root (short) of the ciliary ganglion. Here synapse is made with the cells of postganglionic fibers, which pass with the short ciliary nerves to innervate the ciliary and sphincter pupillae muscles.

Sympathetic nervous system. The sympathetic nervous system (Fig. 1-55) has centers located in the hypothalamus and the medulla: (1) the superior ciliospinal center, and (2) the inferior ciliospinal center (of Budge). The *superior ciliospinal center* is located near the nucleus of the hypoglossal nerve. The *inferior ciliospinal center* (of Budge) is located in the upper portion of the spinal cord. Sympathetic efferent fibers originate in the anterior lateral columns and leave the spinal cord in the ventral roots of thoracic I to lumbar II spinal nerves. These fibers pass with the anterior rami lateral to the vertebral column until they leave the anterior rami in the white ramus communicans. The white rami turn at right angles at the vertebral column to form the sympathetic nerve trunk, which extends from the base of the skull to the tip of the coccyx. Within the trunk are ganglia in which synapse is made with peripheral postganglionic sympathetic nerves.

The ganglia at the level of cervical I, II, and III spinal nerves fuse to form a superior cervical ganglion. Most of the preganglionic fibers that synapse in the superior cervical ganglion have left the spinal cord at the level of the first two thoracic nerves and have coursed upward in the sympathetic nerve trunk.

Postganglionic fibers from the superior cervical ganglion are widely distributed. The internal carotid branch extends intracranially with fibers distributed to the internal carotid artery and the cavernous plexus. These fibers provide almost all of the sympathetic nerve branches to the eye and the orbit. Fibers for sweating of the face, however, are distributed with the external carotid artery.

Sympathetic nerve fibers pass through the ciliary ganglion without synapse. They are mainly vasomotor and are distributed by the short ciliary nerves to the uveal blood vessels.

Fibers to the dilatator pupillae muscle pass to the eye in the two long ciliary nerve branches of the nasociliary nerve and do not pass through the ciliary ganglion.

EMBRYOLOGY

The optic primordium and optic sulcus appear at the eight-somite state (22 to 23 days postovulation), and thereafter any adverse environmental influences cause ocular developmental abnormalities. In general, genetic or exogenous factors that influence development early in embryonic life cause such severe defects that the fetus seldom survives. Thus ocular defects seen clinically occur relatively late in ocular development.

The eye and its appendages originate from neural and surface ectoderm, mesoderm, and the neural crest. The sensory retina, retinal pigment epithelium, and neural portion of the optic nerve develop from the neural ectoderm. The neural ectoderm also forms the optic cup, the anterior portion of which gives rise to the ciliary epithelium, pigment layer of the iris, and its sphincter and dilatator muscles.

The surface ectoderm is the primordia of the lens, the corneal epithelium, the conjunctiva and eyelid epithelium, together with the epithelium of their glandular structures, and the lacrimal gland. Primordial neural crest cells form the corneal stroma, endothelium (mesothelium), Descemet membrane, the iris stroma, the iridocorneal angle, the fibroblasts of the sclera, the vascular pericytes, the connective

Table 1-4. Primordia of ocular structures

I. Surface ectoderm
  A. Lens
  B. Corneal epithelium
  C. Conjunctival epithelium
  D. Cilia
  E. Epithelium, tarsal glands
  F. Epithelium, glands of Zeis and Moll
  G. Epithelium, lacrimal and accessory lacrimal
  H. Epithelium, lacrimal passages
II. Neural crest cells
  A. Corneal stroma
  B. Corneal endothelium (mesothelium) and Descemet membrane
  C. Scleral fibroblasts
  D. Iris stroma and melanophores (not pigmented epithelium)
  E. Iridocorneal angle (trabecular meshwork)
  F. Choroid melanophores, pericytes, and stroma
  G. Orbital bones
  H. Optic nerve meninges
  I. Nerves

III. Neural ectoderm
  A. Sensory retina
  B. Retinal pigment epithelium
  C. Iris pigment epithelium
  D. Sphincter pupillae muscle, dilatator pupillae muscle
  E. Neural portions of optic nerve
IV. Mesoderm
  A. Conjunctival stroma
  B. Episclera
  C. Tenon capsule
  D. Extrinsic ocular muscles
  E. Ciliary muscles
  F. Choroidal endothelium
  G. Vitreous
V. Mixed
  A. Surface ectoderm and mesoderm
    1. Eyelid from ectoderm, mesoderm, and neural crest
    2. Zonule (tertiary vitreous)
  B. Neural ectoderm and mesoderm
    1. Bruch membrane

tissue of the choroid, and all pigment cells except those in the retinal and iris pigment epithelium (but including those in the iris stroma). Neural crest cells form the bones of the orbit, the meninges, Schwann cells, and the autonomic nervous system and peripheral sensory nerves. Mesoderm provides the striated extrinsic muscles of the eye and the endothelium of blood vessels. The eyelid forms from surface ectoderm, mesoderm, and neural crest cells. The tertiary vitreous (zonule) forms from surface ectoderm and mesoderm. The Bruch membrane originates from mesoderm and neural ectoderm (Table 1-4).

The neural crest is the sole source of all pigment cells of the body except those of the retina and iris pigment epithelium, which are derived from the optic cup. Neural crest cells form all of the skeletal and connective tissues adjacent to the medial and lateral parts of the eye, including the corneal endothelium and stroma and much of the orbit. The extraocular muscles are of mesodermal origin, with only a small contribution from neural crest derived cells. The connective tissue associated with the extraocular muscles is of neural crest origin as are the ciliary muscles.

After fertilization of the ovum, a solid cluster of cells forms, the morula (Fig. 1-56, *A*). This develops into the blastula (Fig. 1-56, *B*), a hollow sphere containing a central cavity, the blastocele. The outer wall of the blastula forms the placenta. The cells in one section of the inner wall form the embryo, amnion, and yolk sac (primitive gut or archenteron) (Fig. 1-56, *C*). The embryo develops from the embryonic plate at the area of contact between the amnion and the yolk sac (Fig. 1-56, *D*). It consists of two layers: a dorsal ectoderm and a ventral entoderm connected to the inner wall of the blastula by a body stalk. A primitive streak, followed by a groove, develops on the ectodermal surface and provides an axial symmetry to the embryonic plate.

The ectoderm thickens to form a neural (medullary) plate, the mid portion of which deepens to form a neural groove. The lateral parts of the neural plate proliferate, become raised, and flank the neural groove as the neural folds (Fig. 1-57). The neural folds are first recognizable 18 days post ovulation and are prominent by 3 weeks. The neural folds coalesce to form an enclosed primitive neural tube from which the brain, spinal cord, and peripheral nerves develop.

The optic primordium and optic sulcus appear in the neural fold on each side of the forebrain at about 22 to 23 days, when the embryo

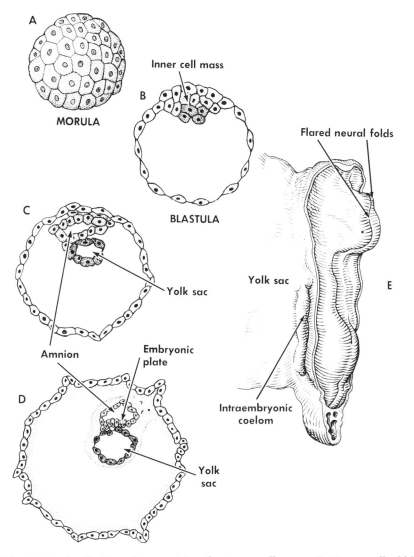

Fig. 1-56. A, Morula. **B,** Blastula containing the inner cell mass. **C,** Outer wall of blastula forms the placenta; the cell mass adjacent to the inner wall of the blastula gives rise to the amnion; the remaining cells form the yolk sac. **D,** Embryo develops in the area of contact between the amnion and yolk sac. **E,** Amnion is cut away to show the neural folds at the anterior extremity of the neural plate.

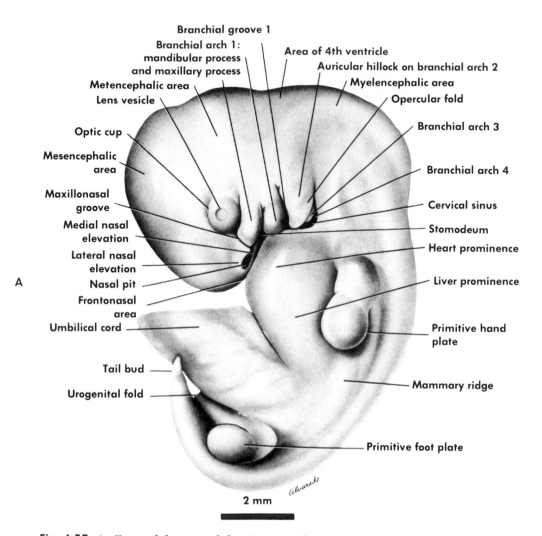

Branchial groove 1
Branchial arch 1:
mandibular process
and maxillary process
Metencephalic area
Lens vesicle
Optic cup
Mesencephalic
area
Maxillonasal
groove
Medial nasal
elevation
Lateral nasal
elevation
Nasal pit
Frontonasal
area
Umbilical cord
Tail bud
Urogenital fold

A

Area of 4th ventricle
Auricular hillock on branchial arch 2
Myelencephalic area
Opercular fold
Branchial arch 3
Branchial arch 4
Cervical sinus
Stomodeum
Heart prominence
Liver prominence
Primitive hand
plate
Mammary ridge
Primitive foot plate

2 mm

Fig. 1-57. A, External features of the 10 mm embryo at 37 postovulation days. The optic cup, lens vesicle, and various areas of the brain can be located on the surface of the head. **B,** Section through the optic stalk lumen and lens vesicle of the 10 mm embryo. (With permission from Gasser, R.F.: Atlas of human embryos, Hagerstown, Md., 1975, Harper & Row, Publishers.)

has eight pairs of somites and is about 2 mm maximum in length. At 24 days the optic sulcus has become the optic vesicle. The anterior portion of the primitive brain consists of a cerebral vesicle separating lateral optic vesicles (Fig. 1-58).

At the time the primitive neural tube is forming, specialized neuroectodermal cells form a longitudinal cap along its dorsal aspect at its point of closure. These cells rapidly proliferate to form right and left neural crests the entire length of the neural tube. Neural crest cells in the cranial region produce autonomic and sensory neuroblasts as well as connective

cells that differentiate into teeth and membranous bones of the head. Neural crest cells in the trunk region also produce sensory and autonomic neuroblasts. Pigment cells, meninges, neurolemma, and neuroendocrine cells also originate in the neural crest. The first brachial arch subdivides into maxillary and mandibular portions. Abnormalities of the maxillary portion result in down and outward slanting palpebral fissures (antimongoloid) and a sunken upper face with depressed cheek bones. Abnormalities of the mandibular branch result in a receding chin. Abnormalities of the second brachial arch may cause nerve deafness.

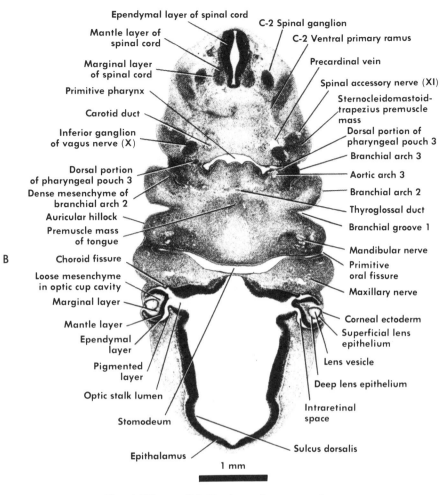

Ependymal layer of spinal cord
Mantle layer of spinal cord
Marginal layer of spinal cord
Primitive pharynx
Carotid duct
Inferior ganglion of vagus nerve (X)
Dorsal portion of pharyngeal pouch 3
Dense mesenchyme of branchial arch 2
Auricular hillock
Premuscle mass of tongue
Choroid fissure
Loose mesenchyme in optic cup cavity
Marginal layer
Mantle layer
Ependymal layer
Pigmented layer
Optic stalk lumen
Stomodeum
Epithalamus

C-2 Spinal ganglion
C-2 Ventral primary ramus
Precardinal vein
Spinal accessory nerve (XI)
Sternocleidomastoid-trapezius premuscle mass
Dorsal portion of pharyngeal pouch 3
Branchial arch 3
Aortic arch 3
Branchial arch 2
Thyroglossal duct
Branchial groove 1
Mandibular nerve
Primitive oral fissure
Maxillary nerve
Corneal ectoderm
Superficial lens epithelium
Lens vesicle
Deep lens epithelium
Intraretinal space
Sulcus dorsalis

B

1 mm

Fig. 1-57, cont'd. For legend see opposite page.

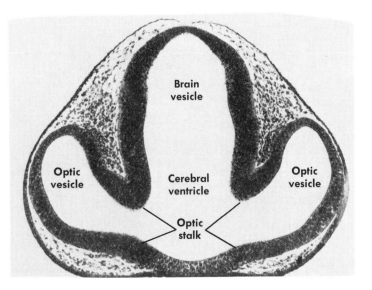

Fig. 1-58. Optic vesicles at 28 postovulation days. (×70.) (With permission from O'Rahilly, R.: Exp. Eye Res. **21**:93, 1975. Copyright by Academic Press Inc. [London] Ltd.)

After about the twenty-eighth postovulation day, the retinal disk appears in the wall of the optic vesicle, and the lens placode appears in the surface ectoderm. Within a few days the retinal disk becomes invaginated to form the optic cup, and the retinal fissure is delineated. The lens placode becomes indented to form the lens pit (Fig. 1-59).

By the thirty-sixth postovulation day the primary vitreous body begins to form, and melanin pigment appears in the outer wall of the optic cup destined to be the retinal pigment epithelium. The lens pit has closed to form the lens vesicle surrounded by its capsule. The restored surface ectoderm constitutes the epithelium of the future cornea. The lens body appears with primary lens fibers, and the hyaloid artery enters the lentiretinalis space through the retinal fissure. By the forty-second postovulation day the thicker inner layer of the optic cup begins to differentiate, and the cavity of the lens vesicle becomes obliterated by primary lens fibers. By the fifty-sixth day (Fig. 1-60) the optic nerve fibers have formed from the retinal ganglion cells. The nerve fiber layer of the retina appears, and nerve fibers grow into the brain. The mesothelium of the anterior chamber, the substantia propria of the cornea (Fig. 1-61), and the pupillary membrane develop. The scleral condensation is more apparent. Secondary lens fibers and the secondary vitreous body are forming. The embryo has a crown length of 30 mm, and the optic cup is approximately 1.5 to 2 mm in diameter.

Failure of the optic vesicle to invaginate results in a congenital cyst in which the orbit contains a large cyst with traces of nerve elements rather than an eye.

Invagination of the optic vesicle involves not only the lateral surface but also its inferior surface and the distal end of the optic stalk, so that a linear cleft or fissure forms on its posterior surface. This cleft is the retinal, or embryonic, fissure and is sometimes called the choroidal fissure. The retinal fissure provides a bypass for blood vessels and optic nerve fibers that enter and leave the optic vesicle so they do not pass around its lateral margin. Defects in the region of the retinal fissure result in colobomas that may involve the 6 o'clock meridian of the optic nerve, the retina, the choroid, the ciliary body, and the iris.

During the 17 to 20 mm stage (7 weeks), the nose develops by fusion of the median nasal process with each other and with the lateral nasal processes to form the frontonasal process. Failure of this fusional process results in the median cleft face syndrome.

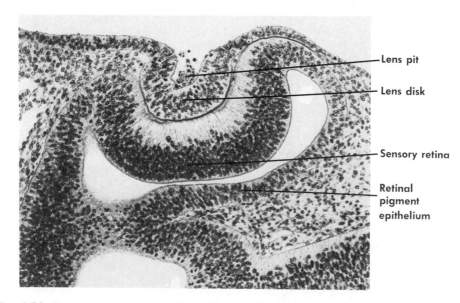

Fig. 1-59. Optic cup at 32 postovulation days. The sensory retina has a nucleus-free zone. Invagination of the lens disk has resulted in the appearance of a linear pit. (×210.) (With permission from O'Rahilly, R.: Exp. Eye Res. **21:**93, 1975. Copyright by Academic Press Inc. [London] Ltd.)

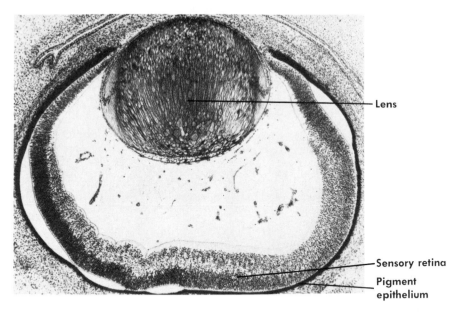

Lens

Sensory retina

Pigment
epithelium

Fig. 1-60. Eye at the end of the embryonic period. (×65.) (With permission from O'Rahilly, R.: Exp. Eye Res. **21**:93, 1975. Copyright by Academic Press Inc. [London] Ltd.)

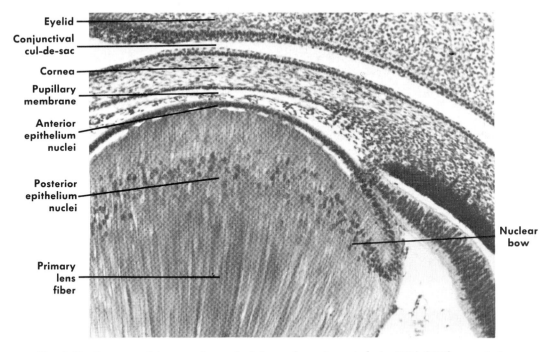

Eyelid

Conjunctival
cul-de-sac

Cornea

Pupillary
membrane

Anterior
epithelium
nuclei

Posterior
epithelium
nuclei

Primary
lens
fiber

Nuclear
bow

Fig. 1-61. Cornea and lens at the end of the embryonic period. (×135.) (With permission from O'Rahilly, R.: Exp. Eye Res. **21**:93, 1975. Copyright by Academic Press Inc. [London] Ltd.)

THE EYE
Outer coat

The sclera. The sclera originates as a condensation of secondary mesenchyme (neural crest cells mainly combined with mesodermal cells) surrounding the anterior portion of the optic cup and then extends posteriorly. During the fourth month, collagenous fibers extend posteriorly, and by the fifth month a fibrous coat envelopes the globe.

The cornea. The corneal epithelium is formed by the surface epithelium, from which the lens placode detaches itself. Neural crest cells form the corneal stroma and later the corneal mesothelium (endothelium) and the Descemet membrane. The cells of the corneal stroma provide the primary pupillary membrane, which is then vascularized by mesodermal cells.

Medial coat

The choroid. The choroid has a complex origin from the secondary mesenchyme surrounding the primary optic vesicle. Its blood vessels are of mesodermal origin, whereas the melanophores, pericytes, and connective tissue originate from the neural crest derivatives. All of its layers can be recognized by the fifth month. Pigment develops relatively late, first near the entrance of the posterior ciliary artery branches and then extending forward. At 6 weeks it is highly vascular, and the tissue is spongy. The choroid corresponds to the pia mater and arachnoid of the brain; anteriorly the neural crest derivatives differentiate into the connective tissue of the ciliary body while the ciliary muscle is of mesodermal origin.

At the anterior edge of the secondary optic cup, the inner sensory and the outer pigmentary layers fuse together to form the following structures: (1) the ciliary epithelium (pars ciliaris retinae), with an inner nonpigmented layer that is a continuation of the sensory layer and a pigmentary layer that is the continuation of retinal pigment epithelium, and (2) further anteriorly, the iris epithlium (pars iridica retinae) together with the sphincter and dilatator pupillae muscles.

The ciliary body. The ciliary body is formed by a fusion of the optic cup and the adjacent secondary mesenchyme. The ciliary processes are derived from the pigmented and nonpigmented epithelium of the primitive retina, and the capillaries are derived from mesoderm. The ciliary muscle grows in from mesoderm located between the sclera and the ciliary ectoderm. Longtiudinal fibers are formed about the fourth month, and the circular portion is formed at the end of the sixth month. The attachment of the longitudinal fibers to the scleral spur establishes an anterior chamber angle. Secretion by the ciliary epithelium and outflow through the trabecular meshwork begin about the sixth or seventh month.

The iris and pupil. The pigment epithelium of the iris, the sphincter pupillae muscle, and dilatator pupillae muscle are derived from the neural ectoderm of the optic cup. The iris stroma and its melanophores originate with neural crest cells. The surface pattern of the iris in postnatal life closely reflects its embryologic origin. The most anterior extremity of the optic cup is visible as the pupillary frill. The sphincter pupillae muscle and dilatator pupillae muscle are derived from neural ectoderm and, with the arrectores pilorum muscles, are the sole muscles in the body of ectodermal origin. Cells of neural crest origin first grow over the surface of the optic cup to form the anterior stromal layers of the iris. Until the third month of embryonic life, the margin of the optic cup extends only a short distance beyond the equator of the lens. About the fourth month the cup grows forward with an attachment to the mesenchyme. The mesenchyme in the pupillary area then atrophies as far back as this attachment, which forms the collarette. The collarette is concentric with the pupillary margin and marks the position of the minor vascular circle of the iris.

Inner coat

Retinal pigment epithelium. The outer layer of the optic cup forms the retinal pigment epithelium. Initially, it is some four to six cells thick (32 postovulation days), but with cytolysis of these cells the pigment epithelium becomes deeply pigmented and a single cell–layer thick. This cytolysis may influence the stratification of the sensory retina. Because the sensory retina grows at a different rate, the two layers are not in apposition until stratification of the sensory retina is complete.

Sensory retina. The sensory portion of the retina develops from the inner portion of the optic cup. It consists, as does the neural tube, of three zones (ependymal, mantle, and marginal) limited by a terminal bar net on the outer side and by a basement membrane on the inner. Because of invagination of the optic cup, the basement membrane is on the surface closest to the vitreous cavity and the terminal bars of Müller fibers on the surface closest to the retinal pigment epithelium. The basement membrane provides the internal limiting lamina of the retina.

The ependymal zone develops cilia that project into the vesicle between the inner and outer walls of the optic cup; these develop into cone and rod outer segments. The marginal zone develops into the nerve fiber layer (and a transient, nonnucleated layer of Chievitz). The central mantle layer develops into the primitive neuroepithelium, which is divided into an outer and inner neuroblastic layer. The outer neuroblastic layer contains nuclei of rods and cones and bipolar and horizontal cells. The inner neuroblastic layer contains ganglion cells, amacrine cells, and Müller cells. Development proceeds from the posterior pole toward the periphery. The specialized area of the macula lutea begins in the third month, but its development proceeds slowly. Not until the sixth month is there a thinning of ganglion cells, and anatomic differentiation continues after birth. Inasmuch as central vision does not fully develop until the third year, it is evident that functional differentiation lags behind anatomic differentiation.

Lens. The tip of the optic vesicle, as it extends laterally, is covered by surface (head) ectoderm. During a brief interval, the ectodermal and vesicular basement membranes adhere to each other, which is followed by elongation of ectodermal cells over the zone of contact to form a lens placode. As the optic vesicle invaginates to form an optic cup, the lens placode invaginates to form a lens cup, the lumen of which is continuous with the surface of the embryo through the lens pore. The lens pore decreases in size until the residual surface ectoderm (the presumptive corneal epithelium) becomes smooth and the lens cup is connected to the surface ectoderm by a solid lens stalk. The stalk attenuates so that the lens cup separates from the surface ectoderm and the basement membrane surrounding the lens cup (enlage of lens capsule) closes completely to envelop the lens cup.

Further maturation of the lens requries a healthy developing neural retina with appropriate positioning of the lens and the rim of the optic cup (presumptive ciliary epithelium). Elongation of the cells on the wall of the lens cup adjacent to the vitreous cavity side of the lens obliterates the lumen of the lens cup. As the apices of the elongating cells (primary lens fibers) approach the presumptive lens epithelial cells on the wall of the lens adjacent to the anterior chamber, they send out processes that are followed by gap junctions between apposed surfaces.

Subsequent fibers (secondary lens fibers) are formed by cells located anteriorly while the primary lens fibers lose their nuclei when the base of the lens fiber loses contact with the posterior capsule. As secondary fibers form their lateral surfaces, they associate with adjacent fibers by gap junctions, desmosomes, and ball-and-socket interdigitations. As additional lens fibers are laid down and then displaced from contact with the posterior capsule, they meet base to base near the posterior pole to form the Y-shaped posterior suture and apex to apex to form the anterior Y-shaped anterior suture.

The nuclei migrate to the equator where secondary lens fibers continue to develop throughout life (see Fig. 1-61).

With the development of the ciliary prosesses, zonular fibers are deposited between the ciliary epithelium and the capsule at the lens equator (12 weeks post ovulation).

Vitreous humor. The vitreous humor consists of primary or hyaloid vitreous, secondary or definitive vitreous, and tertiary vitreous of the suspensory zonule of Zinn. The primary vitreous begins with protein-rich PAS-positive material that forms between the lens placode and optic vesicle about the thirty-sixth post-ovulation day. Vascularized mesoderm enters the optic fissure, and by the seventh week the hyaloid artery is developed and reaches the lens. By the ninth week the hyaloid system is fully developed. The hyaloid system begins to resorb about the fifth month, no longer carries blood after the seventh month, and is absent after birth except for its remnant, the canal of Cloquet.

The secondary or definitive vitreous appears about the seventh week as the retinal fissure closes and gradually fills the vitreous cavity as the hyaloid system resorbs. It is apparently of neuroectodermal origin.

The tertiary vitreous, the zonule of Zinn, begins to form in the sixth month. Eventually fibers insert into the basement membrane of the ciliary epithelium and the lens capsule.

BLOOD SUPPLY

The retinal fissure extends to about the anterior one third of the optic stalk. About the end of the first month (when the fetus is 7 to 8 mm), an arterial plexus below the optic cup consolidates into (1) a hyaloid artery that enters the optic nerve and cup through the fissure, and (2) a small annular vessel that ramifies on the rim of the cup and eventually becomes the choroid.

The hyaloid artery forms a network of vessels covering the back of the lens (tunica vasculosa lentis) and filling the vitreous body (vasa hyaloidea propria). The hyaloid system begins to resorb after the fifth month.

The vascular return of the entire hyaloid system is by the capsulopupillary membrane that covers the lens from the equator to the edge of the pupil. As the hyaloid system atrophies, the pupillary membrane is supplied by the long posterior arteries. It continues to develop until early in the sixth month, when the arteries begin to atrophy and disappear.

At about 14 to 15 weeks of gestational life (70 to 110 mm), mesenchymal cells appear in the vicinity of the hyaloid artery. They proliferate into the optic disk and subsequently invade the nerve fiber layer of the retina. The mesenchymal cells differentiate into endothelial cells that form solid cords, which gradually canalize to become capillaries. Thus arteries and veins arise from capillaries and not the reverse. The growth progresses from the optic disk, and blood vessels reach the ora serrata 39 weeks after gestation, an important factor in the retinopathy of prematurity.

A wide variation in orbital blood vessels occurs, mainly because of failure of early branches to disappear. Portions of the pupillary membrane commonly persist over the pupillary aperture, and persistence of the hyaloid artery is common. It extends a variable distance from the optic disk into the vitreous cavity, sometimes as far as the lens. It may form a small opacity (the Mittendorf dot) on the posterior lens capsule. The Bergmeister papilla is a glial sheath that surrounds the first one third of the hyaloid artery. It may persist in the adult as a small tuft of tissue replacing the physiologic optic cup of the optic disk.

The optic stalk provides the neuroglial supporting structures of the optic nerve. The nerve fibers consist of axons of ganglion cells located in the inner layer of the retina together with fibers extending from the brain to the retina. The sheaths and septa of the optic nerve develop from mesoderm.

THE EYELIDS

The eyelids are derived from both the surface ectoderm and the mesoderm. The upper eyelid develops from the frontonasal process in medial and lateral portions. The mesodermal portion of the lower eyelid originates from an upgrowth of the maxillary process. The surface ectoderm provides both the exterior skin and the internal conjunctiva. The eyelids grow together and fuse at approximately 9 weeks, and they do not reopen again until the seventh month. The tarsal plate, muscles, and connective tissues of the eyelids are derived from mesoderm. The glands and the cilia originate from the ectoderm.

LACRIMAL APPARATUS

The lacrimal gland develops from the ectoderm forming the conjunctival surface of the eyeball. Once formed, it receives connective tissue septa and supporting structures from the mesoderm.

The lacrimal passages develop in a cleft between the lateral nasal and maxillary processes. This cleft is converted into a tube by canalization of a solid rod of ectodermal tissue cells found beneath the surface, and these epithelial cells form the lacrimal passages. The lacrimal puncta do not open into the eyelid margins until just before the eyelids separate during the seventh month. The lower ends of the nasolacrimal ducts frequently do not open into the nose until birth or shortly thereafter.

BIBLIOGRAPHY
Anatomy

Apt, L.: An anatomical reevaluation of rectus muscle insertions, Trans. Am. Ophthalmol. Soc. **78:**365, 1980.

Cogan, D.G.: Neurology of the visual system, Springfield, Ill., 1980, Charles C Thomas, Publisher.

Doxanas, M.T., and Anderson, R.L.: Clinical orbital anatomy, Baltimore, 1984, Williams & Wilkins Co.

Duane, T.D., and Jaeger, E.A., eds.: Biomedical foundations of ophthalmology, vols. 1-3, Philadelphia, 1983, Harper & Row, Publishers.

Fine, B.S., and Yanoff, M.: Ocular histology: a text and atlas, ed. 2, New York, 1979, Harper & Row, Publishers.

Helveston, E.M., Merriam, W.W., Ellis, F.D., Shellhamer, R.H., and Gosling, C.G.: The trochlea: a study of the anatomy and physiology, Ophthalmology **89:**124, 1982.

Jakobiec, F.A., ed.: Ocular anatomy, embryology, and teratology, Philadelphia, 1982, J.B. Lippincott Co.

Miller, N.R.: Walsh and Hoyt's clinical neuro-ophthalmology, ed. 4, vol. 2, Baltimore, 1985, Williams & Wilkins Co.

Nelson, J.D., and Wright, J.C.: Conjunctival goblet cell densities in ocular surface disease, Arch. Ophthalmol. **102:**1049, 1984.

Warwick, R.: Eugene Wolff's anatomy of the eye and orbit, ed. 7, Philadelphia, 1977, W.B. Saunders Co.

Embryology

Bahn, C.F., Falls, H.F., Varley, G.A., Meyer, R.F., Edelhauser, H.F., and Bourne, W.M.: Classification of corneal endothelial disorders based on neural crest origin, Ophthalmology **91:**558, 1984.

Bard, J.B.L., and Hay, E.D.: The behavior of fibroblasts from the developing avian cornea: morphology and movement in situ and in vitro, J. Cell Biol. **67:**400-418, 1975.

Bard, J.B.L., Hay, E.D., and Meller, S.M.: Formation of the endothelium of the avian cornea: a study of cell movement in vivo, Dev. Biol. **42:**334-361, 1975.

Beauchamp, G.R., and Knepper, P.A.: Role of the neural crest in anterior segment development and disease, J. Pediatr. Ophthalmol. Strabismus **21:**209, 1984.

Coulombre, A.J.: Problems in corneal morphogenesis, Adv. Morphogen. **4:**81-109, 1965.

Hay, E.D.: Development of vertebrate cornea, Int. Rev. Cytol. **63:**263-322, 1980.

Hendrickson, A.E., and Yuodelis, C.: The morphological development of the human fovea, Ophthalmology **91:**603, 1984.

Kissel, P., Andre, J.M., and Jacquier, A.: The Neurocristopathies, New York, 1981, Masson Publishing USA, Inc. (Distributed by Year Book Medical Publishers, Chicago.)

le Dourarín, N.: The neural crest, Cambridge, 1982, Cambridge University Press.

Noden, D.M.: The control of avian cephalic neural crest cytodifferentiation. 1. Skeletal and connective tissues, Dev. Biol. **67:**296, 1978.

2

PHYSIOLOGY AND BIOCHEMISTRY OF THE EYE

"Vision is the process that produces from images of the external world a description that is useful to the viewer and not cluttered with irrelevant information." The simplicity of this statement by David Marr is deceptive. The 100 million rods and cones of the human retina, together with three layers of nuclei, perform at least 10 billion calculations per second before the signal reaches the optic nerve. Then the cerebral cortex processes the information in more than a dozen separate vision centers. The process becomes even more complex with the processing of the two-dimensional image from each eye to the three-dimensional world.

The human eye is not the equal of many animal eyes in specific functions. Nonetheless, it provides a wide spectrum of functions that are not duplicated in lower orders. The media are transparent, providing a clear image. The changes in shape of the lens in accommodation make for a clear focus from near to far. Beginning with three different cone pigments, color vision is well developed. The human eye adapts to light and dark over an intensity range of 1 to 100,000. The location of human eyes in the front of the head and the decussation of axons from the nasal half of each retina permits a retinal correspondence so that an object may be seen with depth and solidity (stereoscopic vision).

THE CORNEA

The cornea is a transparent tissue composed mainly of stroma with a regularly arranged stratified squamous epithelium on its outer surface and a single layer of endothelial cells lining its inner surface. The anterior surface is bathed with tears, whereas the apices of the endothelial cells of the posterior surface are bathed in aqueous humor.

The corneal stroma consists of type I collagen fibers of uniform diameter gathered together in lamellae that are at right angles to each other. The lamellae are enmeshed in glycosaminoglycans, a relatively recent term for what was previously termed mucopolysaccharides. Corneal glycosaminoglycans are composed of 60% keratan sulfate (a glucosaminoglycan) and 40% chondroitin sulfates (galactosaminoglycans). These act as anions and bind cations and water. In mucopolysaccharidosis (see Chapter 24), these glycosaminoglycans accumulate in the cornea and cause corneal clouding. Normal corneal transparency requires that both the epithelium and endothelium be intact to prevent corneal edema.

Because the central cornea is avascular, it must derive oxygen from the atmosphere and metabolic materials by diffusion from the pericorneal capillaries, tears, and aqueous humor. Only the peripheral cornea receives adequate nutrients from the bloodstream.

Transparency. The cornea transmits electromagnetic radiation having a wavelength* of between 300 nm in the ultraviolet and 2,500 nm in the infrared. Transmission is about 80% at 400 nm and 100% at 500 to 1,200 nm. There are two areas of absorption beyond 1,200 nm, but transmission of long wavelengths is otherwise high. Radiation of wavelengths of more than 1,000 nm does not stimulate the retinal receptors and is dissipated as heat. Ultraviolet radiation below 365 nm is mainly absorbed by the cornea; the rest is absorbed by the lens and does not reach the retina unless the intensity is very high (lasers can deliver energy at this high intensity).

The transparency of the cornea is the result of the following: (1) anatomic structure, (2) the tight junctions of the epithelial cells that are not permeable to aqueous solutions, and (3) the dynamic balance between ions and water in the stroma that is maintained by an endothelial pump mechanism that controls corneal dehydration (deturgescence).

The anatomic factors include absence of blood vessels and pigment in the cornea, the regular arrangement of the epithelial and endothelial cells, and the few nuclei in the stroma. Additionally, the epithelial cells are not keratinized, and the anterior surface of tears forms a regular refracting surface. The cells of different layers do not reflect light at their interfaces because they all have the same index of refraction. The collagen fibrils of the corneal stroma have an index of refraction of 1.47; that of the surrounding glycosaminoglycans is about 1.34. This difference should produce considerable scattering of light, causing the cornea to be more translucent than transparent. The collagen fibers are, however, oriented in a two-dimensional lattice with the distance between each fiber approximately equal (Fig. 2-1). The fibers have a diameter of less than one wavelength of light, so that the lattice is transparent in the direction of an incident beam. That portion of the light striking the lattice itself is eliminated by destructive interference.

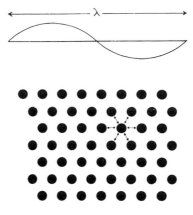

Fig. 2-1. The lattice structure of the cornea explains its transparency. Arrows between the fibrils indicate the system of forces that are supposed to maintain the regularity of the structure. The wavelength of light above is drawn to the same scale as the lattice. (From Maurice, D.M.: J. Physiol. [Lond.] **136**:263, 1957.)

Relative dehydration (deturgescence) of the stroma is necessary for transparency. Each corneal lamella contains about 75% of the water it is capable of binding. A button of cornea with the stroma exposed swells to about three times its normal thickness and becomes translucent. If the endothelium is poisoned with ouabain, cyanide, or iodoacetate, similar swelling occurs. Disease or injury of the epithelium or endothelium causes a corneal edema. The epithelium rapidly replicates itself and the swelling is transient. The endothelium in humans does not replicate although there is mitotic acitivity, but the cells increase in size to cover defects. After disease (endothelial dystrophy) or endothelial injury, a severe swelling of all corneal layers, bullous keratopathy (Chapter 10), may occur.

The endothelium constantly pumps fluid from the corneal stroma to the aqueous humor. The fluid leaks into the aqueous by several routes, predominantly across the endothelium itself. This process generates an electrical potential difference across the endothelium of ImV (aqueous negative) (Fig. 2-2). The negative charge of the aqueous is the opposite of that which would occur if there was an electrogenic transport of Na^+. The polarity may be explained by (1) electrogenic transfer of HCO_3^- from the endothelium to the aqueous; (2) H^+ movement from the endothelium to the

---

*The wavelength of electromagnetic energy is designated as nanometers (one billionth of a meter; m $\times$ 10^{-9}). Old units included Angstrom units (one ten-billionth of a meter; m $\times$ 10^{-10}) and millimicrons, which are the same as nanometers.

lateral intercellular space; (3) Na^+ movement from the endothelium to intercellular space; or (4) a combination of these. The perfused in vitro preparations of the cornea survive longer in a tissue culture medium enriched with oxidized glutathione. Possibly the oxidized glutathione contains cellular adenosine triphosphate (ATP) and protects NaK ATPase.

Permeability. The peripheral cornea maintains its metabolism by means of the capillary network at the corneoscleral limbus. The nutrition of the central cornea, however, depends on substances that enter through either the endothelium or the epithelium. To penetrate the epithelium a substance must be water-soluble to penetrate the film of tears covering the cornea. The epithelium constitutes the principal barrier of the cornea to ions. The zonulae occludentes and adherentes and maculae occludentes and adherentes of the epithelium make

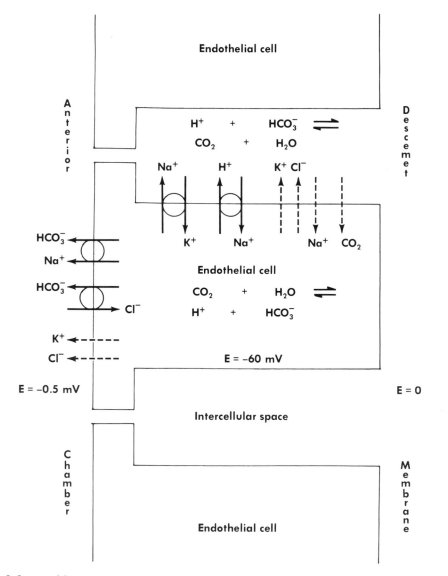

Fig. 2-2. Possible ionic transport mechanisms across the apical and basolateral membranes of the corneal endothelium. Solid lines represent either active transport or coupled movements. Dashed lines represent passive movements. Electrogenic effects could result from the activity of the Na^+ pump shown at the lateral membrane and the bicarbonate-sodium symport shown at the apical membrane. (From Fischbarg, J., and Lim, J.J.: Curr. Top. Eye Res. **4:**201, 1984.)

it impermeable to ions and other lipid-insoluble substances. The corneal epithelium is readily permeable to lipid-soluble substances because the cell membranes are composed of a lipoprotein. To pass through the stroma and endothelium the compounds must be water-soluble. Thus topical medications must be both water- and lipid-soluble to penetrate the normal cornea.

Metabolism. The cornea requires energy to maintain its deturgescence, provide its metabolic needs, and provide for epithelial cell renewal. Energy in the form of adenosine triphosphate is provided by the metabolism of glucose. The central cornea derives glucose from the aqueous humor and oxygen from the atmosphere. The peripheral cornea is nurtured by the corneoscleral vascular arcade. The epithelium is the site of most metabolism, since it contains 15 to 20 times more cells than the stroma and endothelium.

Glucose is first phosphorylated to glucose-6-phosphate so that it may by utilized (Fig. 2-3). This step requires the enzyme hexokinase, which is inhibited by its own product, glucose-6-phosphate. The glucose-6-phosphate is used in one of several metabolic pathways.

1. In glycolysis (Embden-Meyerhof pathway), which requires no oxygen, the glucose-6-phosphate is converted to two molecules of glyceral-dehyde-3-phosphate, which is converted to two molecules of pyruvate. In the absence of oxygen the pyruvate is converted to two molecules of lactic acid and excreted into the precorneal tear film.

2. In the presence of oxygen, the pyruvate is first decarboxylated to acetylcoenzyme A and, by a series of enzymatic reactions in the tricarboxylic acid cycle (Krebs or citric acid), is converted to carbon dioxide and water. This is the major cellular source of energy from glucose and molecular oxygen.

3. Glucose-6-phosphate may be degraded (phosphogluconic acid, phosphogluconate pathway, pentose phosphate pathway, or hexose monophosphate shunt) to 5-carbon sugars. The D-ribose-5-phosphate generated by the pathway is used in the nucleic acid synthesis required by the mitotic activity of the corneal epithelium.

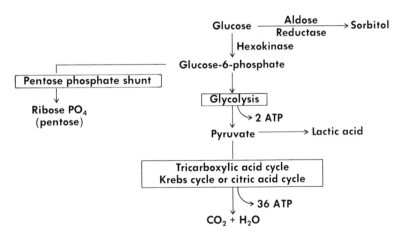

Fig. 2-3. A simplified schema of the metabolism of glucose in tissues. The aldose reductase pathway that forms sorbitol (an alcohol) from glucose is active only in the presence of excess sugar. This mechanism is important in "sugar cataract." Glycolysis (Embden-Meyerhof) does not utilize oxygen and is the major metabolic pathway of lens epithelium which is the major source of lactate in the aqueous humor. The pentose phosphate shunt provides the ribose-6-phosphate for nucleic acid synthesis and reduced nicotinamide adenine dinucleotide phosphate (NADPH) for which both hexokinase and aldose reductase compete. The major energy-producing pathway is the tricarboxylic acid cycle that requires oxygen. The major metabolism of the cornea is in the epithelium, which has 15 to 20 times more cells than the stroma and endothelium.

About 65% of glucose-6-phosphate in the cornea is metabolized by glycolysis and the remainder by way of the pentose phosphate pathway. The enzymes of the tricarboxylic acid cycle are mainly located in the epithelium. Thus, when the corneal epithelium is deprived of oxygen by a large contact lens that is not permeable to oxygen, an epithelial edema develops (Sattler veil). This reflects the inability of glycolysis to support epithelial metabolism and the inadequacy of the oxygen supply from the corneoscleral limbus vasculature. If the corneal epithelium is removed and a contact lens applied, the stroma and endothelium remain transparent almost indefinitely.

Wound healing. After laceration or freezing of the cornea, repair occurs in the epithelium, stroma, and endothelium. Loss of corneal epithelium causes enlargement and flattening of adjacent uninjured epithelial cells within an hour. These cells develop pseudopodia and migrate into the denuded area to provide a new layer one cell thick. Mitosis then occurs, the epithelial cell layer thickens, and after 6 weeks, the epithelium adheres to its underlying basement membrane. The migration is impaired only by severe injury, but mitosis is inhibited by anesthetics and antibiotics. It is stimulated by the epithelial growth factor.

Injury to the Bowman layer causes scar formation. Because the Bowman layer is a condensation of the corneal stroma, its wound repair is similar. Repair is effected by multiplication of undamaged keratocytes together with migration from the blood of either fibroblasts or monocytes transformed into fibroblasts. New glycosaminoglycan synthesis begins after 24 to 48 hours and is well established by the fifth day. Chondroitin sulfate predominates, and only late in the healing process is it replaced with the typical keratan sulfate. Stromal healing is not initiated until the defect is covered with epithelium.

In lower species the endothelium heals by mitotic replication. In humans endothelial cells spread to cover the defect. (Specular photography demonstrates an occasional mitotic figure in human endothelium.) Since damaged cells are not replaced, stromal and epithelial edema occurs (bullous keratopathy) if there are too few remaining cells to cover the injured area.

TEARS

The anterior surface of the eye is moistened mainly by tears secreted by the accessory lacrimal glands of Krause (67%) and Wolfring (33%). The lacrimal glands function mainly in psychic stimulation (crying) and after stimulation of the trigeminal nerve in injury and disease (reflex tearing). The accessory lacrimal glands constitute some 10% of the mass of lacrimal glands. The glands contain many plasma cells that are independent of antigenic stimulation, as is the lymphoid tissue in the gut. The major flow of tears is along the eyelid margin (marginal tear strip) and in the conjunctival fornices. Periodic involuntary blinking spreads the tears over the surface of the globe and causes a pumping action of the lacrimal drainage system.

Orbicularis oculi muscle fibers surround the puncta and insert into the periosteum of the anterior and posterior lacrimal crests. Blinking draws the puncta nasally, shortens the canaliculi, and forces tears into the lacrimal sac. Contraction of the orbicularis oculi muscle expands the lacrimal sac, creating a partial negative pressure to suck in tears. The pumping action of the orbicularis oculi muscle is essential for normal tear drainage.

The corneal epithelium is covered by a relatively stagnant layer of tears, the precorneal tear film. The precorneal tear film is composed of three layers (Fig. 2-4): (1) a thin (0.9 to 0.2 μm), anterior lipid layer derived from the meibomian glands, sebaceous glands of Zeis, and sweat glands of Moll; (2) a thick (6.5 to 7.5 μm), middle aqueous layer derived from the accessory lacrimal glands of Krause and Wolfring; and (3) a thin mucin layer derived from conjunctival goblet cells and minimally from lacrimal gland cells. The lipid layer retards the evaporation of tears and provides a smooth and regular anterior optical surface. The mucin layer wets the microvilli of the corneal epithelium and must be intact to retain the precorneal film. A deficiency of mucin occurs in avitaminosis A and scarring of the conjunctiva. An excess occurs in hyperthyroidism and reflex tear stimulation, and biochemical alterations (acidic glycosaminoglycans become neutral) in keratitis sicca.

The average normal secretion of tears is between 0.9 and 2.2 μl/min. The maximum ca-

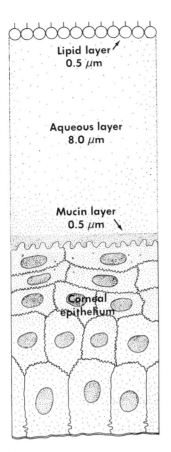

Fig. 2-4. Schema of the precorneal tear film. The mucin is a wetting agent that provides a hydrophilic surface to the hydrophobic corneal epithelium.

pacity of the cul-de-sac is about 30 μl, so that tears overflow if the rate of drainage does not increase with the rate of secretion. Once the rate of tear secretion exceeds 100 μl/min, overflow occurs.

With the eyes open and the precorneal oily film intact, a maximum of 0.85 μl of tears evaporates each minute, and the remainder pass through the lacrimal passages. The evaporation causes the tears to become slightly hypertonic, so that there is a minute osmotic flow of water from the anterior chamber, through the cornea, to the tear film. When the eyes are closed, the precorneal tear film is in osmotic equilibrium with the aqueous humor, no osmotic flow occurs, and the corneal stroma thickens.

The collection of tears to determine their composition is complicated by evaporation and by dilution that follows stimulation. The ante-

rior lipid layer probably reflects the composition of meibomian gland secretion that includes the following: wax esters, 35%; cholesterol ester, 30%; phospholipids, 16%; triglycerides, 4%; free fatty acids, 2%; and free sterols, 2%. The aqueous phase is 98% water and 2% solids. Sodium and bicarbonate levels parallel the plasma, whereas potassium and chloride levels exceed plasma levels. Urea, amino acids, and other small molecules parallel the plasma, whereas the glucose content is markedly less.

There is a large amount of protein, averaging approximately 7 mg/ml. The concentration decreases in aging. The protein includes a unique specific tear albumin that serves as a buffer of the tear system. Immunoglobulins and additional protein anti-inflammatory factors are also present.

Immunoglobulin A (IgA) and secretory (exocrine) IgA are the major immunoglobulins of the tears. Secretory IgA is composed of two IgA molecules synthesized by plasma cells in the main and accessory lacrimal glands and bound together by a secretory piece produced within the epithelial cells of lacrimal glands. IgA neutralizes viruses and inhibits bacterial adherence to the conjunctival surface. IgG is the second major immunoglobulin of tears and probably diffuses through conjunctival vessels. It promotes phagocytosis and complement-mediated bacterial lysis. Both increase in conjunctival inflammations. Immunoglobulin E increases in allergic inflammations.

Periodic blinking and the tear flow provide physical barriers to microbial colonization of the external eye. Many protective substances are present in tears, including immunoglobulins, lymphocytes, and complement, and nonspecific factors such as phagocytic cells, lactoferrin, lysozyme (muramidase), nonlysozyme antibacterial factor, anti-complement factor, and interferon.

Lactoferrin occurs in tears, many mucosal secretions, bile, and human (and bovine) milk. It chelates iron and may deprive microorganisms of iron. It is bactericidal to *Bacillus subtilis*, *Staphylococcus aureus* and *epidermidis*, and *Pseudomonas aeruginosa*. It may extend the lytic action of lysozyme to otherwise insensitive bacteria. Additionally, it may react with specific antibody to produce an antimicrobial system more powerful than either does singly. It modulates complement activity in vitro.

Lysozyme (muramidase) is an antibacterial enzyme that is widely distributed in nature— egg is the commercial source. It causes lysis of the glycosaminoglycan coating of a few nonpathogenic gram-positive bacteria. In the presence of complement it facilitates IgA bacteriolysis.

Basic tear formation has no apparent stimulus or specific innervation. Reflex tearing occurs in response to psychic stimuli (crying) and reflex stimulation of fibers of the ophthalmic division of the trigeminal nerve (NV). Application of heat to the tongue and mouth and uncomfortable retinal stimulation by bright lights also cause reflex tearing. Normal moisture of the eye is maintained entirely by the basic secretion of accessory lacrimal glands; reflex secretion of tears constitutes an emergency or psychic response.

Clinically, tear formation is measured by hooking (see Fig. 12-2) a strip of filter paper 5 mm wide over the middle portion of the lower eyelid. The amount of wetting that occurs in 5 minutes as measured from the fold indicates the volume of tears. Basic secretion is that which occurs after the eye is anesthetized with a topical anesthetic. Reflex secretion is measured without the use of a local anesthetic (there is no reflex wetting with general anesthesia). There is less tear formation after 50 years of age.

AQUEOUS HUMOR

The aqueous humor helps maintain the intraocular pressure and the metabolism of the cornea, trabecular meshwork, and lens. It is formed by secretion and ultrafiltration (dialysis under applied pressure). Specific transport systems of the nonpigmented epithelium of the ciliary body secrete chloride, potassium, chloride bicarbonate, some amino acids, glucose, ascorbic acid, and some organic compounds into the posterior chamber. Large protein molecules, erythrocytes, and leukocytes are excluded. The nonpigmented epithelium of the ciliary body also removes organic ions from the eye through specific transport systems.

The aqueous humor passes from the posterior chamber through the pupil into the ante-

rior chamber. It leaves the eye, mainly through the trabecular meshwork, passing into the canal of Schlemm, and then the deep scleral plexus (Fig. 2-5). In humans some 20% leaves the eye through the suprachoroidal space. The normal rate of flow is approximately 2 µl/min.

Once secreted into the posterior chamber, the composition of the aqueous humor is modified by several factors: (1) reabsorption by the ciliary processes; (2) the uptake of glucose, fatty acids, and amino acids by the lens and cornea; and (3) excretion of metabolic waste products by these tissues. The tight junctions of the pigment epithelium of the ciliary processes and iris, combined with those of the iris blood vessels, constitute the blood-aqueous barrier. Small molecules such as water, urea, and some amino acids enter the aqueous humor by diffusion from the plasma. Diffusion, aqueous flow, metabolism, and interaction with tissues make the composition of anterior chamber aqueous humor different than that of posterior chamber aqueous humor. It is also likely that the aqueous humor immediately adjacent to the ciliary processes differs from that in the posterior chamber.

Most studies concerning the composition of aqueous humor describe that which is obtained from the anterior chamber. Human studies often relate to fluid removed at the time of cataract extraction. Animal studies show wide species variation.

The aqueous humor concentration of sodium, potassium, and magnesium parallel that of the plasma, but calcium is about one half of the plasma level. In humans, goats, and horses, the chloride concentration is higher than the plasma, and bicarbonate is lower. In rabbits bicarbonate is in excess, while in monkeys and dogs both chloride and bicarbonate exceed plasma concentration. The higher bicarbonate concentration presumably buffers the metabolic production of lactic acid, the end product of anaerobic glycolysis, in eyes with a low flow rate of aqueous humor and a large lens.

Ascorbic acid is 10 to 50 times higher in the aqueous humor than in the plasma. Glutathione is higher than plasma but not blood in which virtually all glutathione is present in erythrocytes. Both ascorbic acid and glutathione protect against the damaging oxidative effects of free radicals and peroxides. These injurious effects are enhanced by light, and ocular tissues are at considerable risk of oxidation injury.

In vitro, the ciliary processes transport organic ions out of the eye. There are at least three separate systems: a hippuran, an iodipamide, and an iodide system. Additionally, prostaglandins are actively transported out of the eye, although this transport may utilize one of the first two systems rather than an additional one.

Sodium- and potassium-activated adenosine triphosphatase (NaK ATPase) facilitate electrolyte secretion into the posterior chamber. Inhibition of NaK ATPase by ouabain or vandate decreases the secretion of aqueous humor. Impairment of the sodium transport mechanism,

metabolic poisoning of the ciliary epithelium, and reduction of the temperature of the ciliary body to 19° C also decrease secretory activity.

Inhibition of carbonic anhydrase decreases the secretory activity of the ciliary epithelium. Carbonic anhydrase inhibitors are important compounds in the management of glaucoma.

The low protein concentration of the aqueous humor is the major difference between it and plasma. The aqueous humor of humans contains about 0.25 mg/ml of protein, mainly orosomucoid, transferrin, albumin, and IgG. The concentration of proteins in the aqueous humor varies with their molecular size; thus the blood-aqueous barrier is thought to have a pore diameter of about 104 nm. If the ciliary body epithelium or the blood vessels of the iris are damaged through injury or through

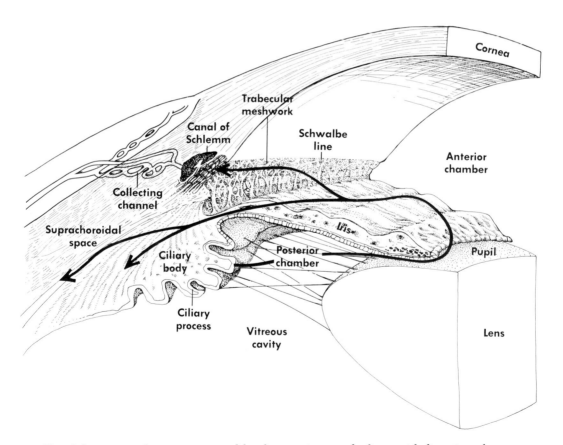

Fig. 2-5. Aqueous humor is secreted by the nonpigmented ciliary epithelium into the posterior chamber. It flows through the pupil into the anterior chamber and leaves the anterior chamber through the trabecular meshwork, which opens into the canal of Schlemm. In humans, about 20% of the aqueous humor leaves the eye through the suprachoroidal space and ciliary muscle spaces.

the release of prostaglandins, the aqueous humor has the same composition as plasma.

INTRAOCULAR PRESSURE

The interior pressure of the eye must exceed that of the surrounding atmosphere to prevent collapse. The normal intraocular pressure is between 10 and 20 mm Hg greater than atmospheric pressure. There is a variation of 1 to 2 mm Hg with each heartbeat caused by fluctuation in the intraocular vascular volume, and there are slower variations with respiration. The intraocular pressure normally fluctuates 2 to 5 mm Hg daily.

The three main factors concerned with the maintenance of intraocular pressure are the rate of formation of the aqueous humor, the ease with which the aqueous humor passes through the trabecular meshwork to the canal of Schlemm, and the pressure in the episcleral veins into which the canal of Schlemm empties. Most (75%) of the resistance to outflow is in that portion of the trabecular meshwork immediately adjacent to the canal of Schlemm.

Many factors modify the intraocular pressure. Most factors are quickly compensated so that the intraocular pressure varies only momentarily. Increased intraocular pressure decreases the rate of aqueous humor inflow (expressed as µl/min/mm Hg: pseudofacility of outflow). Increased intraocular pressure increases the rate of outflow from the anterior chamber. Clinically, in tonography, the intraocular pressure is increased by the weight of the indentation tonometer (see below) upon the eye. The decrease in pressure over a 4-minute interval indicates the amount of fluid that leaves the eye during that period (true facility of outflow). Pseudofacility is 20% to 25% of total facility in normal eyes and is independent of the value of true facility. In glaucomatous eyes, pseudofacility may constitute more than 50% of total facility.

Drainage of aqueous humor to the canal of Schlemm takes place by percolation through the trabecular meshwork tissue adjacent to the canal and vacuoles on the inner wall of the endothelium of the canal of Schlemm. These vacuoles open into the lumen of the canal of Schlemm. In addition to drainage through the canal of Schlemm, aqueous humor also drains into ciliary muscle spaces at the root of the iris

and into the suprachoroidal space (uveoscleral route). In humans some 20% of aqueous humor may exit by this route.

The pressure in the episcleral veins connecting to the canal of Schlemm is approximately 10 mm Hg. If this pressure markedly increases, or if the pressure of the eye falls, there is a reflux of blood into the canal of Schlemm and increased resistance to outflow. The intraocular arterial and venous pressure and the volume of the arteries usually remain constant. Markedly increased venous pressure, as occurs in the Valsalva maneuver, is accompanied by a marked increase in intraocular pressure because of intraocular venous dilation. The intraocular pressure rapidly returns to normal when the Valsalva maneuver is stopped. Increased osmotic pressure of the blood brought about by administration of glycerol, mannitol, or urea decreases the intraocular pressure. Decreased osmotic pressure of the blood induced by rapid intravenous infusion of saline solution or by drinking a large quantity of water on an empty stomach causes a modest increase in intraocular pressure. The elasticity of the cornea and the sclera remains relatively constant but is an important factor in the measurement of the intraocular pressure by tonometry.

The intraocular pressure is directly measured by cannulation of the anterior chamber in a manner that does not disturb the flow of aqueous humor and the vasculature. This type of measurement is done in humans only before enucleation of the eye. Clinically, the ocular tension is measured by means of a tonometer that determines the resistance of the surface of the globe to a change in shape. There are two main types of tonometers: (1) contact types, which measure ocular tension by mechanical indentation (Schiøtz), by electronic indentation (Mackay-Marg), or by flattening of the cornea (Goldmann applanation, requiring a biomicroscope, or the hand-held types of Draeger or Perkins); and (2) noncontact types, which flatten the cornea with a pulse of air. The applanation tonometer of Langham and McCarthy also uses an airstream but touches the eye.

THE LENS

The lens is derived from surface ectoderm. It is surrounded by a typical basement membrane, the capsule, that is secreted anteriorly by epithelial cells and posteriorly by the cortical fibers that have their nuclei in the nuclear bow. It is continuously renewed by the underlying epithelium and lens fibers. The lens capsule is permeable to water and to small molecules, including horseradish peroxidase (40,000 daltons) but not ferritin (500,000 daltons). The capsule has no metabolic or enzymatic activity.

The anterior lens epithelial cells are firmly attached to the anterior lens capsule. No epithelial cells are present normally in the posterior capsule and the nuclei of its cells are in the equatorial region. Epithelial cells originate in the anterior subcapsular region adjacent to the lens equator in the germinative zone (Chapter 1). These cells migrate mainly to the equatorial region and then to the nuclear bow where they increase in size and form lens fibers. Lens fibers are arranged in onionlike layers, with the most recently formed lens fibers located in the superficial, peripheral layers, and the oldest located centrally. Thus the most central lens fibers (embryonic nucleus) were formed in early embryonic life. As the lens fiber differentiates, its nucleus disappears. The nucleus contents, however, are not extruded from the lens.

The fully differentiated lens fiber has anterior and posterior processes. They are composed of a protein matrix surrounded by a lipid bilayer membrane that interdigitates with adjacent fibers through tongue-and-groove and ball-and-socket structures. The most recently formed lens fibers remain attached to their basement membrane, the posterior capsule.

The lens is held in position behind the pupil by means of zonular fibers. These attach to the anterior and posterior lens capsule in the equatorial region and to the valleys between ciliary processes. The fibers relax with contraction of the ciliary muscle, causing the refractive power of the lens to increase as its inherent elasticity causes it to become more spherical (accommodation).

Transparency. The lens transmits almost 80% of electromagnetic energy between 400 and 1400 nm. Small-angle x-ray and light-scattering techniques demonstrate that the spatial correlations between protein molecules of the lens crystallins account for the lens transparency. The nuclei of the single layer of epithelial cells beneath the anterior capsule are not thick enough to impair transparency.

Despite the homogeneity of the lens structure, its total index of refraction is greater than any single portion. This results from a concentric structure of layers in which the older central layers have a greater index of refraction than the surrounding younger layers.

The total refractive power of the lens is thus much greater than one would anticipate from its external curvature, thickness, and the index of refraction of individual layers. In a simplifying assumption in physiologic optics, the lens is considered to be composed of a central core with a high index of refraction that has a layer with a lower index of refraction on either side.

Metabolism. The crystalline lens of the experimental animal is used to study protein synthesis and cataract induction and as a source of membranes. The animal lens differs from the human lens in many respects. The bovine, rabbit, and rat lenses grow fast initially but slow in maturity; thus there is little increase in weight in the second half of the lifespan. In contrast, the human lens grows slowly throughout life. Only humans and some primates accommodate for near and far vision. The concentric layers of the human lens, called "zones of discontinuity," have no counterpart in other mammalian lenses. In middle life the color of the lens slowly yellows, thus decreasing the amount of blue and violet light that reaches the retina. Some of the yellow color may originate from low molecular weight derivatives of tryptophan found only in the human and primate lens. These are fluorescent and absorb ultraviolet light maximally at the 360 to 368 nm wavelength. The bovine, rabbit, and rat lens does not metabolize tryptophan.

The lens fiber proteins are composed of a water-soluble fraction, the crystallins, and a water-insoluble group (albuminoid-obsolete). The crystallins are divided into four fractions: α, β_{Heavy}, β_{Light}, and λ.

Alpha is the largest crystallin and first appears in the lens epithelium in embryonic life. It comprises the embryonic nucleus of the adult lens. It is composed of related proteins of differing size but similar properties. The subunits are designated α_{A1}, α_{A2}, α_{B1}, and α_{B2}. Beta crystallin is the most abundant water-soluble lens protein. It first appears in the lens fiber with a basic structure preserved over eons of vertebrate evolution. Gamma crystallin is the smallest and least abundant water-soluble protein. Their precise role in lens economy is unknown.

Alpha and gamma crystallins are normally found in human aqueous humor. The amount of both increases in cortical cataract, whereas in nuclear cataract the alpha crystallin concentration increases and gamma crystallin decreases.

In aging, macromolecules of protein are formed that have a high molecular weight and contain much calcium. There is an increase in negatively charged components. Protein aggregates of large molecular weight scatter light to produce an opacity. Heavy molecular weight aggregates represent 10% to 15% of the total soluble protein of normal human lenses at 72 years of age. Their molecular weight may be greater than 1.5×10^8.

Sugars enter the lens through a carrier system of facilitated diffusion that constantly brings additional sugar. When present in physiologic amounts, most of the glucose in the lens is converted to glucose-6-phosphate in a reaction catalyzed by the enzyme hexokinase. Hexokinase is present in small amounts in the lens and limits the phosphorylation of glucose. If the sugar content of aqueous humor is increased, the sugar content of the lens remains unchanged until the external concentration reaches 175 mg/ml when control breaks down. Excess sugar (an aldehyde) is then converted to sugar alcohol by the enzyme aldose reductase. The sugar alcohol does not diffuse freely to exit through the lens capsule and the lens accumulates water (see cataract below).

Once formed, glucose-6-phosphate enters one of two metabolic pathways (see Fig. 2-3). About 85% of glucose metabolism is through anaerobic glycolysis in which glucose is degraded to two molecules of glyceraldehyde-3-PO_4, which is converted to pyruvate and then to lactate. This conversion provides two molecules of adenosine triphosphate for each molecule of glucose utilized. It is evident that lens metabolism does not require oxygen but does require a constant supply of glucose.

About 15% of the glucose-6-phosphate formed is degraded through an aerobic pathway (pentose phosphate or hexose monophosphate shunt) to form ribose-5-phosphate and carbon dioxide. The ribose-5-phosphate is available for nucleic acid synthesis. Additionally, this reaction generates reducing power in the cytoplasm in the form of reduced nicotinamide-adenine dinucleotide phosphate (NADPH; also called reduced triphosphopyridine nucleotide [TPNH]). This reducing power is required for glutathione reductase, aldose reductase, and hexokinase reactions.

In many respects the lens behaves as an erythrocyte. Thus it maintains a high intracellular potassium content although surrounded by aqueous humor and vitreous humor, both of which have a high sodium content. The lens epithelium maintains this gradient and actively transports sodium out of the lens by an NaK ATPase pump. Glycolysis provides the necessary ATP energy. The lens transports and accumulates potassium, amino acids, and ascorbic acid. It synthesizes inositol (a completely hydroxylated cyclohexane) and glutathione. With interference in lens metabolism, sodium and water accumulate in the lens, and it loses potassium, glutathione, amino acids, and inositol.

Cataract. Any loss of transparency of the lens is called a cataract. Cataracts are described as nuclear (central) and cortical (peripheral or anterior or posterior subcapsular). The capsule itself remains transparent except when lacerated. Nuclear and cortical cataract may be the result of different mechanisms.

A number of different changes occur in nuclear cataract. Sodium increases, soluble protein decreases, and insoluble protein increases. Bound water decreases, reflecting a loss of binding sites. There are widespread oxidative changes with a decrease in glutathione concentration and oxidation of methionine and cysteine in membrane proteins. This process leads to the formation of membrane-bound, high molecular weight disulfide-linked aggregates and membrane breakdown.

In cortical cataract, crystallin aggregates into high molecular weight components. There are decreased protein concentrations in clefts between lens fibers. Both Mg^2 and NaK ATPase activities decrease.

When excessive glucose is present in the lens, the enzyme aldose reductase coupled to NADPH, derived from the pentose phosphate shunt, reduces the glucose to the alcohol D-glucitol (L-sorbitol). Sugar alcohols (polyols) do not penetrate membranes well and accumulate within the lens, drawing water into the lens and causing swelling of the lens fibers. This in turn leads to stretching of the lens capsule along with secondary electrolyte imbalance and loss of amino acids. Major attention is directed to aldose reductase in the study of experimental cataract since aldose reductase is inhibited by many compounds. These studies, which implicate aldose reductase in experimental sugar cataracts, suggest the possibility that sugar alcohols participate in the neuropathy, nephropathy, and retinopathy of human diabetes mellitus. High concentrations of aldose reductase have been found in the Schwann cells of peripheral nerves, in the pericytes of the retinal blood vessels, and in the kidney papillae. A current clinical study of aldose reductase inhibitors seeks to learn if they will prevent diabetic retinopathy and neuropathy.

In mice with hereditary cataracts, there is a deficiency of NaK ATPase, which leads to electrolyte imbalance.

Two types of cataract occur in galactosemia: (1) galactokinase deficiency, which occurs infrequently, and (2) hexose-1-phosphate uridyl transferase deficiency, which is more common. These cataracts occur as congenital autosomal recessive conditions. Some cataracts in individuals 20 to 40 years of age may be secondary to heterozygosity for one or the other of these enzymes.

THE VITREOUS HUMOR

The vitreous humor is a transparent hydrogel that fills the posterior (vitreous) cavity of the eye. It is composed mainly of water (98% to 99.7%). Collagen provides a framework (Fig. 2-6), and a high level of hyaluronic acid (one molecule of glucuronic acid and one molecule of acetyl glucosamine) provides the gel properties. Its base is firmly attached to the pars plana of the ciliary body and the peripheral retina in the region of the ora serrata. Posteriorly it attaches to the periphery of the optic disk. In

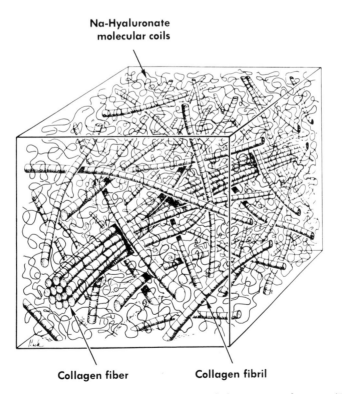

Na-Hyaluronate molecular coils

Collagen fiber **Collagen fibril**

Fig. 2-6. Schema of the macromolecular structure of the vitreous humor. (From Balazs, E.A.: Functional anatomy of the vitreous. In Duane, T.D., and Jaeger, E.A., editors: Biomedical foundations of ophthalmology, vol. 1, Philadelphia, 1983, Harper & Row Publishers.)

some instances it is attached to the sensory retina and to blood vessels. Its anterior condensation, the vitreous face, forms the posterior boundary of the posterior aqueous chamber. This layer sometimes attaches to the posterior lens capsule, the hyaloideocapsular ligament (of Wieger). The vitreous humor is composed of (1) a cortical tissue layer, whose surfaces are condensed to form an anterior hyaloid adjacent to the lens and a posterior hyaloid adjacent to the inner limiting membrane of the retina, and (2) a central vitreous humor proper.

The *cortical tissue* is approximately 100 μm thick and surrounds the vitreous humor proper. It contains fine fibrils composed of collagen, an accumulation of proteins, a high concentration of hyaluronic acid, and a few migrating hematogenous monocytes. The collagen fibrils run approximately parallel to the surface of the vitreous humor. Up to 20 years of age, they attach to the internal limiting lamina of the retina and the ciliary body. After 20 years of age, such attachments are found only in the anterior one third of the eye.

The *vitreous humor proper* is a true biologic and chemical gel. Its framework is composed of fine collagen fibrils. The spaces between the fibrils (the interfibrillar spaces) are filled with hyaluronic acid. It occurs in tissues with a high water content and forms a molecular network in the vitreous. The vitreous humor has no metabolic activities that use glucose.

THE RETINA

The optic cup differentiates as two layers: (1) an outer layer, the retinal pigment epithelium, that at birth is a layer one cell thick, and (2) an inner layer, the sensory layer consisting of the photoreceptor cells, their synaptic connections, and the supporting glia. The microvilli of the retinal pigment epithelium surround the outer segments of rods and cones. The complex is enmeshed in glycosaminoglycans synthesized by the photoreceptor cell. All metabolites of the outer portion of the retina pass through the cells of the retinal pigment epithelium that are tightly bound at their apices. The dendrites in the outer plexiform layer mark the approximate division between metabolic support from the choriocapillaris through the retinal pigment epithelium and support by the central retinal artery branches. The retinal pigment epithe-

lium cell bases have binding sites for retinol-binding protein (pro-albumin) that transports vitamin A. Additionally, the retinal pigment epithelium contains the enzymes necessary for the visual cycle. Its tight junctions (and those of the retinal blood vessels) provide the blood-retinal barrier.

The rods and cones are the light-sensitive elements of the sensory retina. The rods function at low levels of illumination (scotopic vision), whereas the cones are functional at medium and high levels of illumination (photopic vision) and in color vision. The cones are concentrated in the fovea centralis where rods are absent, and they are also scattered in the peripheral retina. The rods are the main photoreceptors in the periphery (Fig. 2-7).

The outer segments of rods and cones are removed diurnally by the phagocytic action of the pigment epithelium cells. For this reason the outer segments must undergo constant renewal by the inner segment. There is a much more active turnover rate of rod outer segments than cone outer segments. Cone disks are shed shortly after the retina is darkened and synthesized thereafter, whereas rod disks are shed shortly after the retina is illuminated and synthesized during light.

The outer segment (adjacent to the pigment epithelium) of each rod and cone contains about 700 to 1,000 plasma membrane disks that contain light-sensitive pigments (Fig. 2-8). The rod disks float free and are surrounded by the cell plasma membrane while the disks of cones are continuous with the surrounding plasma membrane. The inner segment of each photoreceptor cell contains a dense concentration of mitochondria and intracellular organelles that synthesize new outer segment disks.

The axons of rods and cones synapse with horizontal cells and bipolar cells in the outer plexiform layer. Horizontal cells connect photoreceptors (mainly rods) to each other. The axons of the bipolar cells synapse with amacrine cells and with dendrites of the ganglion cells in the inner plexiform layer. The axons of the ganglion cells join to form the optic nerve and extend to the brain.

The human sensory retina contains about 100 million rods and 6 million cones. The optic disk has no photoreceptors and is a blind spot in the field of vision. The fovea centralis contains ap-

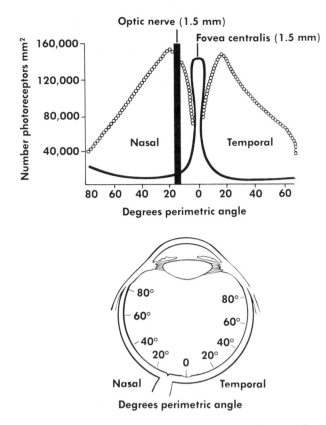

Fig. 2-7. The density of retinal rods and cones as a function of retinal location. The cones are concentrated in the fovea centralis (0°). The rod density peaks at about 20° from the fovea contralis and gradually diminishes to the retinal periphery.

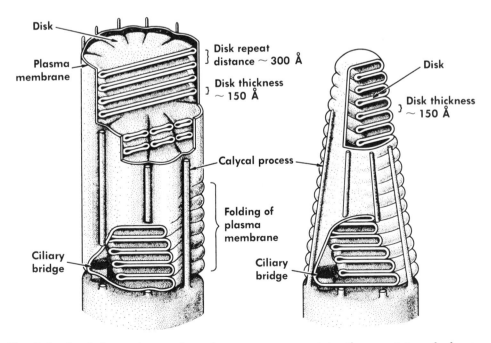

Fig. 2-8. The disk membrane of a rod outer segment contains three proteins, rhodopsin, transducin, and a specific retinal cyclic-GMP phosphodiesterase. These proteins interact after absorption of light to decrease the cyclic-GMP concentration in the disk membrane. (From Fein, A., and Szuts, E.Z.: Photoreceptors: their role in vision, New York, 1982, Cambridge University Press.)

proximately 150,000 cones/mm^2. The remaining retina contains about 4,500 cones/mm^2. The rod density peaks about 3 mm (20°) from the fovea centralis at about 150,000 rods/mm^2 and then falls off less abruptly than the cone population to about 35,000 rods/mm^2 at the temporal periphery and 60,000 at the nasal periphery.

The distribution of optic nerve fibers to receptors is not uniform. In the foveola, the approximately 200,000 cones are connected to at least that many optic nerve axons. In the far periphery, there may be as many as 10,000 rods connected in clusters to a single nerve fiber with considerable overlapping, so that a point of light may stimulate several clusters at once.

Metabolism. The glucose and oxygen required by the inner layers of the sensory retina are derived from the retinal circulation, while the choriocapillaris nurtures the retinal pigment epithelium and photoreceptor cells. Both systems must be intact for normal function. Glucose from the choriocapillaris is converted into glucose-6-phosphate through hexokinase in the pigment epithelium and diffuses to the ellipsoid of the photoreceptor cell. The mitochondria of the ellipsoid cells convert the glucose-6-phosphate rapidly to two molecules of glyceraldehyde (glycolysis), which is converted to two molecules of pyruvic acid. The retina consumes more oxygen than any other tissue. It is used mainly in the mitochondria of the ellipsoid in the tricarboxylic acid cycle, by which pyruvic acid is converted to carbon dioxide and water and produces adenosine triphosphate. Glycolysis provides so much pyruvic acid that some is converted to lactic acid even in the presence of adequate oxygen. The adenosine triphosphate provides the energy required to extrude sodium ions from the inner segment through a NaK ATPase pump. The adenosine triphosphate also provides energy for axonal transport, outer segment renewal, and biosynthesis of cell membranes.

The enzymes of the phosphogluconic acid pathway are concentrated in the rod and cone nuclei and provide the ribose required for RNA synthesis. Müller cells store glycogen, but the quantity is not adequate to support retinal function more than briefly.

Photochemistry of vision. When a portion of the electromagnetic spectrum constituting light (400 to 700 nm) is absorbed by a pigment of the retinal photoreceptor disks, a graded electrical potential is initiated. The potential is amplified and modulated in the inner layers of the retina and is propagated to the brain, where perception occurs. To permit continued stimulation the pigment of the photoreceptor disks must be constantly renewed. To permit the nerve impulse to stop after cessation of the stimulus, the chemical reaction initiating the nerve impulse must cease at the same time.

Human photoreceptor disks contain at least four light-absorbing conjugated proteins (opsins), each tightly bound to 11-*cis*-retinal, the adlehyde of vitamin A$_1$ (Fig. 2-9). Rhodopsin (visual purple [obsolete]) is the photopigment of rods and has a maximum absorption at about 507 nm and an absorption spectrum similar to the light-sensitivity curve of the retina in dim light. The photoreceptor cone disks contain three different photopigments that have a maximum absorption at about 440 nm (short wavelength–sensitive, blue), 535 nm (middle wavelength–sensitive, green), and 570 nm (long wavelength–sensitive, red). In each, the prosthetic group is 11-*cis*-retinal.

Retinol (vitamin A, an alcohol) contains four carbon-carbon double bonds in its side chain (Fig. 2-9). It is utilized in the retina in its aldehyde form (retinal), and only when the 11-12 position is *cis* and the other three positions are *trans* is it able to bind opsin. When the pigment absorbs light, the bound 11-*cis*-retinal undergoes an isomerization to all-*trans*-retinal with a substantial change in shape (Fig. 2-10). This isomerization of retinal is followed by a series of chemical reactions ending in the disassociation of the bleached photopigment to yield free opsin and all-*trans*-retinal (Fig. 2-11).

Visual transduction is the process by which the light absorbed by the light-sensitive disks of the outer segment is converted to electrical energy. The exact mechanism is unknown. The absorption of a single photon by a photoreceptor disk triggers a conformational change of 11-*cis*-retinal to all-*trans*-retinal. This conformational change (or an intermediate in the change) activates the photopigment to reduce the permeability of the outer segment plasma membrane to sodium.

The photoreceptor cell is unique among sensory receptors in that a steady current, the

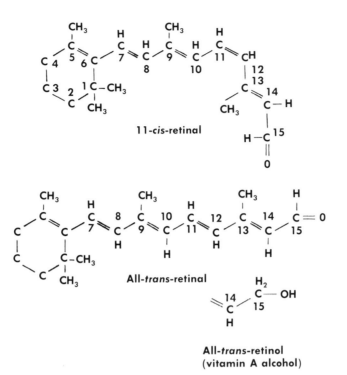

Fig. 2-9. The 11-*cis* isomer of retinal (vitamin A aldehyde). The stereotoxic change from the 11-*cis* isomer to the all-*trans* isomer by light initiates the visual impulse. Vitamin A is an alcohol.

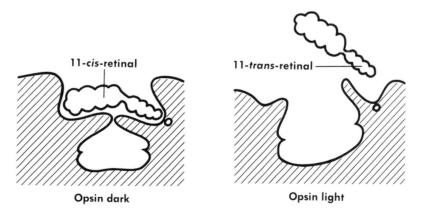

Fig. 2-10. The change in configuration of the rhodopsin molecule as it is activated by absorption of a photon of light.

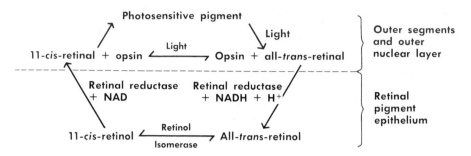

Fig. 2-11. Light absorption by the photoreceptor outer segments isomerizes 11-*cis*-retinal to all-*trans*-retinal, which disassociates it from opsin. New photosensitive pigment requires isomerization of all-*trans*-retinal to 11-*cis*-retinal. This occurs by further exposure to light or by a sequence of reactions in the retinal pigment epithelium. Initially, the all-*trans*-retinal is reduced to all-*trans*-retinol (an alcohol) by the action of retinal reductase and reduced nicotinamide adenine dinucleotide (+NADH + H). The all-*trans*-retinol is converted to 11-*cis*-retinol by the enzyme retinol isomerase. The 11-*cis*-retinol is converted to the 11-*cis*-retinal (aldehyde) by reductase and nicotinamide adenine dinucleotide (+NADH).

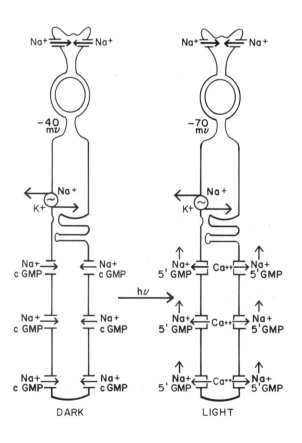

Fig. 2-12. Conversion of light energy to electrical energy in the retinal rod. In the dark sodium chambers of the outer segment plasma membranes are open (as are channels in the synaptic terminal). The channels in the outer segment remain open through the action of cyclic guanosine monophosphate. Light-activated rhodopsin reacts with a disk membrane–bound protein transducin, which activates disk membrane–bound phosphodiesterase. The activated phosphodiesterase hydrolyzes cyclic guanosine monophosphate and the sodium channels close in the plasma membrane, which becomes further hyperpolarized. Intracellular calcium concentration decreases.

dark current, flows along the photoreceptor plasma membrane in the absence of stimulation. Absorption of light by the visual pigments induces a hyperpolarization of the photoreceptor membrane (Fig. 2-12). The dark current flows extracellularly from the inner segment to the outer segment (and less markedly from the inner segment to the synaptic vesicle). The current is generated by an electrogenic NaK-ATPase pump in the inner segment, which actively removes sodium from the cell. The sodium enters the cell passively through the sodium channels in the plasma membrane of the outer segment (and synaptic vesicle), which are open in the dark. Light induces a change in shape (isomerization) of 11-*cis*-retinal with a cascade of biochemical changes that closes the sodium channels in the outer segment so that intracellular sodium is markedly decreased, and the plasma membrane potential changes from -40 mV to -70 mV. This hyperpolarization is propagated to the synapse at the inner end of the cell and communicated to other cells of the retina. The system is so sensitive that the absorption of a single photon of light by a single molecule of rhodopsin reduces conductance through the plasma membrane by 2% to 4%.

The mechanism by which light reduces sodium permeability of photoreceptor outer segment is not known. Presumably the structural change in outer segment photopigment releases a transmitter that diffuses to the outer segment plasma membrane and closes the sodium channels. Calcium was proposed as the internal sodium channel controller, but reduction of intracellular calcium does not abolish the ability of the cell to respond to light.

Current theory suggests that sodium channels in the plasma membrane are kept open in the dark by cyclic-GMP (3'-, 5'cyclic-guanosine-monophosphate). The rod outer segment disk membrane contains a specific protein (G protein or transducin) that binds guanosine triphosphate. When photon-capture activates the rod rhodopsin, the rhodopsin reacts with transducin so that it exchanges bound guanosine diphosphate with guanosine triphosphate. Guanosine triphosphate-bound transducin disassociates from the disk membrane and activates phosphodiesterase. Phosphodiesterase in turn hydrolyzes cyclic-GMP (cGMP), and the sodium channels close. Guanosine triphosphate modulation of light activation of cGMP is analogous to guanosine triphosphate regulation of the adenylate cyclase system.

For additional photosensitive pigment to be synthesized, the all-*trans*-retinal must be isomerized to 11-*cis*-retinal. This occurs either by exposure to light in the photoreceptors or by a sequence of reactions catalyzed by two enzymes in the retinal pigment epithelium and the myoid of the inner segment of the photoreceptors.

All-*trans*-retinal is vitamin A_1 and is transported in the blood bound to a specific retinol-binding protein (pro-albumin). The bases of the retinal pigment epithelium cells have specific protein receptor sites where the vitamin A is released to the cell and the carrier protein excluded. Dietary sources of vitamin A are from both the vitamin and from carotenoids, particularly carotene, which are converted into vitamin A by enzymatic reactions in the intestinal mucosa and liver.

Synaptic transmission. Synaptic transmission in the retina is both by direct contact and neural transmitters released by axons that react with receptors on the outside of the cell membrane of dendrites. These change the electrical potential of the membrane. Among the neural transmitters in the retina, dopamine, γ-aminobutyric acid, glycine, and taurine exert a depressant action on retinal neurons, whereas glutamate and aspartate excite or depress retinal neurons, depending on their concentration.

Axoplasmic transport. Axoplasmic transport is the flow of metabolic substances from the nerve cell body through its axon. There are two components of axoplasmic transport: a slow component at a rate of approximately 1 mm a day and a component 100 times faster. Most materials travel at both rapid and slow rates. Glycoproteins and sulfated glycosaminoglycans are transported almost completely by the rapid component. Rapidly transported material is largely in the membrane or particulate form that includes synaptic vesicles, mitochondria, and smooth endoplasmic reticulum. The slow component consists mainly of soluble protein.

The eyes of birds and goldfish have been used for study because a radioactive amino acid may be injected into the vitreous cavity in close proximity to ganglion cells and because there is a complete decussation of optic fibers at the chiasm. Thus after injection, radioactive-labelled material can be demonstrated in the contralateral optic tract and tectum. Rapid transport is in the circumferential portion of the axons, whereas slow flow progresses within the core of the axon. Rapid transport may be responsible for the movement of substances required at synaptic terminals, including the enzymes necessary for synthesis or destruction of transmitter substances. Slow components maintain and replenish material required for structural integrity of the axon.

Rapid axoplasmic transport is inhibited by anoxia, local anesthetics, and metabolic inhibitors such as sodium cyanide and dinitrophenol. Increased intraocular pressure may impede axonal flow, particularly the slow transport.

The retinal cotton-wool patch (histologically, a cytoid body) follows focal retinal ischemia, which causes localized edema of the axons of ganglion cells. The cotton-wool patch contains aggregations of mitochondria, dense bodies, vesicles, and granules. The cotton-wool patch indicates interrupted axonal transport in the retinal nerve fiber layer. Papilledema (Chapter 18) reflects impaired axonal flow at the optic disk.

Neural activity. Vision is divided into surround (or ambient) vision and focal vision. Surround vision is mediated primarily by the peripheral retina and provides information concerning spatial localization. Focal vision is mediated primarily by the fovea centralis and subserves form perception, identification, and color vision. Cats achieve spatial orientation with large ganglion cells (mainly Y and transient cells) and Y nerve fibers, which are connected not only with the visual cortex but also with the superior colliculus. Focal vision is sustained through the fovea centralis, using cones, small ganglion cells, and neurons (mainly X cells and sustained cells) that mainly extend particularly to the lateral geniculate body and then to the visual cortex.

Ganglion cells may be divided into two types on the basis of their response to a receptive field. A receptive field consists of the information gathered by a group of photoreceptors as transmitted to the ganglion cells. Receptive fields are organized in a concentric manner.

They have a central region surrounded by a ring-shaped outer zone.

There are two types of spatial receptive fields: (1) those in which illumination of the center causes stimulation of the ganglion cell and illumination of the periphery causes inhibition in the ganglion cell (an on-center, depolarizing type of receptive field), and (2) a reverse type of receptive field in which illumination of the center causes inhibition of the ganglion cell and illumination of the periphery causes stimulation (an off-center, hyperpolarizing receptive field). In some ganglion cells in the retina, the "on" and "off" zones are not concentric but are coincidental. There are additional and different receptive fields for color reception. Some receptive fields are most sensitive to moving targets.

Receptive fields are not constant in size, and they are larger in the dark-adapted eye than in the light-adapted eye. They are larger in the peripheral than in the central retina. They change in size and shape and alter in their stimulatory and inhibitory components with the state of light adaptation.

The neural circuitry within the retina is complex. The signal from rods is received by rod bipolar cells and by horizontal cells. Cones stimulate two types of bipolar cells—flat and invaginating—and also a and b horizontal cells. Amacrine cells possibly serve bipolar and ganglion cells and are related solely to rods (Fig. 2-13).

In lower species, neural function is mediated by at least three and perhaps more classes of ganglion cells. The X cells have sustained responses to stimuli, axon conduction velocities of 9 to 14 m/sec, and are in greatest concentration in the fovea centralis. X cells transmit luminance as well as color information. A separate neural channel for red-green information probably does not exist. The Y cells have transient responses to stimuli, axon conduction velocities of 29 to 39 m/sec, and respond to rapid motions. The W cells appear to respond both to the beginning and to the ending of a flash of light throughout their entire receptive field. Other ganglion cells stimulate pupillary constriction.

Retinal neural activity is considerably integrated in lower species. In the frog, some receptive fields are responsive to small, dark, moving objects (bug detectors) but not to large or stationary objects. Thus the frog's retina integrates the signal useful in capturing food. In retinas of higher species there is less integrative function in the retina; most integration is in the brain.

The spiked discharges from retinal ganglion cells are further integrated in the lateral geniculate body. The images from the two eyes may be reinforced in binocularity to cause a more vigorous response or may be inhibited with a diminished response in the absence of binocular vision.

The complexity and capacity of the human visual cortex is emphasized by its size: 6 m by 2.5 mm if flattened out. The major portion of the striate cortex is concerned with form vision.

Form-sensitive cortical cells are described as "simple," "complex," and "hypercomplex." "Simple" cells are arranged into excitatory and inhibitory regions separated by boundaries that are straight and parallel, and they are related to the X (simple) system. Their fields may be mapped with stationary retinal stimuli. "Complex" cells (related mainly to the Y system) appear to be combinations of simple cells that respond particularly to moving edges on the retina with directional sensitivity. "Hypercomplex" cells respond only to moving stimuli on the retina and are most potently stimulated by the ends of lines, line segments, and corners. Again the signal may be inhibited or reinforced. Unlike the retinal receptive fields, which are round, the cortical fields are linear.

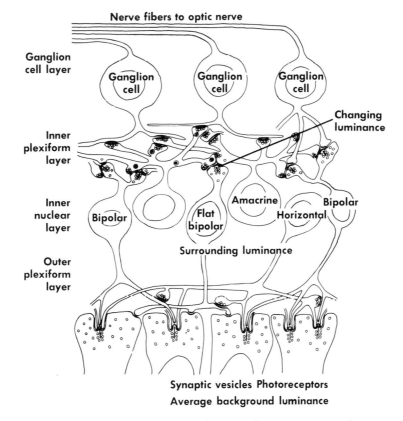

Fig. 2-13. Diagram of synaptic contacts found in vertebrate retinas. In the outer plexiform layer, processes from bipolar and horizontal cells penetrate into invaginations in the receptor terminals. The processes of flat bipolar cells make superficial contacts on the bases of some receptor terminals. Horizontal cells make conventional synaptic contacts on bipolar dendrites and other horizontal cell processes. In the inner plexiform layer, biopolar terminals may contact one ganglion cell dendrite and one amacrine process at a ribbon synapse or may contact amacrine cell processes. Amacrine processes in all retinas make synapses of the conventional type back onto biopolar terminals (reciprocal synapse). (From Dowling J.: Invest. Ophthalmol. **9:**655, 1970.)

Visual information in humans is processed differently than it is in other species. There is much more integrative activity in the retina in lower species than there is in humans and the distribution of ganglion cell axons in the brain may be different.

VISUAL MECHANISMS

Electromagnetic radiation. Energy is transferred through space by means of electrical and magnetic fields in waves that are perpendicular to each other and to the direction of propagation. In a vacuum, electromagnetic radiation has a velocity of 3×10^8 m/sec (186,000 miles/sec). It is characterized by a wavelength and a frequency (the number of vibrations of a wave per unit time). Electromagnetic waves exhibit the properties of wave motion, and processes such as reflection and refraction are best understood by geometric principles.

Electromagnetic energy may be considered as a discrete bundle or quantum that has an energy equal to its frequency ν multiplied by Planck's constant: h. A quantum of electromagnetic energy is a photon. Processes such as absorption and emission of electromagnetic radiation are most easily understood in terms of photons.

The arrangement of electromagnetic radiation according to its wavelength or frequency is called the electromagnetic spectrum. The wavelength varies from a minute fraction of a meter (3×10^{-20} m) for cosmic waves to many thousand meters for long radio waves (3×10^6 m). The energy varies inversely with the wavelength so that the energy of a cosmic ray photon is high (4×10^{17} electron volts) while a radio wave photon has minimal energy (4×10^{-13} electron volt).

Light is that portion of electromagnetic radiation that, when absorbed by the pigment of the photoreceptor disks of the outer segment of the retina, changes the shape of the pigment molecule to initiate a nervous impulse. Light has a wavelength of 380 nm (nm = one-billionth meter) to 770 nm. Electromagnetic radiation with wavelengths greater or lesser than that of visible radiation are either absorbed by the cornea or pass through the eye without absorption. Cosmic rays stimulate photoreceptors and cause flashes of light (in astronauts) while x-rays stimulate rods in the dark-adapted eye.

Laser-generated energy stimulates the retina at extremes of 100 nm (ultraviolet) and 1000 nm (infrared).

Action of light on the eye. When that portion of the electromagnetic spectrum known as visible light (380 to 770 nm) is absorbed by the visual pigment in the rods and cones, a nervous impulse is transmitted to the brain and causes a subjective sensation.

Equal amounts of radiant energy of different wavelengths do not produce equal visual sensations. Thus, 0.001 watt of green light appears bright to an observer, whereas 0.001 watt of blue light appears dim. Luminous units express the amount of radiant light energy in terms of the production of the sensation of brightness in the observer. Luminous energy is radiant energy corrected for the sensitivity of the retina to different wavelengths. Since individual visual sensations differ, luminous units are expressed in terms of the average of many observers (the standard observer). Photopic, or cone, luminosity function (V_ν) indicates the sensitivity of a light-adapted human eye. It has a maximum sensitivity at 555 nm. Scotopic luminosity function ($V^1\gamma$) indicates the sensitivity of the dark-adapted human eye and has a maximum sensitivity at 507 nm (rhodopsin). When viewed in dim illumination, a colored object appears to have no color. As illumination is increased, the object appears colored. This change from achromatic to chromatic vision reflects the change from scotopic (rod) vision to photopic (cone) vision. The change in luminosity function is called the Purkinje shift.

Dark adaptation. The increase in sensitivity of the eye to detection of light that occurs in the dark is called "dark adaptation." The pupil dilates, and there are both neural (largely unknown) and biochemical changes in the retina. In darkness, after exposure to bright light that bleaches the visual photopigments, there is an initial hundredfold increase in sensitivity following an exponential time course that reaches a plateau after 5 to 9 minutes. This initial phase is attributed to regeneration of photosensitive pigments in the cones. Thereafter, there is a 10^3 to 10^5 increase in sensitivity following a slower exponential time course that reaches a plateau in 30 to 45 minutes (Fig. 2-14). This second phase is attributed to regeneration of rhodopsin in the rods. In addition to rhodopsin regeneration, retinal summation and inhibition change to increase sensitivity further. Dark adaptation is delayed by prolonged exposure to bright light (thus the increased danger of driving at night after a day in bright sunshine). When fully dark-adapted, the retina is about 100,000 times more sensitive to light than when bleached.

The dark-adapted retina is most sensitive in the region 2.5 mm from the fovea centralis. In the fully dark-adapted eye, a visual sensation can be evoked by the activity of approximately seven rods, each being stimulated by the absorption of a single photon. The variation in sensitivity in different parts of the retina probably reflects differences in the number of photoreceptors and their neural summation mechanism rather than differences in the sensitivity of the photoreceptor itself.

Light adaptation. Exposure of the dark-adapted eye to bright light results in a marked decrease in sensitivity involving two changes: (1) a neural process that is completed in about 0.05 second and (2) a slower process, appar-ently involving the uncoupling of retinal and opsin in rhodopsin, occurring in about 1 minute. The neural mechanism occurs regardless of the area of the retina stimulated, whereas the photochemical mechanism involves only the region of stimulation. In the light-adapted eye the rhodopsin is bleached, the pupil is constricted, there is a shift of luminosity to the yellow-red end of the spectrum, and hydrogen ion concentration (pH) of the retina shifts from 7.3 to 7.0.

Color perception. This is a complicated topic that involves physical, biological, and psychological mechanisms. The stimuli for color vision are light rays reflected from an object. Their appearance depends on their intensity and on the surrounding colors. The rays are not colored, but those light rays that have a wavelength between 400 nm and 700 nm stimulate retinal cones so that colors are perceived.

Thomas Young (1801) postulated three principal classes of retinal elements responsible for color vision. Trichromatic color vision occurs from stimulation of three classes of cones in the retina. Long wavelength-sensitive cones have a peak sensitivity in the region of 570 nm (red-sensitive cones). Middle wavelength-sensitive cones have a peak sensitivity in the region of 535 nm (green-sensitive cones). Short wavelength-sensitive cones have a peak sensitivity of 440 nm (blue-sensitive cones). Color perceptions are based on differential stimulation of these three types of cones. The sensation of white occurs when all three types are simultaneously stimulated, each to a specified degree. Yellow is produced by the stimulation of green- and red-sensitive cones. When red and blue-green or yellow and blue are mixed, they do not produce an intermediate hue but give the sensation of gray (achromatic). Such pairs of colors are called "complementary colors."

The trichromatic theory does not explain why red matched with green appears yellow or why blue added to yellow appears white. The opponent-color process holds that colors we describe as "red" and "green" are encoded by the same opponent processing channel (Fig. 2-15). The encoding process is such that, if redness is encoded by an increase in electrical activity in this channel, then greenness will be signaled by a decrease in activity. Similar antagonistic encoding of yellow and blue is present. But

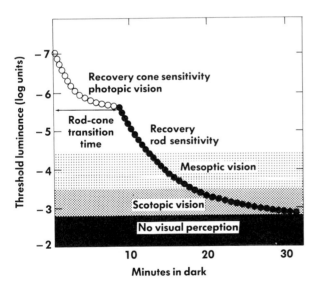

Fig. 2-14. The dark-adaptation curve. There is a plateau between 5 and 9 minutes. The initial portion of the curve indicates the smallest light intensity that will stimulate cones. Rods attain their maximum sensitivity after 30 to 45 minutes. The luminance at -7 is that of sunlight. The luminance at -5 is that of good reading luminance for white paper. The luminance at -4 log units is that at night with city street lighting. The luminance at -3 is mean ground luminance in full moon.

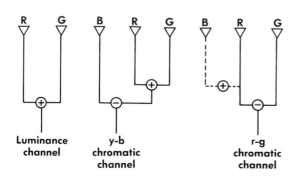

Fig. 2-15. An example of an opponent color model of human color vision. The top shows the three types of cones in the retina. The middle row shows some possible interaction of the cone signals that results in a luminance (summed) channel and two chromatic opponent channels. The y-b channel signals yellowness-blueness, and the r-g channel signals redness-greenness.

Table 2-1. Types of hereditary defective color perception

I. Congenital
  A. Anomalous trichromatism (abnormality of one photosensitive pigment)
    1. Protanomaly (red)
    2. Deuteranomaly (green)
  B. Dichromatism
    1. Protanopsia (absence of red photopigment)
    2. Deuteranopsia (absence of green photopigment)
    3. Tritanopsia (absence of blue photopigment; ganglion cell deficiency?)
  C. Achromatopsia
    1. Typical (reduced visual acuity and nystagmus)
      a. Complete (rod monochromacy)
      b. Incomplete
        (1) Autosomal recessive
        (2) X chromosome-linked (blue cone monochromacy)
    2. Atypical (normal visual acuity)
      a. Complete (cone monochromacy)
        (1) Protanoid
        (2) Deuteranoid (red cone monochromacy)
      b. Incomplete (pseudomonochromacy)
II. Developmental
  A. Progressive cone degenerations
  B. Generalized cone-rod dystrophies
  C. Generalized rod-cone dystrophies

there are no yellow-sensitive cones in the retina and the opponent-processing involves encoding of signals for luminance (brightness) and chromaticity (color).

Output from red and green cones summates and activates a luminance channel. The output from red, green, and blue cones activates two opponent channels: one for yellow-blue (y-b) and the other for red-green (r-g). The red-green channel is activated by red-green cones. The yellow-blue pathway output represents the difference between the output of the luminance channel and the output of blue cones.

Opponent cells have been located in the horizontal cells of cold-blooded animals. The ganglion cell firing pattern of primates indicates that opponent processing must be in the neural network of cells that have their nuclei in the inner nuclear layer, but the neural network is unknown.

Defective color perception. Defective color perception may be hereditary or may be acquired. Acquired color defects are the result of systemic or ocular disease. Hereditary defective color perception occurs because one or more of the retinal photopigments is absent or abnormal. A person with normal color vision has all three cone pigments in a normal proportion (a trichromat). If only two cone pigments are present, the person is a dichromat, or if only one pigment is present, a monochromat (Table 2-1).

X chromosome–linked color defects may be divided into those types in which there is an abnormality but not a complete absence of one of the cone pigments (anomalous trichromacy) and those types in which one of the cone pigments is absent (dichromacy). Visual acuity is normal, the defect is present at birth, and the condition does not progress. The types are designated according to the pigment involved: protan (first), long wavelength-sensitive pigment (red); and deutan (second), middle wavelength-sensitive pigment (green).

In protanomaly there is poor red-green discrimination, and the red end of the spectrum appears dimmer than it does in normal individuals. In deuteranomaly there is poor red-green discrimination, but the red end of the spectrum appears as bright as it does to normal individuals.

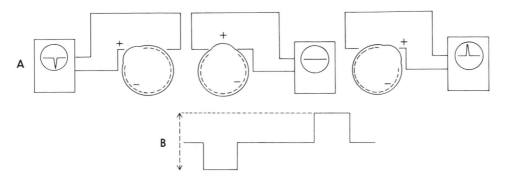

Fig. 2-16. A, Electro-oculography. The electrode closer to the cornea is positive, and when the eye turns, a deflection is induced in the recording system. **B,** The electro-oculography deflection is measured from the trough of the deflection on eyes left to the height of the deflection on eyes right.

A dichromatic individual with an X chromosome-linked defect has only two cone pigments. If the long wavelength-sensitive pigment is absent, the defect is protanopsia. If the middle wavelength-sensitive pigment is absent, the defect is deuteranopsia. These are differentiated from anomalous trichromacy by color and brightness matching.

About 8% to 10% of American and European men have protan or deutan defects in some degree. Less than 1% of women have either defect.

Tritan defects are transmitted as an autosomal dominant defect and may not involve cone pigments.

The term "achromatopsia" describes individuals born with severely deficient color perception. Two types may be present at birth: typical, associated with reduced visual acuity and nystagmus, and atypical, associated with normal visual acuity. Either may be complete or incomplete (Table 2-1).

Resting potential. The electrical potential of the cornea in humans is positive in relation to the back of the eye, and there is a difference in potential of several millivolts. The resting potential is dipole with the cornea positive. The resting potential is dependent on the retinal pigment epithelium, and it is approximately two times greater in the light-adapted eye than in the dark-adapted eye.

Electro-oculography. When electro-oculography is used, the increase in potential with light adaptation is measured to evaluate the condition of the retinal pigment epithelium. Electrodes are placed at each canthus, and the changes in the potential between these electrodes are recorded as the eyes move (Fig. 2-16). The average amplitude of the resting potential in light and dark adaptation is measured as the eyes turn a standard distance to the right and the left. If the light intensity and the period of dark adaptation are adequate, the ratio of the maximum amplitude obtained in the light (light peak) to the minimum amplitude obtained in the dark (dark trough) is normally greater than 2, whereas the ratio is less than 2 in patients with disorders of the retinal pigment epithelium.

Electroretinography. When the retina is stimulated with light, an action potential is superimposed on the resting potential. A record is made by placing an active electrode on the cornea, usually one embedded in a corneal contact lens, with saline solution bridging the gap between the electrode and the cornea, and placing an indifferent electrode on the forehead. The retina is stimulated with light and the small voltage amplified and usually photographed from the face of an oscilloscope (electroretinogram [ERG]) (Fig. 2-17). The retina is stimulated with light after either dark (scotopic) or light (photopic) adaptation. After the stimulus, there is a latent period and then an initial negative deflection known as the a-wave, followed by a positive deflection designated as the

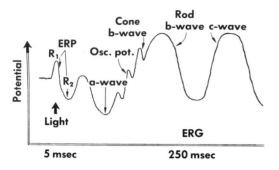

Fig. 2-17. The ocular potentials after a light stimulus in an eye that is adapted to the dark. The initial positive deflection R₁ (early receptor potential) is followed by a negative deflection R₂. These are followed by the a-wave of the electroretinogram that reflects photoreceptor activity. The positive deflection of the b-wave follows and then the c-wave. (Redrawn from Records, R.E.: Physiology of the human eye and visual system, New York, 1979, Harper & Row, Publishers.)

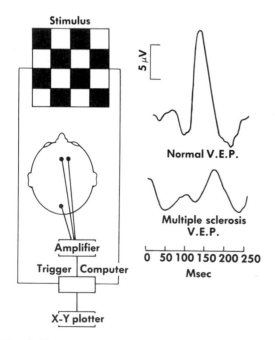

Fig. 2-18. Diagram of the system used to record the visual-evoked potential (VEP). The amplitude of the potential is shown to the right. In multiple sclerosis, the amplitude of the response is reduced and there is a significant delay in the peak-time of the positive wave. (Redrawn from Ikeda, H.: Electrophysiology of the retina and visual pathway. In Rose, F.C., editor: Medical ophthalmology, St. Louis, 1976, The C.V. Mosby Co.)

b-wave. The a-waves reflect photoreceptor activity. The b-wave originates from cells in the inner nuclear layer, most likely from a cell that undergoes depolarization when the retina is stimulated with light. The intracellularly recorded responses of Müller (glial) cells most closely match the b-wave.

The b-wave usually exceeds the largest amplitude of the a-wave by a factor of 1.5 or more. The duration of the entire response is usually less than 250 msec. The value for the b-waves is generally between 75 and 200 mV for photopic response and between 250 and 450 mV for scotopic response. The ERG is a mass response of the outer layers of the retina. The record varies with the state of adaptation of the retina, the color of the light used in adaptation, and the intensity and color of the light used for stimulation. In disorders limited to the ganglion cell layer, the nerve fiber layer, or the optic nerve, the ERG is normal.

Pathologic responses are described as supernormal, subnormal, or nonrecordable. When a large area of the retina is damaged or diseased, the ERG is subnormal. When the entire retina is involved, the ERG is nonrecordable.

Intraretinal microelectrodes record several other electrical potentials not recorded clinically: (1) a steady retinal resting potential from the junction of the photoreceptors and retinal pigment epithelium, (2) an early receptor potential (R_1) from the outer segments of photoreceptor cells corresponding to the isomerization of photopigments, (3) a later receptor potential (R_2) at the inner portion of photoreceptors corresponding to the a-wave of the electroretinogram, (4) a slow, widespread S-potential at the level of horizontal cells, (5) a well-defined positive potential at Müller cells corresponding to the b-wave of the electroretinogram, and (6) an oscillating potential from amacrine cells.

Visual-evoked potential. Stimulation of the retina with light changes the electrical activity of the cerebral cortex. The visual-evoked potential (VEP) (or response [VER]) is the electroencephalogram recorded at the occipital pole (Fig. 2-18). Because the evoked potential is too small to be separated from other cerebral electrical activity, several successive responses are averaged on a computer. Cerebral activity not related to the stimulus occurs randomly and is canceled out in the course of averaging. Electrical activity that is synchronized with a visual stimulus is summed and shown as a measurable electrical wave.

The only consistent recordable response is a large positive deflection occurring about 120 msec after stimulation when a pattern is used and about 100 msec when a flash is used. Pattern VEP is related to visual acuity and to stimulation of foveal cones since the amplitude decreases when the pattern is not in focus. Flash VEP reflects transmission of light from the entire retina, including fast-conducting axons from the retinal periphery.

The amplitude is reduced and the latency increased in patients who have optic neuritis. In patients who have demyelinating disease, there is often decreased amplitude and delayed peak response even though each retina and optic nerve is clinically normal.

IMAGE-FORMING MECHANISMS

Refraction. When a ray of light passes from one transparent medium to another, its velocity is either decreased in a more dense medium or increased in a less dense medium. If the medium is bounded by surfaces that are not perpendicular to the ray of light, then, in addition to the change in velocity, the emerging ray has a different direction than the entering ray. This change in direction of light is called "refraction." It is proportionate to the sine of the angle formed by the light ray to the surface of the refracting medium and the velocity of light in this medium. (The index of refraction is the ratio of the velocity of light in a vacuum to the velocity of light in another medium. The greater the change in the velocity of the light

as it passes from one medium to another, the greater will be its refraction.) Usually, rather than stating this angle and the index of refraction, the refractive power of a lens (Fig. 2-19) is described as the distance from its surface that the rays come to a focus (the focal length) or as the reciprocal of this distance in meters (diopters). Therefore, if the focal length of a lens is 20 cm (1 ÷ 0.2 m), its dioptric power is 5.

Refractive surfaces. A ray of light entering the eye is refracted by the cornea and then, after passing through the aqueous humor, by the lens. The anterior surface of the cornea is the main refractive surface of the eye. The refractive power of the cornea is approximately 43 diopters. The anterior and posterior surfaces of the lens are convex, but since the lens is immersed on either side in fluids with similar indexes of refraction, it has less refractive power than the cornea. Optically the lens behaves as though it were composed of a series of concentric lenses, so that its total index of refraction is greater than any individual portion of the lens. With accommodation, in a youthful eye the refractive power of the lens increases from about 19 to 33 diopters because of the change in its thickness and curvature.

Refractive error. A refractive error is determined by two factors: (1) the refractive power of the cornea and the lens and (2) the length of the eye. Usually the refractive power and the length of the eye are correlated. Most individuals have a refractive power almost exactly required to cause parallel rays of light to fall upon the retina. The normal eye varies in length from about 22 to 27 mm. The total refractive power of the normal eye at rest thus varies

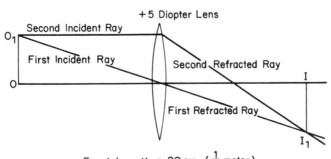
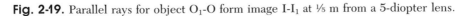

Focal Length = 20 cm. ($\frac{1}{5}$ meter)

Fig. 2-19. Parallel rays for object O_1-O form image I-I_1 at ⅕ m from a 5-diopter lens.

from about 52 to 63 diopters. Failure of the refractive power of the anterior segment to be correlated with the length of the eye results in an error of refraction.

Accommodation. Accommodation is the process by which the refractive power of the anterior lens segment increases so that a near object may be distinctly imaged upon the retina. The increased refractive power results from increased thickness of the lens and increased convexity of the central portion of its anterior

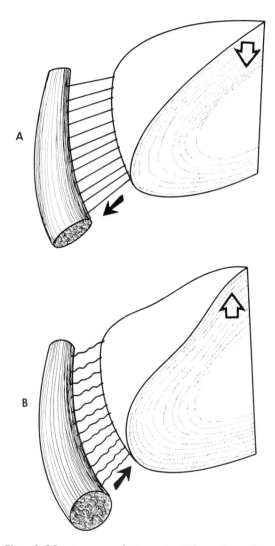

Fig. 2-20. Accommodation. **A,** When the ciliary muscle is at rest, the zonule is contracted, and the refractive power of the lens is minimal. **B,** When the ciliary muscle contracts, the zonule is relaxed, and the inherent elasticity of the lens causes it to increase in thickness and power of refraction.

surface in response to contraction of the circular portion (mainly) of the ciliary muscle. This muscle is attached to the lens capsule through zonular fibers. When the muscle is relaxed its diameter is maximal, the zonular fibers are taut, and the lens is not accommodated. Contraction reduces the diameter of the circular muscle and relaxes the zonular fibers (Fig. 2-20). This relaxation permits the lens to become thicker and more spherical, producing a greater refractive power.

Because of the elasticity of its anterior capsule, the lens tends to assume a more spherical shape. The anterior surface of the lens, particularly its central portion, becomes more markedly curved, and the anterior pole of the lens moves forward so the lens increases in thickness in its center.

The stimulus to accommodation is maintenance of a clear retinal image. One may imagine a continuous feedback mechanism in which the brain signals the amount of accommodation required and, through stimulation of the short ciliary branches of the oculomotor nerve, constricts or relaxes the circular muscle so that the eye almost instantly adjusts to provide clear vision at whatever distance.

With aging, the lens capsule becomes less elastic and the lens nucleus becomes harder and less compressible, so that the lens becomes less spherical with relaxation of the zonule. This causes a gradual loss of accommodation. The process begins shortly after birth and continues thereafter until about 50 years of age, when only one diopter of accommodation remains (presbyopia). The process is mainly the result of changes in the lens, but there may be decreased strength of the ciliary body musculature with aging.

EXTRAOCULAR MUSCULAR MECHANISMS

Each eye is moved by six extraocular muscles. Normally their action is so sensitively adjusted that each eye is directed to the same object in space.

When the eye is directed straight ahead, it is said to be in the primary position. If it is directed upward, downward, laterally, or medially, it is said to be in a secondary position. If it is directed in an oblique position (up and in or down and in), it is said to be in a tertiary position.

The medial rectus muscle (N III) has the single action of turning the eye medially (adduction) (Fig. 2-21). The lateral rectus muscle (N VI) has the single action of turning the eye laterally (abduction). The remaining four extraocular muscles, the cyclovertical muscles, have different actions depending on the position of the globe (Table 2-2). Thus, if the eye is directed straight ahead, the superior oblique muscle (N IV) turns the globe around an anteroposterior axis so that a point on the corneoscleral limbus in the 12 o'clock position turns medially (Fig. 2-22, *A*) (intorsion). If the eye is directed laterally, the superior oblique muscle steadies the globe in this abducted position. If the eye is directed medially, the superior oblique muscle depresses the eye (Fig. 2-22, *B*). The action of the other muscles is shown in Table 2-2 and Fig. 2-21.

Duction. The rotation of one eye from one position to another is called duction (Fig. 2-23). The muscles of one eye that work together in duction are called synergists in that function. In adduction the medial rectus muscle is aided by the superior and inferior recti muscles, whereas in abduction the superior and inferior oblique muscles are synergists of the lateral rectus muscle. In elevation the superior rectus and the inferior oblique muscles are synergistic, and in depression the inferior rectus and the superior oblique muscles are synergistic. In intorsion the superior oblique and superior rectus muscles are synergists, and in extorsion the inferior rectus and inferior oblique muscles are synergists. Each extraocular muscle is opposed by an antagonist that has the opposite action in a particular position. Thus the antagonist of the medial rectus muscle is the lateral rectus muscle. When the eye is elevated by the superior rectus muscle, its antagonist is the inferior rectus muscle.

An innervational impulse flows to the active muscle while the innervational impulse is inhibited to the muscle's antagonist (Sherrington's principle of reciprocal innervation).

Version. The simultaneous movement of eyes from the primary position to a secondary position is called version: (1) eyes right—dextroversion, (2) eyes left—levoversion, (3) eyes up—sursumversion, and (4) eyes down—deorsumversion. The muscles of the eyes primarily responsible for directing the eyes is version movements are yoke muscles. Thus, in turning the eyes to the right, the right lateral rectus

Table 2-2. Action of ocular muscles

Adduction (in)	Abduction (out)	Intorsion	Extorsion
Medial rectus muscle	Lateral rectus muscle	Superior oblique muscle	Inferior oblique muscle
Superior rectus muscle	Superior oblique muscle	Superior rectus muscle	Inferior rectus muscle
Inferior rectus muscle	Inferior oblique muscle		
Elevation in adduction	*Elevation in abduction*		
Inferior oblique muscle	Superior rectus muscle		
Depression in adduction	*Depression in abduction*		
Superior oblique muscle	Inferior rectus muscle		

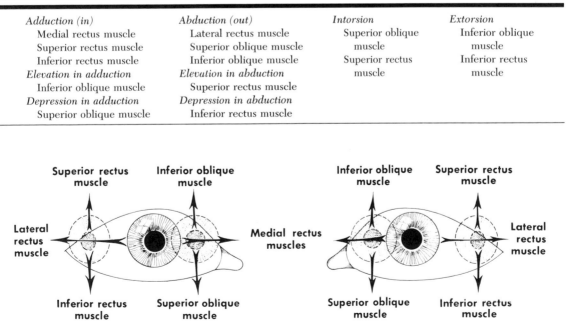

Fig. 2-21. Action of the six extraocular muscles of each eye.

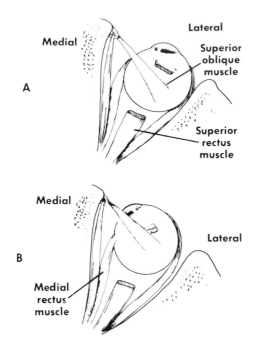

Fig. 2-22. The superior rectus muscle is removed to expose the reflected portion of the superior oblique muscle. **A,** With the eye directed straight ahead (primary position), the main action of the superior oblique muscle is intorsion. **B,** When the eye is turned medially, the main action of the superior oblique muscle is to turn the eye downward. When the eye is turned laterally (not shown), the superior oblique muscle aids in the abduction.

muscle is yoked to the left medial rectus muscle. Each superior rectus muscle is yoked to the contralateral inferior oblique muscle, and each inferior rectus muscle is yoked to the contralateral superior oblique muscle.

In version movements, an equal innervational impulse flows from the cerebral oculogyric centers to each muscle involved in the action (Herring's law). Thus, with both eyes turned to the right, the right lateral rectus and the left medial rectus receive equal innervational stimulus.

This equal innervation is important in the diagnosis of a paretic muscle. Thus, if the paretic muscle is on the right side and the right eye is used for fixing (as might be accomplished by covering the left eye), the nerve impulse required to hold the right eye in position is greater than it would be if the muscle were normal. Since the impulse is directed equally to the left eye, the left eye yoke muscle will receive an excessive innervational impulse and the eye will deviate. The deviation of the left eye will thus be greater when the paretic right eye is used for fixation. If the nonparetic left eye fixes, a normal innervation impulse is relayed to the paretic right eye and its deviation is minimal.

Vergence. Vergence is the term applied to simultaneous ocular movements in which the

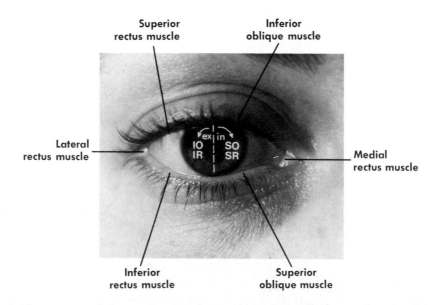

Fig. 2-23. Ductions of the eye showing the main muscle involved in each action. *In* refers to intorsion by superior oblique and superior recti muscles. *Ex* refers to extorsion by the inferior oblique and inferior recti muscles.

eyes directed to an object in the midbody plane, that is, somewhere in front of the nose. The term is applied to convergence, in which the eyes rotate inward toward each other, or to divergence, in which they rotate outward simultaneously. Vertical (sursumvergence) and torsional vergences are uncommon.

The locations of convergence and divergence centers are not known, although convergence and divergence paresis is observed clinically. The nucleus of Perlia has long been considered the center for convergence. Convergence palsy occurs in midbrain disease, and the convergence center is assumed to be located in this region. Divergence paresis may occur after head injury associated with perceptual deafness. The center is postulated to be located in the midbrain near the acoustic nerve nucleus.

Ocular movements. The three basic types of ocular movements are: (1) fast eye movements or saccades; (2) slow eye movements; and (3) vergence eye movements (also of the slow type) (Table 2-3).

Fast eye movements may be reflex, voluntary, or both. They are designed to bring a visual stimulus in the retinal periphery to the fovea centralis. Often the head moves also. Saccades reach an angular velocity of 700° of arc/second after a latency of 200 msec. Saccadic movements occur in reading, in the fast phases of evoked and pathologic nystagmus, and in the rapid eye movements (REM) of sleep.

Slow eye movements are smooth rotations designed to maintain the fovea centralis on a moving target. The maximum velocity is 30° to 50° of arc/second after a latency of 125 msec. If the fovea centralis is fixed on a moving target with an angular velocity of less than 30°/second, the eye follows the target almost exactly (pursuit or tracking movement). With greater velocity, an irregular type of saccadic movement results, with overcorrection and correction.

Vergence eye movements are slow eye movements involving convergence and divergence. They are designed to maintain the fixation of the fovea centralis of each eye upon an object of attention located approximately in front of the eyes.

The eyes maintain a horizontal position, despite movements of the head, by means of postural reflexes originating in the neck muscles and in each labyrinth. Thus, when the chin is depressed on the chest, an innervational impulse stimulates the elevators of the two eyes and inhibits the depressors, and the eyes remain directed ahead. Elevation of the chin causes the opposite reaction (the depressors are stimulated, and the elevators inhibited). If the head is tilted to either shoulder, torsion occurs so that the 12 o'clock meridian rotates and the vertical meridian of the cornea remains vertical, assuming the tilting of the head is less than 20°.

If the fovea centralis is fixed on a *steady target*, three types of movement occur: (1) those with a frequency of 30 to 70/seconds and an amplitude of 20 seconds, (2) those with an irregular frequency of about 1 every second and an amplitude of 3 minutes (saccades, or flick movements), and (3) irregular drifts of about 6 minutes. The fine high-frequency movements permit new retinal receptors to be stimulated

Table 2-3. Classification of eye movements

Version		Vergence
Fast eye movements	**Slow eye movements**	**Vergence eye movements**
Saccade		
Refixation	Pursuit (tracking)	Refixation
Reflex		
Voluntary	Voluntary	Tracking (pursuit)
Corrective saccade		
Saccadic pursuit (cogwheel)	Compensatory	Voluntary
Fast phase of nystagmus (pendular)	Slow phase of nystagmus	
Square wave jerk		
	Afterimage induced	
Sleep		

After Dell'Osso, L.F., and Doroff, R.B.: Aerospace Med. **45:**873, 1974.

during the latent period so that the image does not disappear. The saccadic, or flick, movements tend to correct either drift or previous saccade.

Fusional movements are vergence movements directed toward the maintenance of a single perception by keeping the retinal image on receptors having the same visual direction.

The near reaction is related to convergence involving the visual response to the awareness of the nearness of an object. It may occur without visual clues when an individual converges for the distance he believes the object to be, basing his judgment on sound or touch.

Electrical phenomena. There is continuous electrical activity in the extraocular muscles during a waking state. Moving the eye into the major field of action of a muscle causes a marked increase in the number and frequency of electrical discharges of the muscle involved. Accompanying this is a reduction in activity of the antagonistic muscle (Sherrington's principle).

The ocular muscles do not exhibit the electrical phenomena of fatigue. Sleep, however, reduces the electrical activity of the extraocular muscles to zero. During dreaming there are bursts of electrical activity and ocular movements (rapid eye movements, REMs). During sleep and forced eyelid closure the eyes are usually directed upward and outward in the Bell phenomenon. During general anesthesia, anatomic-mechanical factors position the eyes in the anatomic position of rest in which there is no muscle tone, so that the eyes are divergent.

THE IRIS AND PUPIL

The iris is a diaphragm originating from the anterior extremity of the optic vesicle and the adjacent mesoderm. The iris surrounds a central aperture, the pupil, and contains the sphincter pupillae muscle (N III) and the dilatator pupillae muscle (sympathetics), which are smooth muscles originating from the ectoderm of the primitive optic vesicle.

The pupil regulates the amount of light entering the eye, increases the depth of focus of the eye, and minimizes spherical and chromatic aberrations of the eye and the astigmatism caused by oblique pencils of light.

Pupillary reflexes

Direct light reflex. When the amount of light falling upon the eye is increased, the pupil constricts. There is a latent period of about 0.18 second, and maximum contraction occurs about 1 second after the start of stimulus. There is considerable variability in the state of the pupil thereafter unless the stimulus is maintained. The pupil may dilate again and then constrict, or it may remain constricted.

Light falling upon one eye and causing pupillary constriction also causes the pupil of the other eye to constrict simultaneously and to a similar degree—the *indirect* or *consensual light reflex*.

The pupillary reflex to light (Fig. 2-24) is a true reflex. The receptors for the pupillary response are the retinal photoreceptors. The afferent axons responsible for conducting pupillary impulses from the retina to the brain do not synapse in the lateral geniculate body but pass through its medial border by way of the brachium of the superior colliculus into the pretectal nucleus, which is located at the junction of the diencephalon and the tectum of the midbrain. Axons synapse here and pass to the Edinger-Westphal nucleus on both the same and opposite sides. From the Edinger-Westphal nucleus, pupillary constrictor nerves pass with the inferior division of the oculomotor nerve (N III) to the ciliary ganglion. Here they synapse with the postganglionic nerves, which pass by the short ciliary nerves to the sphincter muscle.

Near reaction (miosis). When an individual directs his eyes to and focuses on a nearby object, there is accommodation (lens), convergence, and pupillary constriction. The near reaction (miosis) is one of synkinesis, or an associated movement involving the common innervation of the medial rectus muscle and the sphincter pupillae muscle by the inferior branch of the oculomotor nerve. The pupil does not constrict with accommodation in the absence of convergence.

Eyelid closure reaction (orbicularis muscle reflex). The eyelid closure reaction does not occur consistently. When an effort is made to close the eyes by contraction of the orbicularis oculi muscle (N VII), the pupil on the side of closure may constrict. This reaction indicates the close association between the third and the seventh cranial nerves.

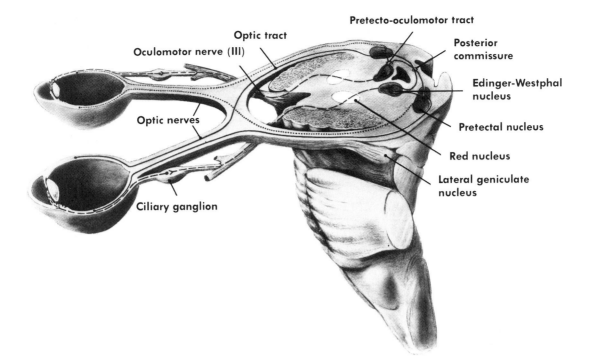

Fig. 2-24. Diagram of the pupillary light reflex. The pupillary impulses originate in the retina and the transmitting axons. Probably a collateral of the visual axons leaves the optic tract before the visual axons synapse in the lateral geniculate body. The pupillary axons synapse in the pretectal nucleus with an intercalated neuron that passes to the Edinger-Wesphal nuclei of the oculomotor nerve (III) on each side. Preganglionic pupillary motor axons (parasympathetic) in the inferior branch of the oculomotor nerve synapse in the ciliary ganglion. Postganglionic fibers extend to the sphincter pupillae muscle in the short ciliary nerves. (From Miller, N.R.: Walsh and Hoyt's clinical neuro-ophthalmology, ed. 4, vol. 2, Baltimore, 1985, Williams & Wilkins Co.)

Trigeminal reflex. Continued stimulation of trigeminal nerve from irritation of the cornea, conjunctiva, or skin of the face causes constriction of the pupil, possibly because of leakage of substance P into the aqueous humor. Reflex dilation of the blood vessels of the iris also causes pupillary constriction.

Psychic reflex. Emotional states, such as fear, may cause dilation of the pupil. There is simultaneous stimulation of the sympathetic nerves and inhibition of the parasympathetic nerves.

BIBLIOGRAPHY
General

Allansmith, M.R., and Gillette, T.E.: Secretory component in human ocular tissues, Am. J. Ophthalmol. 89:353, 1980.

Anderson, R.E., coordinating editor: Biochemistry of the eye (American Academy of Ophthalmology Manuals Program, 1983), San Francisco, 1983, American Academy of Ophthalmology.

Boynton, R.M.: Human color vision, New York, 1979, Holt, Rinehart and Winston.

Davson, H., editor: The eye, ed. 3, New York, 1984, Academic Press.

Duane, T.D., and Jaeger, E.A., editors: Biomedical foundations of ophthalmology, vol. 2, Philadelphia, 1983, Harper & Row.

Marr, D.: Vision, San Francisco, 1982, W.H. Freeman & Co.

Montgomery, R., Dryer, R.L., Conway, T.W., and Spector, A.A.: Biochemistry: a case-oriented approach, St. Louis, 1983, The C.V. Mosby Co.

Morgan, W.W.: Retinal transmitters and modulators, vols. I and II, Boca Raton, Fla., 1985, CRC Press.

Moses, R.A., editor: Adler's physiology of the eye, ed. 7, St. Louis, 1980, The C.V. Mosby Co.

Pokorny, J., Smith, V.C., Verriest, G., and Pinckers, A.J.L.G., editors: Congenital and acquired color vision defects, New York, 1979, Grune and Stratton.

Radius, R.L., and Anderson, D.R.: Rapid axonal transport in primate optic nerve, Arch. Ophthalmol. **99:**650, 1981.

Records, R.E.: Physiology of the human eye and visual system, New York, 1979, Harper & Row, Publishers.

Rose, F.C., editor: Medical ophthalmology, St. Louis, 1976, The C.V. Mosby Co.

Spehlman, R.: Evoked potential primer, Boston, 1985, Butterworth Publishers.

Cornea

Fischbarg, J., and Lim, J.J.: Fluid and electrolyte transports across corneal endothelium. In Zadunaisky, J.A., and Davson, H., editors: Current topics in eye research, vol. 4, New York, 1984, Academic Press.

Huff, J.W., and Green, K.: Characteristics of bicarbonate, sodium, and chloride fluxes in the rabbit corneal endothelium, Exp. Eye Res. **36:**607, 1983.

Maurice, D.: The structure and transparency of the cornea, J. Physiol. **136:**263, 1957.

Tears

Chandler, J.W., and Gillette, T.E.: Immunologic defense mechanisms of the ocular surface, Ophthalmology **90:**585, 1983.

Aqueous humor

Green, K.: Physiology and pharmacology of aqueous humor inflow, Surv. Ophthalmol. **29:**208, 1984.

Lens

Delaye, M., and Tradieu, A.: Short-range order of crystallin proteins accounts for eye lens transparency, Nature **302:**415, 1983.

Duncan, G.: Human cataract formation, Nature **306:**640, 1983.

Lerman, S.: Biophysical aspects of corneal and lenticular transparency, Curr. Eye Res. **3:**3, 1984.

Vitreous

Gardner-Medwin, A.R.: A foot in the vitreous fluid, Nature **309:**113, 1984.

Newman, E.A., and Frambach, D.A.: Control of extracellular potassium levels by retinal glial cell K^+ siphoning, Science **225:**1174, 1984.

Visual mechanisms

Altman, J.: New visions in photoreception, Nature **313:**264, 1985.

Brown, C.M.: Computer vision and natural constraints, Science **224:**1299, 1984.

George, J.S., and Hagins, W.A.: Control of Ca^{2+} in rod outer segments disks by light and cyclic GMP, Nature **303:**344, 1983.

Lewin, R.: Unexpected progress in photoreception, Science **277:**500, 1985.

Schichi, H.: Biochemistry of vision, London, 1983, Academic Press.

Schröder, W.H., and Fain, G.L.: Light-dependent calcium release from photoreceptors measured by laser micro-mass analysis, Nature **309:**268, 1984.

Spiegel, A.M., Gierschik, P., Levine, M.A., and Downs, R.W., Jr.: Clinical implications of guanine nucleotide-binding proteins as receptor-effector couplers, N. Engl. J. Med. **312:**26, 1985.

Sporn, M.B., Roberts, A.B., and Goodman, D.S., editors: The retinoids, vols. 1 and 2, London, 1984, Academic Press.

Stryer, L.: Transduction and the cyclic-GMP phosphodiesterase amplifier protein in vision, Cold Spring Harbor Symp. Quant. Biol. **48:**841, 1983.

3
PHARMACOLOGY

Many different drug actions may be observed in the eye. The effects of cholinergic or adrenergic stimulation or blockade of the pupillary musculature are easily visible, as is the hypersensitivity of denervation. Many anti-inflammatory and anti-infective agents are available for topical administration, and usually high tissue concentrations may be obtained. Toxic reactions range in severity from dermatitis medicamentosa of the eyelids to glaucoma induced by topical corticosteroids or mydriatics to permanent alteration of the fundi with impaired vision induced by phenothiazines.

DRUG ADMINISTRATION
Systemic route

Medications instilled in the conjunctival sac enter the aqueous humor mainly through the cornea, and their effects are limited to the anterior segment. If the lens is absent, minor amounts may be distributed posteriorly. Penetration is sometimes great enough to cause cystoid central retinal edema, as may occur after prolonged topical instillation of epinephrine in the aphakic eye. The ocular tissue concentration of drugs administered systemically parallels that of other tissues with one important difference: the vitreous humor, aqueous humor, central cornea, and lens lack blood vessels.

There are two blood-ocular barriers: the blood-aqueous barrier and the blood-retina barrier. The blood-aqueous barrier is formed by the nonpigmented layer of the ciliary epithelium and by the endothelium of the iris vessels. Both of these tissues have tight junctions that are selectively permeable to water and ions ("leaky" tight junctions). The blood-aqueous barrier is permeable through both transport mechanisms and pressure-dependent osmotic flow (ultrafiltration).

The blood-retina barrier is located in the retinal pigment epithelium and the endothelium of the retinal blood vessels. Both of the tissues have junctions of the tight type. The permeability of the cells to water and solubles is determined by active and passive transport mechanisms of the cell.

Systemic and topical drugs that are either ionized, lipid-insoluble, or both, are mainly excluded from the intraocular intracellular space. Drugs enter the eye in proportion to their lipid solubility. The tight junctions of the endothelium of the retinal and iris capillaries particularly limit the diffusion of lipid-insoluble substances. The fenestrated choriocapillaris and ciliary body capillaries permit the passage of relatively large molecules, but the tight junctions of the retinal pigment epithelium and its anterior extension, the pigmented ciliary body epithelium, prevent further intraocular penetration. Severe inflammation and trauma damage the blood-aqueous barrier, and compounds that do not penetrate the normal eye in high concentrations penetrate easily and are distributed as in other body tissues and fluids.

The ciliary body epithelium transports organic ions from the posterior aqueous humor into the blood by a mechanism similar to that in the renal tubule and choroid plexus. Uric acid and drugs such as the penicillins are actively transported out of the posterior chamber by the nonpigmented ciliary epithelium, and this transport is inhibited by probenecid.

Some drugs, such as the phenothiazines, concentrate in cells containing melanin, leading to a high level in the retinal pigment epithelium. This may damage the sensory retina; alternatively, the stabilization of cell lysosomes by phenothiazines may impair phagocytosis of the photoreceptors of the outer segments.

Local route

Drugs may be applied to the eyelids or anterior globe in aqueous or viscous solutions or suspensions, in ointments, as fine powders, on cotton pledgets, by drug-impregnated contact lenses, by injection, by mechanical pumps, or by membrane release systems. In contrast to systemic administration, the ocular concentration after topical administration is high. Dilution of the drug by tears, overflow onto the cheek, and excretion through the nasolacrimal system limits tissue concentration.

Placing the drug beneath a contact lens or applying a cotton pledget saturated with the drug to the eye ensures prolonged contact and enhances penetration. A soft contact lens may be soaked in a compound, and when the lens is placed in contact with the eye, it gradually releases the drug.

Subconjunctival or sub-Tenon retrobulbar injections are useful for the administration of antibiotics and corticosteroids. Before injection, the conjunctiva is anesthetized with topical 4% cocaine solution or subconjunctival lidocaine. A high tissue concentration is maintained for a long period. Some surgeons inject an antibiotic subconjunctivally at the end of an intraocular operation to ensure a high concentration of antibiotic in the aqueous humor. Injections into the anterior portion of the vitreous body are limited to a few antibiotics and are largely reserved for treatment of infections that threaten destruction of the globe.

Maximal effectiveness of eyedrops requires proper instillation. The patient is instructed to look upward, and the skin of the lower eyelid is grasped and drawn outward to create a pouch between the eyelid and the globe. The

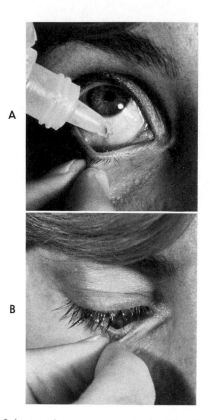

Fig. 3-1. A, The proper method of instillation of eyedrops in the eye. The lower eyelid is drawn away from the globe, the patient is instructed to look upward, and the drop is delivered into the pouch. **B,** The patient is then instructed to look downward, and the skin of the eyelid is slowly released. The patient should be warned not to squeeze the eye. The eyelids may then be gently closed for 2 minutes. Increased concentrations may be provided in a particular region by having the patient tilt the head in the direction of desired effect.

drug is then instilled in the pouch without touching the eyelids with the container (Fig. 3-1). The patient is instructed to look down and to close the eye without squeezing. Pressure by a finger for 2 minutes to the inner cornea of the eye occludes the lacrimal puncta and prevents loss of the drug (and systemic absorption) into the nose. The cul-de-sac retains a single drop, and the excess overflows. Increased viscosity of the vehicle minimizes dilution and prolongs contact. Thus, medications may be prescribed in oils, ointments, methyl cellulose, and other viscous vehicles. The medication must have a greater affinity for the cornea than

Table 3-1. Concentrations of some especially prepared antibiotics for use in severe eye infections

Name	Topical	Subconjunctival	Intravitreal	Systemic
Ampicillin		100 mg	5.0 mg	2-4 g/4 hr
Bacitracin	100 units/ml	10,000 units		
Carbenicillin	4 mg/ml	250 mg	2.0 mg	4-6 g/4 hr
Cefazolin	50 mg/ml	100 mg		1 g/6 hr
Cephaloridine	50 mg/ml	100 mg	0.25 mg	1 g/6 hr
Chloramphenicol	5 mg/ml	500 mg	2.0 mg	50 mg/kg/day
Clindamycin		40 mg		600 mg/8 hr
Colistin	5-10 mg/ml	75 mg	0.5 mg	
Erythromycin	50 mg/ml	100 mg		
Gentamicin	8-15 mg/ml	40 mg	0.4 mg	5 mg/kg/day
Lincomycin		150 mg	1.5 mg	600 mg/8 hr
Methicillin		100 mg	2.0 mg	2 g/4 hr
Nafcillin				2 g/4 hr
Neomycin	8 mg/ml	500 mg		
Penicillin G	100,000 units/ml	500,000 units		2-4 ml/4 hr
Polymixin B	2 mg/ml	20 mg		
Sulfacetamide	300 mg/ml			8 g/day
Tobramycin	11 mg/ml	20 mg	0.5 mg	
Vancomycin	50 mg/ml	25 mg	1.0 mg	1 g/12 hr
Anti-fungal agents				
Amphotericin B	2.5 mg/ml		0.01 mg	1.0 mg/kg/day
Flucytosine	10 mg/ml			Oral only 150 mg/kg/day in divided doses
Miconazole	10 mg/ml	5 mg		30 mg/kg/day
Natamycin	50 mg/ml			
Nystatin	100,000 units/ml			Oral: 500,000 unit tablets

for the vehicle. If the medication has a greater affinity for the vehicle, it will not be released and will remain in the vehicle rather than be absorbed into the eye.

Membrane release systems. These systems provide continuous release of a predetermined amount of drug over a 5- to 7-day period. Ocusert R (pilocarpine) is commonly available for glaucoma treatment. It provides a continuous but lower drug concentration, which produces the same effects as intermittent topical instillation and minimizes side effects of pilocarpine treatment in youthful individuals who have an active accommodation. Daily inspection is required to be certain the device has not been inadvertently lost.

Corneal penetration. Compounds enter the anterior chamber mainly through the cornea. The tight junctions of the intact corneal epithelium are the chief barrier to water-soluble, polar compounds. Lipid-soluble compounds pass through the epithelium. When the epithelium is diseased or damaged, penetration by water-soluble, polar compounds into the anterior seg-

ment is increased. Local anesthetics, wetting agents, massage, and corneal abrasion enhance penetration. To penetrate the stroma, the drugs must be water-soluble. Thus the highest intraocular concentrations follow administration of drugs that are both water- and lipid-soluble.

Topical preparations. Many factors relate to the effectiveness, safety, and comfort of eyedrops and ointments: sterility, hydrogen ion concentration, tonicity, physiologic activity, stability, toxicity, surface tension, and compatibility. Most commonly used medications are prepared commercially and require Food and Drug Administration-approved quality control to ensure sterility.

Concentrated antibiotics. In serious disorders, such as suppurative corneal ulcers, endophthalmitis, and orbital cellulitis, concentrated antibiotics are often used topically and subconjunctivally. They are prepared by mixing a parenteral preparation with sterile artificial tears distributed for topical instillation (Table 3-1) or with sterile saline for injection. These preparations are much more concentrated then commercially prepared solutions. They are not intended for long-term use because of potential toxicity and increased osmolarity.

Sterility. Eyedrops intended for interstate commerce are sterile when released. Once the container is opened the solution is easily contaminated. The physician must regard all solutions in open containers as contaminated.

The adenovirus that causes keratoconjunctivitis may be transmitted by means of contaminated eye anesthetic solutions. Fluorescein solution is liable to contamination by *Pseudomonas aeruginosa,* and it may introduce the organism when used in diagnosis of corneal abrasions. To avoid infection, fluorescein should be instilled only from a sterile individual container or should be applied by means of a filter paper strip that has been saturated with fluorescein and then sterilized. It must never be used from a stock bottle.

Eyecups are usually contaminated and may cause recurrent infections. Eyedroppers are easily contaminated by touching the eyelids or the conjunctiva, and they may then contaminate a stock bottle. Contact lens containers are often contaminated. Plastic "squeeze" bottles in which most commercially available medications are distributed are more difficult to contaminate that the bottles with eyedroppers.

AUTONOMIC DRUGS

The autonomic nervous system may be divided into parasympathetic (or cholinergic) and sympathetic (or adrenergic) systems. Drugs affecting these systems may be divided into cholinergic-stimulating (agonist) and cholinergic-blocking (antagonist) agents and adrenergic-stimulating (agonist) and adrenergic-blocking (antagonist) agents (Table 3-2).

Acetylcholine is the cholinergic neurohumoral transmitter, and norepinephrine (noradrenaline, levarterenol) is the main adrenergic neural transmitter. Acetylcholine is inactivated by the enzyme cholinesterase, whereas norepinephrine is largely inactivated by reuptake by the axon that released it (90%) or by the enzyme catechol-O-methyl transferase. The amount of norepinephrine stored in the axon of the synaptic junction is limited by inactivation of norepinephrine by monoamine oxidase.

The sphincter pupillae and ciliary muscles

are innervated by postganglionic parasympathetic efferent fibers of the short ciliary nerve branches of the oculomotor nerve (N III) that have synapsed in the ciliary ganglion. The dilator pupillae muscle is innervated by the long ciliary nerves that carry postganglionic fibers of the sympathetic nervous system that have synapsed in the superior cervical ganglion. The sphincter pupillae and ciliary muscles belong principally to the cholinergic system, whereas the dilator pupillae muscle belongs to the adrenergic system. Cholinergic stimulation of the sphincter pupillae muscle causes constriction of the pupil (miosis). Cholinergic stimulation of the ciliary muscle increases accommodation. Cholinergic blockade dilates the pupil (mydriasis) and relaxes the ciliary muscle to cause decreased accommodation (cycloplegia).

Adrenergic stimulation causes dilation of the pupil, whereas adrenergic blockade causes pupillary constriction. The ciliary muscle may have minor adrenergic innervation with stimulation decreasing accommodation. The more

Table 3-2. Autonomic nervous system

Cholinergic (parasympathetic)
  Cholinergic-stimulating drugs (agonist)
  Cholinergic-blocking drugs (antagonist)
Adrenergic (sympathetic)
  Adrenergic-stimulating drugs (agonist)
  Adrenergic-blocking drugs (antagonist)

Table 3-3. Acetylcholine transmission

Cholinergic synapses
  Postganglionic parasympathetic innervation
    Smooth and cardiac muscle
  Postganglionic sympathetic innervation
    Sweat glands
    Arrectores pilorum muscles
  Preganglionic autonomic fibers
    Adrenal medulla
    Parasympathetic ganglia
    Sympathetic ganglia
  Some control nervous system synapses
Acetylcholine receptors
  Muscarinic (blocked by atropine)
    Smooth and cardiac muscles
    Exocrine glands
  Nicotinic receptors (blocked by *d*-turbocurarine)
    Autonomic ganglia (blocked by hexamethonium)
    Motor endplates skeletal muscle (blocked by decamethonium)

prominent cholinergic effects obscure adrenergic effects.

Cholinergic system

Acetylcholine is the neurohumoral transmitter for four classes of cholinergic synapses (Table 3-3):

1. Autonomic effector sites innervated by postganglionic parasympathetic fibers (smooth and cardiac muscle) and postganglionic sympathetic fibers (sweat glands and arrectores pilorum muscles). These effector sites are stimulated by muscarine and are muscarinic receptors.
2. The adrenal medulla and sympathetic and parasympathetic ganglia innervated by preganglionic autonomic fibers.
3. Motor endplates of skeletal muscle innervated by somatic motor nerves. These receptors are mainly nicotinic and are stimulated by small doses of nicotine, although in large doses nicotine is a ganglionic-blocking agent.

4. Some synapses in the central nervous system are predominantly nicotonic in the spinal cord and both muscarinic and nicotinic at the subcortical and cortical levels in the brain.

Acetylcholine affects two types of choline receptors: (1) muscarinic receptors (blocked by atropine) located in smooth and cardiac muscles and exocrine gland cells, and (2) nicotinic receptors (initial stimulation and then blockade with large doses of nicotine) in autonomic ganglia cells and the motor endplates of skeletal muscle. *d*-Tubocurarine blocks nicotinic receptors in both locations, but hexamethonium blocks only those located in autonomic ganglia and decamethonium blocks only those located in the motor endplates of skeletal muscle.

Acetylcholine is stored within synaptic vesicles in the nerve and released into the synaptic cleft upon depolarization (Fig. 3-2). It diffuses across the cleft to activate muscarinic receptors, the predominate receptor of smooth and cardiac muscles and exocrine glands, or nico-

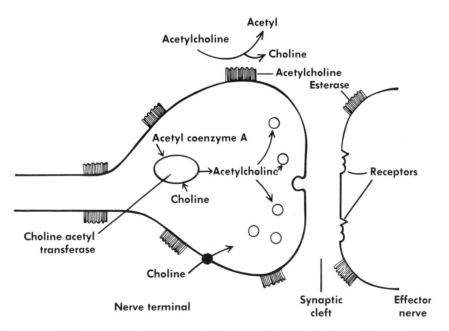

Fig. 3-2. Schema of cholinergic synapse. Acetylcholine is synthesized from choline and acetyl coenzyme A by the enzyme choline acetyltransferase. Acetylcholine is stored within vesicles in the nerve terminal and, upon depolarization, released into the synaptic cleft. It diffuses across the cleft to activate muscarinic or nicotinic receptors. The action is rapidly terminated by hydrolysis by the enzyme acetylcholinesterase, which is located on the surface of cholinergic neurons as well as neurons receiving cholinergic innervation. (Modified from Coyle, J.T., Price, D.L., and DeLong, M.R.: Science **219**:1184, 1983.)

tinic receptors of autonomic ganglia and skeletal muscle. The acetylcholine depolarizes the postsynaptic membrane, causing transmission of the nervous impulse. The action of the released acetylcholine is terminated within 1 μsec to 1 second by hydrolysis mediated by the enzyme acetylcholinesterase located on the surface of the cholinergic membrane. This permits repolarization and transmission of the next impulse.

Acetylcholinesterase, also called specific cholinesterase, occurs mainly in neurons and at neuromuscular junctions. Butyrocholinesterase, also called serum esterase or nonspecific cholinesterase, is found in plasma and liver. Both hydrolyze acetylcholine, but nonspecific cholinesterase also inactivates long-chain choline esters. Specific acetylcholinesterase inactivates acetylcholine only. It is the main cholinesterase of the iris and the lens. The anticholinesterases used clinically inhibit acetylcholinesterase and cause accumulation of endogenous acetylcholine.

Cholinergic-stimulating drugs mimic the action of acetylcholine on effector cells or at synapses. The action may be brought about directly by compounds chemically similar to acetylcholine or by those such as pilocarpine that act directly on smooth muscle. Indirect stimulation occurs when acetylcholine activity is prolonged by inactivating the acetylcholinesterase that normally hydrolyzes it. Such compounds are called anticholinesterases and are commonly classified as reversible if their action is relatively short or as irreversible if it is long.

Cholinergic-stimulating drugs. These compounds (Table 3-4) are not used systemically. When instilled in the conjunctival sac, choline esters dilate the conjunctival and anterior ciliary arteries, constrict the pupil (miosis), and increase the permeability of the blood-aqueous barrier. Most penetrate the intact cornea poorly. Direct-acting ophthalmic cholinergic drugs used in ophthalmology include the following compounds.

Acetylcholine chloride. Acetylcholine chloride (1:100) in mannitol solution (1:20) (Miochol) constricts the pupil when injected into the anterior chamber after cataract extraction. It is rapidly hydrolyzed by cholinesterase. After topical administration, it is inactivated by corneal cholinesterase so that it does not enter the anterior chamber.

Table 3-4. Cholinergic-stimulating drugs

Displacement of acetylcholine from axonal terminal
  Carbachol
  Tetraethylammonium (also a blocking agent)
Mimicking of acetylcholine at postsynaptic receptors
  Muscarinic-type receptors
    Pilocarpine
    Muscarine
    Arecoline
    Methacholine (Mecholyl)
  Nicotinic-type receptors
    Nicotine
    Pilocarpine
    Arecoline
Inactivation of cholinesterase (anticholinesterase)
  Physostigmine (eserine)
  Neostigmine (prostigmine)
    Edrophonium chloride (Tensilon)
  Organophosphates
    Phospholine iodide (echothiophate iodide)
    Diisopropyl fluorophosphate (DFP)
    Demecarium bromide
Reactivation of acetylcholinesterase
  Pralidoxime chloride (Protopam)

Pilocarpine. Pilocarpine, like acetylcholine, acts directly on smooth muscle and glandular receptors innervated by postganglionic cholinergic nerves. It stimulates the sphincter pupillae muscle (miosis), the ciliary muscles (increased accommodation), and increases outflow of aqueous humor through the trabecular meshwork. In some patients, it decreases secretion of aqueous humor. It is used topically in 1% to 4% solution in the treatment of glaucoma. It is prescribed in the minimum concentration that will prevent progression of the glaucoma and is seldom instilled more frequently than once every 6 hours. Increased outflow of aqueous humor is its most useful function in open-angle glaucoma, whereas pupillary constriction is its most useful function in angle-closure glaucoma. Systemic toxicity after topical instillation is uncommon, although long-term use may be associated with lens opacities or contact allergy (type IV hypersensitivity) of the eyelids and conjunctiva.

Carbachol. Carbachol (Carcholin, Doryl), 0.75% to 3.0%, must be combined with a wetting agent to penetrate the cornea. It is not hydrolyzed by cholinesterases and is so potent that it is not used systemically. Frequently this drug is substituted for pilocarpine in patients who have developed a tolerance to pilocarpine.

Anticholinesterase drugs. Anticholinesterase drugs permit the accumulation of exogenous acetylcholine by inactivating cholinesterase. There are three main types of anticholinesterase compounds: (1) physostigmine (eserine), a tertiary amine with a urethane group; (2) neostigmine (Prostigmin), a quaternary ammonium compound; and (3) organophosphates. The first two are classified as reversible cholinesterase inhibitors. The organophosphates inactivate cholinesterase irreversibly.

Systemic administration of anticholinesterase compounds causes widespread cholinergic stimulation. There is constriction of gastrointestinal, urinary, and bronchiole muscles. Skeletal muscle is weakened and fibrillates. Salivation, lacrimation, sweating, and pulmonary secretions increase. Central nervous system symptoms range from giddiness to coma and convulsions.

The sphincter pupillae and ciliary muscles contract so that the pupil is miotic and accommodation is increased. The drugs do not constrict the pupil after retrobulbar anesthesia or if the eye has no parasympathetic innervation and hence no acetylcholine. The organophosphates more markedly dilate the conjunctival and ciliary blood vessels and cause greater permeability of the blood-aqueous barrier than physostigmine or neostigmine.

Physostigmine. Physostigmine (eserine) was the first miotic used in the treatment of glaucoma (1876). It is used in an aqueous solution of the salicylate salt in a concentration of 0.25% to 1% or as a 0.25% ointment. Usually it is given only at bedtime to supplement the instillation of pilocarpine. Prolonged use causes tolerance, conjunctival irritation, or both.

Neostigmine. Neostigmine (Prostigmin) was synthesized as an analogue of physostigmine. It is used in the treatment of glaucoma as a 5% solution every 4 to 6 hours and systemically in the treatment of myasthenia gravis. It penetrates the cornea poorly and is used rarely.

Edrophonium chloride (Tensilon), an analogue of neostigmine, has a systemic action of 2 or 3 minutes. After testing for hypersensitivity, it is injected intravenously in doses of 2 to 6 mg in the diagnosis of myasthenia gravis (Chapter 29).

Organophosphates. Echothiophate iodide (Phospholine Iodide) is an organophosphate in which a quaternary ammonium compound has been substituted. It is active against nonspecific cholinesterases. Echothiophate iodide is used locally in open-angle glaucoma every 12 hours in a 0.06% to 0.25% solution. It causes intense miosis and spasm of the ciliary muscle.

All organophosphates are contraindicated in angle-closure glaucoma, bronchial asthma, gastrointestinal spasm, vascular hypertension, myocardial infarction, myasthenia gravis, and Parkinson disease. Long-term use of echothiophate iodide may cause iris cysts in children. It inactivates the Na^+K^+ ATPase of the specific cholinesterase of the lens capsule and causes water vesicles in the anterior portion of the lens after prolonged use (6 months).

Despite the long list of contraindications, echothiophate iodide has proved to be particularly effective in open-angle glaucoma, aphakic glaucoma, and accommodative esotropia.

Local instillation of echothiophate iodide (and other organophosphates) depletes systemic nonspecific cholinesterases. Thus, if succinylcholine is used as a muscle relaxant in the course of general anesthesia, the succinylcholine is not inactivated, and there may be prolonged apnea. Additionally, the compounds may cause intestinal cramping that may be mistaken for an acute surgical emergency.

Reactivators of cholinesterase. Severe toxicity from anticholinesterase compounds in drugs, chemical warfare agents, and insecticides occurs because of the accumulation of systemic acetylcholine. Atropine (2 to 20 mg, intravenously or intramuscularly) antagonizes acetylcholine at muscarinic receptor sites. Pralidoxime (1 g at maximum rate of 500 mg/min, intravenously) reactivates acetylcholinesterase, particularly at nicotinic receptors in the motor endplate of skeletal muscle.

Cholinergic blocking drugs

Acetylcholine is the neurohumoral transmitter at two major types of neurohumoral effector sites, the muscarinic and the nicotinic. The muscarinic actions are antagonized by the atropine group of drugs, whereas the nicotinic actions are antagonized by ganglionic blocking agents and neuromuscular blocking agents (Table 3-5).

Atropine group. These drugs prevent the action of acetylcholine at postganglionic muscarinic receptors in smooth muscle, cardiac muscle, and exocrine glands. Systemic adminis-

Table 3-5. Cholinergic blocking compounds

Interference with acetylcholine synthesis
  Hemicholinium
Prevention of acetylcholine release
  Botulinum toxin
Blockade of transmitter at postsynaptic receptor
  Muscarinic-type receptors
    Atropine (smooth and cardiac muscles)
  Nicotinic-type receptors
    Nicotine (autonomic ganglia and motor end-
      plates of skeletal muscle)
    d-Tubocurarine (same as nicotine)
    Hexamethonium (autonomic ganglia)
    Decamethonium (motor endplates of skele-
      tal muscle)

tration increases the heart rate and decreases sweating, lacrimation, salivary secretion, gastric secretion, gastrointestinal motility, and tone. Many of the compounds have a depressant effect on the central nervous system and can cause confusional psychosis.

The ocular effects of these drugs are dilation of the pupil (mydriasis) through paralysis of the sphincter pupillae muscle, decreased accommodation through paralysis of the ciliary muscle (cycloplegia), and reduced permeability of the blood vessels of the iris and ciliary body when the blood-aqueous barrier is impaired in uveitis and keratitis.

Systemic administration has less ocular effect than local administration because of decreased concentration of the compounds at the effector sites in the eye. Systemically administered atropine has a greater effect on the pupil and ciliary muscle than the atropine-related compounds used for their antispasmodic action on the gastrointestinal tract.

On local instillation, the atropine-related compounds developed as gastrointestinal antispasmodics have varying degrees of mydriatic and cycloplegic activity. Systemic administration in younger persons may cause an annoying decrease in accommodation. Many patients with ill-defined gastrointestinal complaints for whom such antispasmodics are prescribed also have unsuspected open-angle glaucoma.

Members of the atropine group of drugs used in ophthalmology include atropine, scopolamine, homatropine, eucatropine (Euphthalmine), cyclopentolate hydrochloride (Cyclogyl), and tropicamide (Mydriacyl).

Atropine. Atropine is the principal alkaloid of belladonna. It is used in a 0.125% to 2% aqueous solution topically, in an ointment, or in castor oil base to minimize systemic aborption. It paralyzes the sphincter pupillae muscle and causes pupillary dilation that begins in about 15 minutes, reaches a maximum in 30 to 40 minutes, and persists 7 to 10 days. Paralysis of the ciliary muscle (accommodation) begins 20 to 30 minutes after instillation, reaches a maximum in 1 to 3 hours, and persists 7 to 12 days. Atropine is widely used in the treatment of anterior uveitis and keratitis and for refraction in children, particularly those with esotropia. In inflammatory conditions, it may be used every 1 to 6 hours. For refraction in children, it is commonly instilled in an ointment base three times daily for 3 days, with examination on the fourth day.

Scopolamine. This drug is closely related to atropine but has a shorter duration of action (3 to 7 days) on the sphincter pupillae and ciliary muscles. It is often substituted for atropine, which may cause conjunctival irritation or contact allergy when prolonged mydriasis and cycloplegia are required in conditions such as retinal detachment or uveitis.

Homatropine. This synthetic, atropine-like compound is used mainly for refraction. It is used in a 1% to 5% aqueous solution, and it produces mydriasis and cycloplegia that lasts 24 to 72 hours.

Cyclopentolate (Cyclogyl). This cholinergic-blocking drug is used almost exclusively for refraction in concentrations of 0.5%, 1%, and 2%. It produces mydriasis and paralysis of accommodation with recovery within 24 hours. Premature and young infants are particularly prone to central nervous system and cardiopulmonary side effects and should have no more than one instillation of a 0.5% concentration with pressure over the lacrimal sac to minimize systemic absorption. For mydriasis in neonates, a 0.2% solution combined with 1% phenylephrine is commercially available.

Tropicamide (Mydriacyl). This drug causes more rapid mydriasis and cycloplegia and quicker recovery than any other cholinergic-blocking agent. It is used in a 0.5% (mydriasis mainly) and 1% (mydriasis and cycloplegia) concentration. Cycloplegia is maximal 20 to 30 minutes after instillation and disappears within

6 hours. A 0.5% solution is often combined with 2.5% phenylephrine for mydriasis in ophthalmoscopy in adults.

Botulinum toxin. This toxin interferes with acetylcholine release from the individual motor neurons. It is thus a presynaptic blocking agent of cholinergic junctions. It is injected in small doses (1.25×10^{-5} μg to 6.25×10^{-5} μg) into overactive muscles in strabismus and is used in the treatment of blepharospasm.

Ganglionic-blocking drugs. These agents block the action of acetylcholine at adrenergic and cholinergic autonomic ganglia. They are used in the treatment of hypertensive cardiovascular disease to reduce peripheral resistance by decreasing sympathetic tone to vascular beds. They are also useful in vasospasm therapy and in producing a controlled hypotension in general anesthesia.

The ocular side effects of ganglionic blockade constitute their main ophthalmic interest. The conjunctival blood vessels and the pupil are dilated. The volume of tears and the amount of accommodation decrease. The intraocular pressure decreases slightly, apparently because of a decreased secretion of aqueous humor. The decrease is accompanied by an increased resistance to the exit of aqueous humor through the trabecular meshwork. Increased intraocular pressure does not occur because of the reduced aqueous secretion.

Neuromuscular blocking agents. Pharmacologically the most important effect of these drugs is to block the effects of acetylcholine at the motor endplates of skeletal muscle. There are two types: competitive (stabilizing), of which curare is the classic example; and depolarizing, of which succinylcholine is the classic example.

The main ophthalmic application is in general anesthesia. Curare combines with nicotinic receptor sites on motor endplates of skeletal muscle and thereby blocks the uptake of acetylcholine. Succinylcholine and decamethonium depolarize the motor endplate in the same manner as acetylcholine but for a longer period. The initial depolarization contracts the extraocular muscles with an increased intraocular pressure. Succinylcholine is contraindicated in ocular lacerations. Succinylcholine is synergistic with anticholinesterase agents used in glaucoma and accommodative esotropia and may

cause prolonged apnea after general anesthesia in patients who use such compounds.

Adrenergic system

The catecholamines (norepinephrine, dopamine, and epinephrine) are the neurohumoral transmitters responsible for the stimulation of the majority of structures innervated by postganglionic sympathetic nerves. (The arrectores pilorum muscles and sweat glands are exceptional in having acetylcholine as the postganglionic effector substance.) Norepinephrine (noradrenalin or levarterenol) is the major transmitter at most postganglionic sympathetic impulses; dopamine is the major transmitter in the extrapyramidal system; and epinephrine is the major hormone in the adrenal medulla.

Hydroxylation of phenylalanine to tyrosine (hydroxyphenylalanine) initiates catecholamine synthesis. Tyrosine is hydroxylated to Dopa (dihydroxyphenylalanine), a key compound of certain "false transmitters" used therapeutically. Dopa loses a CO_2 molecule through the action of the enzyme L-aromatic acid decarboxylase (dopa decarboxylase) and is converted to dopamine. Dopamine is converted to norepinephrine by the enzyme dopamine β-hydroxylase. Methylation of norepinephrine yields epinephrine. Norepinephrine is mainly confined to potsganglionic fibers, whereas epinephrine is localized to chromaffin cells of the adrenal medulla.

There are two alpha types and two beta types of adrenergic receptor cells. Alpha$_1$ receptor sites predominate at postjunctional effector sites of smooth muscles and glands. Alpha$_2$ receptor sites are located on presynaptic terminals. Activation of alpha$_2$ receptors results in inhibition of the norepinenephrine release by adrenergic nerve terminals. Beta$_1$

Table 3-6. Comparative effects of different catecholamines on adrenergic receptors

Compound	Type of receptor			
	α_1	α_2	β_1	β_2
Epinephrine	+ + + +	+ + +*	+	+ + +
Norepinephrine	+ + +	+ + + +*	+	+
Isoproterenol	+	– – –	+ + +	+ + +

*Depends on the tissue responsive to catecholamines.

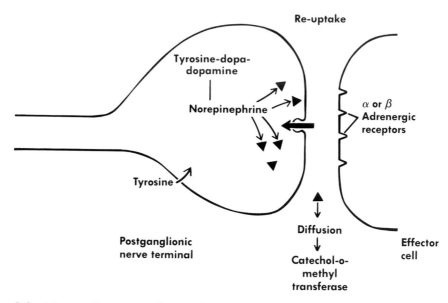

Fig. 3-3. Schema of a postganglionic adrenergic synapse. Norepinephrine is synthesized from tyrosine (tyrosine → dopa → dopamine → norepinephrine). Upon activation, norepinephrine diffuses across the nerve terminal to act on the effector cell. After release the excess is removed from the extracellular space mainly by return to the nerve terminal through active transport. Some diffuses and is inactivated by catechol-O-methyl transferase.

adrenergic receptor sites predominate in cardiac muscle. Beta$_2$ adrenergic receptor sites are present in smooth muscle and glands. The sensitivity of these adrenergic receptors to catecholamines varies considerably. Generally, the effect of sympathomimetic drugs is excitatory on alpha receptors and inhibitory on beta receptors, but this is not always true (Table 3-6).

The norepinephrine released from the sympathetic nerve vesicle is almost completely (90%) inactivated by reuptake by the terminal that released it (Fig. 3-3). The norepinephrine that escapes into the circulation is metabolized by the enzyme catechol-O-methyl transferase.

The action of adrenergic compounds in glaucoma is puzzling. Epinephrine, an adrenergic agonist, decreases the intraocular pressure as does timolol, a beta$_1$ and beta$_2$ (nonselective) antagonist and betaxolol, a beta$_1$ (selective) antagonist. The synergistic action of epinephrine compounds and beta blockers suggests that the pressure-decreasing mechanism may not be directly mediated through the adrenergic nervous system.

The mechanism of action of adrenergic compounds in glaucoma is not understood. An adrenergic receptor-coupled adenylate cyclase converts extracellular messages to intracellular signals. The receptors are functionally coupled to the enzyme by two proteins, the stimulatory and the inhibitory guanine nucleotide proteins. When the inhibiting protein is absent, the effects of the stimulating protein are modest. When the inhibitory protein is present, the effects of the stimulating protein are much more marked. The inhibitory protein may thus be required both for maximal agonist action and for inhibition of adenylate cyclase. Thus epinephrine, an adrenergic agonist, has a relatively mild pressure-lowering effect in glaucoma. When administered with an antagonist, such as timolol or betaxolol, its action is much more marked.

Not all of the adrenergic receptors in the human intraocular musculature have been determined. Both the dilatator pupillae and sphincter pupillae muscles of the monkey eye contain mainly alpha-adrenergic receptors. Thus, stimulation of alpha receptors of the iris musculature produces antagonistic actions, but the larger number of receptors in the dilator muscle causes pupillary dilation. The trabecular meshwork contains mainly alpha receptors, and stimulation increases the facility of outflow. The ciliary epithelium contains mainly beta receptors. Both inhibition and stimulation decrease the secretion of aqueous humor.

Table 3-7. Ocular effects of autonomic drugs

	Effect on secretion	Effect on aqueous outflow	Effect on intraocular pressure	Accommodation (ciliary muscle)	Sphincter pupillae muscle	Dilator pupillae muscle
Cholinergic agonist	±	Increase	Decrease	Increase	Miosis	
Cholinergic antagonist	±	±		Decrease	Mydriasis	
Alpha-adrenergic agonist	±	±	Decrease			Mydriasis
Beta-adrenergic agonist	Decrease	±	Decrease			
Alpha-adrenergic antagonist	± *		Decrease			
Beta-adrenergic antagonist	± †	±	Decrease			Slight my-driasis

*Beta-adrenergic predominance.
†Alpha-adrenergic predominance.

Adrenergic stimulating compounds. Ophthalmic interest in these drugs is concerned with stimulation of alpha- and beta-adrenergic receptors by topical administration. Phenylephrine stimulates alpha receptors, isoproterenol stimulates beta receptors, and epinephrine stimulates both alpha and beta receptors (Table 3-7). The ocular effects (but not the systemic) are minimal after systemic administration.

Topical instillation of adrenergic-stimulating compounds causes (1) pupillary dilation, (2) increased facility of outflow of aqueous humor through the trabecular meshwork, (3) decreased secretion of aqueous humor by the ciliary epithelium, and (4) vasoconstriction of the conjunctival blood vessels.

Epinephrine. Epinephrine (adrenalin) is but slightly lipid soluble and penetrates the corneal epithelium poorly. In the treatment of glaucoma, 0.25% to 2% epinephrine is used to decrease aqueous humor production and to increase the outflow of aqueous humor through the trabecular meshwork. In glaucoma therapy, epinephrine is often combined with a cholinergic-stimulating drug such as pilocarpine or a beta blocker. In ocular hypertension, topical 1% epinephrine may be used without pilocarpine. In young patients in whom pilocarpine causes a spasm of the ciliary body, epinephrine is used alone or combined with timolol.

Pupillary dilation normally does not follow instillation of 1% solution. In denervation hypersensitivity, after the postganglionic sympathetic fibers to the dilatator pupillae muscle have been interrupted, a 0.1% solution will dilate the pupil.

In some individuals, epinephrine produces a black, localized, isolated, subepithelial deposit of adrenochrome in the conjunctiva or corneal epithelium. It is easily removed and may spontaneously peel off. After removal of the lens, topical administration may cause a cystoid macular edema that is reversible on stopping the drug.

Epinephrine conjugated with two pivalic acid groups yields dipivefrin (Propine), a compound that is 17 times more lipophilic than epinephrine. It easily penetrates the corneal epithelium and is converted to epinephrine by hydrolysis within the eye. It is used topically in a 0.1% solution in the treatment of open-angle glaucoma.

Norepinephrine. Norepinephrine (levarterenol) is not as potent when administered topically as it is at the postganglionic nerve terminal. It acts predominantly on alpha-adrenergic receptors and has a feeble effect on beta receptors. Experimental topical administration reduces intraocular pressure but causes severe hypertension in susceptible persons.

Isoproterenol. Isoproterenol (Isuprel) acts almost exclusively to stimulate beta receptors. Although it decreases aqueous humor secretion and reduces intraocular pressure about as effectively as epinephrine, topical application of a 5% solution causes tachycardia and palpitation. Unlike epinephrine, it does not constrict conjunctival blood vessels and is readily absorbed systemically.

Phenylephrine hydrochloride. Phenylephrine hydrochloride (Neo-Synephrine), an almost exclusive alpha receptor stimulator, is effective for pupillary dilation. It penetrates the cornea well and is commonly used to dilate the pupil for examination of the ocular fundus. Marked increase in blood pressure may occur in neonates of low weight, infants, and adults with orthostatic hypotension. Elderly patients have experienced syncope, myocardial infarction, tachycardia, cardiac arrhythmia, and fatal subarachnoid hemorrhage after instillation of a 2.5% solution. A single application of a 2.5% solution in each eye every hour is recommended by the manufacturer. In patients receiving monoamine oxidase inhibitors or tricyclic antidepressants that cause the effects of sympathetic denervation, there may be hypersensitivity to the alpha-adrenergic stimulation. Phenylephrine is sometimes used in combination with cholinergic-blocking agents to enhance pupillary dilation in the treatment of uveitis. It is available in 1% and 2.5% solutions.

Phenylephrine is the preferred agent for dilating the pupil to study the ocular fundus because it can be easily neutralized with cholinergic drugs. It may prevent the formation of cysts of the pupillary pigmented epithelium in children in whom anticholinesterase preparations are used to minimize accommodation in accommodative esotropia. It is often combined with 0.5% tropicamide for mydriasis.

Other adrenergic-stimulating drugs. Hydroxyamphetamine hydrobromide (Paredrine) and other amphetamines variably dilate the pupil when instilled into the conjunctival sac. Except for Paredrine, which is less effective than phenylephrine, they are not used in clinical ophthalmology.

Adrenergic neuron and receptor blockade

Adrenergic neuron–blocking agents inhibit the synthesis, storage, or release of norepinephrine at the presynaptic vesicle. Adrenergic receptor–blocking agents inhibit the action of norepinephrine and other sympathetic amines on alpha$_1$-, alpha$_2$-, beta$_1$-, and beta$_2$-adrenergic receptors. Additionally, blockade of adrenergic autonomic ganglia by ganglionic blockade decreases adrenergic stimulation as do central nervous system depressants.

Interference with the adrenergic nervous system may cause orthostatic hypotension, nasal stuffiness, diarrhea, and sodium retention. Some drugs cause pupillary constriction or dilation and decreased intraocular pressure.

Adrenergic neuron–blocking agents. The enzyme dopa decarboxylase catalyzes the synthesis of dopamine from dopa. Thus inhibition of dopa decarboxylase prevents formation of dopamine and subsequently norepinephrine.

Alpha-methyldopa (Aldomet) is converted by dopa decarboxylase to alpha-methyl norepinephrine, a "false neurotransmitter," and the systemic level of norepinephrine is reduced. Topical administration does not affect the intraocular pressure in experimental animals. Systemic administration reduces the arterial blood pressure, and there is a parallel but transient reduction in intraocular pressure.

Reserpine and guanethidine (Ismelin) interfere with the storage of catecholamine in presynaptic vesicles. These compounds cause an initial release of stored norepinephrine and thereafter prevent its uptake.

Reserpine, one of the alkaloids of rauwolfia serpentine, releases and inhibits the binding of norepinephrine in synaptic vesicles. It thus simulates the systemic effects of a sympathectomy. The tranquilizing effects are the result of a similar effect on serotonin binding. It slightly decreases intraocular pressure by an unknown mechanism.

Guanethidine (Ismelin) initially depletes norepinephrine in the nerve fiber, blocks its neuronal release, and blocks the reuptake of catecholamines by the axon. Additionally, it sensitizes adrenergic receptor sites. After depletion of the catecholamines, denervation hypersensitivity occurs. Guanethidine decreases eyelid retraction in Graves' disease. Combined with epinephrine it reduces intraocular pressure.

Adrenergic receptor–blocking agents. Agents that block adrenergic receptors are used mainly in the management of vascular hypertension, cardiac arrhythmias, and angina pectoris. Most members of the group block predominantly either alpha- or beta-adrenergic receptors.

Many compounds block alpha-adrenergic receptors and are available for clinical study. The main members of the group are phenoxybenzamine (Dibenzyline), ergot alkaloids, tolazoline (Priscoline), phentolamine mesylate (Regitine Mesylate), and Prazosin. Chlorpromazine, haloperidol, and many other neuroleptic drugs cause alpha blockade. Clonidine, an antihypertensive drug, is active in the central nervous system, possibly because of inhibition of alpha$_1$- or alpha$_2$-receptors in the lower brain stem. Dibenamine, which is similar to but less potent than phenoxybenzamine, has been used experimentally in the treatment of angle-closure glaucoma. Retrobulbar tolazoline causes vasodilation, particularly of the central retinal artery in retinal arterial occlusions.

Compounds that block both beta$_1$- and beta$_2$-adrenergic receptors (nonselective) reduce blood pressure and heart rate. The most widely used is propranolol (Inderal), a compound not used to decrease intraocular pressure because of its local anesthetic effect.

Timolol. Timolol is a beta$_1$- and beta$_2$-adrenergic receptor blocking agent (nonselective). It is widely used in chronic open-angle and aphakic secondary glaucoma. It is used topically in a concentration of either 0.25% or 0.5% and should never be used more than once every 12 hours. It decreases the formation of aqueous humor through the inhibition of either the synthesis of or the action of the adenyl cyclase of the nonpigmented epithelium of the ciliary body.

The pressure-lowering effect of timolol may be lost or decreased over a few days or several months of therapy. The most critical period is within the first 3 days of therapy when, after an initial decrease, the intraocular pressure increases, although rarely to the pretreatment level. Evaluation of timolol treatment after 2 weeks suggests its effectiveness during the subsequent 3 months when its action should again be evaluated.

Timolol and acetazolamide seem to provide additive effects in glaucoma, although both have similar effects in reducing aqueous humor formation. The ocular effects of timolol and epinephrine are poorly additive, although adding timolol to epinephrine therapy may substantially reduce intraocular pressure for several weeks. When patients have been receiving maximum therapy for glaucoma (typically a topical cholinergic agent, epinephrine, and an oral carbonic anhydrase inhibitor), the addition of timolol appears to have a pressure-lowering effect in about 75% of the eyes for more than 1 year.

Timolol may have serious side effects. It is contraindicated in bronchial asthma, severe chronic obstructive pulmonary disease, and sinus bradycardia and arterioventricular block. It may cause additive systemic effects in patients being treated with other beta-adrenergic blocking agents. There may be additive effects in patients receiving catecholamine-depleting drugs such as reserpine. Many side effects are those anticipated from systemic administration of beta blocking drugs. The twice-daily instillation must not be exceeded. Bradycardia is common, and postural hypotension with syncope may develop in elderly patients. Depression, fatigue, weakness, memory loss, and somnolence occur. Myasthenia gravis may be aggravated or become symptomatic. Superficial punctate keratopathy, keratitis sicca, and corneal anesthesia have been described.

Betaxolol, a cardioselective beta$_1$-adrenergic receptor blocking agent, reduces intraocular pressure in glaucoma patients. It is administered topically to the eye two times daily in a 0.5% solution. Nonselective beta-adrenergic blocking agents may aggravate obstructive pulmonary disease, but betaxolol has much lower potential for compromising pulmonary function. Studies are as yet underway, but betaxolol may be used in glaucoma with other pressure-lowering medications and may become more effective with long-term administration.

Denervation hypersensitivity

6-Hydroxydopamine destroys aderenergic presynaptic vesicles and chemically produces a sympathectomy. Its initial effect is a release of endogenous norepinephrine followed by destruction of adrenergic presynaptic vesicles. This inactivates the major pathway of norepinephrine reuptake by presynaptic nerves. The structure is thus more sensitive to exogenous catecholamine. Thus, in the Adie pupil, an abnormality that likely involves the ciliary ganglion or postganglionic cholingergic nerves, the pupil is constricted by the instillation of 0.1% pilocarpine, which does not affect the normal sphincter pupillae muscle—it normally constricts only with instillation of a 1% concentration.

If there is interference with the sympathetic pathway between the superior cervical ganglion and the dilatator pupillae muscle, as occurs in Horner syndrome, the pupil dilates on instillation of 0.1% epinephrine. This concentration has no effect on the normally innervated pupil.

PROSTAGLANDINS

Prostaglandins are a group of 20-carbon unsaturated fatty acids synthesized on demand by most cells. They act primarily as local tissue hormones. Synthesis begins with the release of stored arachidonic acid from cellular phospholipids, chiefly by the action of phospholipases. Cyclic oxygenases convert arachidonic acid to unstable cyclic endoperoxidases that are metabolized to tissue-specific end products: prostacyclin (PGI_2) for the vasculature; PGE_2 for transporting epithelia of the urinary and gastrointestinal tracts, and possibly the ciliary epithelium; and thromboxane A_2 (T_xA_2) for aggregating platelets and PGF_{2a}, a potent vasoconstrictor. They differ greatly in their biologic properties and are important in maintaining homeostasis and acting as agents of tissue defense by regulating metabolism, blood flow, and vascular permeability.

Corticosteroids prevent the release of stored arachidonic acid for prostaglandin synthesis by inhibiting phospholipase activity. Aspirin and indomethacin inhibit cyclic endoperoxidases and prevent the formation of endoperoxides causing decreasing prostaglandin and thromboxane synthesis. The cyclic oxygenase of platelets is inhibited for the life of the platelet. The vascular wall can regenerate cyclic oxygenase. Thus, in managing thromboembolic disease, the therapist aims to inhibit platelet aggregation without impairing prostacyclin synthesis by the vascular wall. Aspirin in a dose of not more than 200 mg every third day achieves this. Recurrent hyphema after blunt trauma to the eye may follow administration of oral aspirin.

Removal of the aqueous humor from the anterior chamber (paracentesis), stroking the iris, infrared radiation to the iris, and blunt ocular trauma (in the rabbit) cause local synthesis and release of prostaglandin. The ciliary processes are particularly active. There is a breakdown of the blood-aqueous barrier, with increased protein in the aqueous humor, prolonged constriction of the pupil, and ciliary injection. Aspirin or indomethacin inhibit this ocular response. Stimulation of beta-adrenergic receptors is linked in the chain of reactions that occur before release of stored tissue arachidonic acid.

An ocular response identical to that induced by prostaglandin release follows painful stimuli of the eye or stimulation of the trigeminal nerve. The response is a result of the release of substance P in the aqueous humor. Substance P when injected into the anterior chamber causes an intense miosis, but other irritative effects are dose-related. Substance P is a polypeptide also found in the gut and brain that may be a neurotransmitter.

9^Δ-TETRAHYDROCANNABINOL

Marijuana smoking reduces intraocular pressure in humans as does oral or intravenous administration of 9^Δ-tetrahydrocannabinol, its active principle. Additionally, smoking marijuana dilates conjunctival blood vessels and decreases tearing and the rate of blinking. The mode of action is unknown, but outflow of aqueous humor is increased in humans. Topical instillation of the compounds does not decrease intraocular pressure in humans. The decrease of tears with these compounds may cause contact lens wearers to have uncomfortable eyes and decreased wearing time.

CARBONIC ANHYDRASE INHIBITORS

Carbonic anhydrase is an enzyme that catalyzes the equilibrium between carbonic acid and carbon dioxide. The enzyme is widely distributed in (1) erythrocytes, where it functions in the exchange of carbon dioxide in capillaries; (2) the renal tubule cell, where it functions in the exchange of intracellular hydrogen for tubular sodium; (3) the epithelium of the ciliary body, where it functions in the secretion of aqueous humor; (4) the choroid plexus, where it functions in the secretion of cerebrospinal fluid; and (5) the gastric mucosa and the pancreas.

Inhibitors of carbonic anhydrase were synthesized after it was observed that the systemic administration of sulfonamides caused an acidosis because of loss of sodium bicarbonate to the urine and failure of the exchange of cellular hydrogen for tubular sodium. Despite the widespread distribution of carbonic anhydrase in the tissues of the body, the effects of enzyme inhibition are largely renal. Some of the agents, however, decrease secretion of aqueous humor and cerebrospinal fluid. Decreased secretion of aqueous humor occurs even in the absence of renal effects and is apparently the result of impaired secretion by the ciliary body.

Effective drugs in this group reduce the secretion of aqueous humor from 50% to 60%. There is a concomitant reduction in intraocular pressure. The most commonly used agent is acetazolamide (Diamox). Because of side effects, a number of other compounds have been substituted for acetazolamide.

Acetazolamide. Acetazolamide (Diamox) is the most widely used carbonic anhydrase inhibitor in ophthalmology. In patients with open-angle glaucoma the usual dosage is either 125 or 250 mg orally every 6 hours (not four times daily) or 250 or 500 mg every 12 hours in sustained-release tablets. The ocular effect is observed 1 to 2 hours after oral administration, and the maximum effect persists for 3 to 5 hours. It may be used intravenously in patients with angle-closure glaucoma. The secretion of aqueous humor is reduced but never stopped, and it is evident that only mechanisms of secretory activity involving carbonic anhydrase are concerned. A variety of side effects may occur. Myopia, blood dyscrasias, exfoliative dermatitis, and other reactions observed with sufonamide derivatives occur rarely. Paresthesia, with numbness and tingling in the extremities and mouth, and anorexia are common. There is a slight tendency to renal lithiasis, gout, and depression; confusion may occur in the elderly.

Ethoxzolamide (Cardrase), dichlorphenamide (Daranide), and methazolamide (Neptazane) are carbonic anhydrase inhibitors that may be substituted for acetazolamide. Their side effects are similar to those caused by acetazolamide, but occasionally one may be substituted to provide equal tension-decreasing effects and less patient discomfort.

OSMOTIC AGENTS

If the osmotic pressure of the blood is increased, fluid is drawn from the vitreous body, and the intraocular pressure is decreased. The increased osmotic pressure of the blood is usually maintained for only a short time, and within 4 to 6 hours the intraocular pressure returns to its previous level. Osmotic agents are used to decrease the intraocular pressure and volume for a relatively short period, as in the following: (1) in closed-angle glaucoma to reduce the intraocular pressure so the sphincter pupillae muscle will respond to miotics, (2) immediately before surgery to reduce intraocular pressure, (3) in retinal detachment surgery to reduce intraocular volume to aid in scleral wound closure, and (4) in orbital surgery to reduce orbital volume.

Mannitol. Mannitol is the alcohol of the sugar mannose and is pharmacologically inert. It is excreted by filtration through the renal glomeruli and is minimally reabsorbed by the tubules. It induces osmotic diuresis. Mannitol is administered intravenously in a 20% solution in a dose of 1.0 to 2.0 g/kg of body weight. Often 500 ml of a 20% solution is used in an average adult. Administration time is 3 to 60 minutes. Use before surgery usually requires urinary bladder catheterization because of diuresis. The maximum decrease in intraocular pressure occurs within 1 hour, and it returns to pretreatment levels after about 4 hours. The rapid expansion of extracellular fluid volume may cause cardiac decompensation in vulnerable persons. Hypersensitivity rarely occurs. Reduction of intracranial pressure may cause headache. It is contraindicated in cardiac decompensation and chronic obstructive lung disease.

Glycerol. Glycerol is a trivalent alcohol that contributes to glyceride and phosphatide molecules. It is metabolized to carbon dioxide and water by the tricarboxylic acid cycle. (Insulin is not required in its metabolism.) After oral administration of a 50% solution in lemon juice in doses of 1.0 to 1.8 g/kg of body weight, it decreases intraocular pressure within 30 to 60 minutes; pretreatment levels return within 4 to 5 hours.

Side effects are few. Usually headache does not occur, and diuresis is not marked. Nausea and vomiting may prevent its long-term use.

Topical glycerol does not reduce intraocular pressure but reduces corneal edema in glaucoma to make gonioscopy possible.

Isosorbide. Isosorbide (Ismotic) is a dihydric alcohol formed by the removal of two molecules of water from the glucitol (sorbitol) molecule. It is given orally in a 45% vanilla-mint solution. In oral dosage of 1.5 g/kg of body weight, the intraocular pressure reaches a minimal value 1 to 2 hours after administration and remains depressed for 5 to 6 hours.

Miscellaneous agents. Urea, ascorbate, ethanol, and sucrose produce an osmotic vitreous-blood gradient with reduction of intraocular pressure. Additionally, alcohol inhibits the antidiuretic hormone and induces diuresis. Ingestion of large amounts of ethanol 8 to 12 hours before examination may produce abnormally low tonometric values in glaucoma patients.

Dyes

Fluorescein is used topically to stain the stroma of the cornea (the Bowman zone has affinity for fluorescein). Sodium fluorescein is used topically in 0.25% to 2% alkaline solution. Because of the possibility of contamination with *Pseudomonas aeruginosa,* it should be instilled either from a single-dose container or by means of a strip of sterile filter paper saturated with dye. The dye is instilled in the conjunctival sac, and excess dye may be irrigated with sterile saline. The corneal stroma stains bright green in areas of disease or absent corneal epithelium. The intensity of stain is accentuated if 2% cocaine ophthalmic solution is instilled in the eye or if the eye is illuminated with a cobalt blue filter to stimulate fluorescence.

Fluorescein is instilled in the eye to demonstrate the dilution that occurs when anterior aqueous humor escapes from a postoperative fistula, a penetrating wound, or a conjunctival bleb following glaucoma filtration surgery. It is used to demonstrate areas of contact ("touch") between the lens and the cornea or sclera in the fitting of contact lenses. Applanation tonometry is based on the appearance of the fluorescein pattern when pressure is applied to the eye. The rate of disappearance of fluorescein through the nasolacrimal passages is used to estimate their patency.

Intravenous sodium fluorescein is combined with serial fundus photography to study the dynamics of the retinal circulation. Two to five ml of a 10% to 25% solution is injected rapidly into an arm vein, and fundus photographs are taken. Nausea may occur with the injection. Fluorescein is excreted in the urine for the next 24 to 48 hours (and prevents accurate urine testing for sugar). Anaphylactic reactions vary in severity from urticaria to shock. Coma, cardiac arrest, and myocardial infarction have been reported. The drug should not be used in individuals with a history of drug sensitivity. When angiography is performed, an emer-

gency tray and oxygen should be readily available. Administration of the fluorescein through an indwelling catheter permits the administration of drugs in the event a severe reaction should develop.

Systemic administration is followed by the appearance of fluorescein in the aqueous humor, a method of measuring aqueous flow. The concentration is increased in conditions in which the blood-ocular barriers are impaired. If fluorescein remains in contact with the surface of the globe, it enters the anterior chamber, and its disappearance rate can be used to gauge the rate of outflow of aqueous humor.

Rose bengal (1%) stains devitalized cells better than fluorescein, which has an affinity for the corneal stroma. The principal use of rose bengal is demarcation of devitalized conjunctival epithelium in keratoconjunctivitis sicca.

Both fluorescein and rose bengal stain soft contact lenses, which must be removed before instillation of the drugs.

Artificial tears. A deficiency of either the aqueous or mucin component of tears causes a drying of the conjunctiva and cornea. A deficiency of the aqueous component is seen in keratoconjunctivitis sicca while the mucin component is deficient in conditions that cause loss of goblet cells: chemical burns, Stevens-Johnson disease, hypovitaminosis A, and ocular cicatricial pemphigoid. A variety of artificial tear preparations are available. They are mainly composed of various polymers (methyl cellulose preparations, polyvinyl alcohol, and others) usually combined with a preservative. They have no pharmacologic action and may be instilled as often as necessary for comfort.

Emollients are used mainly at bedtime to protect the eyes from drying. They consist of various amounts of white petroleum combined with mineral oil, lanolin, and similar compounds. Their action is solely mechanical.

LOCAL ANESTHETICS

The small size of the eye and the accessibility of its nerve supply permits most adult ocular surgery to be done under local anesthesia. The conjunctiva and cornea are readily anesthetized by means of topically instilled agents, of which cocaine, the prototype, has been succeeded by tetracaine (Pontocaine, 0.5%), be-

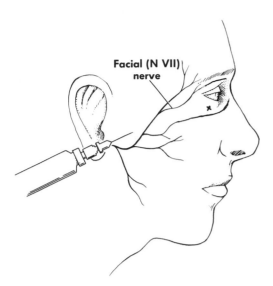

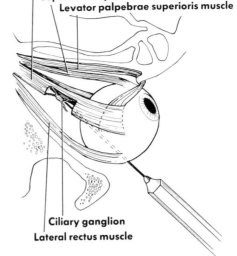

Fig. 3-4. Akinesia of the orbicularis oculi muscle by means of blocking the facial nerve in the preauricular region.

Fig. 3-5. Retrobulbar injection. The eye is adducted and rotated upward. The injection is made through the lower eyelid (X in Fig. 3-4).

noxinate (Dorsacaine, 0.4%), and proparacaine (Ophthaine, 0.5%). Sensory and motor paralysis is readily achieved with skillful infiltration of procaine (Novocaine), lidocaine (Xylocaine), or bupivacaine (Marcaine).

Topical anesthetics are used for procedures such as tonometry or removal of corneal foreign bodies. The severe pain of corneal abrasions, ultraviolet keratitis, and corneal foreign bodies is quickly relieved. Since these agents are potent sensitizers and delay corneal epithelization, they should not be prescribed for analgesia.

Infiltration anesthesia is used mainly in the region of the eyelids for the excision of local lesions. Both motor and sensory block follow injection of the anesthetic agent in the region of the orbital portion of the orbicularis oculi muscle (van Lint technique) to prevent eyelid closure in intraocular surgery.

Blockade of the eyelid musculature is provided by infiltrating fibers of the temporal branch of the seventh nerve as they pass anterior to the temporomandibular articulation (O'Brien technique) (Fig. 3-4). Blockade of the motor nerve supply to the extraocular muscles and sensory block of the nerve supply to the globe follow the retrobulbar injection of anesthetic solution posterior to the globe in the region between the lateral rectus muscle and optic nerve (Fig. 3-5). This blocks the nerve supply to all of the extraocular muscles except the superior oblique muscle; it blocks the ciliary ganglion so the pupil dilates; and it anesthetizes the entire globe. Other sensory blocks follow injections of the anesthetic agents in the region of the supratrochlear and infratrochlear nerves at the superior medial angle of the orbit; the infraorbital nerve, either in its orbital course or as it emerges through the infraorbital foramen to the face; and the lacrimal and zygomaticofacial nerves as they exit from their respective foramina.

Epinephrine (1:100,000) prolongs anesthesia by inducing vasoconstriction in the injected area with slower absorption. Therefore it is contraindicated in patients with coronary artery disease or thyrotoxicosis and in halothane anesthesia.

Hyaluronidase enhances the dispersion and absorption of local anesthesia. The increased dispersion makes possible a more effective motor block. The more rapid absorption limits the effective duration of the local anesthetic.

ANTI-INFECTIVE AGENTS

Several factors modify the use of anti-infective agents in ocular infections. Frequent local instillations of antibiotics or sulfonamides provide unusually high concentrations in the superficial tissue. Compounds that have severe adverse effects when administered systemically often may be useful when instilled locally. Heavy metals such as zinc sulfate are still used in astringent eyedrops, and silver nitrate is used in the prophylaxis of gonorrheal ophthalmia.

Many compounds instilled in the conjunctival sac cause either an allergic or irritative contact dermatoconjunctivitis. Prolonged use of antibiotics combined with corticosteroids predisposes to superinfection, particularly with fungi. A fungal invader must be considered in any persistent conjunctival or corneal inflammation. Local anti-infective agents are diluted rapidly by tears, and they must be instilled at 1- or 2-hour intervals to ensure adequate local tissue concentration.

The blood-ocular barriers limit the penetration of many anti-infective agents into the eye from the systemic circulation. Intraocular inflammation impairs the blood-ocular barriers so that increased amounts of antibiotics enter the eye from the blood. When an infection and inflammation begin to subside, the blood-ocular barriers regain their integrity, although viable microorganisms may persist in the eye. Therefore drug dosage should not be reduced until the intraocular fluids are definitely free of organisms.

Injection of the anti-infective agent into the subconjunctival space, sub-Tenon space, or retrobulbarly is generally limited to those instances in which high local concentration is required. Intraocular injection of antibiotics is limited to endophthalmitis in which the damage that may be caused by the agent is balanced by the damage caused by the disease.

Sulfisoxazole and sulfacetamide are the most useful sulfonamides for topical therapy. These two agents rarely cause local hypersensitivity. Their action is inhibited by pus. The penicillins, cephalosporins, and streptomycin cause hypersensitivity reactions so frequently that topical application is contraindicated. Systemic sulfonamides are useful in trachoma and inclu-

sion conjunctivitis. They are used as an adjunct to pyrimethamine in systemic toxoplasmosis.

Preoperatively, gentamicin, Neosporin, or erythromycin are often used topically to reduce the bacterial content of the conjunctiva. Some surgeons inject subconjunctivally gentamicin, carbenicillin, chloramphenicol, or aqueous penicillin combined with streptomycin at the time of surgery so that the aqueous humor of secondary formation will contain a high concentration of antibiotics. Alternatively, an antibiotic such as ampicillin may be administered before surgery so that it enters the eye in a high concentration when the blood-aqueous barrier is damaged by the opening of the anterior chamber.

Effective management of central corneal ulcers, orbital cellulitis, and endophthalmitis requires prompt diagnosis and treatment. Initial treatment is based on the Gram stain of organisms or smear and the presumable cause. Often a pencillinase-resistant penicillin, such as methicillin or nafcillin, is combined with a beta-lactamase-resistant third generation cephalosporin (cefoperazone, moxolactam, cefotaxime) or combined with gentamicin or chloramphenicol. Intravenous, subconjunctival, topical, and sometimes intravitreal routes may be used. Specific antibiotics are used after a microbial cause is identified.

Antibiotics

Antibiotics are compounds produced by some microorganisms or prepared synthetically that in dilute solutions suppress the growth (bacteriostatic) or destroy (bactericidal) other microorganisms. They are effective through one of several mechanisms. They may (1) inhibit biosynthesis of bacterial cell walls or activate enzymes that destroy them (penicillins, cephalosporins, bacitracin, vancomycin, ristocetin, and cycloserine); (2) affect bacterial ribosomes to inhibit protein synthesis (tetracyclines, chloramphenicol, erythromycin, lincomycin, and clindamycin); (3) alter cell wall permeability with leakage of intracellular contents (polymyxins, colsitimethate, nystatin, and amphotericin B); (4) bind 30 s ribosome subunits with accumulation of synthetic protein initiation complexes that are misread by the mRNA code (gentamicin, tobramycin, amikacin, kanamycin, streptomycin, and neomycin); (5) inhibit DNA-dependent RNA polymerase (rifampin); and (6) block specific metabolic steps (trimethoprim, sulfonamides, and antivirals).

Drugs that are primarily effective against gram-positive cocci and bacilli include penicillin G, semi-synthetic pencillinase-resistant penicillins, bacitracin, erythromycin, lincomycin, vancomycin, and clindamycin. Drugs that are primarily effective against the aerobic gram-negative bacilli include kanamycin, streptomycin, and neomycin. Relatively broad-spectrum drugs that are effective against gram-positive cocci and gram-negative bacilli include broad-spectrum penicillins (ampicillin, amoxicillin, carbencillin, carbencillin indanyl, ticarcillin, and piperacillin), tetracyclines, cephalosporins, chloramphenicol, trimethoprim, and sulfonamides.

The use of antibiotics is complicated by bacterial resistance, hypersensitivity reactions, toxicity, alteration of normal microorganismal flora, peripheral neuritis, and hematologic complications. Staphylococcic penicillinase hydrolyzes the antibiotic. The beta-lactamases of many gram-negative bacteria inactivate the penicillins. In some instances, spontaneous mutations cause enzymatic changes that permit microbial resistance. Many gram-negative bacteria contain a resistance transfer factor that may transmit resistance to other bacteria.

Cutaneous hypersensitivity varies in severity from contact dermatitis to purpura, erythema multiforme, and exfoliative dermatitis. Systemic hypersensitivity may be manifested by fever, serum sickness, and (rarely) anaphylactic shock (mainly with penicillin).

Renal toxicity may be produced by a variety of antibiotics (cephaloridine, neomycin, colistin, gentamicin, tobramycin, kanamycin, vancomycin, and amphotericin). Eighth nerve damage has occurred after administration of streptomycin, vancomycin, kanamycin, neomycin, and gentamicin. Renal impairment with decreased excretion may cause exceptionally high levels of these agents in the blood.

Alteration of normal bacterial flora is particularly common after the use of tetracyclines. Topical antibiotics and corticosteroids are a factor in superinfection of the cornea with fungi. Systemic administration may be associated with overgrowth of *Candida albicans* in the mouth, pharynx, and bowel, and there may be tetracycline-resistant *Proteus, Pseudomonas*, and *Staphylococcus* organisms in the bowel. Tetracyclines stain developing teeth and are contraindicated before emergence of second dentition and in pregnant and nursing women.

Failures with the use of antimicrobial agents result from (1) use in conditions not caused by microorganisms; (2) failure to identify causative organism and to use an appropriate antimicrobial agent in proper dosage; (3) use in conditions caused by organisms not susceptible to agents; (4) continued use after bacterial resistance has developed, toxic or allergic reactions have developed, or superinfection has occurred; and (5) use of improper combinations.

Penicillins. Penicillins may be divided into those prepared by fermentation and those synthesized by conjugation of various side chains to 6-amino-penicillinic acid obtained from penicillin fermentation media. They impair bacterial cell wall synthesis in those organisms accessible to the penicillin agent. Their use is governed by three main disadvantages: (1) degradation by gastric acid so that many cannot be used orally, (2) destruction of some by the enzyme beta-lactamase and (3) relatively high incidence of hypersensitivity reactions. One group of the semi-synthetic penicillins (methicillin, oxacillin, nafcillin, cloxacillin) resists the action of beta-lactamase and is used mainly in the treatment of infections by penicillinase-producing staphylococci. Penicillins are secreted out of the eye by the ciliary epithelium and do not cross the intact blood-aqueous or blood-retina barrier. Semisynthetic penicillins are bound to protein in serum and are not free to cross the blood-aqueous barrier. Methicillin and ampicillin are the least protein-bound.

All of the penicillins cause hypersensitivity reactions that may range in severity from urticaria to anaphylaxis to delayed hypersensitivity reactions. The penicillins are all cross-reactive, and a patient sensitive to one will be sensitive to other penicillins although not always to the same extent. Patients are more sensitive to the natural penicillins than to the semisynthetic derivatives.

Penicillin G is the penicillin of choice in the treatment of syphilis and infections caused by streptococci (including the pneumococci), meningococci, gonococci, anthrax, and actinomycetes. It is available in a crystalline form for intramuscular or intravenous use and in a repository form (procaine penicillin G or penicillin G benzathine). Penicillin V may be given orally.

The beta-lactamase (penicillinase) resistant penicillins available for parenteral use include methicillin, oxacillin, cloxacillin, dicloxacillin, floxacillin, and nafcillin. Cloxacillin is absorbed well after oral administration, whereas nafcillin has variable absorption after oral administration. Oxacillin and nafcillin are most active, but methicillin is less bound to serum protein so that more of the drug may be available to enter the eye. Methicillin may cause reversible bone marrow depression and interstitial nephritis. In severe systemic infection, such as orbital cellulitis, a combination of antibiotics provides broad-spectrum coverage pending identification and susceptibility testing of the microbe.

In hospitals where methicillin-resistant strains of *Staphylococcus aureus* are prevalent, vancomycin or vancomycin and rifampin may be substituted.

Ampicillin and amoxicillin are not penicillinase resistant but are active against *Haemophilus influenzae*, *Proteus mirabilis*, and *Neisseria* species. Amoxicillin may be combined with a beta-lactamase inhibitor to extend its activity. Some *H. influenzae* are resistant to ampicillin, and in life-threatening conditions chloramphenicol is substituted. Carbenicillin, carbenicillin indanyl, and ticarcillin are active against the same organisms and *Pseudomonas* species, *Enterobacter* species, and indole-positive *Proteus*. Azlocillin is active against *Pseudomonas* species of *Klebsiella*. Gentamicin, which is also used in *Pseudomonas* infections, should never be mixed in the same bottle with carbenicillin, which inactivates aminoglycosides.

A history of adverse reactions to penicillin may be more important than the results of various tests to anticipate allergic reactions. Skin testing may be hazardous, but test material is available to learn if anaphylactic-type allergy is present. If the results are positive, penicillin should be used cautiously, if at all. Additionally, there may be cross allergy to the penicillins and the cephalosporins.

Cephalosporins. A number of cephalosporins classified mainly by "generations" are available for systemic use. The first generation—cephalothin (Keflin) and cefazolin (Ancef and Kefazol), cephalexin (Keflex), and others—have good activity against gram-positive bacteria and modest activity against gram-negative microorganisms. They are not active against enterococci, methicillin-resistant *Staphylococcus aureus* and *Staphylococcus epidermidis*.

Second generation cephalosporins—cefamandole (Mandol), cefoxitin (Mefoxin), and others—have more activity against gram-negative organisms than do first gneration cephalosporins, but are much less active than third generation cephalosporins.

Third generation cephalosporins—cefotaxime (Claforan), moxalactam (Moxam), and others—are exceptionally active against gram-negative organisms.

Cephalosporins are often drugs of choice for patients sensitive to penicillin, although they too may cause sensitivity reactions and cross-reactions with penicillin. Cephalosporins may cause a positive Coombs test for erythrocyte antibodies. Concurrent administration of cephalothin (Keflin) and gentamicin or tobramicin synergistically cause nephrotoxicity.

Cephalosporins are effective systemic therapeutic and prophylactic agents. Many pass the blood-ocular barriers and are used in the treatment of endophthalmitis. First generation cephalosporins are used prophylactically before and after intraocular surgery. Third generation cephalosporins may be useful in infections caused by nosocomial infections by organisms resistant to first generation cephalosporins, ampicillin, and some aminoglycosides.

Aminoglycosides. This group of antibiotics includes gentamicin, neomycin, tobramycin, amikacin, kanamycin, debekacin, netilmicin, and streptomycin. They act on the bacterial ribosomes of aerobic gram-negative organisms. They are poorly absorbed after oral administration, do not penetrate the blood ocular barrier, and may cause auditory nerve (VIII) and renal toxicity. Gentamicin- and tobramycin-resistant strains of *Enterobacter*, *Klebsiella*, *Proteus*, and *Pseudomonas*, particularly in burn units and intensive care units, limit their usefulness. Netilmicin may be active against such organisms.

Gentamicin. Gentamicin is bactericidal against most strains of *Pseudomonas, Klebsiella, Aerobacter, Proteus, Staphylococcus,* and *Escherichia coli.* It is used topically in ophthalmology in a 0.3% solution or ointment.

Tobramycin. Tobramycin has a bactericidal activity similar to gentamicin but it is more active against many, though not all, strains of *Pseudomonas aeruginosa* than gentamicin. It should be used concurrently with an anti-pseudomonal cephalosporin for ocular *Pseudomonas* infection. It is used in a 3 mg/ml concentration as an eyedrop.

Neomycin. Neomycin is bactericidal against staphylococci and gram-negative bacteria, but not most *Pseudomonas* species. It is widely used topically in ophthalmology, often combined with polymyxin B. Localized hypersensitivity occurs frequently (8%) and may be masked by corticosteroid given concurrently.

Tetracyclines. The tetracyclines are bacteriostatic agents that inhibit microbial ribosomal protein synthesis in a broad range of gram-negative and gram-positive bacteria. Additionally, they are active against *Rickettsia, Mycoplasma, Chlamydia,* some atypical mycobacteria, and protozoa. They are the preferred agents in chlamydial infections. In patients intolerant of penicillin, tetracyclines may be used to treat syphilis. *Pseudomonas, Proteus,* and many strains of *Staphylococcus* are resistant to tetracyclines. A number of compounds are available.

In general, tetracycline (Achromycin) and oxytetracyline (Terramycin) are the least effective, while doxycycline (Vibramycin) and minocycline (Minocin) are the most effective. Milk, antacids containing aluminum, magnesium hydroxide or silicate, and iron impair gastrointestinal absorption. The compounds penetrate the intact blood-ocular barriers poorly. Resistant strains develop during therapy. After suppression of susceptible microflora, an overgrowth of resistant organisms may cause a superinfection. Declomycin and Vibramycin may cause mild to severe erythema in the skin of individuals exposed to sunlight.

Tetracyclines are usually administered orally and may cause nausea, vomiting, and diarrhea. Outdated tetracycline may cause reversible renal tubular dysfunction indistinguishable from the Fanconi syndrome. Developing, unerupted teeth may be discolored. The compounds should not be given to pregnant women or before the eruption of all secondary dentition. Demeclocycline causes photosensitivity in some individuals. Pseudotumor cerebri may occur in adults. All potentiate the effects of dicumarol-type anticoagulants. A number of tetracyclines are available for topical use.

Miscellaneous antibiotics. The most valuable members of this group are chloramphenicol, erythromycin, bacitracin, clindamycin, and vancomycin.

Chloramphenicol. Chloramphenicol (Chloromycetin) is a potent inhibitor of microbial protein synthesis. It blocks the polypeptide linkage and messenger RNA-ribosome complex. It has a wide spectrum of bacteriostatic activity that includes gram-negative bacteria, all anaerobic bacteria, gram-positive cocci, *Clostridium* species, and gram-negative rods. It is rapidly and completely absorbed from the gastrointestinal tract and is not impaired by simultaneous administration of food or antacids. It penetrates well into all tissues, including the brain, cerebrospinal fluid, and aqueous humor. High intraocular concentrations follow systemic administration.

Bone marrow toxicity restricts the use of systemic chloramphenicol to life-threatening infections for which no other antimicrobial drug is as effective. Aplasia of the bone marrow with fatal pancytopenia may be an idiosyncratic reaction with a genetic predisposition. It occurs more commonly in individuals who have repeated exposure to the drug or who undergo prolonged therapy. Dose-related bone marrow suppression regularly occurs with large dosage, prolonged treatment, or both. Persistent bone marrow hypoplasia has been reported after prolonged use of chloramphenicol eyedrops or ointment.

Peripheral neuritis, retrobulbar neuritis, and acute encephalopathy have been reported. Patients with cystic fibrosis who receive long-term parenteral chloramphenicol may develop optic atrophy secondary to optic neuritis.

Erythromycin. This is a systemic well-tolerated antibiotic used particularly in the treatment of streptococcal infections, syphilis, and the prophylactic treatment of rheumatic fever in patients sensitive to the penicillins. In children it is used topically and systemically against infection caused by *Chlamydia trachomatis*. Oleandomycin, carbomycin, spiramycin, and ristocetin have antibacterial spectra similar to erythromycin.

Bacitracin. Bacitracin has an antibacterial spectrum similar to penicillin with which it is markedly synergistic. Bacterial resistance is rare and its potency is not reduced by blood or pus. It is used topically in an ointment or solution particularly in the treatment of staphylococcal blepharoconjunctivitis. It is often combined with neomycin and polymyxin in topical preparations. Bacitracin causes hypersensitivity but rarely.

Clindamycin. Clindamycin is active against gram-positive cocci and gram-positive and gram-negative anaerobic pathogens except *Clostridium* species. It is used orally coupled with sulfadiazine in the treatment of active toxoplasmosis retinochoroiditis. It frequently causes diarrhea and, in some patients, a severe pseudomembranous colitis (antibiotic-associated colitis). The drug must be stopped at once.

Vancomycin. Vancomycin is highly effective against gram-positive cocci. It is used intravenously in severe staphylococcal infections and endocarditis when the causative agent is resistant to the usual antibiotics. It is synergistic with gentamicin or tobramycin. It is locally irritating and causes thrombophlebitis and (in large doses) ototoxicity and nephrotoxicity. It is used orally in antibiotic-associated colitis and diarrheas.

Sulfonamides

The sulfonamides are bacteriostatic agents that prevent susceptible microorganisms from synthesizing folic acid from para-aminobenzoic acid by substrate competition. They act against a variety of gram-positive and gram-negative bacteria. Sulfonamides have a limited usefulness in ophthalmology as topical agents. When resistance develops to one sulfonamide, then cross-resistance to all derivatives is observed. Similarly, cross-sensitivity occurs, and therefore no sulfonamide is safe once a patient demonstrates a hypersensitivity reaction to any derivative.

Most sulfonamides are nearly insoluble and do not provide therapeutic concentrations when used locally. Two compounds are used locally in ophthalmology: sulfacetamide (Sulamyd) and sulfisoxazole (Gantrisin).

Sulfacetamide. Sulfacetamide (Sulamyd) is used in 10% and 30% solutions and 10% ointment. It is the most useful of the sulfonamide compounds for local use. It is minimally antigenetic, and hypersensitivity reactions are rarely observed.

Sulfisoxazole. Sulfisoxazole (Gantrisin) is used locally in a 4% solution. A white precipitate of the drug may gather at the canthus. Other sulfonamides should not be used topically.

Corticosteroid combinations

A variety of antibiotics for topical use are combined with corticosteroids for the treatment of conjunctival and eyelid infections. The antibiotic-corticosteroid preparations are used for the treatment of (1) mixed staphylococcal marginal blepharitis, (2) blepharoconjunctivities with primary or secondary replicating organisms, (3) marginal corneal ulcers related to staphylococcal infection, and (4) postsurgical trauma.

Such combinations are often contraindicated. The corticosteroids reduce local tissue immunity and induce increased resistance to the outflow of aqueous, which may lead to glaucoma in susceptible eyes. The combination may facilitate the development of a fungal keratoconjunctivitis. Fixed combinations do not permit the administration of the two drugs in different concentrations or at different time intervals. The effects of the antibiotic on the microorganism may also be obscured by the anti-inflammatory action of the corticosteroid.

Virus chemotherapy

Effective chemotherapy of ocular virus disease is concerned mainly with keratitis caused by herpes simplex virus type 1 and, uncommonly, type 2. Vidarabine, trifluorothymidine, and acyclovir are equally effective in topical administration for epithelial keratitis. With stromal infection, trifluorothymidine is more effective than vidarabine or acyclovir. Idoxuridine, the initial topical agent used for herpes keratitis, is therapeutically inferior to all.

Vidarabine (adenosine arabinoside, Ara-A, Vira-A). Vidarabine is a purine nucleoside analog with antiviral activity against several DNA viruses, such as herpes simplex virus types 1 and 2, varicella-zoster virus, and cytomegalovirus. It inhibits DNA-dependent DNA polymerases of DNA viruses 40 times more than host cells. It is incorporated into the terminal positions of herpes virus DNA and prevents completion of the chain. It is relatively insoluble and penetrates the cornea poorly. Herpes simplex epithelial keratitis is treated with a 3% ophthalmic ointment applied topically every three hours. Topical therapy of stromal herpes is not practical with vidarabine because the cornea deaminates the compound.

Trifluorothymidine (F_3T, trifluridine, Viroptic). Trifluorothymidine is a synthetic fluorated pyrimadine that inhibits viral DNA synthesis more than cellular DNA synthesis. It penetrates the cornea well and is effective in a 1% ophthalmic solution in stromal infections and in patients resistant to topical vidarabine and acyclovir. It penetrates the aqueous humor well and is used systemically in herpesvirus iritis.

Acyclovir (Zovirax). Acyclovir is a synthetic nucleoside analog with a high degree of specificity against herpes simplex 1 and 2 and varicella-zoster viruses. Cells infected with herpesvirus code for a specific viral thymidine kinase that phosphorylate acyclovir, which in turn inhibits viral DNA polymerases. Acyclovir is relatively nontoxic, but thymidine-kinase deficient mutants have developed. It is not effective against latent infections, since the virus is not replicating.

Acyclovir is effective topically against epithelial herpes. It has excellent corneal penetration and attains therapeutic levels when applied topically. It is not effective against stromal herpes, possibly because the lesion is not the result of virus replication. Oral acyclovir is effective in the treatment of genital herpes, recurrent mucocutaneous herpes in the immunologically impaired host, and varicella-zoster infections.

Dihydroxy propoxymethyl guanine is an investigational nucleoside analog similar to acyclovir that completely inhibits viral DNA polymerase. It has in vitro activity against the cytomegalic virus that is 30-fold greater than that of acyclovir in cytomegalovirus retinitis in patients with AIDS or immunosuppression from chemotherapy. Therapy with the compound results in the disappearance of the virus from the bloodstream and, in some patients, resolution of the virus retinitis. There is relapse within a short time after stopping therapy in patients with AIDS. Possibly continuous therapy is necessary.

Idoxuridine (Herplex, Stoxil). Idoxuridine is the first clinically effective nucleoside. Structurally it resembles thymidine and is incorporated into viral DNA during DNA synthesis. A faulty DNA results that cannot produce virus particles. It penetrates the stroma poorly and is used solely in epithelial keratitis.

Oculomycosis chemotherapy

Antifungal drugs (Table 3-8) work as fungistatic and not as fungicidal agents, and their

Table 3-8. Principal agents used in ocular and systemic fungal infections

Drug	Route	Principal mycoses affected in vivo
Polyenic macrolides		
Tetraenes		
Nystatin	Oral, topical	*Candida*
Natamycin	Topical	*Candida, Aspergillus, Fusarium*
Heptaenes		
Amphotericin B	Oral, intravenous, intrathecal (irritating topically)	Deep mycoses (candidiasis, cryptococcosis, histoplasmosis, coccidioidomycosis, aspergillosis)
Imidazole derivations		
Ketoconazole	Oral	Candidiasis, coccidioidomycosis
Miconazole	Topical, intravenous, oral, subconjunctival	Cryptococcosis, coccidioidomycosis, paracoccidioidomycosis
5-Fluorocytosine	Oral, intravenous	Candidiasis, cryptococcosis, aspergillosis, chromomycosis, cladosporiosis
Chemical agents		
Sulfonamides	Oral	Paracoccidioidomycosis, histoplasmosis, actinomycotic mycetoma

penetration into tissues is poor. Fungi, as vegetables, grow slowly and persistently. The object of treatment is to inhibit growth over a long period until the host's immune mechanism excludes the fungus. The drugs used in therapy may damage tissues. Often antifungal chemotherapy is combined with removal of infected tissue by vitrectomy or keratoplasty. Debilitation, trauma, corticosteroid therapy, or immunosuppression may each limit the effectiveness of chemotherapy.

Three groups of agents are used in antifungal therapy: (1) polyenes (amphotericin B, nystatin, natamycin [pimaricin]); (2) imidazoles (ketoconazole, miconazole); and (3) pyrimidines (5-flucytosine).

Amphotericin B. Amphotericin B disrupts the cellular mechanisms and inhibits *Histoplasma capsulatum*, *Blastomyces dermatitidis*, *Coccidioides immitis*, *Cryptococcus neoformans*, *Candida albicans* and other *Candida* species, *Torulopsis glabrata*, *Aspergillus fumigatus*, and other species of *Aspergillus*, *Spinthrix*, *Schenckii*, and *Mucor* species. Treatment with amphotericin B is often hazardous, and most patients develop an azotemia necessitating reduction of dosage or cessation of treatment. It is used topically (0.1% solution) in the treatment of some fungal ulcers (Table 3-9).

Nystatin (Mycostatin). Nystatin is administered topically in a concentration of 100,000 units/ml of commerical diluent in demonstrated fungus infections of the anterior ocular segment. Its main value is in the treatment of superficial *Candida* infection, and it is ineffective in cutaneous dermatophyte infections. It is not absorbed from the gastrointestinal tract, and its toxicity is such that it cannot be used intrave-nously. It is insoluble in saline solution and is administered as a suspension.

Natamycin (Pimaricin). This drug is used topically as a 5% suspension in propylene glycol or as an ointment. It has a fairly broad spectrum and is more useful in superficial fungus infections than amphotericin B. Systemically it may be administered orally in doses of 400 mg daily. Doses in excess of this cause diarrhea and vomiting. It is effective against *Fusarium solani*.

Flucytosine. 5-Flucytosine is related to 5-fluorouracil, to which it is converted within cells of sensitive fungi. It has a narrow spectrum of activity, which includes mainly strains of *Cryptococcus neoformans*, various *Candida* species, and rarely *Aspergillus* species. It penetrates the aqueous humor well. It is recommended as an adjunct to treatment with amphotericin B.

Ketoconazole (Nizoral). Ketoconazole inhibits the synthesis of ergosterol by the cell membrane of susceptible fungi. It is active by oral administration against most dermatophytes, *Candida* species, *B dermatitidis*, *H capsulatum*, *P brasiliensis*, and *P boydii*. It is used orally in a dosage of 200 to 400 mg at mealtime. The concentration in the central nervous system and presumably in ocular tissues is low.

Miconazole (Monistat). Miconazole is an imidazole with a broad spectrum of activity against gram-positive bacteria and many fungi. In low doses it is fungistatic, while in high doses it is fungicidal. It is well tolerated topically and subconjunctivally.

Heavy metals

Mercuric salts are used locally to inhibit sulfhydril enzymes. Nitromersol (Metaphen) is

Table 3-9. Concentration of especially prepared antifungal agents used in ophthalmology

	Topical instillation	Subconjunctival injection	Intravitreal
Amphotericin B	2.5-10 mg/ml (water or 5% dextrose solution)	750 mg/ml	5-10 µg
Nystatin	100,000 units/g ointment		
Pimaricin (Natamycin)	50 mg/ml suspension		
Flucytosine	10 mg/ml		
Miconazole	10 mg/ml		

used in a 1:2,500 ointment in the conjunctival sac. Thimerosal (Merthiolate) is used as an antiseptic and as a preservative in eye products. It commonly causes hypersensitivity reactions. Silver nitrate is used as a 1% solution in Credé prophylaxis of ophthalmia neonatorum and to treat superior limbic keratoconjunctivitis. It precipitates proteins, including those of microbes, and reacts with the sodium chloride of tissues to form insoluble silver chloride. Silver protein preparations are seldom used. Zinc sulfate has been used to treat conjunctivitis caused by the diplobacillus of Morax-Axenfeld (*Haemophilus*), but antibiotics are superior. Zinc sulfate is used as an astringent in many collyria and nonspecific over-the-counter eye preparations.

MAST CELL INHIBITION

Cromolyn sodium. Disodium cromolate is thought to prevent calcium transport across mast cell membranes and thereby to inhibit the release of IgE mediators of immediate hypersensitivity (histamine, serotonin, slow-reactive substance of anaphylaxis, and eosinophil chemotactic factor). A 4% solution is used topically four to six times a day in the treatment of atopic disease of the conjunctiva (vernal keratoconjunctivitis, giant papillary conjunctivitis, and allergic keratoconjunctivitis).

IMMUNOSUPPRESSIVE AGENTS

Cyclosporine. Cyclosporine inhibits the activities of both B and T lymphocytes. Its predominant effect is interference with the release of interleukin-2 that stimulates the initiation of DNA synthesis in antigen-activated helper and cytotoxic T cells. Cyclosporine does not grossly interfere with activation of antigen-specific suppressor T cells. It appears to induce a nephrotoxicity. This may be reversible if the drug is stopped prior to severe structural and functional changes. Low doses may minimize or prevent changes. It has been used in uveitis and corneal transplant rejection when other immunosuppressives have failed.

CORTICOSTEROIDS

The adrenal gland consists of the medulla and the cortex. The medulla secretes mostly epinephrine and a small amount of norepineph-

rine. In response to stimulation by the adrenocorticotropic hormone (ACTH), the adrenal cortex synthesizes three types of steroids: (1) the androgenic steroids, which are important in the development of secondary sex characteristics; (2) the mineralocorticosteroids, mainly aldosterone and desoxycorticosterone, which partake of fluid and electrolyte metabolism, the secretion of which is largely independent of ACTH; and (3) the glucocorticosteroids, cortisol and corticosterone, which act on the metabolism of carbohydrates, proteins, fats, electrolytes, and water. The glucocorticosteroids are strongly anti-inflammatory, inhibit the manifestation of cell-mediated immunity in humans, and stabilize lysosomal enzymes.

Corticosteroids are mainly effective in suppressing the manifestations of inflammation without affecting its cause. Thus the drugs are most useful in self-limited or intermittent disease processes by decreasing inflammation until remission occurs. Relatively high doses and long-term administration may be required to suppress inflamation. Long-term systemic administration is associated with numerous side effects that limit their usefulness. Ocular complications may be seen following topical, retrobulbar, or systemic administration of the compounds.

The most common ocular complication of topical administration is secondary open-angle glaucoma, which may cause loss of vision combined with typical excavation of the optic disk and visual field defects. Posterior subcapsular cataracts may occur after topical administration, but they are more common in patients with connective tissue disorders who receive systemic corticosteroids for a long period. Patients with rheumatoid arthritis are particularly prone to cataract formation. Cataracts rarely occur in patients with ulcerative colitis or asthma who receive similar doses. Retrobulbar administration of corticosteroids may cause progression of toxoplasmosis retinochoroiditis after initial improvement.

Local tissue immunity restricts most herpes simplex inflammation of the cornea to the corneal epithelium. Topical corticosteroids reduce local tissue immunity, and the virus infects additional epithelium and may cause stromal necrosis. The anti-inflammatory effect of the corticosteroids is such that the eye is less injected and more comfortable. Unwittingly the patient may use excessive amounts of corticosteroid, which results in eventual rupture of the cornea.

Fungus infections of the cornea were rare until the widespread use of topical corticosteroids combined with antibiotics. A mycotic infection must be suspected in any corneal ulceration that persists after long-term treatment with these compounds.

Topical instillation of corticosteroids impairs wound healing by delaying fibroblastic regeneration. After systemic administration, the local tissue concentration is usually inadequate to interfere with wound healing. The abdominal striae seen in Cushing disease are evidence that systemic corticosteroids impair wound healing. Topical corticosteroids in small amounts after cataract extraction and corneal transplant do not appear to affect wound healing adversely. Topical corticosteroids may also cause a mild blepharoptosis and pupillary dilation.

Long-term systemic administration may suppress immunity to *Candida* species, toxoplasmosis, cytomegalic inclusion, and *Herpesvirus hominis*. These organisms may cause widespread intraocular inflammation, necrotizing angiitis, and loss of vision. Similar disorders after immunosuppression are seen in the course of Hodgkin disease, lymphatic leukemia, AIDS, and tumor radiation therapy.

Considerable caution must be exercised in the treatment of ocular disorders with corticosteroids for a long period. A maintenance dose of 200 mg or less of prednisone every other morning does not seem to have as serious side effects as daily administration. Side effects associated with long-term corticosteroid administration include peptic ulcer, perforation of the stomach and intestine, gastrointestinal hemorrhage, osteoporosis, psychosis, nitrogen depletion, diabetes mellitus, myopathy, sodium retention with edema, vascular hypertension, potassium depletion, and avascular bone necrosis. Side effects also include gain in weight, fat distribution of the Cushingoid type, acne, hirsutism, amenorrhea, cutaneous striae, and increased tendency to bruise. Retinal microaneurysms as well as papilledema have been described.

CHELATING AGENTS

Chelating agents form complexes with heavy metals and reverse their binding to body tissues. Those of ophthalmic interest include edathamil, deferoxamine, and penicillamine.

Edathamil (Ethylenediaminetetraacetate [EDTA]). The calcium in band keratopathy or alkalis may be removed from the cornea by bathing in 1.7% (0.05 M) disodium EDTA for 15 to 20 minutes. The corneal epithelium must be removed initially, since EDTA does not penetrate.

Deferoxamine. Deferoxamine (desferrioxamine mesylate) is specific for iron and may remove corneal rust stains. It is applied topically in a 10% solution in methylcellulose. Deferoxamine is not effective in the removal of blood staining the cornea.

Penicillamine. Penicillamine chelates copper, mercury, zinc, and lead and promotes their excretion in the urine. It is well absorbed in the intestinal tract and is used in the treatment of hepaticolenticular degeneration and rheumatoid arthritis. Additionally, systemic penicillamine is valuable in the therapy of scleromalacia perforans. In rheumatoid arthritis, but not in Wilson disease, penicillamine may enhance the severity of an underlying autoimmune disorder such as myasthenia gravis.

COMPLICATIONS OF TOPICAL ADMINISTRATION OF DRUGS

A surprising number of ocular conditions are either induced, persistent, or aggravated because of overtreatment with drugs used locally. Inasmuch as many eye diseases are self-limiting, there is no indication for the local instillation of medication in the absence of exact diagnosis.

Mechanical injury. Patients and attendants instilling medications into the eye by means of an eyedropper or squeeze bottle should be instructed to place the long axis parallel to the eyelid margin so that if the patient lunges forward, the tip of the dropper will not strike the eye. Patients should be reassured that the conjunctival sac holds but a single drop and the exact measurement of a single drop is not necessary because the excess medication overflows. Because medications are costly, patients should be taught how to instill them correctly.

Pigmentation. Prolonged instillation of various compounds may cause pigmentation of the conjunctiva and the eyelids. Repeated instillation of silver preparations causes argyrosis. Metallic silver is deposited in the conjunctiva, particularly in the fornices, where it causes a slate-gray color. Microscopically, it results from minute, closely packed dots of gray-black matter of metallic silver. There is no effective treatment.

Mercury preparations such as ammoniated mercury or yellow oxide of mercury may cause a similar type of pigmentation from mercury deposition after long use.

Epinephrine used locally may cause a black pigmentation of the eyelid margins that looks like eye makeup. More common is a sharply defined, rounded black area of adrenochrome pigmentation caused by the oxidation of epinephrine to adrenochrome in the conjunctiva or cornea. There are no symptoms, and the deposits may be wiped off.

Ocular injury. Many compounds may cause direct ocular injury on instillation. Silver nitrate in concentrations greater than 5% may cause necrosis of the cornea. To be assured of using only 1% silver nitrate in Credé prophylaxis, one should use the wax ampules distributed for this purpose. Physicians who cauterize granulation tissue with silver nitrate find silver nitrate sticks safer than strong solutions.

Many compounds may cause punctuate defects of the corneal epithelium, which result in a foreign body sensation. Compounds that denature the protein of the corneal epithelium, such as ethanol and benzalkonium chloride (Zephiran), are common offenders. These may be brought to the eye on instruments used for minor ocular surgery. Local anesthetics are often dispensed in a stronger solution for use on nasal and oral mucous membranes rather than for the eye. Instillation of these stronger solutions may cause a white precipitate in the superficial corneal epithelium; the precipitate usually disappears when irrigated with distilled water.

Cocaine solutions are markedly hypotonic to the tears and cause desiccation of the corneal epithelium, which may then be removed easily. Cocaine is an excellent local anesthetic, and its use in surgery is sometimes desirable because it produces local vasoconstriction and moderate dilation of the pupil.

Sensitivity reactions. The skin of the eyelids and the conjunctiva may be the locus of atopic inflammation (type I hypersensitivity) or the site of cell-mediated (type IV) hypersensitivity reactions. Any drug or cosmetic that is repeatedly applied to the ocular tissues (or any other tissue) may be the causative agent.

Delay of corneal epithelization. Small defects in the cornea heal by sliding of adjacent epithelium; large defects heal by mitosis and sliding of adjacent epithelium. Many of the compounds used in ocular therapeutics delay mitosis but have no effect on epithelial sliding. Local anesthetics delay wound healing markedly.

Pupillary constriction. Drugs that constrict the pupil may cause minor and major symptoms. The extreme miosis produced by the organophosphates combined with edema of the ciliary body may cause closed-angle glaucoma in susceptible individuals. Extreme miosis has been considered a cause of retinal detachement because of traction by the zonular fibers that insert into the anterior retina.

Constriction of the pupil in patients with minor lens opacities may impair vision.

The use of beta-receptor blockers instead of miotics allows useful vision in many patients with minor cataract and glaucoma. Miotics are used in children for the treatment of accomodative esotropia and may cause pupillary cysts. Instillation of 2.5% phenylephrine immediately after instillation of the miotic prevents the cysts. Contraction of the ciliary muscle in young individuals after instillation of a miotic causes an accommodative spasm. In children in whom miotics are used in the treatment of accommodative strabismus, cysts may form at the pupillary margin involving the pigmented epithelium. The use of phenylephrine immediately following the instillation of the miotic prevents the development of cysts. In young individuals, spasm of accommodation occurs with compounds that cause miosis and may result in a severe myopia.

Systemic reactions to local instillation. Atropine, pilocarpine, phenylephrine, and timolol may be absorbed through the conjunctiva or pass through the lacrimal passages to be absorbed by the nasal mucous membranes. They may cause characteristic pharmacologic actions because a single eyedrop (0.15 µl) may exceed the systemic therapeutic dose (Table 3-10). Commercial eyedroppers and squeeze bottles deliver between 50 and 75 µl, which is two to

Table 3-10. Therapeutic dose of eye medications

	Dose	
Medication	1 drop (0.15 µl)	Therapeutic systemic dose
1% atropine	1.5 mg	0.6 mg
4% pilocarpine	6.0 mg	5.0 mg
0.25% echothiophate iodide (Phospholine Iodide)	0.375 mg	Too toxic for systemic therapy
2.5% phenylephrine	3.75 mg	5.0 (IM)

seven times more than the cul-de-sac can hold. Systemic absorption can be minimized by having the patient close the eyes and compress the lacrimal puncta with a finger for 2 minutes after instillation.

Drugs should be prevented from entering the nasolacrimal duct by maintaining pressure over the inner corner of the closed eyelids for 2 minutes after instillation. Atropine and scopolamine are often administered either in an oily solution or in an ointment to minimize systemic absorption. Even though this is done, systemic absorption from the conjunctiva and anterior chamber may cause toxicity.

Atropine poisoning develops quickly, causing agitated behavior, hallucinations, and disorientation. The mouth is dry, and speech and swallowing are difficult. The pupils are dilated and accommodation is paralyzed. The skin is dry, red, and hot, and body temperature increases. Treatment is symptomatic: stop the medication and reduce the fever with ice packs or sponging. A cholinergic drug, such as physostigmine, may provide more prompt relief.

Cyclopentolate hydrochloride (Cyclogel) may cause hallucinations, dysarthria, ataxia, and temporary behavioral changes suggestive of schizophrenia. The 0.5% solution should be used in infants and small children.

Timolol, a nonselective beta-adrenergic receptor blocking agent is the most widely used anti-glaucoma drug in the United States. It should be instilled no more than twice daily. It is contraindicated in bronchial asthma, severe chronic pulmonary disease, and in nursing mothers. It blocks exercise tachycardia and may lead to cardiac failure. Impotence, personality disorders, depression, muscle fatigue, and aggravation of myasthenia gravis have been described. Betaxolol, a selective beta-receptor blocker, may be used in many patients with reactive pulmonary disease and not aggravate symptoms.

Pilocarpine toxicity may occur after frequent instillation of the drug in patients with closed-angle glaucoma. Some patients are exceptionally sensitive and develop gastrointestinal overactivity and sweating when given small doses. More severe signs include salivation, nausea, tremor, bradycardia, and decreased blood pressure.

Anticholinesterase agents, particularly the organophosphates, significantly depress the erythrocyte cholinesterase levels. Systemic absorption may cause diarrhea, abdominal cramps, and the signs and symptoms of an acute abdominal or other gastrointestinal disturbance. On occasion, these signs have led to unnecessary laparotomy. Children receiving these compounds, particularly echothiophate iodide (Phospholine Iodide), may become irritable and cross; their behavior problems result from chronic cholinesterase poisoning. Children with Down syndrome are particularly sensitive to echothiophate iodide. Patients using organophosphates should be advised to inform their other physicians of the drug they are using. The use of succinylcholine during general anesthesia in a cholinesterase-depleted individual may lead to prolonged apnea.

Phenylephrine is widely used as a nasal decongestant (0.125% to 0.5%), as a mydriatic (2.5%), and in some vasoconstrictor eyedrops. It is a powerful postsynaptic alpha-receptor agonist and increases systolic and diastolic pressure. Cerebrovascular accidents and cardiac arrhythmia with extra systole occur. There may be the sensitivity of denervation in individuals with alpha-adrenergic blockade.

OCULAR REACTIONS TO SYSTEMIC ADMINISTRATION OF DRUGS

The eye may be involved in a variety of reactions resulting from the systemic administration of drugs. Occasionally, ocular reactions do not occur in experimental animals, and severe eye lesions may be produced before the relationship between the eye abnormality and the drug is suspected.

Alcohol. Alcohol intoxication causes nystagmus, esophoria, and diplopia. Intraocular pressure decreases chiefly through alcohol diuresis. Alcohol amblyopia is a vitamin B deficiency commonly associated with a peripheral neuritis and may cause a toxic optic neuropathy (see Chapter 18). Vision is reduced, and there are cecocentral scotomas. Adequate diet and large doses of vitamin B correct the condition even though alcoholism continues.

Accidental ingestion of methanol causes a severe acidosis, nausea, vomiting, abdominal pain, failing vision, and coma. Those who recover from the coma may have no light perception. These patients initially have edema of the optic nerve and surrounding retina followed by severe optic atrophy. The acidosis must be corrected with alkalyzing therapy. Renal dialysis removes methanol from the blood, and large doses of systemic ethanol compete successfully with methanol for metabolic sites.

Most central nervous system depressants may cause muscle weakness along with diplopia and, on occasion, blurred vision. In some instances, these compounds aggravate preexisting ocular defects or cause nystagmus. The ocular signs are usually reversible after reduced intake of the medication.

Chloroquine. Chloroquine is an antimalarial agent commonly used for the treatment of lupus erythematosus, arthritis, and other connective tissue disorders. Prolonged administration of high doses may cause keratopathy, myopathy, or retinopathy. Generally, the total chloroquine dose must exceed 100 g, and the drug must be used for more than a year before a retinopathy develops. The drug may be retained in the body for years after its use has been discontinued, and the retinopathy may develop several years later.

Chloroquine keratopathy is a reversible deposition of chloroquine in the cornea. Minute whitish dots distributed in a whorl pattern can be observed with the slit lamp. Patients complain of "glare," ill-defined blurring of vision, and irridescent vision, the halo surrounding lights being identical to that in glaucoma. The condition is entirely reversible on discontinuation of the drug, and it may disappear spontaneously even if the drug is continued.

Chloroquine retinopathy is a severe pigmentary degeneration of the retina that may progress to blindness. Initially there is a minute degree of pigment clumping in the central retinal area. A characteristic "bull's eye" or "doughnut" retinal lesion develops that may be incomplete. This is followed by stippling or hyperpigmentation of the fovea centralis, surrounded by a clear zone of depigmentation, which in turn is circled by another ring of pigment. In the end stages there is widespread retinal atrophy, pigment clumping, and threadlike retinal vessels.

Quinine. Quinine in excessive doses has long been known to cause damage to the retinal ganglion cells and associated constriction of the retinal arterioles. Idiosyncratic reactions may follow administration of even minute amounts of quinine (as little as that contained in quinine water), and constriction of the visual field to a central area 5° to 10° in diameter may also occur. There may be associated deafness and other signs of central nervous system damage. Quinine is often mixed with heroin, and drug users may develop typical quinine poisoning. The abnormality is usually reversible, but continued ingestion of quinine may cause irreversible constriction of the visual fields, impaired dark adaptation, and loss of visual acuity.

In rare instances severe atrophy of the pigment epithelium of the iris may follow quinine amblyopia. The pupils do not react to light in the area of iris atrophy. The condition is presumably caused by ischemia of the anterior uvea.

Ethambutol. Ethambutol is an oral chemotherapeutic agent widely used in therapy of pulmonary tuberculosis. The main ocular complication of long-term use is an optic neuropathy that occurs in about 2% of those treated. Visual acuity should be measured before treatment is started and then monthly during the first months of treatment. Patients must be alerted to note any loss of vision. The optic neuropathy causes reduced visual acuity and color vision as well as a central scotoma. The neuropathy is reversible when the drug is discontinued, and vision improves over a period of weeks. After recovery, the use of the drug may be reinstituted without immediate recurrence of the optic neuropathy.

Digitalis. Digitalis toxicity may be associated with disturbed vision in which objects may appear to be covered with frost or have a pale yellow color or in which flashing lights may be present. Usually, visual symptoms are associated with nausea, vomiting, and bradycardia at high dosage levels, but they may occur in patients using the drug in a therapeutic range. A similar xanthopsia has been attributed to systemic effects of chlorothiazide and also to aspidium (male fern).

Oral contraceptives. The agents most commonly used for oral contraceptive therapy are progesterone and estrogen in combination or in sequence. These may cause occlusive vascular disease in susceptible patients. Women who smoke or who have vascular hypertension, migraine, or vascular disease are thought to be especially vulnerable. Brain infarction may be associated with ocular signs, depending on the area of the brain involved. Papilledema and optic neuropathy appear to occur more commonly in women using contraceptive therapy than in others. Retinal hemorrahages may be seen. The indications for using oral contraceptives must be carefully weighed. A patient should not receive them for long periods without medical supervision. They should be discontinued in the event of thromboembolic disease, neurologic disease, or suggestion of liver damage.

Some contact lens wearers develop an intolerance to the contact lenses while taking oral contraceptives. Often this is characterized by photophobia, increased irritation caused by the contact lenses, and prolonged recovery from the corneal edema that may occur when wearing the contact lenses.

Induced refractive errors. Drugs may increase the refractive power of the eye by one of three mechanisms: (1) sustained contraction (spasm) of the ciliary muscle, causing increased refractivity of the lens; (2) increased refractive power of the lens contents as the result of water imbibition; and (3) swelling of the ciliary processes, causing forward displacement of the lens. The sulfonamides and related compounds,

particularly acetazolamide (Diamox), may cause edema of the ciliary processes. All of the anticholinesterase compounds may cause ciliary spasm and miosis. Many insecticides are anticholinesterases, and spasm of accommodation combined with pupillary constriction has been described. Increased refractive power of the lens or sustained accommodation reduces hyperopia or increases myopia.

The ganglionic-blocking agents used in the treatment of vascular hypertension decrease accommodation that many patients in the younger age groups find extremely annoying. There may be dilation of the conjunctival blood vessels, giving the appearance of conjunctivitis. The loss of accommodation may have to be corrected by means of bifocal lenses. The conjunctival injection may be alleviated slightly by local instillation of a vasoconstrictor, such as 1:1000 epinephrine.

Optic atrophy. Many compounds have been reported to cause optic atrophy. These include chloramphenicol, streptomycin, sulfonamides, and isoniazid. Tryparsamide, a pentavalent arsenical previously used in the therapy of central nervous system syphilis, has a direct toxic effect on the optic nerve.

Vitamin A. Vitamin A (retinol) and its naturally occurring relatives, retinaldehyde (retinal) and retinoic acid, are members of a class of over 1500 naturally occurring and synthetic compounds, the retinoids. Vitamin A is required for vision, reproduction, mucous secretion, and maintenance of differentiated epithelia. Different retinoids exhibit some, but not necessarily all, of the biologic activities of vitamin A. All-*trans*-retinoic acid supports normal growth and epithelium but cannot replace vitamin A as a visual pigment precursor and will not support reproduction.

The major natural sources of vitamin A are dietary plant carotenoid pigments, such as β-carotene, and retinyl esters in meat. They are converted to retinol in the intestine.

Vitamin A deficiency, usually in association with general malnutrition, is a leading cause of blindness in many underdeveloped countries. The array of signs and symptoms grouped under the term xerophthalmia progress from night blindness (XN) to conjunctival xerosis (XIA), Bitot spots (X1B) to corneal xerosis (X2), and finally to keratomalacia (X3). Hypovitaminosis A in developed countries usually reflects inadequate absorption as the result of small bowel surgery, malnutrition, particularly alcoholism, or a dietary faddism. Low serum retinol may be associated with an increased risk of cancer.

Prolonged intake of dietary carotenes may lead to yellowing of the skin and conjunctiva that resembles jaundice. Chronic intake of 10 to 20 times more vitamin A than required may lead to increased intracranial pressure (with headache, nausea, and papilledema), skeletal pain, and mucocutaneous signs. Isotretinoin, a retinoid, is used in the treatment of cystic acne. Papilledema may develop, particularly when combined with tetracyclines.

All-*trans*-retinoic acid ointment in concentrations of .01% to 0.1% (weight/weight) has been instilled one to three times daily in patients with conjunctival squamous metaplasia. Treatment minimized symptoms and reversed squamous metaplasia in patients with keratoconjunctivitis sicca, Stevens-Johnson syndrome, ocular cicatricial pemphigoid and drug-induced pseudopemphigoid, and surgical- or radiation-induced dry eye. The treatment is experimental and is still being evaluated.

Rifampin. Persons who use systemic rifampin, which is used in the treatment of tuberculosis and in pharyngeal carriers of *Neisseria* meningitis, may have (5% to 14%) orange, light pink, or red tears. The tears may stain contact lenses or cause a painful exudative conjunctivitis or blepharoconjunctivitis.

BIBLIOGRAPHY
General

Ellis, P.P.: Ocular therapeutics and pharmacology, ed. 7, St. Louis, 1985, The C.V. Mosby Co.

Fraunfelder, F.T.: Drug-induced ocular side effects and drug interactions, ed. 2, Philadelphia, 1982, Lea & Febiger.

Fraunfelder, F.T., Roy, F.H., and Meyer, S.M.: Current ocular therapy, Philadelphia, 1985, W.B. Saunders Co.

Gilman, A.G., Goodman, L.S., Rall, T.W., and Murad, F., editors: Goodman and Gilman's the pharmacological basis of therapeutics, ed. 7, New York, 1985, Macmillan Publishing Co.

Grant, W.M.: Toxicology of the eye, ed. 2, Springfield, Ill., 1974, Charles C Thomas, Publisher.

Havener, W.H.: Ocular pharmacology, ed. 4, St. Louis, 1983, The C.V. Mosby Co.

Sears, M.L., editor: Pharmacology of the eye (handbook of experimental pharmacology, vol. 69), New York, 1984, Springer-Verlag.

Sears, M.L., and Tarkkanen, A., editors: Surgical pharmacology of the eye, New York, 1985, Raven Press.

Tripathi, R.C., and Tripathi, B.J.: The eye. In Riddell, R.H., editor: Pathology of drug-induced and toxic diseases, New York, 1982, Churchill Livingstone.

Autonomic nervous system

Bensinger, R.E., Keates, E.U., Gofman, J.D., Novack, G.D., and Duzman, E.: Levobunolol, Arch. Ophthalmol. **103**:375, 1985.

Berry, D.P., Jr., Van Buskirk, E.M., and Shields, M.B.: Betaxolol and timolol: a comparison of efficacy and side effects, Arch. Ophthalmol. **102**:42, 1984.

Feghali, J.G., and Kaufman, P.L.: Decreased intraocular pressure in the hypertensive human eye with betaxolol, a β_1-adrenergic antagonist, Am. J. Ophthalmol. **100**:777, 1985.

Mellanby, J.: Comparative activities of tetanus and botulinum toxins, Neuroscience **11**:29, 1984.

Reiss, G.R., and Brubaker, R.F.: The mechanism of betaxolol, a new ocular hypotensive agent, Ophthalmology **90**:1369, 1983.

Spiritus, E.M., and Casciara, R.: Effects of topical betaxolol, timolol, and placebo on pulmonary function in asthmatic bronchitis, Am. J. Ophthalmol. **100**:492, 1985 (correspondence).

Zimmerman, T.J., Baumann, J.D., and Hetherington, J.R.: Side effects of timolol, Surv. Ophthalmol. **28**(suppl.):243, 1983.

Anesthetics

Bruce, R.A., Jr., McGoldrick, K.E., and Oppenheimer, P.: Anesthesia for Ophthalmology, Birmingham, 1982, Aesculapius.

Chin, G.N., and Almquist, H.T.: Bupivacaine and lidocaine rebrobulbar anesthesia: a double-blind clinical study, Ophthalmology **90**:369, 1983.

Anti-infectives

Fedukowicz, H.B., and Stenson, S.: External infections of the eye: bacterial, viral, mycotic with noninfectious and immunologic diseases, ed. 3, Norwalk, Conn., 1985, Appleton-Century-Crofts.

Handbook of antimirobial therapy, New Rochelle, N.Y., 1985, The Medical Letter.

Hermans, P.E., and Keys, T.F.: Antifungal agents used for deep-seated mycotic infections, Mayo Clin. Proc. **58**:223, 1983.

Hirsch, M.S., and Schooley, R.T.: Treatment of herpesvirus infections. Pt. 1 and 2, N. Engl. J. Med. **309**:963, 1034, 1983.

Jeffries, D.J.: Clinical use of acyclovir, Br. Med. J. **290:**177, 1985.

Johnson, A.P., Scoper, S.V., Woo, F.L., Caldwell, D.R., and George, W.J.: Azlocillin levels in human tears and aqueous humor, Am. J. Ophthalmol. **99:**469, 1985.

Leopold, I.H., editor: Anti-infective agents. In Pharmacology of the eye, vol. 69, Berlin, 1984, Springer-Verlag.

Leopold, I.H.: Update on antibiotics in ocular infections, Am. J. Ophthalmol. **100:**134, 1985.

Palestine, A.G., Stevens, G., Jr., Lane, H.C., Masur, H., Fujikawa, L.S., Nussenblatt, R.B., Rook, A.H., Manischewitz, J., Baird, B., Megill, M., Quinnan, G., Gelmann, E., and Fauci, A.S.: Treatment of cytomegalovirus retinitis with dihydroxy propoxymethyl guanine, Am. J. Ophthalmol. **101:**95, 1986.

Salamon, S.M.: Tetracyclines in ophthalmology, Surv. Ophthalmol. **29:**265, 1985.

Sanitato, J.J., Asbell, P.A., Varnell, E.D., Kissling, G.E., and Kaufman, H.E.: Acyclovir in the treatment of herpetic stromal disease, Am. J. Ophthalmol. **98:**537, 1984.

Strom, T.B., and Loertscher, R.: Cyclosporine-induced nephrotoxicity: inevitable and intractable? N. Engl. J. Med. **311:**728, 1984.

Torres, M., Mohamed, J., Cavazos-Adame, H., and Martinez, L.A.: Topical ketoconazole for fungal keratitis, Am. J. Ophthalmol. **100:**293, 1985.

Van Voris, L.P.: Antiviral chemotherapy. In Belshe, R.B., editor: Textbook of human virology, Littleton, Mass., 1984, PSG Publishing Co.

Washington, J.A., II, and Wilson, W.R.: Erythromycin: a microbial and clinical perspective after 30 years of clinical use (second of two parts), Mayo Clin. Proc. **60:**271, 1985.

Carbonic anhydrase inhibitors

Fraunfelder, F.T., Meyer, S.M., Bagby, G.C., Jr., and Dreis, M.W.: Hematologic reactions to carbonic anhydrase inhibitors, Am. J. Ophthalmol. **100:**79, 1985.

Shrader, C.E., Thomas, J.V., and Simmons, R.J.: Relationship of patient age and tolerance to carbonic anhydrase inhibitors, Am. J. Ophthalmol. **96:**730, 1983.

Smith, J.P., Weeks, R.H., Newland, E.F., and Ward, R.L.: Betaxolol and acetazolamide, Arch. Ophthalmol. **102:**1794, 1984.

Vitamin A

Fraunfelder, F.T., LaBraico, J.M., and Meyer, S.M.: Adverse ocular reactions possibly associated with isotretinoin, Am. J. Ophthalmol. **100:**534, 1985.

Goodman, D.S.: Vitamin A and retinoids in health and disease, N. Engl. J. Med. **310:**1023, 1984.

Sommer, A.: Effects of vitamin A deficiency on the ocular surface, Ophthalmology **90:**592, 1983.

Sommer, A.: Nutritional blindness: xerophthalmia and keratomalacia, New York, 1982, Oxford University Press.

Tseng, S.C.G., Maumenee, A.E., Stark, W.J., Maumenee, I.H., Jensen, A.D., Green, W.R., and Kenyon, K.R.: Topical retinoid treatment for various dry-eye disorders, Ophthalmology **92:**717, 1985.

PART TWO

HISTORY TAKING AND EXAMINATION OF THE EYE

4

HISTORY AND INTERPRETATION

All well-trained practitioners, whatever their specialty, should be able to examine the eye quickly and be assured that the eyes do not cross, the pupils are equal and constrict to light, the visual fields are intact, and the optic disk is not swollen or atrophic.

Some elementary principles should reassure the practitioner (see boxed text). Faulty glasses may blur vision and cause discomfort but cannot harm the eyes. The eyes are meant to be used, and there is no way that they can be worn out by use. Reading in dim light may be difficult and uncomfortable and may cause headache, but this does not harm the eyes. The distance at which material is held has no effect on the eyes, although it may be related to discomfort. Headache is usually not caused by the eyes, and certainly organic types of headaches, such as migraine, cluster headaches, and other specific types, never originate from the eyes.

There are a number of important recommendations. Any child who has an eye that constantly crosses after 6 months of age requires specialized examination with pupillary dilation. There should be no delay because the child is not old enough to cooperate in the examination. An enlarged eye or persistent tearing in an infant requires immediate attention. A vari-

---

SOME ELEMENTARY PRINCIPLES OF EYE CARE

Reading in dim light does not harm eyes.
Excessive use of eyes does not harm them, and "bad eyes" are not the result of overuse.
Sitting too close to television does not harm eyes.
Too strong, too weak, or wrongly ground glasses do not harm eyes.
Contact lenses neutralize refractive errors but do not eliminate them.
The eyes clean themselves. Healthy eyes do not require eyedrops.
Organic headaches such as migraine and cluster headaches do not occur because of eyestrain.
Healthy eyes do not require annual examination.
An eye with open-angle glaucoma does not look abnormal.
Cataract extraction is indicated only if the opacity interferes with activities.
Persistent watering of an infant's eye suggests either congenital glaucoma or blocked tear
    duct.
Chemicals in the eye must be diluted with water immediately.

ety of symptoms signal the need for immediate attention (see boxed text).

The eye is a remarkably sturdy organ. The pupil constricts when excess light enters it. Thus sunglasses may make vision more comfortable, but no harm comes from not wearing them. Similarly, tears function so efficiently that it is not necessary to use eyedrops. Once it has been determined that a pair of eyes are healthy, annual examinations are not necessary unless symptoms such as severe pain in the eyes, loss of vision, double vision, or sudden showers of floaters occur.

Contact lenses neutralize refractive errors but do not eliminate them. Contact lenses may change the shape of the eye temporarily so that there may be a period in which vision seems to have been improved by the contact lens. Without the contact lens, the eye gradually reverts to its original shape and vision. The conjunctiva prevents contact lenses from getting behind the eye.

With age, each person loses accommodation (presbyopia). Those who were myopic (nearsighted) before the onset of presbyopia will be able to read without glasses, even though presbyopic. Similarly, if an individual develops a nuclear sclerosis (cataract), there may be a period of being able to see near work without corrective lenses.

A cataract is located behind the pupil and develops in nearly everyone. The indication for its extraction is the effect of the impaired vision on the normal activities of the individual. Because the lens is located behind the iris, it is not peeled off but is surgically removed.

Eyes with open-angle glaucoma, a common cause of visual loss, do not appear to be abnormal. There is no way of diagnosing open-angle glaucoma without measuring the intraocular pressure, although in advanced glaucoma the characteristic excavation of the optic disk (cupping) will indicate the cause.

Visual impairment refers to limitation of one or more basic functions of the eye: visual acuity, dark adaptation, color vision, or peripheral vision. Visual disability refers to inability of an individual to perform specific visual tasks, such as reading, writing, orientation, or traveling unaided. Visual disability is a socioeconomic indication of an individual's capacity to perform

---

IMPORTANT SIGNS AND SYMPTOMS OF OCULAR DISEASE DEMANDING IMMEDIATE OPHTHALMIC EVALUATION

Sudden loss of vision
Flashes of light (lightning streaks) before the eyes
Sudden occurrence of strings, spots, or shadows before eyes
Colored rays or circles surrounding lights (halos)
Double vision
Intermittent dimming of vision
Marked difference in vision between the two eyes
Pain in the eyes
Redness, discharge, crusting, or excessive tearing of the eye
Curtain or veil blocking vision
Swelling, tumor, or mass of the eyelids, conjunctiva, eyeball, or orbit
Difference in size of the eyes
Wandering or turning of the eye (strabismus)
Jerky movements of the eye (nystagmus)
Diabetes mellitus

---

particular tasks. Visual handicap refers to a decrease in the physical, social, and economic function of an individual.

The main symptoms of ocular abnormality include (1) disturbances of vision, (2) pain in one or both eyes or in the head, and (3) abnormal secretion from the eyes.

DISTURBANCES OF VISION

An abnormality of visual function may include decreased central or peripheral vision, deficient color vision, or faulty adaptation to light or dark (Table 4-1). Even if these functions are normal, a patient may complain of abnormal perception that may originate in the eye, its central connections, or in the higher cortical or motor centers.

Visual defects may originate because of (1) a defect in formation of a clear image on the retina; (2) an abnormality in retinal processing of the image; (3) an interference with impulse transmission between the retina and occipital cortex; or (4) abnormal visual perceptual cen-

Table 4-1. Abnormalities of vision

A. Decreased visual acuity
   1. Near
   2. Distance
B. Abnormal color vision
   1. Hereditary: bilateral
   2. Acquired: often unilateral
C. Abnormal visual field
   1. Unilateral asymmetric defects in retinal and optic nerve diseases
   2. Bilateral symmetric defects in diseases at or posterior to chiasm
D. Defective dark adaptation
E. Iridescent vision ("halos")
F. Floaters
G. Photopsia
   1. Unilateral: retinal stimulus other than light
   2. Bilateral: visual hallucination
      a. Unformed: occipital lobe origin
      b. Formed: temporal lobe origin
H. Objects appear smaller (micropsia) or larger (macropsia) than they actually are
   1. Fovea centralis abnormality
I. Cortical blindness: bilateral lesions of occipital cortex
J. Perceptual blindness: lesions of angular gyrus of parieto-occipital fissure
K. Diplopia (double vision)
   1. Physiologic
   2. Monocular: local disturbance of one eye
   3. Near only: convergence abnormality
   4. Distance only: divergence abnormality
   5. Varying with eye or head movements: ocular muscle weakness

ters with faulty processing by the brain. A defect in image formation is caused by an abnormality within the eye itself. One or both eyes may be affected, but often one eye is affected more severely.

The cause is a refractive error and not organic disease if vision is corrected to normal with lenses or improved with a pinhole. Formation of a clear retinal image requires a clear cornea, lens, and vitreous (the ocular media).

The sensory retina must be intact, must line the interior of the eye regularly, and be in contact with the retinal pigment epithelium throughout. Its blood supply from the choriocapillaris and retinal vasculature must be intact. Photoreceptors must signal changes in light intensity (adaptation) and wavelength (color) correctly.

The nerve impulse generated in the photoreceptor must be processed correctly by the inner retina and transmitted from the retina to the brain. If transmission of the impulse is interrupted in the retina or optic nerve, only one eye is involved. Interference at the optic chiasm or posterior to the chiasm affects both eyes.

Visual perceptual defects often produce bizarre patterns or inability to recognize or describe objects.

The physician must learn, therefore, whether the defect involves one or both eyes, if it is corrected with lenses, and if it involves distance or near vision, or both. Additionally, the physician must determine if the visual loss is transient or permanent, if it involves central or peripheral vision, and if the vision itself is normal with visual phenomena such as floaters superimposed. If the visual defect disappears when the patient wears corrective lenses, then a refractive error is the most likely cause of symptoms. There are many people who require corrective lenses but do not wear them. They describe a variety of unusual, apparently inexplicable ocular symptoms, all of which would be relieved by corrective lenses. Attempts to provide relief by other means are seldom successful.

Some individuals who have neurotic ocular symptoms have accumulated many spectacles, none of which relieve their symptoms. They may be convinced that another pair of glasses will help and are reluctant to recognize the psychologic basis of their complaints.

Symptoms that involve near vision when the distance vision is normal (or vice versa) are most suggestive of a refractive error. One or both eyes may be involved.

Diagnosis of the cause of sudden, persistent, unilateral decrease of vision is based on the appearance of the external eye. The external eye is abnormal in keratitis, iridocyclitis, and closed-angle glaucoma. In vitreous hemorrhage, retinal artery or vein closure, or optic neuritis, the external eye appears normal, but the pupillary reactions may be abnormal. Periodic visual loss, varying from slight haziness to no light perception and lasting for a few seconds to minutes (amaurosis fugax; transient blindness; transient ischemic attack), may result from spasm of the ophthalmic artery in occlusive disease of the internal carotid artery or from abnormalities of the aortic arch. Gradual unilateral loss of vision occurs with corneal opacities, glaucoma, cataract, vitreous opacities, retinal detachment, central retinal degeneration, or intraocular inflammation.

Sudden loss of vision involving both eyes is uncommon. Inquiry usually indicates that vision failed first in one eye and that the sudden loss described was noted by the patient when vision in the fellow eye decreased. Both eyes may be involved in the diseases that cause sudden unilateral loss of vision, but this occurs rarely. A sudden bilateral decrease of vision is most suggestive of a conversion reaction, the toxic effects of drugs, or poor observation.

Gradual loss of vision in both eyes may result from nearly any ophthalmic disorder. Generally, if visual acuity is decreased and peripheral vision is intact, the disorder is anterior to the chiasm. If peripheral vision is decreased in each eye, the disorder may be at or posterior to the chiasm.

Color vision. Color vision is a cone function. A deficiency in color perception is inherited in approximately 7% of men and 0.5% of women. The most common type is transmitted as an X-chromosome-linked abnormality. Visual acuity in these individuals is normal, but color perception is depressed to a varying degree. Acquired unilateral depression of color sense occurs in diseases affecting the cone function of one eye, such as central retinal degeneration and optic nerve disease. Loss of visual acuity parallels the loss of color discrimination. Bilateral acquired depression in color vision may occur in malnutrition and after the ingestion of toxic drugs. Opacities of the ocular media, particularly those involving the cornea (leukoma) or lens (cataract), may cause depression but not loss of color vision.

Color perception is disturbed in a variety of diseases of the optic nerve and fovea centralis as well as in nutritional disturbances. Glucose-6-phosphate dehydrogenase deficiency is associated with hemolytic anemia and red-green color blindness in the inhabitants of Sardinia.

Peripheral vision. The retinal periphery contains rods mainly, but cones are scattered throughout. A visual field defect may occur in many abnormalities of the retina, optic nerve, and optic pathways. If the abnormality is anterior to the chiasm, the defect is unilateral. Disorders affecting the chiasm or visual pathways involve both eyes. When one eye is involved in retinal or optic nerve disease, the patient frequently describes the sensation of a curtain falling over a portion of the visual field. When both eyes are involved, the patient may be unaware of the defect.

Defects in the visual fields are usually described as central (within 30° of fixation point) or peripheral. Localized areas of defective vision surrounded by areas of normal vision are called scotomas. Peripheral defects are described as temporal, nasal, superior, and inferior (Fig. 4-1). It should be recalled that the visual field reflects the visual function in the opposite areas of the retina involved. A temporal visual field defect reflects light stimuli to the nasal retina. A superior field defect involves the inferior retina. Thus a superior temporal field defect indicates failure to see objects that stimulate on the inferior nasal retina.

Night blindness. Patients who have an organic disease with night blindness often do not complain of this defect. Conversely, some patients who do not have organic ocular disease may have many complaints concerning poor vision in reduced illumination. Night blindness is caused by pigmentary degenerations of the retina, optic nerve disease, glaucoma, or vitamin A deficiency occurring in cirrhosis of the liver or because of inadequate nutrition. It may occur after panretinal photocoagulation. The patient often complains of poor recovery of vision during night driving after the headlights of a passing car shine in the eyes. Vision that is poorer in bright illumination than in dim illumination occurs in cone degenerations and in toxic optic neuropathy.

Iridescent vision. This term is applied to the halos or rainbow seen surrounding bright lights when there is diffusion by the ocular media. The most common cause is subepithelial edema of the cornea, which may follow a rapid increase in intraocular pressure. Prolonged wearing of hard contact lenses and swimming in fresh water with the eyes open also cause corneal edema. Pus floating across the cornea in conjunctivitis may cause iridescent vision that is corrected by rapid blinking. Corneal degeneration (dystrophy) and cataract may also cause the symptom.

Entoptic phenomena. This is the visualization of structures within the eye, usually in the

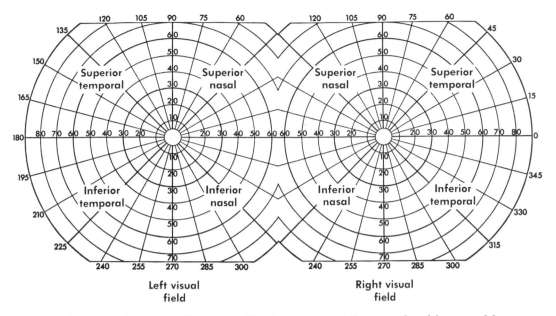

Fig. 4-1. A standard visual field chart. The intersection of the vertical and horizontal lines corresponds to the foveola of the retina and the point of fixation of vision. The concentric circles mark their distance in degrees from the fovea. The temporal quadrants correspond to the nasal retinas, which have axons that decussate at the optic chiasm. The nasal quadrants correspond to the temporal retinas. The superior quadrants correspond to the inferior retinas and the inferior quadrants to the superior retinas.

vitreous cavity. Floaters are translucent specks of various shapes and sizes that float across the visual field. They can be seen only when the eye is open. Commonly the patient observes them when looking at a bright blue sky or a brilliantly illuminated pastel-colored wall. All individuals have small fixed remnants of the hyaloid vascular system in the vitreous humor (muscae volitantes) seen as small dots that dart away as one tries to fix them. Liquefaction (syneresis) of the vitreous humor occurs in aging, in myopia, and after ocular injuries. It is a common cause of floaters; for example, in vitreous degeneration lens opacities may cause floaters that do not move (fixed). Leukocytes from inflammation of the retina or uvea may cause floaters, but usually such large numbers are present that vision is generally depressed. A sudden shower of floaters may occur in the periphery of the visual field with a vitreous hemorrhage. This may be the initial symptom of hole formation preceding retinal separation. The location of the floaters may be helpful in locating the retinal hole. The sudden appearance of a moderately large floater is the main

symptom of vitreous detachment. Rarely, a patient learns inadvertently to observe the leukocytes in his own capillaries and becomes concerned about the flecks that disturb his reading.

Photopsia. These are visual perceptions that form in the absence of light stimuli. The term is applied to such visual phenomena as specks, rings, lightning flashes, and luminous bodies that are observed when the eyes are closed. When monocular, the condition is caused by a retinal stimulus (inadequate stimulus) other than light. It occurs in traction of the vitreous upon the retina or with pressure upon the closed eye. Visual hallucinations (bilateral photopsia) are divided into formed and unformed types. Visual hallucinations from the occipital cortex and association areas produce static light and stars, whereas hallucinations from the parastriate area 18 may produce luminous sensations of colored flashes and rings. Hallucinations from the parieto-occipital cortex center on objects, people, and animals. In addition to the visual illusions, there may be preservation of the visual image in time (palinopia) or in space (visual illusory spread), impaired visual recognition (visual agnosia), defective visual localization, errors in naming color, or defective perception of color.

Hallucinations from the temporal cortex may be scenes recalled from experience or may consist of landscapes, prairie fires, or seascapes, usually with repetitive activity and a minimum of detail. Visual hallucinations may be associated with auditory hallucinations.

Micropsia and macropsia. Micropsia, or perceiving images to be smaller than actual size, is caused by an abnormality of image formation at the fovea or by disorders of the temporal cortex. Edema, tumors, and hemorrhages in the central retinal region may cause the cones to be spread farther apart and cause micropsia.

Macropsia is an abnormality in which objects appear larger than they actually are. It results from edema, tumors, and hemorrhages in the foveal region that may cause the cones to be pressed closer together.

Cortical blindness. Cortical blindness is an abnormality in perception caused by bilateral impairment of the visual centers of the occipital cortex (area 17). It is characterized by a loss of the visual sensation with retention of the pupillary reaction to light. The patient may not be conscious of the loss of vision.

Perceptual blindness. Perceptual blindness is an abnormality caused by lesions in the angular gyrus of the parieto-occipital fissure in which individuals are unable to recognize objects visually (agnosia) but are able to recognize objects by touch or other sensory portals. An individual so afflicted will be unable to recognize a key when looking at it but will readily recognize it when touching it. Defects related to this condition include alexia (inability to read), agraphia (inability to write), and dyslexia (disturbance in the ability to read). These abnormalities may be highly selective so that the patient recognizes numbers but not letters, or recognizes printed matter but not written script, and the like.

Blindness. The definitions of blindness differ, but generally a person is considered legally blind when best visual acuity with corrective lenses in the better eye is 20/200 (6/60) or less or when the peripheral visual field is constricted to within 20° (Table 4-2). The chief causes of blindness in the United States are glaucoma, unoperated cataract, and retinal disorders, mainly proliferative diabetic retinopathy and macular (central retinal) degeneration.

The physician managing a blind patient must avoid any hint of condescension and must learn that the patient's interpretation of the physi-

Table 4-2. Visual acuity in visually handicapped persons (better eye with possible correction)*

Common definition	Snellen index	Practical test	Legal significance
No light perception (total blindness)	—	Cannot see light	Totally blind
Light perception only	Less than 3/200 (1/60)	Unable to see hand movement at 1 meter	Satisfies all criteria for legal blindness†
Form and motion	Less than 3/200 (1/60)	Hand movement visible, but unable to count fingers at 1 meter	Total disability for Social Security Administration
Travel vision	Less than 10/200 (3/60)	Unable to read newspaper headlines	Legal blindness
Minimal reading	Less than 20/200 (6/60)	Reads headlines, but not 14-point (4.7 mm) type	Maximum acuity for legal blindness for Internal Revenue Service and most state industrial commissions
Partially seeing (borderline)	More than 20/200 (6/60) but less than 20/70 (6/24)	Cannot read 10-point (3.4 mm) type without marked difficulty	Not legally blind, but eligible for some services

*After Wheeler, P.C.: Mo. Med. **64:**315, 1967.
†Legal blindness also present if visual field is constricted to 20° or less.

cian's voice and actions are the major factors in reassurance. A person talking to a blind individual should identify himself by name, should not shout, should always give detailed verbal directions and not visual signals, and should always warn the patient before touching him. Blind persons prefer to grasp the arm of a guide rather than having their own arm grasped.

Some blind individuals are not aware of the agencies and services available to promote their adjustment and independence. Information may be obtained from the American Foundation for the Blind, 15 West 16th Street, New York, NY 10011.

Diplopia. Diplopia, or double vision, occurs whenever the visual axes are not directed simultaneously to the same object. Unilateral diplopia is a curiosity in which light rays are split by an opacity in the cornea or lens so that a single object is imaged twice on the retina. Frequently the images are so blurred that the patient notices the defect only under exceptional visual conditions.

Physiologic diplopia is a normal phenomenon in which objects not within the area of fixation are seen double. Usually it does not impinge on the consciousness. It is easily demonstrated by looking at a near object with attention directed to a distant object, which then appears doubled. Such physiologic diplopia contributes to parallax, which enables a person to judge the distance of objects.

Diplopia is a cardinal sign of weakness of one or more of the extraocular muscles. Characteristically, the separation of images increases in the field of action of the extraocular muscle(s) involved. Diplopia can occur only if binocular vision has developed. The absence of diplopia thus does not guarantee that a paresis of an extraocular muscle is not present. Diplopia may also occur without muscle weakness if there is displacement of the globe, as in proptosis or with restrictive muscle disease, so that the visual lines cannot be directed simultaneously to the same object.

PAIN

Pain and aches in the region of the eye or in the head (Table 4-3) may be difficult to interpret and require considerable clinical skill in evaluation. Some patients are phlegmatic about pain, while others would be disabled by pain of the same severity. Moreover, pain is a subjective sensation, and considerable insight into a patient's temperament is required for evaluation.

A superficial foreign body sensation may be caused by several conditions: a lesion in the eyelid, a foreign body on the cornea or the conjunctiva, inflammation of the cornea or the conjunctiva, or loss of conjunctival or corneal epithelium. A local anesthetic instilled in the conjunctival sac usually eliminates the sensation of a superficial foreign body but not that caused by inflammation of the conjunctiva and the cornea. If the eyelid is drawn away from the globe, the sensation caused by a foreign body on the tarsal conjunctiva will be eliminated, whereas the sensation caused by a foreign body on the cornea will continue. Patients invariably localize a foreign body sensation to the outer portion of the upper eyelid irrespective of its location.

Deep, severe pain within the eye may be present in a variety of disorders. The most important causes, since they require immediate attention, are inflammations of the ciliary body

Table 4-3. Miscellaneous ocular symptoms other than visual

I. Pain in one or both eyes or in the head
   A. Superficial foreign body sensation
   B. Deep pain within the eye
   C. Headache
   D. Burning, itching, "tired" eyes (asthenopia)
   E. Photophobia (abnormal ocular sensitivity to light)
II. Abnormal secretion from eyes
   A. Lacrimation (excessive tear production)
   B. Epiphora (defective tear drainage)
   C. Mucus
   D. Pus
   E. Dry eyes
III. Physical signs described by the patient as symptoms
   A. Red eye
      1. Conjunctival injection
      2. Ciliary injection
      3. Subconjunctival hemorrhage
   B. New growths
   C. Abnormal position of eyes or eyelids
   D. Protrusion of globe
   E. Widened palpebral fissure
   F. Narrowed palpebral fissure
   G. Pupillary abnormality

---

and rapid increase in the intraocular pressure, such as that occurring in angle-closure glaucoma. In each of these instances the eye is red and vision is decreased.

Many relatively minor ocular abnormalities manifest themselves by burning, itching, and uncomfortable eyes. These symptoms may originate from an inadequately corrected refractive error, fatigue, keratoconjunctivitis, sicca, and chronic conjunctivitis. Mild, nonspecific inflammation of the eyelids or the conjunctiva without obvious signs may cause ocular discomfort, particularly when the eyes are used extensively. Minor ocular irritation caused by prolonged use of the eyes is mainly without significance.

The interpretation of headache as a symptom of ocular disease requires familiarity with its causes. Headaches that are relieved by salicylates are usually not caused by serious organic disease. Uncorrected errors of refraction or wearing the wrong corrective lenses do not cause severe incapacitating headaches. Headaches that are present on awakening in the morning are not caused by excessive use of the eyes the previous night.

One should determine whether a headache is intermittent or continuous, its location in the head, and other associated signs. An aura followed by severe unilateral headache (hemicrania), nausea, and vomiting is suggestive of migraine (Chapter 26). A headache aggravated by straining and associated with vomiting without nausea is suggestive of increased intracranial pressure. A severe frontal headache associated with paralysis of ocular muscles is suggestive of an infraclinoid aneurysm of the internal carotid artery.

Tic douloureux causes a characteristic excruciating pain in the region of distribution of the sensory branches of the trigeminal nerve. Usually the history of episodic pain of a similar type alerts one to the nature of the disorder. In young patients, it may be related to multiple sclerosis.

Zoster ophthalmicus may cause severe retrobulbar pain, which may precede the cutaneous vesiculation by several days. Often the cause of the pain is not recognized until the typical eruption occurs in the area of distribution of the ophthalmic nerve. Postzoster neuralgia may be extremely disabling in the elderly.

Photophobia is a reflex in which light stimulating the retina causes constriction of the pupil and pain. The term is widely used to indicate any discomfort arising from bright light, such as the reflection of a great amount of light from the sky or an unpleasant contrast between light and dark areas. Glare is the term given to excessive light directed into the eyes from a reflecting surface.

Patients with cone degenerations often have an aversion to bright light that is first noted by the examiner when attempting ophthalmoscopy. Inquiry will then indicate that the patient prefers activities in dim illumination. There may be a reduction in visual acuity as the amount of illumination increases.

ABNORMAL SECRETION

It is sometimes possible to diagnose an ocular disease by observing the nature of an abnormal secretion from the eyes. Pus is found in the conjunctival sac in mucopurulent conjunctivitis. The eyelashes are frequently agglutinated to each other by drying pus, and it may be difficult to open the eyes in the morning. A foamy secretion at the inner canthus is produced by *Corynebacterium xerose*, which lives solely on desquamated epithelium. A stringy secretion with excoriation of the canthus characterizes the inflammation caused by the diplobacillus of Morax-Axenfeld. A tenacious, stringy secretion occurs in allergic inflammation of the conjunctiva.

A distinction is made between lacrimation, in which there is an excessive production of tears, and epiphora, in which there is overflow of a normal volume of tears. Lacrimation occurs in those diseases that cause reflex secretion of tears, whereas epiphora results from an abnormality of the drainage system. Persistent tearing of one or both eyes of an infant is a cardinal sign of congenital glaucoma. There is an associated corneal edema. Tearing shortly after birth may occur because of failure of the nasolacrimal duct to open as it normally does about the third week of life. Tearing also occurs in photophobia, in inflammations of the cornea and conjunctiva, and reflexly in inflammations of the ciliary body.

Decreased tear formation causes drying of the eyes (keratoconjunctivitis sicca). This occurs in Sjögren syndrome, in vitamin A deficiency, and in scarring of the conjunctiva that closes the orifices of the lacrimal glands or destroys goblet cells. Erythema multiforme, trachoma, ocular cicatricial pemphigoid, and chemical burns are the chief causes of such scarring.

LEARNING DISABILITIES

Learning disabilities is a generic term that describes a significant and persistent difficulty in the acquisition and use of reading, writing, mathematical, and reasoning skills. There is an associated difficulty in listening and speaking abilities. These are caused by a dysfunction of the higher nervous system in basic psychologic processes. They are not caused by ocular disease, vision handicaps, poor teaching, hearing problems, motor handicaps, emotional disturbances, or environmental disadvantage. Those affected are of normal or above average intelligence, but there is a discrepancy between the individual's potential for learning and what is actually learned.

Dyslexia is a type of learning disability in which there is impairment in the ability to read. (Discussion is complicated by a vocabulary that adopts neurologic terms that relate symptoms of specific brain lesions to learning disabilities.) Reading is an integrated skill that is important in intellectual maturation. Inasmuch as children develop at different rates, not all are ready to begin reading at the same age. Thus some children learn to read slowly but read well at an older age. Defective vision, refractive errors, defective fusion, and muscle imbalance have no causative role except insofar as reduced visual acuity makes it difficult for the child to interpret symbols.

Basically there are two main types of reading disorders: (1) general reading backwardness and (2) primary or specific language disability, or developmental dyslexia. General reading backwardness affects both boys and girls and is found in children who have other learning problems. Abnormal neurologic findings are common, and disorders of motor, constructional, and speech function are frequent. The condition is often seen in children from large families and deprived social classes. Specific language disability is three times as common in boys as girls, is rarely associated with a neurologic or other abnormality, and occurs in children who are average or superior in other areas of learning, such as mathematics. Essentially, the reading skills and related areas of vocabulary and speech function are disproportionately lower than their other learning skills and their chronologic age.

Individuals with reading problems are characterized by (1) poor word recognition with inability to pronounce words or identify unfamiliar words, (2) poor comprehension with difficulty in deriving literal and implied meanings and drawing conclusions and then following directions, and (3) difficulty in developing vocabulary and a slow reading rate. In addition to the defect in reading, there may be delay in learning to tell time, gross inaccuracy in spelling, and muddled serial thinking. Words are perceived as reversed, printed backward, or upside down. In later life there is a relatively restricted vocabulary, great difficulty in fluent expression of ideas on paper with acceptable standards of syntax and punctuation, and often a lifelong reluctance rather than an incapacity to read.

There are many causes of reading problems (Table 4-4). The family physician plays a key role in managing the disorder. Early recognition of a condition by the teacher is of importance inasmuch as it is much more easily corrected if special teaching is begun at 6 or 7 years of age. The physician may wish psychologic consultation to be certain intelligence is not impaired; an auditory screening test is desirable. A neurologist may be enlisted to exclude mild forms of neurologic abnormalities. There is no evidence to indicate that visual training, such as ocular muscle exercises, ocular pursuit, or neurologic organizational training (for example, laterality training and balance board or perceptual training), is of value. Intense, specialized, structured instruction in reading skills in an uncluttered, unornamented, nondistracting classroom aids all but a few if instruction is begun early enough.

A reading problem may occur because of a deficiency in memory skills, in processing not only letters but geometric forms and abstract forms. The large amount of information perceived by the visual system persists in a raw perceptual form called *visual information storage* for about 0.25 second. During this period, subjects actively code and transfer this infor-

Table 4-4. Reading deficiencies

I. Learning disabilities
  A. General reading retardation
    1. Delayed intellectual maturation
    2. Developmental hyperactivity (short attention span, impulsivity)
    3. Minimal brain dysfunction (premature birth, infantile injury)
    4. Familial
  B. Specific language disability
    1. Reading
    2. Spelling
    3. Word recognition
  C. General language disability
    1. Arithmetic (dyscalculia)
    2. Writing (dysgraphia)
II. Sociopsychologic
  A. Defects in teaching
  B. Deficiencies in cognitive stimulation
  C. Deficiencies in motivation
    1. Poverty
    2. Cultural deprivation
III. Psychophysiologic
  A. Mental retardation
  B. Cerebral palsy
  C. Seizure disorders
  D. Hearing deficits
  E. Progressive neurologic disorders
  F. Acquired alexia (right hemiplegia, left hemisphere lesions)
IV. Psychologic
  A. Receptive language disorders (auditory agnosia)
  B. Articulatory disorders
  C. Audiophonetic disorders

mation into more permanent storage called *short-term storage*. Testing of 12-year-olds with reading defects indicates a normal visual information storage, but a gross defect in processing visual information into short-term storage. This suggests that those with a reading disability have some problem in the encoding, organizational, or retrieval skills that normally follow the initial stage of visual information storage. It appears not to involve verbal and linguistic processes primarily, although inability to recognize and pronounce words follows from the reading defect.

Cerebrovascular disease affecting the angular and supramarginal gyri on the opposite side of the dominant hand may cause loss of ability to read in previously normal individuals. If all ability is lost, the condition is classed as alexia; if the difficulty is partial, the condition is classed as neurologic dyslexia or acquired dyslexia. The severity and nature of the defect vary markedly in ability to read letters while retaining ability to read numbers, ability to recognize words in large type but not in small type, and the like. Color perception may be affected (acquired dyschromatopsia). Often there is severe involvement of large areas of the brain, and exact diagnosis is not possible.

PERIODIC EYE EXAMINATION

Examination of the newborn infant should include inspection of the eyelids and the external eye. The pupils should react to light, and ophthalmoscopic examination should indicate a red reflex with no opacities of the media. A careful practitioner will view the optic disk and the area immediately adjacent to it. In eyes that are not constantly parallel after 6 months of age or that cross thereafter, a complete eye examination including cycloplegic refaction is indicated.

Vision should be measured in each eye no later than 3 years of age inasmuch as strabismic or anisometropic amblyopia may be corrected if detected at this age. A complete eye examination with cycloplegic refraction is desirable before beginning grammar school, in the fourth grade, and before beginning high school, college, and graduate school. If an abnormality is discovered, more frequent examinations may be necessary. Young adults who are without symptoms and who do not have a refractive error may be examined every 5 years. If corrective lenses are worn, the patient should be examined every 2 years. After 45 years of age, examinations should be done every 2 years.

A complete eye examination should include examination of the anterior segment of the eye and the eyelids with a biomicroscope, the ocular fundus should be inspected with a direct ophthalmoscope, and the peripheral fundus should be studied with an indirect ophthalmoscope by means of scleral depression. The intraocular pressure should be measured with a tonometer. The visual fields should be estimated by confrontation or other screen method, and if there is any question of an abnormality, they must be carefully measured with a perimeter. The muscle balance, including convergence and divergence, must be measured for both near and far. The visual acuity should be measured for near and far and the refractive error determined.

Particular attention must be directed to ocular signs of systemic disease. Effective treatment is available for many ocular conditions in their early stages, and it is disheartening to see individuals who have reduced vision caused by abnormalities not detected in their early stages. Similarly, many systemic diseases are first evident in the eyes. In the Framingham Study, over 25% of those who were found to have retinal changes characteristic of diabetes had no previous diagnosis of or treatment for diabetes.

BIBLIOGRAPHY
General

Burde, R.M., Savino, P.J., and Trobe, J.D.: Clinical decisions in neuro-ophthalmology, St. Louis, 1985. The C.V. Mosby Co.

Roy, F.H.: Ocular differential diagnosis, ed. 3, Philadelphia, 1984, Lea & Febiger.

Disturbances of vision

Hirst, L.W., Miller, N.R., and Johnson, R.T.: Monocular polyopia, Arch. Neurol. **40:**756, 1983.

Spector, R.H.: Migraine, Surv. Ophthalmol. **29:**193, 1984.

Learning disabilities

Committee on Children with Disabilities of the AAP and Ad Hoc Working Group of the American Association for Pediatric Ophthalmology and Strabismus and American Academy of Ophthalmology: Learning disabilities, dyslexia, and vision, Pediatrics **74:**150, 1984.

Foundation for Children with Learning Disabilities: The FCLD guide for parents of children with learning disabilities, New York, 1984, Education Systems.

Hynd, G., and Cohen, M.: Dyslexia—neuropsychological theory, research, and clinical differentiation, New York, 1983, Grune and Stratton.

Goldberg, H.K., Schiffman, G.C., and Bender, M.: Dyslexia: interdisciplinary approaches to reading disabilities, New York, 1983, Grune and Stratton.

Gordon, N., McKinlay, I., and Rosenbloom, L.: Medical contribution to the management of dyslexia, Arch. Dis. Child. **59:**588, 1984.

Kirshner, H.S.: Word and letter reading and the mechanism of the third alexia, Arch. Neurol. **39:**84, 1982.

5

FUNCTIONAL EXAMINATION OF THE EYES

The different functions of the eye are evaluated by many tests. The cone function of the fovea centralis is assessed usually by measurement of the ability to distinguish the shape of symbols such as letters. This is designated as visual acuity. It is measured for both near and far, with and without the best possible correction of any refractive error. Because only cones participate in color vision and because they are concentrated in the fovea, the measurement of color recognition also measures foveal function. The function of the peripheral retina, which contains mainly rods, is measured by estimation of the peripheral visual field. Dark adaptation, which is never part of a routine examination, measures recovery of photoreceptor function after exposure to light.

Any reasonably complete physical examination should indicate that (1) vision when corrected with glasses, if necessary, is normal in each eye for near and far, each eye being measured separately; (2) the peripheral visual field of each eye is intact on gross testing; (3) the ocular movements are normal; (4) each pupil constricts when the retina of each eye is stimulated by light; and (5) the optic disks are flat and of normal color. Such an examination is not a complete eye examination but can be performed quickly and will exclude many different serious diseases.

VISUAL ACUITY

Measurement of visual acuity assesses the function of the fovea centralis and its central connections. The measurement involves several components. Detection measurements consist of recognizing one or two objects, a break in a line, or an opening in a ring. Objectively, one may determine if the eye follows a moving target. Descriptive measurements consist of describing the location of a break in a ring, indicating the direction in which lines point, or drawing what is seen. Interpretive

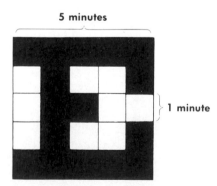

Fig. 5-1. Construction of the Snellen letter (1862) to subtend an angle of 5 minutes; each part subtends an angle of 1 minute. Letters constructed without serifs are recommended. The above letter measures 1.4375 in. (0.12 ft) and subtends an angle of 5 minutes at 991.4 in. (82.6 ft) (1.4375 ÷ tangent 5 minutes [.00145] = 991.38).

154

measurements consist of stating what letter, picture, number, or object is seen.

Visual test objects (optotypes) are constructed so that at a particular distance the whole object subtends an angle of 5 minutes of an arc, and different parts of the object are separated by a distance of 1 minute of an arc (Fig. 5-1.).

Visual acuity is ordinarily designated by two numbers. The first indicates the distance separating the test object from the patient. The second indicates the distance at which the test object subtends an angle of 5 minutes. To denote visual acuity, both numbers are recorded.

The most familiar test objects are letters or numbers (Figs. 5-1 and 5-2). Test letters require a literate and cooperative observer. The letters vary in their recognizability. Thus L is the easiest letter in the alphabet to recognize and B is the most difficult. The Landolt broken ring (Fig. 5-3), in which the break in the ring subtends a 1-minute angle and the entire ring subtends a 5-minute angle, eliminates this variability. Similarly, the letter E may be arranged so that it faces in different directions (the illiterate E) (Fig. 5-3). The checkerboard design (Fig. 5-3) is so arranged that when the target is too small for the checkerboard to be discriminated, all four squares appear uniformly gray. These test objects may be used to test illiterate individuals and persons not familiar with the Western alphabet. A variety of pictures have been designed for testing children.

The measurement of visual acuity involves many complex factors not necessarily related to the ability to see test objects. Visual acuity varies with motivation, attention, intelligence, and physical variants. Lighting, adaptation, contrast, and other factors differ considerably (as does the patience of both the examiner and the patient).

An isolated letter is recognized more easily than a series of letters. This is particularly true in individuals with amblyopia, who may have a visual acuity as good as 20/50 when measured with isolated letters and as poor as 20/200 when the letters are placed in a series. The visual acuity scores improve if the individual is given an unlimited time to recognize the letters, and they decrease when the letters are presented rapidly.

The measurement of visual acuity in a manner that may be consistently reproduced involves attention to a number of complex physical and psychic details that are controlled only in experimental situations. The maximum visual acuity is that in which the individual correctly recognizes 51% of the test symbols within a definite time period. If a portion of the test objects is not recognized, it is customary to indicate the best vision minus the number of

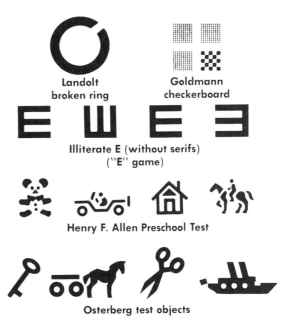

Landolt broken ring **Goldmann checkerboard**

Illiterate E (without serifs) ("E" game)

Henry F. Allen Preschool Test

Osterberg test objects

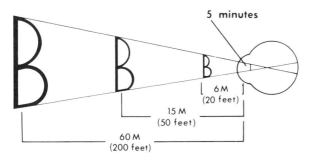

Fig. 5-2. Test letters that subtend an angle of 5 minutes at different distances from the eye. The letter size is equal to the distance from the eye multiplied by the tangent of 5 minutes (50 m × tangent 5 minutes [.00145] = .0725 m).

Fig. 5-3. Symbols used in testing distance visual acuity in preschool children and illiterates. The Landolt broken ring and the Goldmann checkerboard are used in research studies.

letters missed, such as $20/30^{-2}$. Because the number of letters on the 20/30 line is not indicated, this is not particularly meaningful.

Visual acuity should be measured with the patient wearing any corrective lenses appropriate for the test distance. It is nonproductive to measure near vision without glasses if the patient requires them. Similarly, distance vision is not measured with the patient wearing glasses for near vision. If vision is reduced, a pinhole (see below) may be used. Normal visual acuity with a pinhole, with correction or without correction, indicates that (1) the cornea, lens, and ocular media are relatively clear in the visual axis, permitting an image to be formed on the retina; (2) the fovea centralis is relatively intact, as are its nervous connections to the brain; and (3) perception by the higher visual centers is intact.

The largest symbol used clinically in the United States subtends an angle of 5 minutes at a distance of 200 ft (60 m). Symbols then subtend a 5-minute angle at distances of 100 (30), 60 (20), 30 (10), and 20 (6) ft (m). If the individual is unable to recognize the largest test smbol, he should be brought closer to it, and the distance at which he recognizes it should be recorded. Thus if he recognizes the test symbol that subtends a 5-minute angle at 200 ft when he is 6 ft away, the visual acuity is recorded as 6/200 (2/60). This is not a fraction but indicates two measurements: the test distance and the size of the test object.

Accurate measurements of visual acuity can be made down to the range of 3/200 (1/60). Below this level, visual performance is evaluated by learning if the patient can see the examiner's hand move in front of his eyes (hand movements). This measurement should be combined with a notation as to the extent of the confrontation field: hand movements combined with a full visual field, or hand movements combined with a restricted visual field. If the patient is unable to recognize hand movements, a small penlight is used to indicate whether the patient can project the direction from which light is entering the eye. This is recorded as light perception with projection. If the patient is unable to project the direction of light, the patient indicates whether a light can be seen. (To avoid confusion, the examiner must spell out percep-

tion or projection and not use the abbreviation LP.) Only in the absence of perception of light is the eye recorded as blind. Because blindness has a variety of legal and sociologic definitions, many examiners record such an eye as having no light perception rather than blind.

The preceding discussion unfortunately suggests that the measurement of visual acuity is a complicated, time-consuming, difficult-to-interpret maneuver. Rather, it is rapidly performed, simple, and requires minimal equipment.

Measurement of near vision is by no means as accurate as that of distance vision. For the most part, the distance at which near vision is tested is not recorded, and one records the smallest type that can be recognized irrespective of the distance. The standard test distance is considered to be 14 inches (35 cm). Test symbols subtending a 5-minute angle at various distances are used or different size types (Fig. 5-4).

Normal near vision may be recorded as 14/14 (35/35) or 4 point at 14 inches (35 cm). Near optotypes (letters of decreasing size) were first described by Jaeger and thus the designation may be J.4.

Many individuals have never had visual acuity measured in each eye separately. Sometimes decreased vision in one eye is first de-

CM	IN	
353	140	**L**
176	70	**F P**
118	47	**T O Z**
88	35	L P E D
71	28	P E C F D
59	23	E D F C Z P
44	17	F E L O P Z D
35	14	D E F P O T E C

Fig. 5-4. Near vision optotypes designed to subtend an angle of 5 minutes at various distances. Usually the examiner records the smallest optotype seen and does not record the distance of the material from the eye. If distance is recorded, it is measured in inches or centimeters. A patient who reads the smallest optotype, at a reading distance of 14 in., would have near vision of 14/14.

tected when visual acuity is measured after a minor eye injury. If the examiner has not measured the vision before inspecting or manipulating the eye, the patient may mistakenly blame the examiner for causing the decreased vision. In an emergency it is not necessary to have specific testing equipment available. One may gauge the visual acuity by using a telephone book or a newspaper and recording the smallest print that can be recognized with each eye.

It is desirable to measure the visual acuity of children sometime during their third year to detect strabismic or sensory amblyopia and to recognize the presence of severe refractive errors. Picture charts, the illiterate E, or the Landolt broken ring may be used. A rotating drum with alternating strips of black and white that induce rhythmic back-and-forth movement of the eyes (opticokinetic nystagmus) is used to measure vision objectively. A strip of cloth 66 by 7 cm may have a series of 5 cm circles of a different color sewn on it. Movement of the strip in front of the eyes induces an opticokinetic nystagmus in infants and indicates vision adequate for subsequent normal schooling.

In preferential looking, a calm, alert infant is held in front of two screens of matching luminance, one of which displays a grating pattern (Fig. 5-5), the other of which displays a blank field. Infants prefer to look at the pattern rather than the blank field, and visual acuity can be estimated by the stripe width (spatial frequency).

Pinhole test. Measurement of visual acuity with the patient viewing test symbols through a small opening in an opaque shield (Fig. 5-6) rapidly indicates whether reduced vision is caused by an error of refraction (and is thus correctable with lenses) or by some other abnormality. Vision is improved when a refractive error is present, because only rays that are nearly parallel to the visual axis, and thus not refracted, are seen. Usually, if vision is improved using a pinhole, a corrective lens will provide even better vision. Exceptionally, in keratoconus the visual improvement cannot be duplicated. In cataract and vitreous opacities, the pinhole may reduce rather than improve vision.

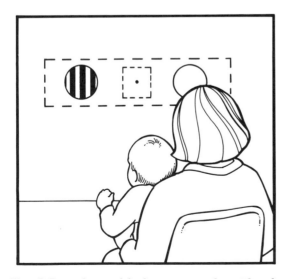

Fig. 5-5. Preferential looking in an infant. The observer is concealed behind the grating target and observes the infant's eyes.

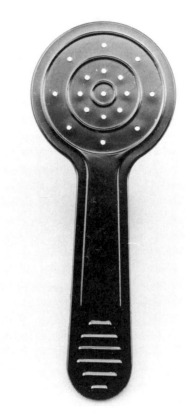

Fig. 5-6. A multiple pinhole shield. Only rays of light that are parallel to the visual axis and are thus not refracted are seen.

VISUAL FIELDS

The ability to recognize optotypes diminishes rapidly in all directions away from the fovea centralis. The function of the extrafoveal retina is assessed by measurement of the visual field, in which the individual detects targets that stimulate the retina at varying distances from the fovea. This function may be measured accurately by means of several instruments, or it may be estimated by means of the confrontation test. The confrontation test grossly measures the visual field, and even though the results are normal, a defect may still be detected by more sensitive methods of examination. The confrontation test is carried out as follows (Fig. 5-7).

The examiner faces the patient at a distance of 1 m in an area with good illumination. The patient is asked to close one eye, usually by holding the eyelid closed with the fingers. The examiner closes his own opposite eye. Thus, if the patient closes his right eye, the examiner closes his left eye. The examiner then places his hand midway between the subject and himself, bringing his hand slowly in from the periphery with one, two, or three fingers extended. The patient is instructed to tell the examiner when he can see and count the number of fingers in his field of vision. When the patient and the examiner have normal vision, each should recognize the number of fingers at the same time. Usually one tests the temporal and nasal fields and the superior and inferior fields in turn. Confrontation testing may also be carried out by substituting a hat pin with a 3 or 5 mm white tip. When testing a child, the examiner may stand behind the child, who has one eye occluded, and bring his hand into the nasal and temporal fields from behind the child's head.

Alternatively, with the patient having one eye closed and situated 1 m in front of the examiner, the examiner may hold both hands in front of the eyes, first above the horizontal plane and then below. The patient is asked if the hands look similar, if they are the same color and distinctness (Fig. 5-8).

The patient may be asked to observe two small color objects (such as the red tops of an eyedropper bottle). One is placed centrally and the other to one side. The patient is then asked to describe any difference in color intensity (Fig. 5-9).

Visual field screening. Visual field screening may be performed conveniently by means of a Harrington-Flocks Multiple Pattern Visual Stimulus. This consists of a screen on which dots of various sizes in different parts of the visual field are flashed for one-tenth second. The device is valuable in detecting visual field defects but has high false-positive rate.

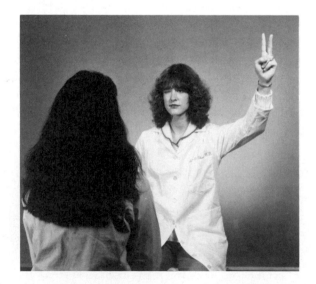

Fig. 5-7. Confrontation fields in which the ability of the subject to see the outstretched fingers is compared with that of the examiner.

Perimeters. Visual fields are quantitated by means of kinetic or static perimetry. In kinetic perimetry a test object of fixed size and illumination is moved from a nonseeing area to an area where it can just be seen by the subject. In static perimetry the test object is of fixed size and position, but the illumination increases until the subject can just detect it.

Perimeters are constructed in such a manner that the eye is at the center of rotation of a hemisphere that has a radius of curvature of 33 cm. Some consist of an arc of a circle that is

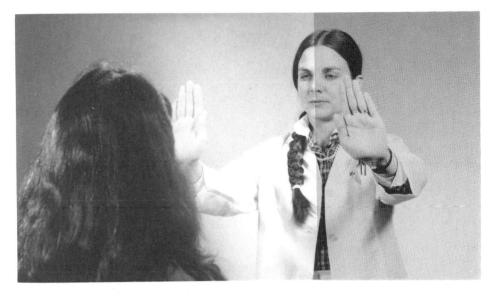

Fig. 5-8. Confrontation fields in which the subject compares the clarity with which the hands are seen in the temporal and nasal visual fields. Each eye is tested separately.

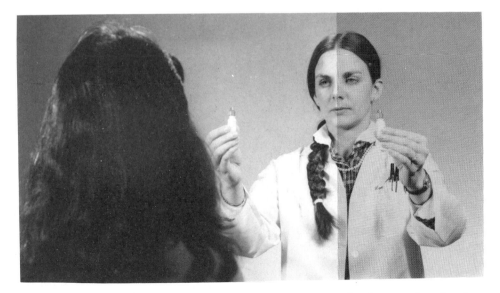

Fig. 5-9. Confrontation test in which the subject compares the brightness of a colored test object used for fixation with the color of a test object in the periphery.

rotated, whereas others are constructed as a half-bowl (Fig. 5-10). In the simplest devices the test object is moved on the end of a wand into the field of view, and in more elaborate perimeters it is projected. The testing distance of 33 cm remains constant. The size and color of the test object as well as the contrast of a projected test object and the surrounding background may be varied. The line connecting the points at which a test object may be just recognized is called the peripheral isopter. The test object is recorded as the size and intensity. The size, but not the intensity, remains the same with most of the computerized static suprathreshold perimeters. The test distance may be 1 or 2 m with a tangent screen, but is fixed at 33 cm with a bowl or arc perimeter. Automated perimeters often record in numbers in which 40 (0.1 apostilb) is the dimmest stimulus and 0 (1000 apostilb) is the brightest (1 apostilb = 0.318 cd/m^2).

Accurate measurement of the visual field may be time-consuming and not performed accurately. Conversely, the disorder that necessitates the examination may impair the patient's attention and awareness so that only the grossest responses can be obtained. In many intracranial lesions, computed tomography has made perimetry unnecessary. Conversely, in many optic nerve disorders, particularly glaucoma, perimetry can be more sensitive and accurate than ever before. To standardize testing, several automated and computerized perimeters are available. They are particularly valuable in glaucoma testing (see Chapter 20). Irrespective of the instrument used, the test is subjective and the results depend on the skill of the examiner and the attentiveness of the patient.

Automated and computer-assisted perimeters provide a testing program to determine the threshold for light sensitivity for each spot tested. Instruments are evaluated in their detection of defects (sensitivity) and their failure (false-positive) in normal subjects (specificity). If there are few false-positives, then early visual field defects are missed (high specificity–low sensitivity). If the aim is detection of the earliest visual field defect, then many normal subjects fail (high sensitivity–low specificity).

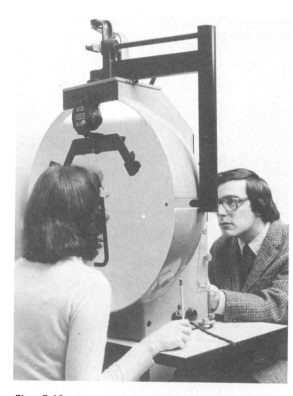

Fig. 5-10. Measurement of the visual field using a bowl perimeter (Goldmann). Although new automated computer perimeters are available, the Goldmann bowl perimeter remains the standard reference instrument.

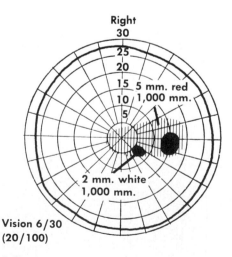

Fig. 5-11. A tangent screen record showing a centrocecal scotoma with an absolute scotoma (in black) surrounded by a relative scotoma (in lines).

The instruments are particularly valuable in the evaluation of the optic nerve function in glaucoma.

One system records the response to 76 fixed spots within a central field of 30° with each spot separated by 6°. The intensity of the illumination for each spot increases until it is just detected. If the response is unreliable, the earlier responses are deleted. The computer printout gives a numeric or a grayness value for each spot tested, which indicates the threshold for that spot. From time to time the threshold for light detection varies significantly in normal eyes. The instruments reduce error caused by technique and the examiner's skill but not the subject's attentiveness.

Tangent screens. Because photoreceptors are concentrated near the fovea centralis and the optic disk contains the ganglion cell axons, determination of field defects within 30° of the fixation point is important. Visual fields within this area may be measured using a tangent screen (tangent because it is a plane tangent to the arc of a perimeter). A tangent screen is usually covered with black felt, and the test is conducted 1 or 2 m from the subject. Test objects varying in size from 1 to 50 mm are used. The peripheral isopter, the blind spot, and various scotomas may be demonstrated (Fig. 5-11).

The Amsler Grid. This test permits patients to monitor central field defects. It is recommended for individuals with retinal disorders, chiefly retinal drusen, that threaten central vision. It consists of 400 squares, each measuring 5 mm × 5 mm (Fig. 5-12), and at the reading distance encompasses the central 20° of the field of vision. The test is performed on each eye separately with the patient in good light and, if necessary, wearing glasses for near vision. The patient fixes the black dot at the center and indicates any lines that appear wavy or curved or any squares that appear to be missing. The test is sensitive and should be carried out before pupillary dilation or ophthalmoscopy. In ocular conditions in which subretinal neovascularization may disturb the sensory retina, patients at risk may test themselves daily.

Visual field defects. Visual fields are charted to represent the visual space as the patient sees it. Thus the left visual field is on the lefthand side and the right visual field is on the righthand side. The blind spot is on the temporal side of each eye (see Chapter 4). The temporal visual field of each eye reflects stimulation of the nasal retina and visual fibers that decussate in the chiasm. The nasal visual field reflects the temporal retina. A vertical line through the fovea centralis divides the retina functionally

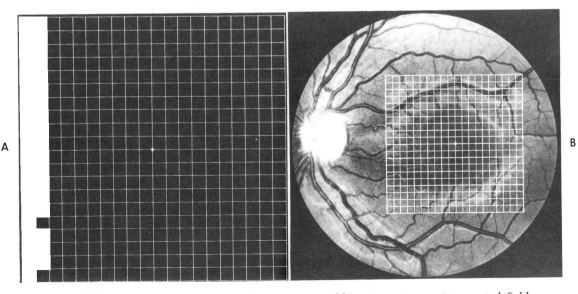

Fig. 5-12. A, The Amsler (1930) grid pattern to enable patients to monitor central field defects. **B,** The Amsler grid superimposed on area of retina tested.

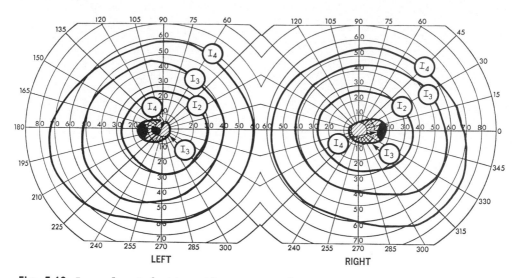

Fig. 5-13. Loss of central vision with a cecocentral scotoma (involving the blind spot and fovea). A scotoma is an area of blindness in the field of vision. The blind spot mirrors the optic nerve that has no photoreceptors. The roman numerals indicate the size of the projected test target (I [0.25 mm^2] is the smallest and V [64 mm^2] the largest). The arabic numeral indicates the density of a filter that decreases the brightness of the test object (1 is the densest and 4 the least dense). Thus, an I$_4$ test object is the brightest in the sequence shown. (From Burde, R.M., Savino, P.J., and Trobe, J.D.: Clinical decisions in neuro-ophthalmology, St. Louis, 1985, The C.V. Mosby Co.)

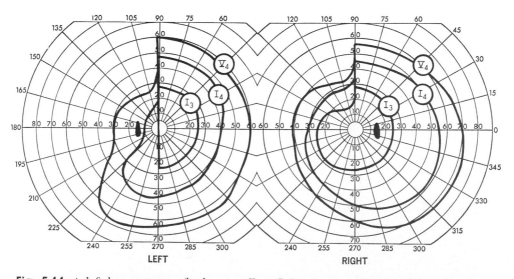

Fig. 5-14. A left homonymous (both eyes effected) hemianopsia (half-blindness; half, even though the left superior quadrant is mainly involved). The defect is not exactly the same in each eye and is termed "incongruous." The lesion causing it is located in the optic tract. (From Burde, R.M., Savino, P.J., and Trobe, J.D.: Clinical decisions in neuro-ophthalmology, St. Louis, 1985, The C.V. Mosby Co.)

into nasal and temporal portions. A horizontal line extending from the fixation point nasally reflects the temporal raphe of axons. It is particularly important in nerve fiber defects in glaucoma. Defects in the visual field are usually described as central or peripheral. A central field defect, a scotoma, is surrounded by a seeing area. Central scotomas involve the fixation point, and paracentral scotomas involve an area adjacent to the fixation point. Central scotomas characterize diseases involving the fovea centralis and the papillomacular bundle of nerve fibers in the optic nerve. Centrocecal scotomas (Fig. 5-13) involve both the physiologic blind spot and the fixation point and are characteristic of toxic diseases of the optic nerve. Annular scotomas form a circular defect around the fixation point and are particularly common in diseases that first manifest themselves at the equator of the eye, particularly retinal pigmentary degenerations. Arcuate (arched) scotomas involve a bundle of nerve fibers and characterize the field defect of glaucoma.

Reference is always to the blind portion of the visual field. Hemianopsia means half-blindness (Gr. *hemi*, half; *an*, negative; *opsi*, vision). A left hemianopsia indicates a left half-blindness (Fig. 5-14) and must involve impulses from the right half of the retina. Homonymous hemianopsia indicates involvement of the right or left portion of each visual field and thus interference with impulse transmission posterior to the optic chiasm. (The term "heteronymous" is not used; a bitemporal hemianopsia such as that in chiasmal disease is heteronymous.)

COLOR VISION TESTING

Good color vision is especially important in industry, school, and vehicle operation, but often color vision testing is neglected. The tests used clinically are relatively gross and too insensitive to detect small changes but nonetheless are helpful to the individual. Color vision deficiencies occur as a hereditary defect in about 7% of men and 0.5% of women. They are usually transmitted as an X chromosome–linked abnormality.

Autosomal defects in color vision occur in congenital achromatopsias and in cone degenerations. In retrobulbar neuritis, there may be early severe depression of color vision. In foveal degeneration caused by vascular disease, retinal separation, and other acquired disorders, the decrease in color vision parallels the loss of visual acuity. The least accurate test for detecting color deficiency involves the matching of yarns (Holmgren test) or recognizing red and green lanterns. Colorplates are available in which numbers are outlined in the primary colors and surrounded by confusion colors. The color-deficient individual is unable to see the figure that is recognized quickly by a person with normal color appreciation. More sensitive tests of color vision involve the use of the Nagel anomaloscope, in which the hue and saturation of yellow are matched by mixtures of red and green. The Farnsworth-Munsell test of hue discrimination consists of 84 chips of color that are matched in terms of increasing hue.

Color perception is disturbed in a variety of diseases of the optic nerve and fovea centralis as well as in nutritional disturbances. Testing has an important role in the diagnosis of total color blindness. Sensitive color vision tests are now used routinely in the clinical evaluation of cone degenerations and other foveal disorders.

BIBLIOGRAPHY
Visual acuity

Helveston, E.M., Weber, J.C., Miller K., Robertson, K., Hohberger, G., Estes, R., Ellis, F.D., Pick, N., and Helveston, B.H.: Visual function and academic performance, Am. J. Ophtalmol. **99:**346, 1985.

Mayer, D.L., and Dobson, V.: Visual acuity development in infants and young children, as assessed by operant preferential looking, Vision Res. **22:**1141, 1982.

Mayer D.L., Fulton, A.B., and Rodier, D.: Grating and recognition acuities of pediatric patients, Ophthalmology **91:**947, 1984.

Simons, K.: Visual acuity norms in young children, Surv. Ophthalmol. **28:**84, 1983.

Thompson, H.S.: Functional visual loss, Am. J. Ophthalmol. **100:**209, 1985

Visual fields

Anderson, D.R.: Testing the field of vision, St. Louis, 1982, The C.V. Mosby Co.

Easterbrook, M.: The use of Amsler grids in early chloroquine retinopathy, Ophthalmology **91:**1368, 1984.

Harrington, D.O.: The visual fields: a textbook and atlas of clinical perimetry, ed. 5, St. Louis, 1981, The C.V. Mosby Co.

Keltner, J.L., and Johnson, C.A.: Automated and manual perimetry—a six-year overview, Ophthalmology **91:**68, 1984.

Parrish, R.K. II, Schiffman, J., and Anderson, D.R.: Static and kinetic visual field testing, Arch. Ophthalmol. **102:**1497, 1984.

Trobe, J.D., and Glaser, J.S.: The visual fields manual: a practical guide to testing and interpretation, Gainesville, Fla., 1983, Triad Publishing Co.

Wilensky, J.T., and Joondeph, B.C.: Variation in visual field measurements with an automated perimeter, Am. J. Ophthalmol. **97:**328, 1984.

Yannuzzi, L.A.: A modified Amsler grid, a self-assessment test for patients with macular disease, Ophthalmology **89:**157, 1982.

Color vision

Smith, V.C., Pokorny, J., and Pass, A.S.: Color-axis determination on the Farnsworth-Munsell 100-hue test, Am. J. Ophthalmol. **100:**176, 1985.

6

PHYSICAL EXAMINATION OF THE EYES

A skilled physician studies patients constantly and unobtrusively for the physical basis of their symptoms. In the initial meeting the physician should note the diameter and shape of the head and the position of the eyes. Gross variations in the insertion of the canthal ligaments are observed easily, and the obliquity of the palpebral fissure is readily evident. Simple observation shows wrinkling of the forehead because of photophobia or an attempt to elevate the upper eyelid in blepharoptosis. Good illumination is necessary, but close inspection is not necessary to disclose injection of the conjunctival vessels or jaundice. The position of the eyelid margins in relation to the eye as well as any discomfort in holding the eyes open should be evident.

Entropion or ectropion may be evident without formally inspecting the eyelid margins. In the course of visiting with the patient, the physician should observe whether the eyes move in unison and whether the movements are full.

More careful inspection may be carried out by means of a small penlight, which provides a concentrated beam of light upon the eye. Better visualization of details may be obtained if good illumination is combined with inspection through a +20 diopter convex lens (Fig. 6-1). This lens may also be used for indirect ophthalmoscopy and for inspection of skin lesions. Better magnification is provided by a binocular loupe that magnifies 1.8 to 5 times.

EXTERNAL EXAMINATION

Examination is carried out in a systematic manner beginning with the skin of the eyelids and continuing inward. The examiner first notices the symmetry and width of the palpebral fissures and the position of the eyes. The eyelids usually conceal the corneoscleral limbus in the 12 and 6 o'clock meridians. Proptosis or retraction of the upper eyelid in thyroid ophthalmopathy is often first manifested by exposure of a narrow rim of sclera above or below the corneoscleral limbus. Keratoconus and subtle proptosis are most easily detected by viewing the contact of the cornea with the lower eyelid from above and behind the patient. The examiner stands behind the seated patient and looks over his brow (Fig. 6-2). By drawing the upper eyelids upward, any difference in prominence of the two eyes is easily noted. In keratoconus, the cornea distorts the lower eyelid outward (Munson sign).

Eyelid margin

The eyelashes (cilia) and the eylid margin are inspected for the characteristic scaling of squamous blepharitis. Abnormalities in position of the eyelid margin are also noted at this time. Intermittent entropion may be demonstrated if the patient squeezes his eyelids closed and then opens them. Particular attention is directed to the position of the puncta in relation to the lacrimal lake at the inner canthus. The inferior punctum should not be seen when the eyes are rotated upward. A frequent cause of tearing is slight eversion of the puncta. Sties involve the eyelid margin, whereas chalazia usually appear in the deeper substance of the eyelid.

Conjunctiva. The bulbar conjunctiva may be inspected directly. The caruncle is evident as a minute pink mass of tissue at the inner can-

thus. The similunar fold is not grossly evident unless the conjunctiva is inflamed. The superior and inferior portions of the bulbar conjunctiva are inspected easily by having the patient look upward and downward while the eyelids are drawn apart.

Eversion of the upper eyelid. Inspection of the upper tarsal conjunctiva requires eversion of the upper eyelid. While the patient looks

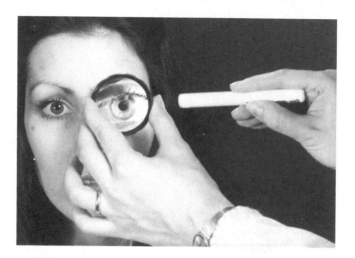

Fig. 6-1. Use of a penlight and a +20 diopter convex lens to study details of the anterior segment.

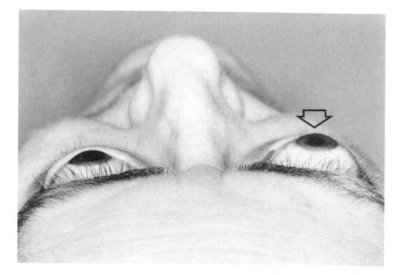

Fig. 6-2. Inspection of prominence of eyes by standing behind the patient, looking over the brow from above and behind, and elevating the upper eyelids. Note the proptosis of the right eye. The abnormal cornea profile in keratoconus may also be demonstrated this way.

downward, the lashes of the upper eyelid are grasped by the examiner between the thumb and the index finger. The eyelid is drawn gently outward to break the suction between the eyelid and the globe. The eyelid is then everted on a toothpick or applicator placed on the palpebral sulcus (Fig. 6-3). The tarsal con-

junctiva is exposed, and the meibomian glands perpendicular to the eyelid margin may be seen through the transparent tarsal conjunctiva. Sometimes the palpebral portion of the main lacrimal gland may be seen at the outer canthus.

Eversion of the lower eyelid. Inspection of the lower eyelid is performed easily. The patient looks upward, and the eyelid is drawn downward by the examiner's index finger applied to its orbital portion (Fig. 6-4). The lower tarsus is not nearly as wide as the upper tarsus. With the exception of trachoma and vernal catarrh, nearly all conjunctival inflammations are more marked in the inferior fornix than in the superior fornix.

Cornea. Attention is directed to the diameter and the clarity of the cornea. A cornea with a horizontal diameter of more than 12 mm may suggest congenital glaucoma or megalocornea (see Fig. 10-2). Extremely small corneas in the adult are suggestive of microcornea, with which hyperopia and angle-closure glaucoma occur.

The evaluation of corneal clarity involves several factors. The anterior surface of the cornea should be smooth, regular, and mirrorlike. The iris pattern should be distinctly seen in all regions. Corneal blood vessels should not be present. In corneal edema, the cornea has a diffuse ground-glass appearance. Marked opacities are usually evident, but magnification is required for less severe defects. Corneal vascularization may be superficial or deep and may involve the entire cornea or merely a seg-

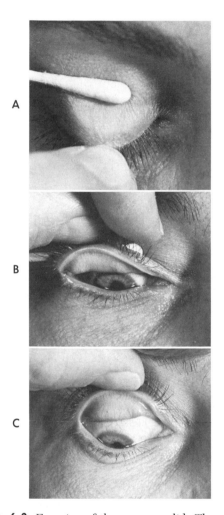

Fig. 6-3. Eversion of the upper eyelid. The patient is instructed to look downward, and the lashes of the upper eyelid are grasped between the thumb and index finger. **A,** A cotton-tipped applicator is placed at the level of the tarsal fold. **B,** The eyelid is then folded back on the cotton-tipped applicator while the patient continues to look downward. **C,** The applicator is then removed, and the details of the tarsal conjunctiva are inspected. The superior conjunctival fornix can be further studied if the eyelid is doubled over a speculum applied to the skin after single eversion.

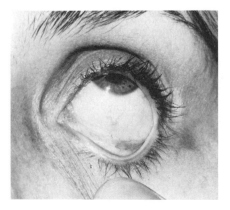

Fig. 6-4. Eversion of the lower eyelid by drawing the margin downward as the subject looks upward.

ment of it. Deep vascularization may be manifested solely as a loss of corneal clarity; magnification is required to see the individual blood vessels. The corneoscleral limbus may be involved in corneal arcus, particularly in elderly individuals or in those with lipid disturbances. Staining of the cornea with fluorescein solution (sterile) may be used to demonstrate areas where epithelium is absent.

Corneal sensitivity. The sensory innervation of the cornea is derived from the nasociliary branch of the ophthalmic division of the trigeminal nerve (NV) through the long ciliary nerves. Corneal sensitivity is tested clinically by means of a cotton-tipped applicator with a wisp of cotton twisted to a point. The patient is instructed to look directly ahead, and the cornea is touched with the cotton wisp. With normal innervation, an eyelid closure reflex follows almost immediately. Care must be taken not to touch the eyelashes or the eyelid margins with the cotton wisp and not to stimulate eyelid closure by allowing the patient to see the wisp. A different cotton-tipped applicator should be used for each eye.

Corneal sensitivity is reduced in herpes simplex inflammations of the cornea. It is also reduced after zoster involving the nasociliary branch of the ophthalmic division of the trigeminal nerve, in adenovirus disease of the cornea, in congenital alacrima, and in many corneal dystrophies. Corneal sensitivity may be reduced in lesions at the apex of the orbit, which may also be associated with impaired ocular movements. Corneal anesthesia is an important sign in cerebellopontine angle tumors.

Anterior chamber. The normal aqueous humor is acellular and transparent. Even in severe uveal inflammations, good magnification is required to see inflammatory cells and a Tyndall phenomenon (flare) in the anterior chamber. Blood in the anterior chamber (hyphema) obscures the view of the iris. A severe leukocytic reaction may cause pus to collect in the inferior portion of the anterior chamber (hypopyon).

The depth of the anterior chamber is estimated as the distance between the posterior surface of the cornea and the front surface of the iris. Usually it measures 3 mm or more. If the iris appears to be convex and to parallel the posterior corneal surface and if the depth of the anterior chamber is less than 2 mm, there is a danger of angle-closure glaucoma. Directing the beam of a penlight from the temporal side of the eye across the anterior chamber may demonstrate a narrow angle, since the iris may bow forward and cast a shadow on the opposite nasal side.

If a shallow anterior chamber is present, attention should be directed particularly (1) to episodes of blurring or fogging of vision or severe pain in an eye after watching movies, television, or prolonged darkness and (2) to occasional halos around lights (iridescent vision). Migraine, impending cerebral aneurysm rupture, or other diseases causing hemicrania may be erroneously diagnosed in patients who have periodic attacks of angle-closure glaucoma.

Iris and pupil. The iris crypts and collarette should be clearly visible. Inability to see them suggests a corneal opacity, cells in the aqueous humor, or an iritis. A difference in color of the irises of the two eyes (heterochromia iridis) suggests the possibility of uveal inflammation, tumor, or an anomaly in the sympathetic innervation of the dilatator pupillae muscle, as occurs in congential Horner syndrome. A retained intraocular foreign body containing iron causes the iris to become brown. An absence of some portion of the iris (coloboma) may be surgical or congenital. Absence of the cystalline lens removes support from the iris, which becomes tremulous, a condition known as iridodonesis.

Attention is directed to the shape, size, reaction, and equality of the pupils. If the pupil is adherent to the cornea (adherent leukoma) or to the lens (posterior synechiae), it will not be circular.

Pupillary reactions should be observed in an environment just bright enough to observe the pupils. The patient should fix on a distant target to prevent the pupillary constriction of the near reaction. A flashlight with fresh batteries is used for testing. The pupils are first inspected for size, shape, and symmetry. If there is a defect in the efferent parasympathetic innervation on one side, the affected pupil will be smaller than its fellow (see Chapter 14). If an afferent defect is present in one eye, the pupils are equal in size.

To observe pupillary constriction to light the flashlight is directed from below to minimize the corneal light reflection and the shadow from the nose, and to prevent activation of the near reaction. Direct the light into one eye for 1 second and observe the pupillary reaction. Then do the same with the fellow eye. The pupils should constrict equally and promptly.

Observation of the pupillary reaction that accompanies unilateral or asymmetric optic nerve disease or extensive retinal disease requires a slightly different technique.The light is directed into one eye for 3 seconds and the pupillary reaction observed. The light is then directed into the fellow eye. Since the pupil is already constricted as a result of the consensual reflex, the pupil does not further constrict. If the pupil dilates rather than remaining the same size when stimulated with light, a relative pupillary defect is present in that eye. When the affected eye is stimulated for 3 seconds, the fellow eye receives less consensual stimulus. When the light is quickly directed to the normal eye, the pupil will further constrict. This inequality of pupillary reaction is a valuable sign of monocular extensive retinal disease or optic nerve disease more advanced or confined to one side.

Lens. The transparent lens is observed by the image reflected from its anterior surface. Cataract may cause a gray, opaque appearance in the pupillary aperture. The lens is evaluated by means of the biomicroscope, but opacities are evident on ophthalmoscopic examination.

Ocular movements. The patient is instructed to look to the right, left, up, and down. Full movements indicate integrity of the third, fourth, and sixth cranial nerves. The patient is then directed to look at a penlight held about 13 inches in front of his eyes. Normally the image reflected from the cornea is approximately in the center of the pupil. The presence or absence of a phoria or tropia is determined by the cover-uncover test and by using a small figure instead of a penlight (see Chapter 21).

Biomicroscopic examination. The ophthalmic slit lamp consists of a microscope that has approximately the same power as a laboratory dissecting microscope. The light source projects a slit of light that illuminates a thin section of the cornea and lens. When the light source is placed at an acute angle to the microscope, the examiner can recognize the depth at which abnormalities occur.

MEASUREMENT OF INTRAOCULAR PRESSURE

Intraocular pressure is directly measured by means of a cannula within the eye that is connected to a suitable transducer and amplifier. Such testing has been carried out in humans before removal of an eye because of disease. It must be done so as not to disturb the normal pressure equilibrium of the eye by the loss of aqueous humor around the cannula or by excessive manipulation of the eye.

Clinical testing of the ocular tension is carried out by means of indentation tonometry, as is done with a Schiøtz tonometer (Fig. 6-5, A; see also Chapter 20), or by applanation tonometry that requires a biomicroscope (Fig. 6-5, B). Noncontact tonometers measure tension by means of the deformation of the light reflex from the cornea caused by a puff of air.

The examiner palpates the eye through closed eyelids to estimate whether the eye is extremely hard or unusually soft (tactile tension). In practice the patient is instructed to look downward. The examiner then rests the third, fourth, and fifth fingers of both hands on the forehead and gently exerts alternate pressure on the globe through the upper eyelids with each index finger. The pressure should be directed to the globe and not to the orbit. The tension is estimated by the resistance encountered. An extremely soft eye occurs with the dehydration of diabetic acidosis, phthsis bulbi, choroidal detachment, and penetrating injuries of the eye (in which tactile tension measurement is contraindicated because of the danger of prolapse of the intraocular contents). High tension occurs in closed-angle and secondary glaucoma. Usually vision is markedly reduced because of corneal edema. Accurate tension cannot be estimated in the intermediate ranges, and palpation is not recommended for determining the ocular tension.

CORNEAL STAINING

Epithelial defects of the cornea may be demonstrated by instillation of a 2% fluorescein solution. The stroma in areas not covered by epithelium stains a brillant green color. Fluorescein is a valuable agent in the diagnosis

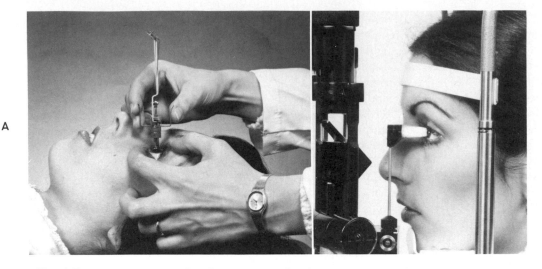

Fig. 6-5. A, Measurement of ocular tension with Schiøtz tonometer. The examiner must be careful not to exert pressure on the globe through the eyelids. **B,** Measurement of the ocular tension with a Goldmann applanation tonometer. This method is more sensitive than Schiøtz tonometry, but it requires an expensive biomicroscope.

Table 6-1. Red eye

	Conjunctival injection	Ciliary injection
Blood vessels	Posterior conjunctival arteries	Anterior ciliary arteries
Location	Superficial conjunctiva orginating from marginal arcade in eyelids	Deep conjunctiva extend anterior from recti muscle insertions to superficial and deep corneal plexus
Appearance	Vessels superficial, red, removable with conjunctiva, most numerous in fornix, fade toward corneoscleral limbus	Vessels deep, violet, immovable, most numerous at corneoscleral limbus, fade toward fornix
1:1,000 Epinephrine	Constricts vessels, "whitens" conjunctiva	No effect
Diseases	Conjunctivitis	Keratitis, irridocyclitis, angle-closure glaucoma
Associated signs	Cornea clear, pupil and iris normal, vision undisturbed, eye uncomfortable	Cornea cloudy, pupil distorted, iris pattern muddy, vision reduced, eye painful

of foreign bodies, abrasions, and inflammations of the cornea, but it must be used solely as a sterile solution or as a sterile strip of filter paper stained with fluorescein solution and then dried.

Bengal Rose (2%) is valuable for demonstrating loss and degeneration of conjunctival and corneal epithelium in keratoconjunctivitis sicca.

Both dyes stain soft contact lenses and should not be used while contact lenses are worn.

RED EYE

A red eye is a cardinal sign of ocular inflammation. It is customarily divided into ciliary and conjunctival injection (Table 6-1).

Ciliary injection involves branches of the anterior ciliary arteries that become congested in inflammations of the cornea, iris, and ciliary body and in closed-angle glaucoma. Each of these conditions is associated with decreased vision and frequently with pain deep within the eye.

Conjunctival injection involves mainly the posterior conjunctival blood vessels that extend from the peripheral marginal arcade in the eyelid and anastomose with the anterior ciliary arteries at the corneoscleral limbus. The posterior conjunctival vessels are most numerous in the conjunctival fornix and are congested in conjunctival inflammations. There is never a loss of vision, and there is ocular discomfort rather than frank pain. Because the posterior conjunctival blood vessels are superficial, they are more red than the ciliary arteries, which are violet. The posterior conjunctival blood vessels move with the conjunctiva and are bleached by topical instillation of 1:1,000 epinephrine.

Subconjunctival hemorrhage occurs with the rupture of a small blood vessel beneath the conjunctiva and causes a bright red blotch of blood beneath the conjunctiva that frequently alarms the patient. The condition is nearly always unilateral, and the hemorrhage absorbs spontaneously within 2 weeks. It is caused by the same mechanisms that cause black-and-blue spots elsewhere. A subconjunctival hemorrhage that involves the entire bulbar conjunctiva after head injury is a serious sign and suggests either rupture of the posterior globe or a fracture of one of the bones of the orbit.

OPHTHALMOSCOPY

Inspection of the interior of the eye with the pupil dilated is fundamental to diagnosis and permits visualization of the optic disk, arteries, veins, retina, choroid, and media. There are three methods of viewing the ocular fundus: (1) direct ophthalmoscopy, by which a magnification of about 15 diameters is obtained; (2) indirect ophthalmoscopy, by which a larger field is obtained, but with magnification of 4 to 5 diameters; and (3) biomicroscopy combined with a lens to neutralize corneal refracting power.

Pupillary dilation. Adequate ophthalmoscopic examination of the ocular fundus requires dilation of the pupils. Without pupillary dilation, the optic disk and surrounding area (about 15% of the fundus) may be visualized (often with difficulty). With direct ophthalmoscopy and pupillary dilation, about half the fundus may be seen. Examination of the entire fundus requires indirect ophthalmoscopy combined with pupillary dilation and scleral indentation.

Soft contact lenses should be removed before instillation of mydriatics.

Selecting drugs to dilate the pupils for examination must be done with great caution. Systemic absorption is decreased by pressure over the inner corner of the orbit to occlude the canaliculi. Phenylephrine should not be used in concentrations of more than 2.5%. It should not be used in patients with vascular hypertension or administered simultaneously or up to 21 days after use of monamine oxide inhibitors. Tricyclic antidepressants potentiate the vascular response of phenylephrine. It should not be used in children or infants with cardiac disease. Cyclopentolate drops should not be used in children with a history of seizures. Pupillary dilation in patients with shallow anterior chambers may precipitate an attack of closed-angle glaucoma. There is a greater danger, however, of neglecting significant ocular or systemic disease by failure to dilate the pupils than there is of precipitating glaucoma by dilation.

Pupils in brown and deeply pigmented irises are more difficult to dilate than pupils in blue and hazel eyes. Often adequate dilation follows one instillation in patients with a fair skin and light hair, while two instillations are required in dark-skinned patients. Suggested dosage varies with age and skin color.

The schedule of instillation varies with different physicians. In neonates, 0.1% cyclopentolate is combined with 1% phenylephrine. In infants 1 to 6 months of age, 0.5% cyclopentolate is combined with 2.5% phenylephrine. Thereafter, 1% cyclopentolate is combined with 2.5% phenylephrine. In dark, unresponsive irises, 0.5% atropine solution may be added if the patient is between the ages of 6 months and 12 years. After the age of 12 years, often 1% tropicamide is used with 2.5% phenylephrine. Except in patients with shallow anterior chambers, tropicamide may be substituted whenever cyclopentolate or phenylephrine are contraindicated.

Direct ophthalmoscopy. Direct ophthalmoscopy (Fig. 6-6) provides an upright image of the retinal structures that is magnified about 15 times. Maximal pupillary dilation makes it possible to study the ocular fundus as far as an area slightly anterior to the equator—the area between the equator and the ora serrata cannot be seen. The maximum resolving power is about 70 μm, and objects smaller than this, such as capillaries, small hemorrhages, or microaneurysms, are not seen. The illumination by the modern direct ophthalmoscope is so bright that some translucent structures, particularly opacities in the media, may not be seen, and other features, such as copper-wire arteries, do not have the color described before electric light illumination.

Technique. The patient is examined in a dimly lighted or dark room. The patient fixes on an object other than the ophthalmoscope light. It is preferable to perform the examination while the patient is seated. The examiner who wears corrective lenses constantly should become accustomed to wearing them when learning to do ophthalmoscopy. Patients who have more than 5 diopters of refractive error ease visualization if they wear their lenses during ophthalmoscopy.

The examiner examines the patient's right eye with his own right eye and the patient's left eye with his own left eye. The ophthalmoscope is held in the corresponding hand. The examiner sits or stands to the side of the eye to be examined. The head of the ophthalmoscope is steadied in the mediosuperior margin of the examiner's bony orbit. The index finger is used to

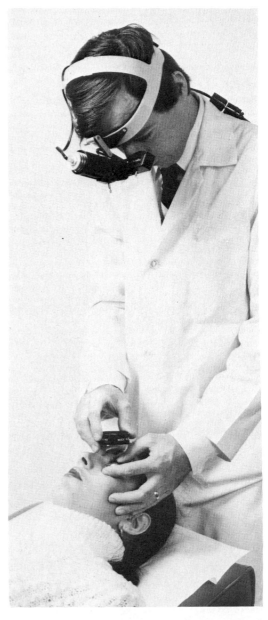

Fig. 6-7. Indirect ophthalmoscopy using a binocular ophthalmoscope. This method provides visualization of the ocular fundus as far as the ora serrata.

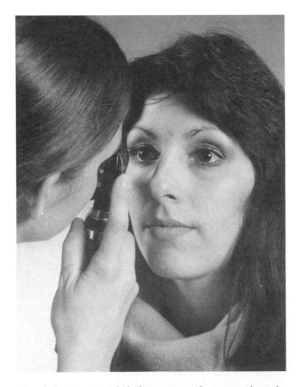

Fig. 6-6. Direct ophthalmoscopy of a patient's right eye. The examiner uses the right eye to study the right eye and the left eye to study the left eye. The ophthalmoscope head is held steady in the bony margin of the examiner's orbit. The index finger of the hand on the side of the ophthalmoscope is used to change the lenses.

change lenses. The examiner's free hand rests at the side. Usually it is not necessary to elevate the patient's eyelid for an adequate view of the eye.

The texture and detail of the retina and the blood vessels are evaluated by constantly focusing the opthalmoscope lens for superficial and deep views, much as one adjusts a microscope when studying a tissue section.

Initially, a +10 diopter lens is rotated onto the viewing aperture of the ophthalmoscope, and the patient looks at a fixation object. The examiner directs the ophthalmoscopic light into the eye at a distance of about 20 cm. A red fundus reflex will be observed. Any opacities in the ocular media will stand out as black silhouettes against a red background. Keeping attention directed to the red reflex, the examiner gradually approaches the patient's eye while steadily decreasing the power of the ophthalmoscope lens. Once fundus details are seen, a blood vessel is followed to its origin at the optic disk, and the systematic examination usually begins with the optic disk.

Indirect ophthalmoscopy. Indirect ophthalmoscopy (Fig. 6-7) is usually performed by means of a binocular ophthalmoscope that directs light into the patient's eye. The image formed by the emerging rays is observed by means of a convex lens of +14 to +30 diopter power. Wearing a binocular indirect ophthalmoscope on the head allows the examiner to use the hands freely to depress the sclera near the ora serrata to observe the extreme retinal periphery and ciliary body. Thus, the entire retina from the optic disk to the ora serrata may be inspected. The indirect ophthalmoscope has an inverted image that is magnified about five times. The field of observation is much larger than that seen with the direct ophthalmoscope, and a stereoscopic image may be seen with the binocular instrument. The maximum resolving power is about 200 μm, and small hemorrhages or microaneurysms cannot be seen. The stereoscopic image of the binocular instrument permits detection and evaluation of minimal elevations of the sensory retina and retinal pigment eptihelium not evident with the direct ophthalmoscope. Because of the bright light, this method of ophthalmoscopy is particularly useful when there are opacities in the media.

Biomicroscopy. The biomicroscope may be combined with a −55 diopter concave contact lens to neutralize the corneal refraction for study of the vitreous and retina. Its increased magnification combined with oblique illumination and stereoscopic view allows for more accurate estimation of the depth of lesions. The contact lens may be fitted with mirrors so that, with adequate pupillary dilation, the retinal periphery may be examined. Alternatively, a +60 diopter handheld lens may be used and the fundus and vitreous inspected as in indirect ophthalmoscopy.

THE OCULAR FUNDUS

The red background of the ocular fundus results from the blood in the choriocapillaris of the choroid, the visibility of which varies with the amount of melanin in the retinal pigment epithelium. The pigment density usually parallels the complexion of the individual. Choroidal veins can be seen in lightly pigmented persons and in the retinal periphery of most individuals. The arteries supplying the choroid go almost directly to the choriocapillaris, and the major portion of the choroid is composed of freely anastomosing veins that are the ophthalmoscopically visible choroidal vessels. In some patients, the contrast between choroidal pigment and blood vessels causes a tessellated or tigroid fundus.

The optic disk is about 1.5 mm in diameter. The diameter of the disk is the standard unit of measurement in the fundus. The disk is approximately the same size in most patients. Marked enlargment of the disk rarely occurs, but its occurrence suggests a conus, myopia, or posterior staphyloma. The disk is smaller than normal in hypoplasia of the optic nerve and appears smaller than normal in severe hyperopia and when the crystalline lens is absent (aphakia).

The disk is pale pink, except for the physiologic cup (see Chapter 20), which is nearly white. The edges of the disk are usually flat and sharp, but not uncommonly the nasal margin is less distinct than the temporal margin. Pigment may be visible, particularly on the temporal side, sometimes as a continuous arc and at other times as linear streaks concentric with the disk. This is called the choroidal ring and is of no pathologic significance. Slightly more uncommon is an arc of stark white tissue on the temporal side of the disk, a scleral ring or conus, which may occur in degenerative myopia. It is often combined with a choroidal ring.

The physiologic cup of the optic disk is a funnel-shaped depression that varies in size and shape. In some cases it is located almost at the center of the disk, and grayish areas of the lamina cribrosa are evident. In other eyes the cup has a more oblique arrangement and its bottom cannot be seen. The ratio of the horizontal diameter of the cup to the horizontal diameter of the disk is important in glaucoma. Irrespective of the position of the physiologic cup, there is always a rim of nerve tissue between the cup and the edge of the disk in the healthy eye.

Occasionally the area usually occupied by the physiologic cup is filled with glial tissue (Bergmeister papilla) that may extend for a short distance over the arteries and the veins. The glial tissue should not be mistaken for vascular sheathing.

The bifurcation of the central retinal artery into its superior and inferior (papillary) branches is visible on the surface of the optic disk or slightly within the optic cup. The central vein usually bifurcates a little deeper within the optic nerve and often has a pulsation synchronous with the central retinal artery. When this physiologic pulsation is not present, it may be elicited by a very slight increase in intraocular pressure induced by pressing the globe with the index finger through the eye-

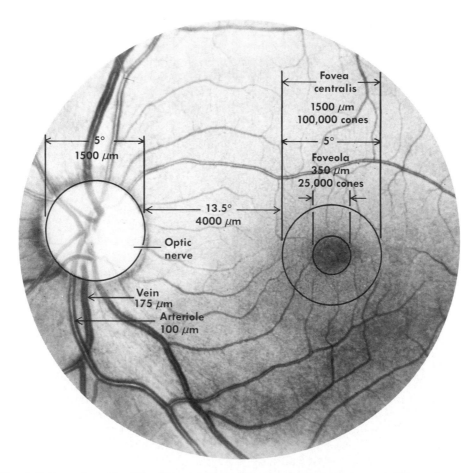

Fig. 6-8. Posterior pole of the left eye. The optic nerve and the fovea centralis are the same diameter. The macula lutea (yellow spot) is not precisely demonstrated. It extends from the foveola almost to the optic disk and about the same distance in other meridians.

lids. In the healthy eye the central retinal artery does not pulsate, and the occurrence of pulsation indicates either an extremely high pulse pressure, as occurs in aortic regurgitation, or an increased intraocular pressure. The superior and inferior papillary branches of the central artery divide into nasal and temporal branches. The muscular coat and internal elastic lamella of these vessels are incomplete and they are thus arterioles. In the healthy eye the walls of the vessels are never visible. Instead the column of blood is observed through the transparent vessel wall.

The retinal arterioles have a smaller diameter than the venules, the usual ratio of arteriole to venule being 3:4 or 2:3. A broad, bright streak is reflected from the convex surface of arterioles. The reflection from venules is narrower, not nearly as bright, and restricted to the major branches near the optic disk. The oxygenated blood is much brighter red in the arterioles than in the veins. In an examination of the fundus, the superior and inferior temporal and nasal arteries are followed as far to the periphery as they can be seen.

In the usual ophthalmoscopic examination, final attention is directed to the central retina (Fig. 6-8). This is about 5 mm in diameter and anatomically corresponds to an area in which the ganglion cell layer is more than one cell nucleus thick. The fovea centralis is situated about 2 disk diameters (3 mm) temporal to the optic disk. Its center is slightly below the center of the optic disk. Usually pupillary dilation is required for careful examination of this area since pupillary constriction is marked when the fovea centralis is illuminated. Within the fovea centralis is the foveola, which measures 400 μm to 500 μm in diameter and corresponds to the capillary-free area of the central retina. The major temporal blood vessels arch above and below the central retina (macula).

The area surrounding the fovea centralis extending to the temporal vessels above and below and about 3 mm (2 disk diameters) on either side has a yellowish pigment xanthophyll in primates. It is best observed in a sectioned eye. It persists for about 15 minutes after the eye has been deprived of its blood supply. The area is called the macula lutea (yellow spot), and thus the posterior pole is frequently loosely called the "macula."

FLUORESCEIN ANGIOGRAPHY

Fluorescein angiography plays an important role in ophthalmoscopic diagnosis. Unlike light ophthalmoscopy, in which light is reflected from the column of blood within the blood vessel, the fluorescein emits light so that the entire diameter of a vessel can be seen. After the intravascular injection of a solution of 10% sodium fluorescein, ophthalmoscopy using a blue filter to excite the fluorescence (fluorescein angioscopy) is useful in detecting leaking capillaries, but the absence of a permanent record limits its value. Photography of the ocular fundus after fluorescein injection (fluorescein angiography) provides much information concerning vascular obstructions, neovascularization, microaneurysms, abnormal capillary permeability, and defects of the retinal pigment epithelium.

For fluorescein angiography, sensitive (usually 400 ASA) black-and-white film is used, and a filter is placed in front of the light source to furnish blue light, which excites the fluorescence. The emitted light is green, and a green filter is placed in front of the film carrier. A control photograph is first made to record intrinsic fluorescence of the fundus. Then 5 ml of a 10% solution of sodium fluorescein solution is rapidly injected into a vein of the arm. Patients experience a hot flash and sometimes nausea; equipment must be on hand to manage the rare anaphylactic reaction. The fluorescein is excreted mainly in the urine during the subsequent 48 hours. It may discolor the skin and conjunctiva, giving a jaundiced appearance, and interfere with urine tests for sugar.

The fluorescein may be seen in the retinal arteries 10 to 13 seconds after injection (Fig. 6-9, A). If the patient is blond or albino, the filling of the choriocapillaris gives a background mottled appearance except in the central retina, where the lipofuscin of the retinal pigment epithelium blocks choroidal fluorescence. During capillary filling, there is an almost simultaneous laminar type of flow in the veins, so that the dye first appears to be in the peripheral portion of the vessels (Fig. 6-9, B). Finally the veins and arteries are both filled with the dye. One minute after injection the vessels still fluoresce slightly, and choroidal veins may be seen as black segments against a slight scleral fluorescence (Fig. 6-9, C).

Abnormal vascular permeability results in the pooling of fluorescein in the choroid, retina, or vitreous. Such areas may fluoresce for several hours after the injection. The accurate localization of such "leaks" may allow treatment by means of laser photocoagulation. Pooling of fluorescein may occur in the choroid, and the sclera may be stained for several hours after administration of fluorescein.

ULTRASONOGRAPHY

Sound waves with frequencies of 5,000 to 20,000 KHz are used in the diagnosis of both intraocular and orbital tumors. The ultrasound is reflected toward its source when it encounters a change in elasticity or density of the medium through which it is passing. This reflected vibration (echo) is converted into an electrical potential by a piezoelectrical crystal and displayed on a cathode ray oscillograph.

Two types of ultrasonography are used in ophthalmology. The A-scan measures the distance of changes in acoustic impedance from a stationary transducer. The change in acoustic density is shown as spikes on the tracing. The distance between the spikes indicates the distance from the transducer. The height of the spike depends upon the acoustic density of the tissue, which varies with the cellular composition. This makes A-scan particularly useful in differentiating benign and malignant intraocular tumors. The A-scan is used to measure the length of the eye to determine the power of an intraocular lens to be used in cataract surgery. The B-scan moves in a linear fashion across the eye, and any increase in acoustic impedance is shown as an intensification on the line of the scan that builds up a picture of the eye and the orbit (Fig. 6-10). In many instances, computed tomography provides a superior image of an abnormality.

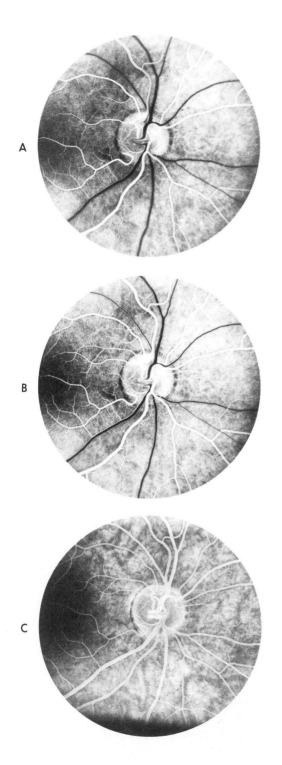

Fig. 6-9. Fluorescein angiography of the right fundus. **A,** The arterial phase after fluorescein injection. The mottled background fluorescence results from filling of the choroid. **B,** The early venous phase. There is filling of some capillaries of the retina, and a laminar flow is evident in the veins. The choriocapillaris is filled, causing a background fluorescence. **C,** The mid-venous phase. The retinal vessels fluoresce less markedly and contain fluorescein diluted by mixing in the blood. The choroidal veins may be seen as black lines contrasting with scleral fluorescence.

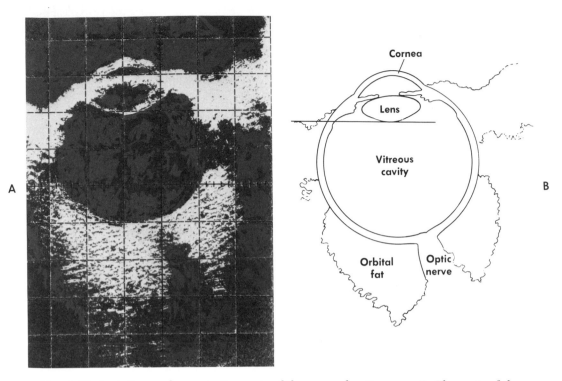

Fig. 6-10. A, A B-scan demonstrating parts of the eye and optic nerve. **B,** The parts of the eye demonstrated.

COMPUTED TOMOGRAPHY

Computed tomography (Fig. 6-11) has generally supplanted conventional roentgenography in the diagnosis of orbital disease. Additionally, intraocular masses can be detected, which is of value in eyes that have opaque media. A detector is substituted for conventional film, and the skull is scanned through 180° in a path from 0.1 to 1.0 cm wide. The signal from the detector undergoes computer analysis to produce a picture 100 times more accurate than conventional roentgenograms. The orbits can be contrasted, and the globe, optic nerve, fat, and various tumors are outlined because of their differences in tissue density. The examination is augmented by the intravenous injection of soluble contrast material that increases the density of inflammatory or vascularized orbital lesions.

Nuclear magnetic resonance imaging. This technique provides detailed images of internal organs without ionizing radiation or injection of contrast material. The patient is placed within a strong magnet and exposed to intermittent stimuli from a radiofrequency coil. The patient's atomic nuclei absorb the radiofrequency pulses and change the direction of their own magnetic field. When the radiofrequency ceases, the nuclei return to their equilibrium state, releasing energy. This released energy produces radio signals that can be detected by a radiofrequency-receiving coil. The signals come mainly from hydrogen nuclei (protons) in tissue, water, and fatty acids. The origin and density of the signals can be learned by applying a nonuniform magnetic gradient field to produce a computer-generated image. Calcium does not produce a signal, and bone does not interfere with imaging. With the use of surface coils, the eye and orbit may be imaged (Fig. 6-12). The method promises to be useful in delineating primary and solid types of retinal detachment, optic nerve abnormalities, and orbital vascular lesions. The procedure is contraindicated in eyes containing ferromagnetic foreign bodies and in patients with pacemakers and those who wear ferromagnetic prostheses.

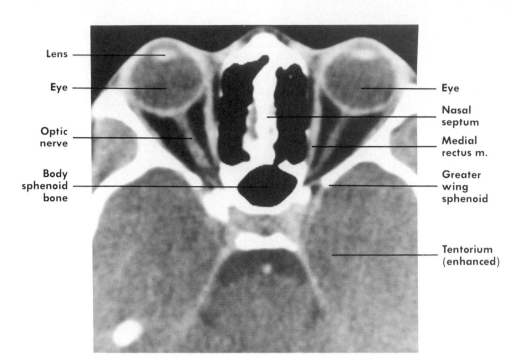

Fig. 6-11. Computed tomography of the orbits. (Courtesy Professor Eugene A. Duda, M.D., Department of Radiology, The University of Chicago.)

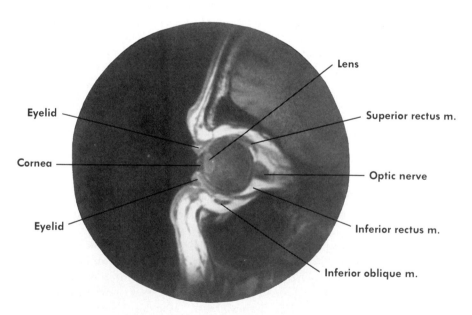

Fig. 6-12. Sagittal magnetic resonance image of the orbit of a healthy man. (Reproduced with permission from the General Electric Co., June 1984.)

BIBLIOGRAPHY

Anderson, D.R.: Testing the field of vision, St. Louis, 1982, The C.V. Mosby Co.

Atychsen, L., and Hoyt, W.F.: Occipital lobe dysplasia. Magnetic resonance findings in two cases of isolated congenital hemianopia, Arch. Ophthalmol. **103**:680, 1985.

Crawford, J.S., Morin, J.D., editors: The eye in childhood, New York, 1983, Grune and Stratton.

Harrington, D.O.: The visual fields: a textbook and atlas of clinical perimetry, St. Louis, 1981, The C.V. Mosby Co.

Hoty, C.S., Nickel, B.L., and Billson, F.A.: Ophthalmological examination of the infant: developmental aspects, Surv. Ophthalmol. **26**:177, 1982.

Jalkh, A.E., Avila, M.P., El-Markabi, H., Trempe, C.L., and Schepens, C.L.: Immersion A- and B-scan ultrasonography, Arch. Ophthalmol. **102**:686, 1984.

Koplin, R., Gersten, M., and Hodes, B.: Real time ultrasonography and biometry: a handbook of clinical diagnosis, Thorofare, N.J., 1985, Charles B. Slack.

Loewenstein, J.I., Palmberg, P.F., Connett, J.E., and Wentworth, D.N.: Effectiveness of a pinhole method for visual acuity screening, Arch. Ophthalmol. **103**:222, 1985.

Sassani, J.W., and Osbakken, M.D.: Anatomic features of the eye disclosed with nuclear magnetic resonance imaging, Arch. Ophthalmol. **102**:541, 1984.

Shammas, H.J.: Atlas of ophthalmic ultrasonography and biometry, St. Louis, 1983, The C.V. Mosby Co.

PART THREE

DISEASES AND INJURIES
OF THE EYE

7

INJURIES OF THE EYE

Prompt and appropriate care of many common eye injuries may prevent much visual disability and, in some instances, the necessity for major corrective surgery. When examining a severely injured patient, one should learn if the eyes are grossly distorted and, if possible, if vision is present. Every effort must be made to prevent marked squeezing of the eyelids by the patient or pressure on the globes by the examiner.

Except in chemical burns, when immediate dilution is imperative, vision should be measured in each eye as carefully as conditions permit. Many patients do not realize they have defective vision in one eye until there is injury, and they may wrongfully accuse the physician of damage that has existed for many years. It is not necessary to use a testing chart—a newspaper or a telephone book will indicate how much vision is present. If the vision is markedly impaired, hand motion and light projection and perception may be tested.

If the cornea is lacerated and the pupil is distorted, if the iris is not visible, or if scleral lacerations are present, both eyes should be covered by a large dressing with no pressure on the globe. The patient should be given parenteral analgesics for pain (aspirin should not be used because it increases the risk of intraocular bleeding). The patient should be moved supine on a litter to a facility for special care.

If the globes are intact, additional treatment is indicated.

If the patient is anesthetized for nonocular injuries, eyelid and conjunctival debris may be carefully irrigated away by using a sterile irrigating solution, preferably Ringer or normal saline solution. This should be followed by the generous topical application of sterile solutions of an ophthalmic antibiotic. Wounds of the face and eyelids should not be debrided.

In open wounds a booster dose of tetanus toxoid, 0.5 ml, is given if the patient has received a booster dose within 10 years or, if the wound is severe and conducive to anaerobic infection, within 3 years. Depending on the severity of the wound, an inadequately immunized person should be given 250 to 500 units of tetanus immune globulin intramuscularly and 0.5 ml of tetanus toxoid. The tetanus toxoid should be repeated twice more at monthly intervals.

FOREIGN BODIES
Cornea

Foreign bodies on the surface of the cornea constitute about 25% of all ocular injuries. A history of the injury and the probable character of the foreign body aid in its detection and removal.

The symptoms vary from little or no discomfort to severe pain. Usually there is a sensation of a foreign body that the patient localizes, inaccurately, to the outer portion of the upper eyelid. There may be associated tearing, photophobia, and ciliary injection.

The foreign body may be seen by careful inspection of the cornea, preferably aided by magnification with a loupe or a magnifying glass. Sterile 2% fluorescein solution instilled in the eye stains the corneal stroma and demarcates the foreign body in the cornea. Corneal foreign bodies should be removed entirely to permit reepithelization and to relieve pain. Topical anesthesia must be used to prevent pain and eyelid closure during removal.

An attempt should be made to remove the foreign body by means of irrigation. A bulb-type syringe or a hypodermic syringe without a needle is used with sterile saline solution as the irrigating fluid. Foreign bodies that are not hot when they strike the eye usually may be removed by directing a stream of fluid against the foreign body to float it off the cornea. This method is often used by physicians' assistants.

If the foreign body cannot be removed by irrigation, it usually cannot be removed by means of a cotton-tipped applicator, which removes much normal epithelium and is, therefore, undesirable. Less injury is caused if the foreign body is lifted gently out of the corneal substance by means of a sharp instrument. Ophthalmologists often use a biomicroscope to provide adequate illumination and magnification, but good visualization can be obtained with a binocular loupe. A sterile spud designed for this purpose or, in an emergency, a 25- to 27-gauge hypodermic needle fitted to a tuberculin syringe may be used. The instrument is held tangent to the cornea so that the cornea will not be perforated if the patient lunges forward. The spud gently elevates the foreign body off the cornea. If a ferrous metal has been embedded for several days, a rust ring may remain after the removal of the main portion of the foreign body; this is removed in the same manner as the foreign body. If it cannot be removed easily at the first attempt, frequently it can be lifted out entirely 24 hours later when leukocytes have softened the surrounding corneal tissue.

After removal of a corneal foreign body, a solution (not ointment) of a sulfonamide such as sulfacetamide or an antibiotic such as gentamicin is instilled. To prevent blinking, which causes discomfort, a dressing is applied to the eye to immobilize the eyelids. The dressing should not be used if it causes discomfort. If there is no keratitis, local medications to cause pupillary dilation are not used. If marked ciliary congestion and photophobia are present or if the removal of the foreign body has been particularly difficult, a cycloplegic such as 5% homatropine is instilled. Atropine causes prolonged pupillary dilation and paralysis of accommodation and is usually not indicated. Since a foreign body may introduce microorganisms into the cornea, the eye should be inspected for infection each day until the area no longer stains with sterile fluorescein. Foreign bodies that damage only the corneal epithelium do not cause a scar. Scarring results from injuries to the Bowman zone or to the substantia propira.

Conjunctiva

Foreign bodies of the conjunctiva can always be removed with irrigation, a spud, or a cotton-tipped applicator.

Foreign bodies frequently lodge on the upper tarsal conjunctiva at its peripheral margin. The upper eyelid must be everted to remove them. The physician must be prepared to remove the foreign body when he everts the eyelid because the foreign body may be dislodged and difficult to locate again if the eyelid is released.

Intraocular

Intraocular foreign bodies are present in injuries in which small particles penetrate the cornea or the sclera. Large foreign bodies cause marked disruption of the globe and so much associated injury that the eye is destroyed and eventually enucleation may be required. Foreign bodies composed of vegetable material such as wood or plants may introduce infection that causes a severe purulent panophthalmitis to occur within hours. Many intraocular foreign bodies are small and are sterilized by the heat caused by their high velocity. They mainly consist of small bits of metal, glass, plastics, and similar material. Their nature varies with the types of industry and recreation of the locality.

Diagnosis and treatment depend on the following factors.

1. *Size of the foreign body.* A foreign body must have a minimal density and size to be demonstrated by means of roentgen-ray examination. Ultrasound or computed tomography will show foreign bodies that are not demonstrable with conventional roentgenography.

2. *Magnetic properties.* Only nickel and iron may be removed by means of a magnet, and

for this reason it is important to determine whether the tool or other material from which the foreign body originated is magnetic.

3. *Tissue reaction.* Many plastics, stainless steel, and glass do not oxidize, and other materials such as aluminum oxidize slowly and if retained cause minimal damage to the eye. Iron slowly oxidizes within the eye and combines with the protein of the intraocular tissues (siderosis) to form an irreversible ferrous compound that results in gradual loss of vision of the eye. The electroretinographic response of the eye is reduced before there is a decrease in visual acuity or a change in the appearance of the retina and foreign body. Unlike siderosis, the tissue reaction caused by retention of copper particles (chalcosis) is reversible if the source is removed. Copper, however, is much more rapidly injurious to the eye. Retention of an intraocular foreign body must always be considered in any patient with uveitis in whom there is a history of injury. Rarely, a foreign body is enmeshed in scar tissue, metallic ions are not released within the eye, and retention of the foreign body causes no symptoms.

4. *Location within the eye.* Foreign bodies in the anterior chamber may be directly observed, although gonioscopy is required to see them in the chamber angle recess. Small metallic foreign bodies within the lens may be tolerated for a long period. However, severe injury to the lens capsule leads quickly to cataract formation. Foreign bodies in the vitreous humor and retina are often obscured by hemorrhage but sometimes may be demonstrated by means of ophthalmoscopy, particularly by using the indirect ophthalmoscope.

Retained foreign bodies must be suspected in all instances of perforating wounds of the eye. If the point of entry is extremely small, high magnification may be required to see the wound in the cornea or the iris. Transillumination of the iris may demonstrate a small hole. Minute wounds in the sclera are almost invisible. Roentgenography, ultrasonography, or computed tomography of the orbit are indicated in such injuries to ensure absence of foreign bodies.

When the presence of a foreign body has been established within the eye, removal is indicated unless the trauma of surgery would be more severe than the damage caused by reten-

tion of the foreign body. The foreign body is initially localized by direct visualization, ophthalmoscopy, ultrasonography, soft tissue roentgenograms, or computed tomography. Foreign bodies in the anterior and posterior chamber and the lens are removed through an incision at the corneoscleral limbus. Sometimes foreign bodies are not removed immediately from the lens but are removed when the subsequent cataract is removed. Foreign bodies in the vitreous cavity are removed through a scleral incision at the pars plana. When removed through the sclera, the foreign body is first localized and the sclera is exposed in the quadrant nearest the foreign body. A scratch incision is then made over the pars plana of the ciliary body. A suture is placed in the incision but left untied and looped out of the field. A magnet is then applied, and the foreign body is removed. The suture is tied. The incision is then surrounded by cryotherapy.

Nonmagnetic foreign bodies are removed by a combination of vitrectomy and suction or by foreign body forceps through a pars plana incision.

Early removal is desirable because foreign bodies may become enmeshed in fibrin and may be difficult to remove after a long period. It is probably better to delay treatment until specialized facilities are available than to attempt removal without the benefit of complete diagnosis.

LACERATIONS
Eyelids

Lacerations of the eyelids are divided into two groups: (1) those that are parallel to the eyelid margin and hence do not gape and (2) those that involve the eyelid margin and are drawn apart by traction of the fibers of the orbicularis oculi muscle (Fig. 7-1, *A*). Eyelid margin lacerations that involve the inner one sixth of the eyelid sever the canaliculus and are particularly troublesome to repair. Children's eyelids are often severely lacerated by dog bites and scratches. If no tissue is missing, surgical correction can be surprisingly effective (Fig. 7-1, *B*).

All wounds of the eyelid must be carefully cleaned with soap and water. Care must be taken not to irritate the conjunctiva and the cornea. Even though markedly contused and damaged, skin is not excised from the lacera-

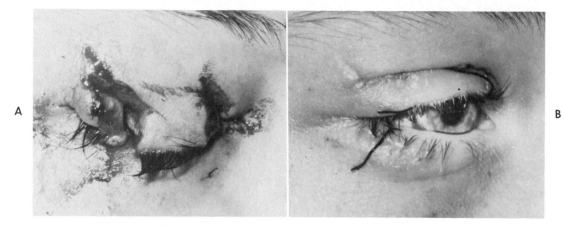

Fig. 7-1. A, Multiple lacerations of the upper eyelid 3 hours after a dog bite. There was no loss of tissue. **B,** Repaired eyelid 7 days later. The long sutures are in the gray line of the eyelid margin. Dog bites of the medial portion of the upper eyelid may damage the trochlea, which subsequently results in palsy or restriction of the superior oblique muscle.

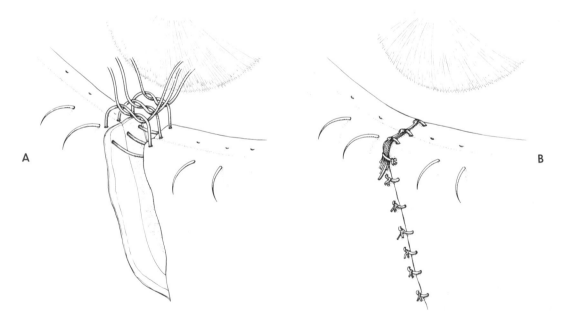

Fig. 7-2. A, The repair of a vertical laceration of the lower eyelid. The first suture is through the gray line. Sutures are then passed through the anterior and posterior portions of the margin of the eye. **B,** The skin is then closed with interrupted sutures.

tion, because the excellent blood supply ensures survival.

Lacerations parallel to eyelid margins require no specialized treatment and are closed with fine sutures. The laceration is parallel to the normal skin folds, and no conspicuous defect results.

Vertical lacerations are divided into those involving the outer five sixths of the eyelid (ciliary) margin and those involving the inner one sixth of the eyelid (lacrimal) margin, which avulse the canaliculi leading to the tear sac.

Ciliary margin. In those lacerations involving the outer five sixths of the eyelid margin, the key to successful repair is the placement of the first suture through the gray line of the eyelid to unite both edges of the laceration with the eyelid margin in the proper plane (Fig. 7-2). Once the eyelid margin is closed properly, the remainder of the eyelid can be closed in layers, using catgut sutures for the tarsus and silk for the skin. The sutures are not tied on the conjunctival surface of the tarsus where their knots will irritate the cornea. Unless other injuries are so serious that treatment must be delayed, it is better not to procrastinate, for a delay of even 24 hours may be followed by retraction of the wound edges, and major plastic surgery may be required for repair.

Lacrimal margin. Lacerations of the inner one sixth of the eyelid in which the canaliculus is severed require (1) placement of a stent through the canaliculus in the hope that it will remain patent, (2) closure of the laceration, and (3) prevention of traction by the orbicularis oculi muscle located lateral to the laceration. The stent, usually silicone tubing, must be left in place 10 to 21 days. Simple apposition of an eyelid laceration causes a typical notched defect of the eyelid margin and constant tearing. Even with highly expert repair, it may not be possible to unite the avulsed ends of a lacerated canaliculus, and additional surgery may be required to correct tearing (epiphora).

Lacerations of the inner one third of the upper eyelid may damage the trochlea of the superior oblique muscle. This may be followed by either paresis of the superior oblique muscle or a muscle contracture that impairs elevation of the eye when abducted.

Conjunctiva

Lacerations of the bulbar conjunctiva that do not involve the globe are rarely severe enough to require surgical closure. With such injuries, the physician must be certain there is no associated laceration of the sclera. Usually the lacerated conjunctiva is surrounded by an area of subconjunctival hemorrhage, and the laceration is evident as a white, crescentic area. Fluorescein will stain the margins of the laceration. The eye is uncomfortable, but there is no loss of vision.

Cornea

Lacerations of the cornea, unless of a puncture type or beveled, are followed by prolapse of the iris, which closes the wound. A characteristic teardrop distortion of the pupil is present. In severe lacerations, there may be frank prolapse of the iris, ciliary body, lens, vitreous humor, and retina, causing a completely disorganized globe.

When a perforating wound of the globe is diagnosed, further examination should be made only by those responsible for surgical correction. Corneal lacerations are frequently associated with retained intraocular foreign bodies, traumatic cataract, secondary glaucoma, infection, and late complications, so that treatment should be carried out by those able to manage the responsibility of the aftercare. First aid is limited to the diagnosis of the condition. A delay of up to 24 hours is preferable to inexpert examination. A broad-spectrum antibiotic is administered systemically in large doses.

The history of the injury and examination of the eye frequently suggest whether a foreign body is retained. Careful roentgen-ray study may indicate metallic foreign bodies. Local anesthesia may be adequate for repair, but if there has been severe trauma, general anesthesia is preferable. Rapid induction is necessary so that there will be no struggling, which increases the intraocular pressure and enhances prolapse of intraocular contents. Succinylcholine must not be used as a muscle relaxant, because it causes a transient increase in the intraocular pressure.

The method of repair depends on the severity of the injury. Direct appositional sutures are used to close lacerations with well-defined margins. When the wound edges are contused or when there has been a loss of corneal tissue, immediate corneal transplantation is done by using either fresh donor tissue or preserved cadaver cornea if necessary.

The corneal wound edges are sutured after the prolapsed iris is either excised or replaced in the eye. Because the tissue may introduce infection into the eye, many surgeons favor iridectomy despite the resulting cosmetic defect. More severe injuries involving the lens and vitreous are treated by immediate reconstruction of the anterior segment with lens removal and excision of vitreous. The laceration is then meticulously repaired with fine sutures. Such an eye must be carefully observed, and if the potential for vision does not outweigh the danger of sympathetic ophthalmia, it must be enucleated.

Sclera

Careful inspection of corneal lacerations is necessary because extension into the sclera may be concealed by intact conjunctiva. Scleral lacerations are much more likely to produce severe damage to the eye than those involving only the cornea. To repair, the lacerated area is exposed by dissecting the cut edges of the conjunctiva and Tenon capsule from the scleral laceration. The first suture is placed exactly at the corneoscleral limbus. Prolapsed uveal tissue is excised and vitreous removed until the wound is entirely free of prolapsed vitreous. If the lens is damaged, it is removed with a suction-aspirator cutting instrument. The sclera is closed with interrupted sutures. Diathermy or cryotherapy may be applied to prevent retinal detachment. An inert gas or air may be injected into the vitreous cavity. The conjunctiva is closed separately.

SYMPATHETIC OPHTHALMIA

Sympathetic ophthalmia (sympathetic uveitis) is an uncommon, diffuse, granulomatous inflammation of the entire uvea (uveitis), usually bilateral, which occurs days, months, or years after penetrating ocular injury or intraocular surgery. Damaged or incarcerated uveal tissue causes a localized (or regional) T lymphocyte-mediated delayed hypersensitivity (type IV hypersensitivity). There are no quantitative abnormalities in circulating peripheral lympho-

cytes and no autoantibodies. Histologically, a diffuse infiltration of the choroid occurs with small lymphocytes, rare plasma cells, macrophagic histiocytes with clumped phagocytosed retinal epithelial cell pigment, and large epithelioid histiocytes. The majority of inflammatory cells are cytotoxic-suppressor T lymphocytes. Dalen-Fuchs nodules occur between the retinal pigment epithelium and Bruch membrane. They contain retinal pigment epithelium cells that have undergone epithelioid transformation together with histiocytes of bone marrow origin. Coalescence of these nodules may cause an inflammatory serous retinal detachment and a granulomatous retinitis.

Most (80%) cases develop within 3 months of injury, although the onset has been reported as early as 9 to 10 days and as late as many years. The injured eye (the exciting eye) has a torpid, persistent, granulomatous type of uveitis that is followed by a similar uveitis in the fellow eye (the sympathizing eye). The inflammation may be suppressed by corticosteroids or other immunosuppressive agents, which may have to be continued for many months or years. Enucleation of the exciting eye is of no benefit once the fellow eye has become inflamed, but blind, exciting eyes should be enucleated. Sympathetic ophthalmia does not occur if the injured eye is removed within 7 days after the injury. Because sympathetic ophthalmia does not occur immediately after an injury, irrespective of the severity of the ocular damage, it is never necessary to enucleate an injured eye before skilled evaluation of the potential for repair with restoration of some function.

CONCUSSION INJURIES

Apparently minor blunt trauma to the eye and orbit may result in surprisingly severe injury. Hemorrhage into the eyelids is in itself usually of little import but may be associated with fractures of the orbital bones. A severe subconjunctival hemorrhage and a persistently soft globe after a severe contusion suggest the possibility of a rupture of the posterior sclera. If the hemorrhage involves the entire conjunctiva with bleeding into the eyelids, there may be a basal skull fracture or ruptured sclera.

The cornea may be abraded in contusion injuries, but this is usually not serious and heals quickly. The sphincter pupillae muscle may be ruptured, resulting in a semidilated pupil that does not react to light (iridoplegia). In relatively minor contusion injuries there may be minute ruptures of the sphincter so that the pupil is no longer round. In more severe injuries the outer edge of the iris may be torn from its insertion to the scleral spur, causing iridodialysis. This may be so minute as to be visible only with a gonioscope, or it may involve a major portion of the insertion of the iris. An extensive iridodialysis is repaired by suturing the peripheral edge of the iris into a corneoscleral wound. Correction is not indicated unless the iridodialysis is extensive or if diplopia is present because of the additional pupil.

Contusion of the globe may rupture a portion of the lens zonule, causing the lens to become subluxated. The vitreous body bulges into the anterior chamber through the ruptured area. The lens is seldom markedly displaced, and it is rarely necessary to remove it. Curiously, lens subluxation is most common after trauma in individuals with syphilis. As years pass, the lens may become opaque. A transient lens opacity may also occur immediately after a blunt injury to the globe.

Glaucoma may develop 10 to 20 years after ocular contusion. The glaucoma resembles open-angle glaucoma except that it is monocular. Gonioscopic examination indicates that a sector of the anterior chamber angle is much deeper (angle recession) than other regions. Often the patient no longer recalls the injury.

Contusion may cause the release of a large amount of pigment into the anterior chamber, which may give the appearance of iritis. There are no keratic precipitates, and posterior synechiae do not form.

Choroidal and retinal hemorrhage, edema, and scarring following blunt trauma are discussed elsewhere.

TRAUMATIC HYPHEMA

Contusion of the globe is frequently followed by frank bleeding into the anterior chamber. This blood usually does not clot and, with bed rest, settles at the most dependent portion of the anterior chamber, and a fluid meniscus forms (Fig. 7-3). The original hyphema, which may be relatively minor, may be followed by more severe bleeding 24 to 48 hours after the original injury. A secondary glaucoma may occur immediately or many years later. Aspirin, which impairs blood clotting, should never by used to relieve pain. Acetaminophen is given instead.

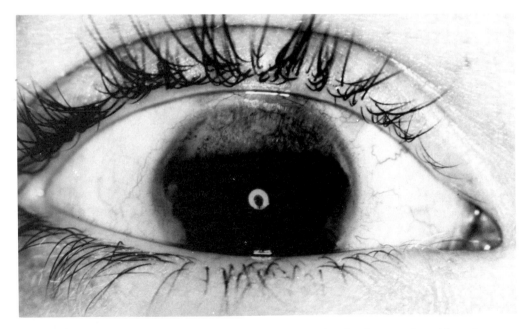

Fig. 7-3. Traumatic hyphema. The blood in the anterior chamber has not clotted but, during rest, forms a fluid meniscus.

Spontaneous recovery is usual if the anterior chamber is not entirely filled with blood. The potential damage caused by secondary hemorrhage is so severe that hospital bed rest without ambulation for at least the first 5 days after injury is desirable. The injured eye should be protected with a shield for 1 to 2 weeks after injury. Ocular tension should be measured daily using an applanation or air tonometer. Systemic amniocaproic acid (Amicar), an inhibitor of fibrinolysis, may prevent early clot retraction within damaged intraocular blood vessels and reduce the possibility of secondary hemorrhage. Double-masked prospective studies indicate that the incidence of secondary hemorrhage is not reduced by topical administration of atropine, pilocarpine, estrogens, or corticosteroids.

Secondary glaucoma may cause optic atrophy, corneal blood staining, and adhesions between the peripheral iris and anterior chamber angle (peripheral anterior synechiae). Minor rises of intraocular pressure are treated with topical timolol and systemic acetazolamide. An increase of pressure to more than 50 mm Hg, a persistently (5 to 7 days) high pressure, or early blood staining of the cornea necessitates surgical treatment.

Simple removal of a small amount of aqueous humor (anterior chamber paracentesis) may be effective. A corneoscleral incision, similar to that of cataract extraction, may be used to express the clot. Clots should never be removed by means of forceps because of the difficulty in distinguishing between the clots and iris. A vitrectomy irrigator-aspirator instrument inserted through the corneoscleral limbus may be used to aspirate the blood. Extreme care must be taken not to injure the corneal endothelium, iris, or lens. General anesthesia is usually desirable because of the difficulty in anesthetizing the congested eye. If the intraocular pressure is increased, it is usually reduced by using intravenous mannitol before the incision into the anterior chamber is made.

When the anterior chamber is filled with blood, prolonged secondary glaucoma causes blood staining of the cornea. The corneal stroma is infiltrated with hemosiderin, which causes a deep yellowish-greenish opacity of the cornea. Clearing occurs at the periphery, but a central corneal opacity remains. In aphakia, blood in the anterior chamber may cause corneal blood staining without concomitant intraocular pressure increase.

Rarely after a corneoscleral incision for cataract or glaucoma, blood vessels in the wound may bleed and cause a microscopic hyphema with blurring of vision. The blood vessels may be sealed with laser photocoagulation.

FRACTURE DISLOCATION OF ORBITAL BONES

Blunt trauma to the orbital region may cause fractures and dislocations of the walls of the orbit, its margins, or both. Many of these injuries are associated with other fractures, head injury, and severe concussions and lacerations and cannot be treated until shock, coma, and life-threatening injuries have been managed.

Fractures that involve the walls only are termed internal and those that involve the margins and possibly the walls are external. There may be associated cerebrospinal rhinorrhea resulting from fracture of the cribiform plate or fontal sinus, orbital emphysema, or nosebleed caused by ethmoidal or frontal sinus fractures that require immediate care. Conversely, orbital hemorrhage and soft tissue contusions may appear as bony fractures but improve quickly. The Waters' view shows the orbital floor and roof and the zygomatic bone. The Caldwell frontal view demonstrates the orbital margins, superior orbital fissure, sphenoidal ridges, and nasal accessory sinuses. Polytomography or computed tomography in axial and coronal views may indicate fractures not otherwise evident.

Fractures of the medial margin of the orbit are usually associated with nasal fractures. The medial canthal ligament may be severed, causing widening of the medial canthus (telecanthus), relaxation of the eyelids, and ectropion. The lacrimal canaliculi may be lacerated. The nasolacrimal duct may be sheared, predisposing to dacryocystitis, as the bony nasolacrimal canal is displaced.

Fractures of the inferior orbital margin are often comminuted and associated with eyelid lacerations. The infraorbital nerve is severed or contused in its canal, and there is anesthesia in its area of distribution. The zygomatic bone is often fractured with inferior or lateral margin fractures. The bony fragments may often be placed in a better position, and depressed fractures may be elevated by forceps introduced through a concomitant laceration.

Fracture dislocation of the zygomatic bone and arch occurs commonly. The lateral canthus is depressed, and the prominence of the cheekbone disappears. Relatively minor blows may be a cause. The temporal and superior zygomatico-frontal suture and the nasal and inferior zygomatico-maxillary sutures are the weakest portion of the orbital margin and may be fractured simultaneously, a tripod fracture.

Fractures of the supraorbital rim often accompany severe head trauma and cerebral injury. The trochlea of the superior oblique muscle may be selectively involved. This causes the signs of paresis of this muscle and a diplopia that is most marked when looking down and in, as in reading. The trochlea tends to reattach itself spontaneously, and does not require treatment.

Orbital rim fractures are repaired surgically only if there is a marked functional impairment or severe cosmetic defect. Delayed treatment may result in fibrosis, contracture, and malunion, and early surgery is desirable.

Bony wall fractures. The walls of the orbit, unlike the margins, are thin. Blunt trauma to the orbit by an object of greater diameter than its anterior dimension may markedly increase the intraorbital pressure and cause a fracture of the wall.

Relatively minor trauma to the medial wall may fracture the thin lamina papyracea of the ethmoid bone and permit air to enter the orbit or the subcutaneous tissue of the eyelid. On palpation there is a peculiar crepitation of the involved tissues. Violent blowing of the nose forces air into the tissue and, if the orbit is involved, may cause double vision. The condition is self-limited and requires no treatment.

Fracture of the floor of the orbit causes prolapse of the ocular contents into the maxillary sinus (Fig. 7-4), and the entire globe may disappear from sight. The palpebral fissure is narrowed. There is slight enophthalmos and inability to rotate the eye upward. In most cases roentgenograms show cloudiness of the maxillary sinus. There is anesthesia in the area of distribution of the infraorbital nerve, including the skin of the lower eyelid, side of the nose, and cheek. A blowout fracture of the orbit

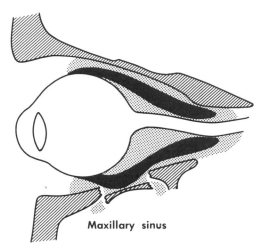

Maxillary sinus

Fig. 7-4. Blowout fracture of the orbit with prolapse of the orbital tissue and the inferior rectus muscle into the maxillary sinus, where the muscle may become entrapped.

should be repaired only if there is permanent diplopia and restriction of ocular movement and if there is enophthalmos after the first 2 weeks of injury indicating entrapment of muscle in the fracture, severe prolapse of tissue into the maxillary sinus, or both. The defect may be exposed through a skin incision over the medial or lateral orbital margin, and the fracture opening may be bridged with bone or plastic.

BURNS
Chemical burns

Chemical burns of the eye are difficult to manage, and even with good care vision may be severely impaired and the eye may be unsightly. The end result is related to maintenance of the blood supply to the peripheral cornea, adequacy of the drainage from the canal of Schlemm, and reepithelization of the cornea. Deep burns, which give the cornea a marbled appearance and destroy conjunctival and scleral blood vessels, may lead to glaucoma and perforation of the globe.

The immediate treatment is dilution of the chemical with water. There should be no delay in learning the history, examining the eyes, measuring vision, or seeking the appropriate chemical neutralizer. The eye should be copiously irrigated with water. In most industries, employees are routinely taught how to do this. An effective method is to plunge the entire face into a container of water and then to open the eyes under water. Immediate dilution is the most important therapy. The fluid used need not be sterile, at body temperature, or even clean, provided the chemical is diluted properly.

After dilution and transport to medical care, the irrigation may be repeated using sterile saline or Ringer solution. Irrigation should be continued until litmus paper touched to the inferior fornix indicates neutrality. Solid particles of lime, lye, or other material should be removed from the superior and inferior conjunctival cul-de-sacs. The upper eyelid should be double everted to make certain all particles are removed. If edema prevents double eversion, the cul-de-sac should be swept with a moistened cotton-tipped applicator. Sodium ethylenediaminetetraacetic acid may be used to chelate calcium hydroxide. Infection is prevented by use of topical antibiotic solutions and ointments. The associated anterior uveitis is treated with topical atropine to dilate the pupil and paralyze the ciliary muscle. Topical corticosteroids may be used the first week; thereafter they are contraindicated unless the cornea has reepithelized. The eye is patched initally to encourage corneal reepithelization. If patching is not effective, a soft contact lens may be used. Symblepharon may be minimized by passing a lubricated probe between the inner surface of the eyelids and the globe.

Necrosis of the sclera and the collecting veins of the anterior chamber angle may lead to secondary glaucoma that can be detected by using a noncontact air tonometer. Timolol, epinephrine, and acetazolamide are used to reduce intraocular pressure.

There is danger of necrosis of the corneal stroma if epithelization is not completed after 1 week. Collagenase and other proteolytic enzymes are inhibited by acetylcysteine, penicillamine, or ethylenediaminetetraacetic acid instilled hourly. The failure of collagen synthesis in the alkali-burned cornea resembles that seen in scurvy. In experimental animals with alkali burns, the systemic administration of ascorbate has minimized corneal perforation. Medroxyprogesterone blocks collagenase formation and

has been used topically and parenterally in experimental animals to limit alkali damage.

Chemical burns cause severe scarring and induce marked corneal neovascularization. Keratoplasty or a keratoprosthesis may be required. Visual results after keratoplasty may be poor because of graft reactions in the highly vascularized cornea.

Thermal burns

Thermal burns of the eyelids usually do not involve the globe, since the blinking reflex provides natural protection. Additionally, tightly closed eyelids usually prevent involvement of the eyelid margins themselves.

Burns of the eyelids require prompt care to prevent severe ectropion. First-aid measures consist of application of sterile dressings and systemic control of pain. Definitive treatment should be carried out within 12 hours of the injury. If dirty, the burned eyelids are cleaned gently with sterile saline solution and a sterile soap. Fluid blebs are left intact. The most important step is suturing the upper to the lower eyelid with 4-0 black silk sutures or, if not available, with other suture material. A mattress suture is placed through the margin of the lower eyelid and through the margin of the upper eyelid, care being taken not to penetrate the globe. The sutures bring the two eyelids together in the closed position, preventing gross contracture and subsequent ectropion formation. Such sutures, if unnecessary, are easily removed. Early skin grafting in severe second- and third- degree burns may speed convalescence and prevent late deformities. Skin for this purpose may be obtained from behind the ear, the inner side of the forearm, or preferably, provided it is uninjured, from the opposite upper eyelid region.

Severe body burns are often associated with smoke inhalation and carbon monoxide poisoning. There are retinal hemorrhages, hyperemia of the optic disk, and venous and arterial congestion. The ocular changes resemble those seen in altitudinal hypoxemia.

INJURIES CAUSED BY RADIANT ENERGY

Only energy that is absorbed causes a reaction. Ultraviolet radiation is almost entirely absorbed by the cornea, and a small band causes ultraviolet keratitis. Radiant energy with wavelengths between 400 nm (blue) and 700 nm (red) is absorbed by the photopigments in the disks of the outer segments and is perceived as light. Excess light energy is absorbed by the retinal pigment epithelium. That portion of the energy not absorbed by the photopigments is absorbed by the melanin of the retinal pigment epithelium and the energy transmitted to the choriocapillaris.

Ultraviolet burns of the cornea occur in arc welders, mountain climbers, persons exposed to snowfields (snow blindness is ultraviolet keratitis), and persons who expose themselves unwisely to sun lamps. Like sunburn, ultraviolet radiation is cumulative; symptoms occur some time after exposure. A marked foreign body sensation in the eyes, lacrimation, and photophobia are present. Symptoms are entirely relieved by a local anesthetic, which, however, delays epithelization of the cornea. The condition is entirely self-limited.

There are three main types of retinal injury from radiant enery: (1) mechanical disruption resulting from energy engendered by extremely short pulses of radiation at high power density levels, (2) thermal insult resulting from absorption of energy in the retinal pigment epithelium and choroid that increases temperature more than 10° C in the tissues, and (3) actinic insult resulting from absorption of energy by the photoreceptors after extended exposure to wavelengths between 400 nm and 500 nm.

Mechanical disruption occurs when the melanosomes of the retinal pigment epithelium absorb radiant energy from Q-switched and mode-locked lasers. The input is so rapid (nanoseconds) and the power so dense (terawatts/cm^2) that heat dissipation cannot take place and the melanin granules become miniature fireballs.

Thermal insult results from exposure of the retinal pigment epithelium to radiant energy that exceeds the cooling capacity of the choriocapillaris. Transmission through the ocular media decreases so much at wavelengths below 550 nm that most thermal injury occurs at wavelengths between 600 nm and 1400 nm.

The amount of energy absorbed by the retina depends on the (1) duration of exposure, (2) pupillary size, since pupillary constriction limits the amount of light that can enter the eye, and (3) refractive error that governs the size of retinal image. The retina is more sensitive in vitamin A depletion and may be sensitized by some drugs.

The retina is damaged by increase of the temperature of the retina by more than 10° C and its proteins are coagulated by an increase to 57° C, the principle underlying photocoagulation therapy with the laser or xenon arc. Accidental damage to the foveola with a photocoagulator reduces vision. Panretinal photocoagulation, as required in some instances of diabetic retinopathy, damages many of the retinal rods and impairs dark adaptation.

Observation of a solar eclipse with the unaided eye causes a photic retinopathy because the pupil is dilated as the result of low light intensity and infrared rays are focused on the fovea centralis. The cones of the fovea centralis are destroyed and replaced with a scar of glia and retinal pigment epithelium. Similar damage may occur in those who gaze at the sun as part of sun worship or psychosis. Marked pupillary constriction may prevent injury.

Infrared energy absorbed by the iris is transmitted to the lens and causes cataract (glassblower's cataract).

Actinic insult results in "color-blinding" lesions after cumulative exposure to intense narrow-band spectral light applied for a few seconds or up to 1 hour for several days. Short-wave-length-sensitive cones are irreversibly destroyed by radiant energy with a wavelength near 400 nm. Middle-wavelength-sensitive cones are damaged by energy with a wavelength of 500 nm, but they recover in a few weeks. Long-wavelength-sensitive cones are not affected.

The use of fluorescent lighting to lower the bilirubin level in low-birth-weight infants who suffer from hyperbilirubinemia is a cause for concern. Infants' eyes should be protected by intermittent patching during phototherapy. In addition, some form of ultraviolet-absorbing material, such as a sheet of glass, should be placed between the infant and the fluorescent bulbs to protect the infants from ultraviolet radiation and to prevent injury from bulb breakage.

Infants should not spend days and nights under the bright room lights of a nursery. It is advisable to protect them from lights periodically to permit visual cell renewal.

Electromagnetic energy of long wavelengths in the range of radar can cause cataract when focused on the eye for several minutes. Presumably the changes are caused entirely by increased temperature of the lens and not specifically related to the type of energy. Electromagnetic energy of short wavelengths (roentgen rays, gamma rays) may damage any part of the eye. Radiation cataract is produced through interference with mitoses at the equator of the lens.

THE BATTERED CHILD SYNDROME

The battered child syndrome includes nonaccidental trauma as well as other problems resulting from lack of reasonable care and protection of children by their parents, guardian, or other caretaker. Many cases are first suspected because of the implausible history offered to explain a child's injury, a discrepancy in the history provided by the two parents, or a delay in seeking medical care. Ocular injuries include cigarette burns of the eyelids, acute hyphema, chemical burns of the eyes, dislocated lenses, and retinal dialysis. Subdural hematomas are often the result of violent shaking and may cause coma and convulsions. Retinal hemorrhages are usually present in these children.

Any child who is a victim of physical abuse requires the protection of admission to a hospital. Further management includes telling those involved the diagnosis, reporting the diagnosis to a protective agency, and seeking social service assistance. The child must not be returned to the caretakers until after adequate intervention.

ALTITUDINAL HYPOXEMIA

Acute mountain sickness occurs within 8 to 24 hours after rapid ascent to altitudes above 8,000 ft. Most individuals show symptoms at elevations of more than 15,000 ft. These symptoms occur within 8 to 24 hours after arrival and clear over a 4- to 8-day period. They include headache, lassitude, insomnia, and gastrointestinal upset. Ocular hemorrhages frequently occur in individuals who ascend to 17,500 ft. There is no association between the

retinal hemorrhages and concomitant sickness. A prior history of migraine as well as rapid ascent and increased physical exertion places the climber at higher risk.

Other ocular changes include increase in the diameter, tortuosity, and cyanosis of the retinal arteries and veins together with cyanosis of the optic disk. There may be increased retinal blood flow and retinal blood volume while the mean retinal circulation time decreases. The concomitant hypoxia and Valsalva maneuvers required in physical exertion along with the hyperviscosity of the blood occurring at high altitudes may play a role. Similar changes occur in carbon monoxide poisoning in humans. Slow ascent to permit acclimatization as well as ingestion of acetazolamide for 48 hours before ascent to prevent cerebral edema appears to be beneficial.

BIBLIOGRAPHY
Lacerations

Hutton, W.L., and Fuller, D.G.: Factors influencing final visual results in severely injured eyes, Am. J. Ophthalmol. 97:715, 1984.
Kaplan, H.J., Waldrep, J.C., Chan, W.C., Nicholson, J.K.A., and Wright, J.D.: Human sympathetic ophthalmia, Arch. Ophthalmol. 104:240, 1986.

Concussion

McGetrick, J.J., Jampol, L.M., Goldberg, M.F., Frenkel, M., and Fiscella, R.G.: Aminocaproic acid decreases severe hemorrhage after traumatic hyphema, Arch. Ophthalmol. 101:1031, 1983.
Thomas, M.A., Parrish, R.K., II, and Feuer, W.J.: Rebleeding after traumatic hyphema, Arch. Ophthalmol. 104:206, 1986.

Fractures

Leone, C.R., Jr., Lloyd, W. C., III, and Rylander, G.: Surgical repair of medial wall fractures, Am. J. Ophthalmol. 97:349, 1984.

Burns

Pfister, R.R.: Chemical injuries of the eye, Ophthalmology 90:1246, 1983.
Pfister, R.R.: The effects of chemical injury on the ocular surface, Ophthalmology 90:601, 1983.

Radiant injury

Fechner, P.U., and Barth, R.: Effect on the retina of an air cushion in the anterior chamber and coaxial illumination, Am. J. Ophthalmol. 96:600, 1983.

8

THE EYELIDS

The eyelids are thin, movable curtains composed of skin on their anterior surface and mucous membrane on their posterior surface. They contain striated and smooth muscle and two tarsal plates, which are noncartilaginous formations of dense connective tissue containing meibomian glands. The eyelids protect the eye, distribute tears over its anterior surface, and limit the amount of entering light. The eyelids are divided by the orbitopalpebral sulcus into two portions: (1) the palpebral portion, adjacent to the eyelid margin, which ends at the margin of the tarsus and is involved in reflex blinking, and (2) the orbital portion, the peripheral portion of which merges into the cheek below and the brow above.

The free margin of each eyelid is about 2 mm wide and has an anterior and posterior border. The cyelashes (cilia) extend from the anterior border. Glands of Zeis (rudimentary sebaceous glands) are attached to each cilium and glands of Moll (sweat) are parallel to the hair bulbs of cilia and open between two lashes or into a duct of a Zeis gland. The ducts of meibomian glands open on the posterior portion of the free borders (Fig. 8-1) of the eyelids. The superior and inferior puncta, the openings of the superior and inferior lacrimal canaliculi, are located medially. The mucocutaneous junction of skin and conjunctiva is at the level of meibomian gland openings. The intermarginal sulcus (gray line) is along the middle of the free margin. The margin is divided into two parts: (1) the lateral five sixths is called the ciliary portion and contains eyelashes, and (2) the medial one sixth, without eyelashes, contains the puncta and is called the lacrimal portion. The lateral junction of the eyelid margins, the lateral canthus, forms a 60° angle located about 2 mm higher than the rounded medial margin, the medial canthus.

The eyelids are covered by a thin, elastic, easily distensible skin that contains no subcutaneous fat. The skin is, of course, subject to the same diseases as skin elsewhere and is rapidly responsive to noxious or allergic stimuli. The orbicularis oculi muscle (N VII) originates from the medial orbit and medial palpebral ligament, circles the orbit covering the orbital margin and the eyelids, and inserts into the lateral orbit and lateral palpebral ligament. The orbicularis oculi muscle is separated from orbital structures by the orbital septum, which limits the extension of inflammation, effusions, and fat between the orbit and into the eyelids.

The upper eyelid is elevated by the levator palpebrae superioris muscle (N III). Müller smooth muscle (sympathetics) provides tone to the elevated eyelid. The eyelids are closed by the orbicularis oculi muscle (N VII). Only the palpebral portion is involved in reflex blinking, whereas both the orbital and palpebral portions are involved in forcible closure of the eyelids.

The eyelids contain numerous glands: sebaceous (Zeis) and sudoriferous (Moll) glands associated with the eyelashes, meibomian glands in the tarsal plates, and accessory lacrimal glands of Krause and Wolfring located in the

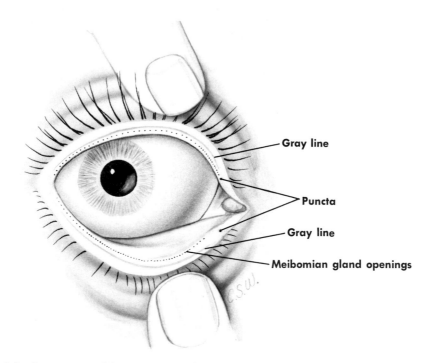

Gray line

Puncta

Gray line

Meibomian gland openings

Fig. 8-1. The upper and lower puncta, the openings of the lacrimal canaliculi, divide the eyelids into ciliary and lacrimal portions. The openings of the meibomian glands are visible inside the gray lines. The gray lines mark the anterior surface of the tarsal plates at the eyelid margins.

conjunctival fornices. Additionally, the skin of the eyelids contains sweat and sebaceous glands subject to the same disorders as elsewhere in the body.

SYMPTOMS AND SIGNS OF EYELID DISEASE

The variety of structures forming the eyelids, their importance in facial expression and appearance, and their function in the protection and health of the eye provide the basis for a wide variety of abnormalities.

The palpebral apertures are normally similar in size, shape, position, and movement, and the eyelids just conceal the corneoscleral limbus in the 12 and 6 o'clock meridians. The obliquity of the aperture varies in different races, being more slanted in Orientals. The upper eyelid is highest at the junction of the medial one third with the lateral two thirds, whereas the lower eyelid is lowest at the lateral one third. Retraction of the eyelids or forward protrusion of the globe exposes the sclera (scleral rim) above or below the corneoscleral limbus.

When the eyelids are closed, the palpebral aperture becomes a fissure and the eye turns up and out (Bell phenomenon), protecting the cornea.

The eyelid margins are normally in close apposition to the globe, and the lashes are directed outward. The lashes are darker and more rigid than body hair, and they do not gray nor are they lost with age but may be lost in disease. The inferior punctum turns slightly inward to dip into the lacrimal lake at the inner canthus. The lacrimal papillae, small prominences surrounding the punctum, become more obvious with age.

The skin of the eyelids is thin and often translucent, so that a delicate tracery of blood vessels gives a slightly bluish cast to the eyelids. The skin is thrown into fine folds, and the superior and inferior palpebral furrows form folds.

Periodic contraction of the tarsal portion of the orbicularis oculi muscle causes involuntary blinking. During attempts to squeeze both eyes closed, contracture is normally equal on

Table 8-1. Some abnormalities of the eyelids

Abnormalities	Characteristic
Ankyloblepharon	Adhesion between upper and lower eyelid margins
Blepharochalasis	Relaxation of skin of eyelids (dermatolysis palpebrarum)
Blepharophimosis	Decreased dimensions of palpebral fissure
Blepharoptosis	Drooping of upper eyelid
Blepharospasm	Tonic spasm of orbicularis oculi muscle
Coloboma	Absence of some ocular tissue
Distichiasis	Accessory row of eyelashes
Ectropion	Outward turning eyelid margin
Entropion	Inward turning eyelid margin
Epiblepharon	Extra fold of skin, lower eyelid
Epicanthus	Extra fold of skin, medial eyelid (palpebronasal fold)
Lagophthalmos	Inability to close eye completely
Madarosis	Loss of eyelashes
Myokymia	Fascicular tremor muscle
Symblepharon	Adhesions between palpebral and bulbar conjunctivae
Telecanthus	Widely separated medial canthal ligaments
Trichiasis	Misdirected eyelashes

both sides. The levator palpebrae superioris and Müller muscles elevate the eyelids to a similar height on the two sides.

The eyelids may be involved in many different abnormalities (Table 8-1). The symptoms vary widely. Inturning of the eyelid margins (entropion) causes the lashes to irritate the cornea and bulbar conjunctiva. Failure of the eyelids to cover the globe, as in lagophthalmos or ectropion, may expose the conjunctiva and cornea, causing inflammation. If the eyelids cover one or both pupils, there may be interference with vision. If one pupil is covered early in life, amblyopia may develop. When both eyelids cover the pupils, the individual often compensates by throwing the head back to expose the visual axis.

Pain, swelling, and redness of the eylids occur with a variety of inflammations. Inflammatory or neoplastic disease may extend from the eyelids to involve the eye. Suppurative infection of the upper eyelid or the lateral one third of the lower eyelid may cause enlargment of the preauricular (parotid) lymph nodes. Involvement of the medial two thirds of the lower eyelid may cause a submaxillary lymphadenopathy.

Tearing may occur because of irritation of the eye or because the eyelids are not in apposition with the globe. Constant tearing may cause excoriation of the skin at the lateral and medial canthi.

CONGENITAL ABNORMALITIES

Failure of an eye to develop may result in ablepharon, which is absence of the eyelid. The eyelid is imperfectly separated in ankyloblepharon, resulting in a horizontally narrowed palpebral fissure. Failure of a portion of the eyelid to develop, which causes a notching defect of its margin, is called a coloboma of the eyelid. Retention of a developmental supernumerary row of lashes, which are frequently directed backward and irritate the cornea, is known as distichiasis. In blepharophimosis, the horizontal and vertical interpalpebral fissure is congenitally narrowed. There is often an associated blepharoptosis with an autosomal dominant inheritance. In blepharoptosis, the height of the palpebral fissure is decreased by drooping of the upper eyelid.

Epicanthus is by far the most common congenital variation. A vertical skin fold occurs in the medial canthal region that conceals the medial angle and the caruncle. Such an epicanthal fold occurs normally in Orientals and is often combined with a fold of skin overhanging the palpebral fissure (mongolian fold), giving it an almond shape (Fig. 8-2). It is present in many infants until growth of the nose and face obliterates it. An epicanthal fold may conceal the medial sclera and may simulate the appearance of esotropia (pseudostrabismus). The presence or absence of esotropia is quickly determined by means of the cover-uncover test (see Chapter 21).

ABNORMALITIES OF SHAPE AND POSITION

In entropion the eyelid margin, usually the lower, is turned inward, and the eyelashes irritate the eye. In ectropion, the eyelid margin, usually the lower, is turned outward so that the conjunctival surface is exposed and becomes keratinized. In blepharoptosis the upper eyelid is not elevated properly so that the palpebral fissure is narrowed. Blepharoptosis and epicanthal folds may occur simultaneously. In lagophthalmos the eyelids fail to cover the globe.

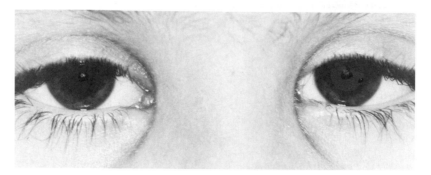

Fig. 8-2. A 5-year-old boy with bilateral epicanthus that is more marked on the left side. The concealment of the left sclera by the extra fold of skin simulates the appearance of an esotropia (pseudostrabismus).

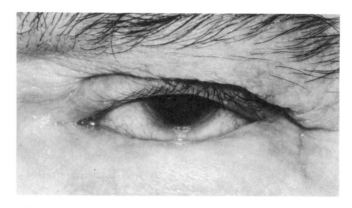

Fig. 8-3. Spastic entropion with the eyelids causing irritation of the eye.

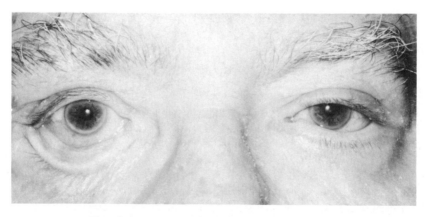

Fig. 8-4. Atonic ectropion in a 74-year-old man.

Entropion

Entropion (Fig. 8-3) is a condition in which the eyelid margin is turned inward so that the lashes irritate the eye, causing corneal epithelial defects, conjunctival injection, tearing, leading sometimes to secondary infection of the cornea or conjunctiva. The lower eyelid is usually involved. Entropion occurs in four main forms: (1) atonic (involutional), the most common type, (2) cicatricial, which may involve the upper or lower eyelid, (3) spastic, and (4) congenital.

The atonic type results from involutional atrophy of the lower eyelid retractors (the aponeurosis of the capsulopalpebral head of the inferior rectus muscle and the inferior tarsal muscle, both of which insert into the lower tarsal margin). These changes reduce the stability of the lower tarsal border, permitting contraction of the orbicularis oculi muscle to rotate the eyelid margin inward. Laxity of the orbital septum also contributes but to a lesser degree. Surgical correction is often necessary. In minor cases temporary relief may be obtained by drawing the skin of the outer canthus down and temporally by means of an adhesive tape strip. The surgical procedures involve a resection of the orbicularis oculi muscle and tarsus to shorten the eyelid horizontally and prevent the inferior margin of the tarsus from rotating outward.

Cicatricial entropion follows scarring of the palpebral conjunctiva, which may be caused by chemical injuries, lacerations, surgical procedures, radiant energy, trachoma, and erythema multiforme. Frequently the tarsus is deformed. The globe is irritated by the lashes. Several surgical procedures have been devised to evert the eyelid margin and the eyelashes. It may be necessary to transplant mucous membrane from the mouth to replace scarred conjunctiva.

Spastic entropion results from excessive contraction of the orbicularis oculi muscle (blepharospasm) combined with atrophy of the eyelid retractors. Ocular irritation from chronic conjunctivitis, keratitis, or ocular surgery is a common cause. Excessive contraction occurring after surgery is sometimes corrected by removing eye dressings. Temporary relief may be provided by alcohol injection into the orbicularis oculi muscle. Surgical correction is the same as that for atonic entropion.

Congenital entropion is usually caused by deformity of the tarsal plate in which the eyelashes are directed toward and irritate the cornea. Resection of the abnormal portion of the tarsal plate and placing the remainder in its normal position corrects the condition. Inepiblepharon, which may occur with congenital entropion, an abnormal fold of skin, usually at the medial one third of the eyelid, turns the eyelid margin inward. Usually the condition disappears as the face grows. If not, the excess skin may be excised.

Ectropion

Ectropion (Fig. 8-4) is a condition in which the eyelid margin is turned away from the eye so that the bulbar and the palpebral conjunctiva is exposed. Symptoms result from exposure of the conjunctiva and the cornea. When the lower eyelid is involved, the inferior punctum is not adjacent to the lacrimal lake, and tearing may occur. Ectropion occurs in several forms: (1) atonic, (2) cicatricial, (3) spastic, and (4) conjunctival. Only the lower eyelid is involved in the atonic type, but the cicatricial and conjunctival types may affect either the upper or the lower eyelid.

Atonic ectropion is the usual type. Mild types occur in aging and weakening of the orbicularis oculi muscle and cause tearing and excessive wiping of the eyes. Treatment is directed to inverting the lacrimal puncta into their normal position. More severe ectropion follows paralysis of the orbicularis oculi muscle (N VII) in facial nerve palsy (Bell). The medial portion sags outward and there is marked tearing. Ophthalmic lubricating agents and methyl cellulose eyedrops are used in early treatment. Persistence after 3 to 6 months requires one of several types of eyelid shortening procedures.

Cicatricial ectropion follows burns, lacerations, and infections of the skin of the eyelids. With most thermal burns, the eyelids close tightly and the eyelid margins are not involved, there being an intact 1 or 2 mm margin present. Subsequent plastic surgery to correct contracture may be unnecessary if the eyelids are sutured together as early as possible. Early skin grafting is desirable in most instances of cicatricial ectropion. Skin of the opposite upper eyelid is ideal for this purpose, or skin may be obtained from over the mastoid region. The plastic surgery required for established cicatricial ectropion may be difficult and may necessitate skilled and prolonged care.

Blepharoptosis

An abnormality in the innervation or musculature of the levator palpebrae superioris muscle causes blepharoptosis (Fig. 8-5), in which the upper eyelid droops and the palpebral fissure is narrowed.

Blepharoptosis is divided into congenital and acquired types. The congenital type, apparent at birth, is usually the result of interference with the superior division of the oculomotor nerve (N III), which innervates only the levator palpebrae superioris muscle and the superior rectus muscle. There may also be weakness of the superior rectus muscle. A superior palpebral sulcus, which marks the insertion of the levator palpebrae superioris aponeurosis into the skin to the upper eyelid, is present in the acquired but not the congenital type. If the muscle has never functioned, the sulcus is absent. Both the congenital and the acquired type may be hereditary or occur sporadically.

Congenital blepharoptosis. Congenital blepharoptosis may involve one or both eyelids. The degree of severity varies. If the visual axes of both eyes are covered by the drooping eyelids, the child acquires a characteristic posture with the head thrown back and forehead furrowed in a perpetual frown as he uses his frontalis muscle to elevate the eyelids. If only one eye is involved, the child may develop a sensory amblyopia so that earlier surgical treatment is required than with bilateral blepharoptosis.

Treatment is based on the degree of severity. If the pupils are not covered by the eyelids, treatment may be deferred for a long period. If only one eye is involved and the visual axis is covered, surgery should be carried out before 1 year of age, and major attention should be directed toward the development of normal visual acuity in the affected eye. When the condition is bilateral, surgery is usually done between 3 and 5 years of age.

Jaw-winking. Unilateral blepharoptosis may be associated with a paradoxical (synkinetic) retraction of the drooping eyelid when the ipsilateral pterygoid muscle is stimulated, usually as a result of chewing, opening the mouth, or sucking (Robert Marcus Gunn syndrome). Amblyopia (35%) and strabismus (30%) are common; amblyopia occurs in all patients in whom the superior rectus muscle is paretic. The jaw-winking can be corrected only by disinsertion of the levator palpebrae superioris muscle and substitution of a fascial sling. To maintain symmetry, both eyes must be operated on. Some patients improve spontaneously and treatment must be individualized.

Acquired blepharoptosis. Acquired blepharoptosis may result from any affection of the nerve supply of the upper eyelid musculature, from disease of the muscles themselves, or from mechanical interference in elevating the eyelid by the weight of a tumor. The most common acquired causes of oculomotor nerve involvement are diabetes mellitus neuropathy and intracranial disorders such as aneurysms, neoplasms, injuries, inflammations, and toxins. Aneurysms of the internal carotid artery within

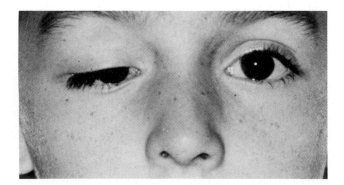

Fig. 8-5. Right blepharoptosis. The absence of a superior palpebral furrow indicates paralysis of the levator palpebrae superioris muscle.

the cavernous sinus may cause a complete ophthalmoplegia from involvement of nerves III, IV, and VI combined with anesthesia in the area of distribution of the ophthalmic and maxillary divisions of the trigeminal nerve (N V).

Interference with the sympathetic innervation of the smooth muscle (Müller) which provides tone to the upper eyelid, causes 1 to 2 mm of drooping, as is seen in Horner syndrome. Blepharoptosis occurs in chronic progressive external ophthalmoplegia, myotonic dystrophy, and myasthenia gravis. It has also been observed in patients who have used topical corticosteroids for long periods. With aging, loss of tone of the levator palpebrae superioris muscle and Müller muscle, together with loss of support caused by enophthalmos from atrophy of orbital fat, may cause some eyelid sagging. Disinsertion or dehiscence, or both, of the aponeurosis of the levator palpebrae superioris muscle from the tarsus may cause a narrowed palpebral fissure in individuals who have had injection of local anesthetic into the eyelid for ocular surgery.

Myasthenia gravis. Paresis of the levator palpebrae superioris muscle may be the initial sign of myasthenia gravis (see Chapter 29). Frequently the disease is limited to the upper eyelid and does not become more generalized. Most commonly only one side is affected. Since the disease may be treated medically, it is most important to exclude myasthenia gravis before surgical correction of an acquired blepharoptosis.

Surgical correction of blepharoptosis. There are several procedures used in the correction of blepharoptosis.

1. Resection of the conjunctiva, tarsus, Müller muscle, and aponeurosis of levator palpebrae superioris muscle (Fasanella-Servat) corrects up to 3 mm of blepharoptosis if the muscle function is good.

2. For moderate blepharoptosis (3 to 4 mm) with moderate levator palpebrae superioris function, the muscle may be resected through either a skin or conjunctival incision. It is the procedure of choice when levator palpebrae superioris muscle function is present. Reattachment of the aponeurosis of the levator palpebrae superioris muscle to the tarsus corrects blepharoptosis that follows local injection of anesthetic agents into the eyelid for surgery.

3. When no levator palpebrae superioris muscle function is present, the upper eyelid is suspended to the frontalis muscle by means of fascia lata or other material. This provides mechanical elevation, but the cosmetic result may be less pleasing than with a levator palpebrae superioris muscle resection. If no muscle function is present, however, the procedure must be used.

Several devices, known as "ptosis crutches," attached to the frame of spectacles elevate the eyelid. They are not particularly well tolerated and, in individuals with unilateral ophthalmoplegia, a drooping eyelid may prevent diplopia.

Lagophthalmos

Lagophthalmos is an abnormality in which inadequate closure of the eyelids results in exposure of the eye. It may occur because of seventh cranial nerve weakness, proptosis, eyelid retraction, or enlargement of the globe. Exposure of the cornea causes drying and secondary infection. Treatment is directed toward the cause. Surgery to prevent exposure keratitis should be carried out as soon as it is evident that the cornea is threatened. Permanent or temporary adhesions may be created between the upper and the lower eyelids (tarsorrhaphy). These may be either lateral, medial, or central. In mild lagophthalmos only the central portion of the cornea may be exposed, and the instillation of an ointment base at bedtime may be all that is required to prevent corneal drying during sleep. Plastic wrap held in position with gummed cellophane tape may be used to cover the exposed eye and create a moist chamber. Alternatively, a soft contact lens and artificial tears may prevent corneal drying in a cosmetically more acceptable manner. Craniofacial surgery is necessary in many bony deformities, whereas orbital decompression may be needed in orbital tumors and thyroid disease.

DISORDERS OF THE ORBICULARIS OCULI MUSCLE
Blinking

Blinking spreads tears over the surface of the eyeball and limits the amount of light entering the eye. It may be involuntary or voluntary. Involuntary blinking occurs as a periodic contraction of the tarsal portion of the orbicularis oculi muscle at a rate peculiar to each individual. It normally occurs about once every 5 seconds and lasts about 0.3 second. Involuntary blinking is absent in infants. Infrequent blinking is seen in progressive supranuclear palsy, Parkinson disease, and hyperthyroidism (Stellwag sign). Infrequent blinking or incomplete closure of the eyelids may aggravate the symptoms of keratoconjunctivitis sicca.

Reflex blinking may follow peripheral stimulation of the trigeminal, optic, or auditory nerves. Irritation of the cornea, conjunctiva, or eyelashes is followed by eyelid closure. Bright lights or glare may initiate blinking through a reflex arc that begins in the retina. It is mediated through the superior colliculus, not the visual cortex, and thus such reflex blinking is not a sign that vision is present. A sudden loud noise may cause reflex closure of the eyelids.

Blepharoclonus

Blepharoclonus is an exaggerated form of reflex blinking in which either the frequency of blinking is increased or the closure phase is excessive. There is often marked contraction of the orbital portion of the eyelids. Blepharoclonus may be initiated by irritation or inflammation of the conjunctiva or the cornea. Even after removal of the cause, blepharoclonus may continue as a tic, and other muscles of the face may be involved. When the stimulus cannot be found, effective treatment is difficult. A variety of surgical procedures have been described that aim at interrupting the facial nerve supply to the orbicularis oculi muscle or interrupting the muscle fibers themselves.

Children 5 to 10 years of age may develop episodes of rapid blinking. Apparently the child is unaware of blinking, but the parents may be distressed. Almost invariably, examination of the eyes indicates no ocular abnormality.

Orbicularis oculi muscle tremor

Involuntary contraction of a few fibers of the orbicularis oculi muscle (myokymia) causes the patient to sense an annoying twitching of the eyelid that the patient feels is conspicuous, although examination discloses a barely perceptible contraction of a few fibers of the orbicularis oculi muscle. Often no cause is found, but fatigue, alcohol and coffee consumption, smoking, and ocular irritation are implicated. Reassurance is usually all that is required. Quinine

sulfate in doses of 200 to 400 mg increases the latent period of skeletal muscle contraction with relief of symptoms. It may be combined with systemic antihistamines.

Local or systemic administration of anticholinesterase compounds may cause myokymia. If the entire muscle is involved, a search must be made for organic causes such as hyponatremia, multiple sclerosis, Parkinson disease, myasthenia gravis, tabes dorsalis, hyperthyroidism, and disorders of the dorsal pons.

Blepharospasm

Blepharospasm is an involuntary, tonic, spasmodic, bilateral contraction of the orbicularis oculi muscle that may last from several seconds to several minutes. It occurs mainly in individuals over 45 years of age. It may be limited to the eyelids or may involve other muscles of the face. It causes a severe cosmetic deformity as well as failure to see because of persistent eyelid closure. It may occur in postencephalitic states, in hemiplegia from various causes, and after Bell palsy. In such patients the blepharospasm may not disappear during sleep. Relief may follow dissection of the seventh nerve just anterior to the parotid gland with interruption of each nerve identified by a muscle stimulator as going to the orbicularis oculi muscle. Some patients have been treated with psychotherapy and others with levodopa when blepharospasm has been considered to be a limited form of Parkinson disease. Injection of botulinum toxin into the affected muscle may be helpful.

Many patients require extensive periorbital surgery with extirpation of the orbicularis oculi muscles of the upper eyelids, the muscles of the eyebrows, and the facial nerve fibers around the zygomatic regions. Additionally, lateral canthal tendon plication and reinsertion of the levator aponeurosis may be required. There is partial anesthesia of the forehead after the procedure. The operation may take up to 3 hours to perform.

MISCELLANEOUS CONDITIONS
Blepharochalasis

Blepharochalasis is an abnormality in which there is atrophy and loss of elasticity of the skin of the eyelids. It occurs most commonly in aged persons. There is a loss of skin turgor, and a fold of skin may hang down over the eyelid margin. Treatment is usually not indicated. If the fold of skin interferes with vision by covering the pupillary area, the excess skin may be excised.

Orbital fat herniation

Puffiness or swelling of the eyelids (baggy eyelids) results from localized edema or protrusion of fat into the eyelids from the orbit. Systemic causes of edema include hyperthyroidism, nephrosis, and angioneurotic edema. In premenstrual edema, fluid retention as well as vasodilation may be conspicuous in this area, with the abundant vasculature of the eyelid evident through the nearly translucent skin.

Fat escapes from the orbit into the upper eyelid (Fig. 8-6) through the opening in the orbital septum for the aponeurosis of the levator palpebrae superioris muscle. Fat escapes in the lower eyelid through the opening for the capsulopalpebral fascia. Fat may also escape through the openings provided for major blood vessels and nerves. Removal of the fatty tissue from the eyelid and orbit is a frequently performed cosmetic procedure.

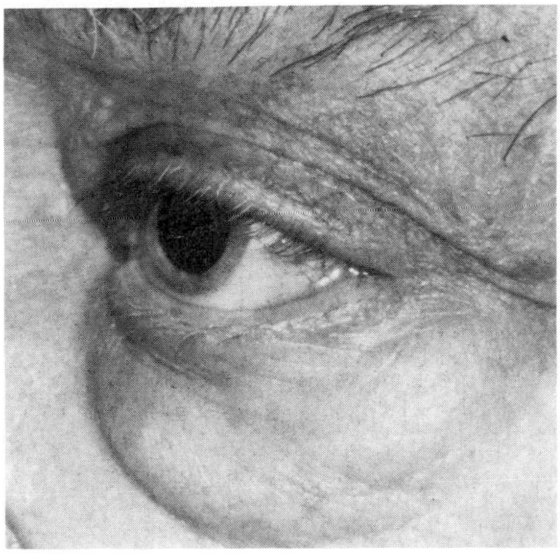

Trichiasis

In this condition the eyelashes are directed toward the globe and irritate the cornea and the conjunctiva, causing secondary infection. The condition usually follows blepharitis but may also be associated with trachoma, cicatricial pemphigoid, alkali burns, and injuries. The cornea and conjunctiva may be protected by a soft contact lens, but usually treatment is directed toward destruction of the irritating lashes. Eyelashes removed by epilation regrow to full size in 10 weeks. Electrolysis may be used to remove lashes permanently but is seldom practical for more than a few. Reducing the temperature of the hair follicles to $-15°$ C, using liquid nitrogen applied to the anesthetized palpebral conjunctiva, may be used to treat extensive trichiasis. Small areas may be treated with direct application to the cilia. The cornea and skin must be protected. Depigmentation of the treated area may contraindicate the process in deeply pigmented individuals.

Distichiasis

Distichiasis is a congenital abnormality in which the meibomian glands atavistically revert

Fig. 8-6. Herniation of orbital fat into the lower eyelid.

to hair follicles to form an accessory line of lashes. Other congenital malformations may be present. If the lashes are numerous and cause irritation of the globe, the area must be excised and a graft substituted.

Hypertrophy of the eyelids

Immense overgrowth of the eyelids may occur in neurofibromatosis, hemangiomas (particularly in infancy), lymphangioma, and a variety of infections. Treatment is directed toward the cause.

INFLAMMATION

The glands in the eyelids may be involved in acute suppurative infections such as those occurring with sties that involve the glands of Zeis or Moll. The meibomian glands may be involved in an acute or chronic inflammation called chalazion.

The eyelid margins may be involved in inflammations (blepharitis) caused by bacteria, seborrheic dermatitis, or localized hypersensitivity reactions. The skin of the eyelids may be involved in a large variety of inflammations that may be more conspicuous than similar lesions elsewhere in the body because of the looseness of the skin, its exposed position, and secondary involvement of the eye. Contact dermatitis and reactions secondary to the application of drugs or cosmetics to the eyelids or conjunctival sac are common.

Blepharitis

Blepharitis is a chronic inflammation of the eylid margins. It begins early in childhood and frequently continues throughout life, becoming more symptomatic in the sixth and seventh decades. Staphylococcal infection and seborrheic dermatitis, often in combination, are its principal causes.

There are two forms of blepharitis: (1) squamous blepharitis and (2) ulcerative blepharitis (uncommon). The squamous type has hard, brittle, fibrinous scales surrounding the cilia (collarette). The ulcerated type has matted hard crusts surrounding individual cilia, and removal discloses small ulcers. Both types are associated with dilated blood vessels in the eyelid margins, white eyelashes (poliosis), loss of lashes, and thin, broken, and small lashes. Chalazia and styes may be recurrent. Almost invariably there is an associated chronic papillary conjunctivitis. Keratitis may occur, as may phlyctenulosis. *Pityrosporum ovale* and *Demodex folliculorum* mites may serve as vectors of staphylococci. *Pityrosporum ovale* possibly produces the disease by splitting lipids into irritating fatty acids.

Squamous blepharitis. Simple squamous blepharitis is characterized by a hyperemia usually limited to the eyelid margins. It is associated with scaling of the skin that may cause fine flakes and scales surrounding the lashes. In severe cases the eyelid margins may become thickened and everted. Most commonly, however, redness of the eyelid margins is the chief complaint. There may be burning and discomfort of the eyes and an associated chronic conjunctivitis or keratoconjunctivitis sicca that further contributes to discomfort.

The disorder may be infectious (mainly *Staphylococcus aureus*) or secondary to a seborrheic dermatitis of the scalp that may also affect the eyebrows and cause an erythema of the cheeks. Patients with acne rosacea and atopic disease have a greater than normal predisposition. Irritation of the eyelid margins by cosmetics, chemical fumes, smoke, and smog may aggravate the hyperemia as may frequent rubbing of the eyelids.

Ulcerative blepharitis. Ulcerative blepharitis is caused by acute and chronic suppurative inflammation of the follicles of the lashes and the associated glands of Zeis and Moll. *Staphylo-coccus aureus* is usually the causative organism, but some strains of *Staphylococcus epidermidis* may be responsible. The eyelid margins are red and inflamed. There are multiple suppurative lesions surrounded by yellow pus that crusts and is removed with difficulty, bringing with it eyelashes. Loss of lashes and the necrotizing inflammation cause distortion of the eyelid margin, leading to ectropion, epiphora, and chronic conjunctivitis.

Treatment of both the squamous and ulcerative types is difficult, and recurrences are common. Coexisting seborrheic dermatitis is treated with frequent (daily to twice weekly) selenium sulfide shampooing of the scalp and eyebrows. Excessive meibomian gland secretions must be expressed using a glass rod. The eyelids should be scrubbed with a moist, cotton-tipped applicator to remove scales. This may be followed by scrubbing with a cotton-tipped applicator moistened with baby shampoo (Johnson & Johnson Baby Shampoo). After shampooing, the eyelids are closed for 5 minutes and the excess shampoo removed with a wet, cotton-tipped applicator.

Antibiotic ointment may be applied to the eyelid margins at bedtime or more frequently in severe inflammation. Bacitracin, erythromycin, or sulfisoxazole (Gantrisin) ointments are usually effective. Systemic tetracycline (erythromycin in children and pregnant women) may be used in acne rosacea and severe inflammation.

Infestation of the eyelashes by lice may cause blepharitis or skin infection. Primary treatment is directed to concomitant treatment of head lice through shampoo with 1% lindane (Kwell), or 0.5% malthion (Prioderm), or piperonyl butoxide (Rid, A-200 Pyrinate, Vonce). A 1% physostigmine ointment kills the lice through its anticholinesterase action. The eyelashes may be treated twice daily with application of heavy petrolatum, and after 8 days the nits and lice may be mechanically removed.

Meibomianitis

In the middle years a passive retention of secretion by the meibomian glands may deposit a white, frothy secretion on the eyelid margins and at the canthi. The glands may be massaged to express an oily secretion, and eversion of the eyelids may show vertical yellowish streaks

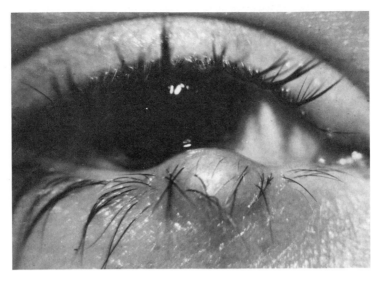

Fig. 8-7. Acute hordeolum of the lower eyelid.

shining through the tarsal conjunctiva. Occasionally cellular debris or calcium is deposited in a gland. If this material penetrates the conjunctiva, it causes a foreign body sensation and must be removed.

Meibomianitis is often associated with blepharitis and chronic conjunctivitis and may cause recurrent chalazia. Treatment consists of tarsal massage and removal of the secretion with a moist, cotton-tipped applicator.

Hordeolum

Hordeolum, or sty (Fig. 8-7), is an acute suppurative inflammation of the follicle of an eyelash or the associated gland of Zeis (sebaceous) or Moll (special apocrine sweat gland). Like pustules elsewhere, the usual cause is staphylococcal infection. The initial symptom is tenderness of the eyelid that may become marked as the suppuration progresses. The initial sign is edema of the eyelid, followed by the development of a red, indurated area on the eyelid margin that may rupture. The main differential diagnosis involves an acute chalazion that tends to point on the conjunctival side of the eyelid and does not involve the eyelid margin unless the opening duct of the meibomian gland is involved. The chalazion is preceded and followed by a minute tumor in the substance of the eyelid that feels like a small buckshot. Sties tend to occur in crops, because the infecting organism spreads from one hair follicle to another,

either directly or by the fingers. Treatment is the same as for that of acute suppurative infection elsewhere in the body. Hot compresses applied at frequent intervals hasten resolution of the lesion. When pointing occurs, incision and drainage are indicated. Frequently a topical sulfonamide or an antibiotic prevents involvement of adjacent glands. The associated blepharitis must be treated.

Chalazion

Chalazion is a chronic inflammatory lipogranuloma of one of the meibomian glands. It is characterized by a gradual painless swelling of the gland without gross inflammatory signs. Palpation indicates a small swelling resembling buckshot in the substance of the eyelid, and this may be its only evidence. With increase in size, it may cause astigmatism by distortion of the globe or it may be evident beneath the skin as a small mass (Fig. 8-8). It may become secondarily infected and cause an acute suppurative inflammation that usually points on the inside of the eyelid. The lesion is a lipogranuloma resembling that seen in sarcoidosis or tuberculosis with giant cells but without caseation.

Asymptomatic chalazia do not require treatment and usually disappear spontaneously within in a few months. Acute suppuration is treated with local hot compresses and a topical antibiotic or sulfonamide. Local injection from

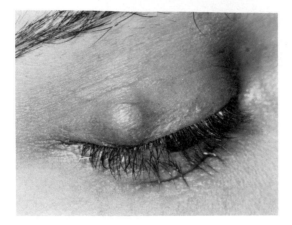

Fig. 8-8. Chronic chalazion (lipogranuloma) of meibomian gland of the upper eyelid.

the conjunctival surface of 0.5 ml of triamcinolone acetoxide into the center of the chalazion may be rapidly effective. Excision, usually through a conjunctival incision, is indicated when persistent or large. Some individuals tend to have a series of chalazia, apparently because of inspissation of the meibomian gland contents in the excretory ducts. If pressure on the eyelid expresses a viscous secretion from the glands, massage of the eyelids, sometimes with a glass rod, may be helpful. Recurrence of what is believed to be a chalazion at the site where it has been excised should make one suspicious of a meibomian gland carcinoma.

Rarely, a hard contact lens migrates to the supratarsal region of the upper eyelid, becomes imbedded, and causes an orbital mass, a chalazionlike swelling, or a blepharoptosis.

Dermatitis

Infection of the skin of the eyelids may occur with a variety of microbial organisms, and it includes nearly the entire range of dermatitides. The thinness of the skin and its good blood supply allow enormous distension and injection, but, more important, secondary infection of the conjunctiva, cornea, and intraocular contents may occur by direct extension from the skin. Conversely, inflammatory skin lesions may originate in the conjunctiva, orbit, nasal accessory sinuses, lacrimal apparatus, or the glands of the eyelids.

Impetigo, erysipelas, anthrax malignant pustule, tuberculosis, chancre, leprosy, yaws, and tularemia may all involve the eyelid on occasion, often with enlargement of the parotid and submaxillary lymph glands.

Herpes zoster ophthalmicus causes a vesicular eruption of the eyelid that is less important than the frequent keratitis and uveitis. Verruca vulgaris and molluscum contagiosum infection of the eyelid margins are important because of the resulting viral conjunctivitis and keratitis.

Fungus infections of the eyelid may occur either as a local infection or in the course of widespread systemic disease.

Contact dermatitis. There are two types of contact dermatitis of the eyelids: (1) primary irritant and (2) T lymphocyte-mediated. Primary irritant contact dermatitis is caused by defatting of the skin by excessive moisture or from substances (acids, alkalis, resins, chemicals) that injure the skin. The T lymphocyte-mediated (delayed hypersensitivity; type IV hypersensitivity) requires the sensitizing substance to combine with a protein in order to sensitize. Sensitization requires 5 to 10 days for potent sensitizers and months for weak sensitizers. Common sensitizers include nickel (in spectacle frames and jewelry), eyedrops with names ending in "-caine," thimersol (a common ingredient in eyedrops), atropine, chloramphenicol, penicillin, sulfonamides, neomycin sulfate, and corticosteroids (rarely). After sensitization, re-exposure to the substance, not necessarily at the same site, produces a contact dermatitis at the original site.

The skin reacts with a recurrent, weeping, enzymatous lesion. Itching is severe. When chronic, the skin becomes indurated and brawny with moderate swelling.

Treatment is unsatisfactory until the cause is removed. This may be difficult to determine but is sometimes aided if the patient keeps a diary to record each day's activities and the severity of the inflammation. Rubbing of the eyes after handling soaps, detergents, or chemicals may cause the reaction. Cosmetics, perfumes, and nail polish may be offenders. The patient should never touch the eyelids. All topical medications should be stopped. Perfumed and colored soaps should not be used. Sometimes a bland ointment such as Aquaphor will relieve symptoms. Systemic corticosteroids are not necessary. Sometimes topical corticosteroids provide relief.

TUMORS

The eyelids are subject to the usual tumors of the skin. If the eyelid margin is not involved, excision is simple. Involvement of the eyelid margin necessitates skilled surgery to ensure complete excision and satisfactory closure.

Cutaneous horns

A cutaneous horn is a small, cylindric, protruding, keratic growth of epidermal cells. Its cause is unknown. It may occur near the eyelid margins in middle-aged or older people. It may be solar, seborrheic, inverted follicular keratosis, verucca vulgaris, or, rarely, sebaceous cell carcinoma in origin. Cutaneous horns are easily excised.

Milia

Milia are small, white, round, slightly elevated cysts of the superficial dermis. They tend to occur in crops localized in a small area of the skin, sometimes on the eyelid. They may be derived from a hair follicle or its associated sebaceous gland. Excision may be desirable for cosmetic reasons.

Xanthelasma

Xanthelasma is a cutaneous deposition of lipid material that occurs most commonly at the inner portion of the upper or the lower eyelid. The lesion appears as a yellowish, slightly elevated area with sharply demarcated margins tending to be approximately parallel to the eyelid margin. The condition occurs with primary and secondary systemic lipid anomalies, but more commonly it occurs spontaneously without evident cause. It produces a cosmetic defect, and treatment is indicated only to remove the defect. The lesion may be excised surgically or destroyed by means of diathermy, photocoagulation, or chemicals. Recurrence is common.

Keratoacanthoma

Keratoacanthoma is a cup-shaped, elevated, benign tumor that has an umbilicated apex. It develops on exposed (usually hairy) areas of the skin of middle-aged and elderly individuals. Sometimes it involves the eyelids. It grows rapidly for 2 to 6 weeks and reaches a maximum size of 1 to 2 cm. It involutes several months after onset, leaving a depressed scar. Histologically, a central crater filled with keratin, acanthosis, and benign cellular structure distinguishes the whole tumor from a well-differentiated squamous cell carcinoma. This differentiation may be impossible to discern with a partial biopsy specimen. Its initial rapid growth and umbilicated necrotic center distinguishes it clinically from squamous cell carcinoma.

Carcinoma

Basal cell carcinoma is the most common neoplasm of the eyelids, occurring almost twenty times more often than squamous cell carcinoma. Both have a similar nodular appearance with elevated, irregular surfaces and sharply demarcated, pearly margins. The squamous cell tumor produces keratin and may appear more pearly white. The centers may be excavated or ulcerated. Extensive ulceration of basal cell tumors occurs with growth (rodent ulcer). The basal cell tumor may, in about 5% of the cases, be pigmented, although pigmentation may indicate nevus or malignant melanoma. Generally, the lower eyelid is involved (Fig. 8-9), particularly its outer portion. The patient may neglect the lesion for a long period because it does not cause symptoms. There is a gradual increase in size of a typical tumor that has pearly margins and an excavated center. If the eyelid margin is not involved, excision in the early stages provides cure. When the eyelid margin is involved, surgical excision may necessitate a major plastic procedure.

Radiation therapy may cause keratinization of the conjunctiva and chronic keratitis. This condition is most likely to occur after treatment of lesions that affect the middle portion of the upper eyelid. When the eyelid margin is involved, surgical excision is preferred to radiation. Excision more fully ensures removal, and inadequate radiation may be followed by metaplasia of basal cell tumors to the squamous cell.

Cryotherapy is frequently indicated in tumors involving the inner canthus since damage to the lacrimal drainage apparatus may be minimized. A thermistor is inserted into the tumor, and liquid nitrogen is sprayed onto the tumor until the temperature within the tumor is reduced to $-30°$ C. Recurrent tumors may have the freeze-thaw cycle repeated several times. Noninfiltrative tumors of the eyelid that measure less than 10 mm in diameter have a 5-year cure rate of 97%; the rate for infiltrative tumor is 94%.

Hematoporphyrin derivative after intravenous administration binds and is retained by neoplastic cells. When tumor cells containing hematoporphyrin derivative are exposed to light, cytotoxic singlet oxygen is formed that leads to cellular destruction. Seventy-two hours after administration of hematoporphyrin derivative tumor areas (that fluoresce in ultraviolet light) are treated with red light (630 nm) that penetrates the tissue about 2 cm. Sunlight must be avoided for 1 month. A posttreatment biopsy of the center and periphery of the treatment field assesses the efficacy of the treatment, which should be repeated if there are residual tumor cells.

Neglected or mismanaged basal cell carcinoma may invade the orbit and the cranial cavity, causing a widespread destructive lesion.

The sweat glands (of Moll) of the eyelids are apocrine glands and, like such glands elsewhere (axilla, surrounding the nipples, and perianal and perigenital regions), may develop a special type of carcinoma, extramammary Paget disease. The diagnosis is usually based on the histologic appearance of the tissue, which may be resected in the belief that the lesion is a basal cell carcinoma.

Adenocarcinoma may develop in the glandular portion of a meibomian gland. Most commonly, patients are treated for recurrent chalazion before the neoplastic nature of the lesion is evident. Such a delay may permit fatal metastasis. The tissue excised in every recurrent chalazion should be examined histologically.

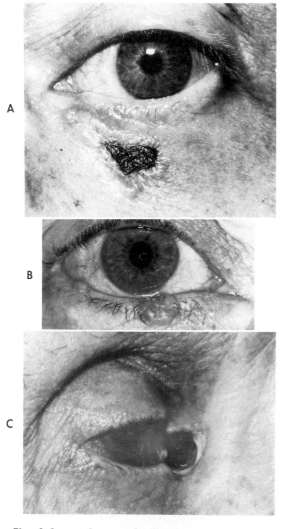

Fig. 8-9. A and **B,** Basal cell carcinomas of the lower eyelid. **C,** Extension of a basal cell carcinoma of the inner canthus into the nose in an 83-year-old man.

BIBLIOGRAPHY
General

Fraunfelder, F.T., and Roy, F.H., editors: Current ocular therapy, ed. 2, Philadelphia, 1985, W.B. Saunders Co.

McCord, C.D., Jr., editor: Oculoplastic surgery, New York, 1985, Raven Press.

Congenital abnormalities

Doucet, T.W., and Crawford, J.S.: The quantification, natural course, and surgical results in 57 eyes with Marcus Gunn (jaw-winking) syndrome, Am. J. Ophthalmol. **92:**702, 1981.

Pratt, S.G., Beyer, C.K., and Johnson, C.C.: The Marcus Gunn phenomenon, Ophthalmology **90:**27, 1984.

Blepharospasm

Frueh, B.R., Felt, D.P., Wojno, T.H., and Musch, D.C.: Treatment of blepharospasm with botulinum toxin, Arch. Ophthalmol. **102:**1464, 1984.

Jones, Jr., T.W., Waller, R.R., and Samples, J.R.: Myectomy for essential blepharospasm, Mayo Clin. Proc. **60:**663, 1985

Scott, A.B., Kennedy, R.A., and Stubbs, H.A.: Botulinum A toxin injection as a treatment for blepharospasm, Arch. Ophthalmol. **103:**347, 1985.

Shorr, N., Seiff, S.R., and Kopelman, J.: The use of botulinum toxin in blepharospasm, Am. J. Ophthalmol. **99:**542, 1985.

Abnormalities of shape and position

Beard, C.: Ptosis, ed. 3, St. Louis, 1981, The C.V. Mosby Co.

Stefanyszyn, M.A., Hidayat, A.A., and Flanagan, J.C.: The histopathology of involutional ectropion, Ophthalmology **92**:120, 1985.

Tumors

Caya, J.G., Hidayat, A.A., and Weiner, J.M.: A clinicopathologic study of 21 cases of adenoid squamous cell carcinoma of the eyelid and periorbital region, Am. J. Ophthalmol. **99**:291, 1985.

Fraunfelder, F.T., Zacarian, S.A., Wingfield, D.L., and Limmer, B.L.: Results of cryotherapy for eyelid malignancies, Am. J. Ophthalmol. **97**:184, 1984.

McCord, C.D., Jr.: Recurrence of sebaceous carcinoma of the eyelid after radiation therapy, Am. J. Ophthalmol. **96**:10, 1983.

Tse, D.R., Kersten, R.C., and Anderson, R.L.: Hematoporphyrin derivative photoradiation therapy in managing nevoid basal-cell carcinoma syndrome, Arch. Ophthalmol. **102**:990, 1984.

Inflammation

Dua, H.S., and Nilawar, D.V.: Nonsurgical therapy of chalazion, Am. J. Ophthalmol. **94**:424, 1982.

9

THE CONJUNCTIVA

The conjunctiva is a thin, translucent mucous membrane that lines the posterior surfaces of the eyelids and covers the noncorneal portion of the anterior segment of the eye ("the white of the eye"). It is divided into the palpebral and bulbar portions and the regions connecting them, the superior and inferior fornices. Its epithelium is continuous with that which covers the corneal stroma and lines the lacrimal passages and glands. It varies in thickness from two layers of nonstratified columnar epithelium at the tarsal plate to 5 to 7 layers at the corneoscleral limbus. Goblet cells are scattered throughout with lymphocytes and melanocytes in the basal layers. The stroma is closely adherent to the tarsal plate but thrown into many folds in the fornices and loosely adherent to the globe. The stroma comprises loosely arranged bundles of coarse collagenous tissue containing numerous fibroblasts. Fibroblasts, macrophages, mast cells, and leukocytes are found extravascularly in the tissues. After 3 or 4 months of age, the superficial stroma in the fornices contains lymphoid tissue.

Inflammation may result from exogenous microorganisms, chemical and mechanical foreign material, or radiant energy. Infection may extend from the areas adjacent to the conjunctiva or may be blood-borne, as in measles and chickenpox. Conjunctival allergic reactions may be conspicuous, as in hay fever or vernal conjunctivitis. Vascular abnormalities are readily apparent and may constitute an obvious part of systemic disease.

SYMPTOMS AND SIGNS OF CONJUNCTIVAL DISEASE

The main symptoms of conjunctival disorders are ocular discomfort or burning and sometimes exudation. Severe pain suggests corneal involvement rather than conjunctival disease. Itching is common in hypersensitivity. Inflammatory exudates may excoriate the skin, particularly at the outer canthus, or aggluttinate the eyelids during sleep. Copious exudate may float across the cornea and blur vision or may even cause halos that surround lights and disappear with rapid blinking.

The most serious symptoms of conjunctival disease originate from secondary corneal involvement. This may occur by extension of inflammation from the conjunctiva or by irritation of the cornea because of continued contact with keratinized epithelium of the tarsal conjunctiva. Corneal disease may be secondary to exposure in cicatricial conditions that limit eyelid mobility, or it may be caused by secretory failure of goblet cells or accessory lacrimal glands resulting in an abnormal tear film. Visual loss from corneal scarring is common, and indeed trachoma, a chlamydial infection involving the conjunctiva initially, is probably the chief cause of blindness in the world.

The signs of conjunctival disease are mainly related to abnormalities of appearance, vascular changes, and edema (chemosis). The bulbar conjunctiva is easily inspected, but the tarsal conjunctiva can be seen only by eversion of the upper and lower eyelids. Inspection of the su-

210

perior fornix requires elevation of the upper eyelid by means of a retractor.

CONJUNCTIVAL BLOOD VESSELS
Injection

The normally inconspicuous posterior conjunctival arteries are dilated and engorged in conjunctival inflammations. Conjunctival injection is characterized by superficial bright red blood vessels, which are most conspicuous in the fornices and fade toward the corneoscleral limbus. These blood vessels move with the conjunctiva and are constricted by 1:1000 epinephrine solution instilled in the conjunctival sac (see Table 6-1).

Both the conjunctival and ciliary vascular beds are usually injected in inflammations of the cornea, iris, and ciliary body, although the ciliary injection is more marked. To distinguish conjunctival diseases from deeper diseases of the eye, it is wiser to direct attention to signs of corneal and iris involvement, pupillary reaction to light, and visual acuity than to emphasize vascular engorgement.

Conjunctival hyperemia is a dilation of the conjunctival blood vessels that occur without exudation or cellular infiltration. Symptoms may be absent, but often a gritty foreign body sensation is aggravated by prolonged near work. Many patients are distressed because of the conjunctival redness, which becomes more severe with wakefulness and fatigue.

Hyperemia is caused by the following: (1) irritation caused by tobacco smoke, smog, and chemical fumes; (2) exposure to wind and sun; (3) inadequate ocular protection from ultraviolet radiation; (4) uncorrected refractive errors and ocular muscle imbalance; (5) prolonged topical instillation of drugs, including vasoconstrictors; (6) acne rosacea; (7) blepharitis and excessive meibomian gland secretion; and (8) ganglionic blockade in the treatment of hypertension. Chronic conjunctivitis may be caused by many of the same entities.

Treatment is directed toward removal of the cause. Temporary relief may be obtained by cold compresses or by local instillation of weak solutions of vasoconstrictors. Many commercial preparations containing epinephrine or phenylephrine are available and may provide temporary relief. Products containing corticoste-roids should not be used because of the danger of inducing infection or glaucoma.

Subconjunctival hemorrhage

Rupture of a conjunctival blood vessel causes a bright red, sharply delineated area surrounded by normal-appearing conjunctiva. The hemorrhage is located beneath the bulbar conjunctiva and gradually fades in 2 weeks. There are no symptoms, but many patients become alarmed by its appearance. A subconjunctival hemorrhage is caused by the same factors responsible for a black-and-blue spot elsewhere in the body: trauma, hypertension, blood dyscrasias, and the like. Usually no cause is found. Treatment is ineffective in hastening the absorption of the blood.

Subconjunctival hemorrhage involving the entire conjunctiva may follow fracture of one of the orbital bones or rupture of the posterior sclera. Adenovirus conjunctivitis is sometimes associated with severe subconjunctival hemorrhage.

Systemic disease

Typical involvement of the conjunctival blood vessels has been described in (1) sickle cell disease, (2) diabetes mellitus, (3) cryoglobulinemia, and (4) Fabry disease. The changes are frequently evident only with biomicroscopic examination. Since the conjunctival blood vessels often show dilation and tortuosity with advancing age and exposure to wind, the changes that accompany diabetes and riboflavin deficiency may be difficult to differentiate from aging changes.

Conjunctival vascular stasis may be present in hemoglobin SC disease and in blood hyperviscosity conditions. Biomicroscopic examination indicates isolated, sharply defined, twisted segments of capillaries with both the efferent and afferent connections empty of blood. The vessels are most involved in the bulbar conjunctiva adjacent to the inferior fornix. There are also nonspecific changes of microaneurysms, telangiectasis, and segmental dilation. The typical vascular stasis disappears with the local application of heat and is accentuated by cholinergic blockade or by cold.

Cryoglobulinemia is associated with stasis of blood flow in conjunctival vessels that have a clumping of erythrocytes. Ice water irrigation of the conjunctival sac slows the bloodstream and causes increased segmentation of the blood column.

Venous congestion, microaneurysms, and venous dilation have been noted in the conjuctival vessels in diabetes mellitus. The changes are nonspecific and may be seen with aging, arteriosclerosis, and vascular hypertension.

Pigmentation

The dull, white sclera accentuates conjunctival pigmentation. A dull, grayish discoloration involving the conjunctiva in the lower fornix may occur after repeated instillation of silver and mercury salts. The pigmentation results from the deposition of the metallic ion and cannot be reversed. Prolonged instillation of epinephrine salts may cause deep black subconjunctival deposits of adrenochrome (oxidized epinephrine).

A yellowish discoloration of the conjunctiva may result from an excess of plant pigment (carotene) in food faddists who eat many carrots. It must be distinguished from jaundice. Ochronosis and Addison disease also cause pigmentation of the conjunctiva. The conjunctiva and not the sclera is stained with bilirubin in jaundice.

CONJUNCTIVITIS

Conjunctivitis is an inflammation of the conjunctiva characterized by cellular infiltration and exudation. Classification is unsatisfactory but is often based on the cause (bacteria, viral, fungal, parasitic, toxic, chemical, mechanical, irritative, allergic, or lacrimal), the age of occurrence (ophthalmia neonatorum), the type of exudate (purulent, mucopurulent, membranous, pseudomembranous, or catarrhal), or course (acute, subacute, or chronic). There is often an associated corneal inflammation (keratoconjunctivitis).

Diagnosis

The diagnosis of conjunctivitis is based on (1) the history and clinical examination, (2) Gram and Wright stains of conjunctival scrapings, and (3) culture of conjunctival scrapings and identification of the cause.

The history of the inflammation may be helpful. Infectious disease (see Chapter 23) is often bilateral and may involve other members of the family or community. Unilateral disease sug-

Table 9-1. Clinical findings in conjunctivitis

I. Preauricular adenopathy
  A. Palpable: inclusion conjunctivitis, most adenoviruses, herpes simplex, sties, acute suppurative chalazion
  B. Gross enlargement with suppuration: Parinaud oculoglandular syndrome
II. Blepharitis and meibomianitis: *Staphylococcus* sp.
III. Excoriation of skin of medial and lateral canthus: *Staphylococcus* sp., diplobacillus of Morax-Axenfeld
IV. Conjunctival injection
  A. Red: infectious disease
    1. Intense with petechial hemorrhages: *Streptococcus pneumoniae* or *Haemophilus aegyptius* (Koch-Weeks)
    2. Subconjunctival hemorrhage: adenovirus or acute hemorrhagic conjunctivitis (picornavirus)
  B. Pale whitish: allergy
V. Chemosis: gonococcus, trichinosis, orbital infections, atopic disorders
VI. Exudate
  A. Stringy, white: allergy
  B. Purulent: gonococcus, meningococcus
  C. Mucopurulent: pyogenic bacteria
  D. Scanty: virus
  E. Foamy, whitish secretion: *Corynebacterium xerose*
  F. Pseudomembrane: *Corynebacterium diphtheriae*, *Streptococcus*, erythema multiforme, APC type 8, vernal conjunctivitis
VII. Follicle formation (lymphatic hypertrophy)
  A. Lower eyelid: follicular conjunctivitis, APC viruses, inclusion conjunctivitis, molluscum contagiosum, hypersensitivity to pilocarpine, eserine, and other topical medications
  B. Upper eyelid: trachoma
VIII. Papillary hyperplasia: vernal conjunctivitis (neovascularization with lymphocyte infiltration)
IX. Conjunctival scarring
  A. Upper eyelid: trachoma
  B. Lower eyelid: erythema multiforme, alkali burns, radiation burns, ocular cicatricial pemphigoid
  C. General: diphtheria, infectious membranous conjunctivitis (herpes simplex, adenovirus, *Streptococcus* sp.)
X. Corneal involvement
  A. Purulent: gonococcus, *Pseudomonas aeruginosa*
  B. Marginal infiltrates: *Staphylococcus*, diplobacillus of Morax-Axenfeld *(Haemophilus* sp.)
  C. Punctate epithelial defects: *Staphylococcus* (lower half), trachoma (upper half)
  D. Generalized epithelial defects: Sjögren syndrome
  E. Superior vascularization: pannus of trachoma, phlyctenular disease
XI. Unilateral inflammation: Parinaud syndrome, adult gonococcus, contact allergy, lacrimal occlusion, viral infection

Table 9-2. Cytologic findings in conjunctivitis

I. Polymorphonuclear leukocytes
  A. Neutrophilis
    1. Bacterial and mycotic infections
    2. Erythema multiforme
    3. Chlamydial infections
  B. Basophils and eosinophils
    1. Allergies
      a. Vernal conjunctivitis (often fragmented)
      b. Hay fever
      c. Sensitivity to drugs, cosmetics, and so on
II. Monocytes
  A. Lymphocytes
    1. Virus infections
  B. Plasma cells
    1. Trachoma
  C. Phagocytes (Leber cells)
    1. Trachoma
III. Inclusion bodies
  A. Basophilic
    1. Upper tarsal: trachoma
    2. Lower tarsal: inclusion conjunctivitis
  B. Acidophilic
    1. Molluscum contagiosum
    2. Herpes simplex
IV. Epithelial cells
  A. Keratinized
    1. Sjögren syndrome
  B. Multinucleated
    1. Virus infection

junctiva fornix without prior topical anesthesia. Sheep blood and mannitol agar plates are used routinely. If *Haemophilus* or *Neisseria* species are suspected, chocolate agar is used; Sabouraud agar is used for suspected fungi. A transport medium should not be used. Viral material for culture is collected in a sterile swab and transferred immediately to a tissue culture medium. The *Chlamydia* group may be cultured in HeLa 229 or McCoy cells that have been pretreated.

Conjunctival scrapings are preferred for cytologic examination. The conjunctiva is anesthetized, the site of maximum involvement is lightly scraped with a sterile spatula, and the material spread on a glass slide to cover an area approximately 1 cm in diameter. The Gram stain demonstrates most bacteria and fungi. A micro-immunofluorescent assay detects IgG or IgM antibodies to *Chlamydia*. An enzyme immunoassay uses a spectrophotometer to detect organism antigen. Giemsa-stained material is read for the predominant cell type present (Table 9-2). Direct microscopic examination of Giemsa-stained material for inclusion bodies has a low yield, except in neonatal inclusion conjunctivitis.

Clinical types

The clinical manifestations of conjunctivitis vary with the cause. The onset is often insidious. The patient notices a fullness of the eyelids and a diffuse, gritty, foreign body sensation. Examination indicates diffuse conjunctival injection, a clear cornea, a distinct iris pattern, and normal pupillary reaction. Within several hours of the onset, there is exudation. There may be swelling of the eyelids and edema (chemosis) of the conjunctiva.

To determine if papillary hypertrophy or follicles are present, the tarsal border must be examined. Papillary hypertrophy is characterized by folds or projections of hypertrophic epithelium that contain a core of blood vessels surrounded by edematous stroma infiltrated with lymphocytes and plasma cells. It is basically a vascular response with secondary monocytic infiltration. All conjunctival inflammations have some degree of papillary hypertrophy. Large papillae occur characteristically in vernal conjunctivitis and in exceptionally severe or prolonged conjunctival inflammation.

Follicular hypertrophy is characterized by

gests a toxic, chemical, mechanical, or lacrimal origin. A copious exudate suggests a bacterial inflammation. A stringy, sparse exudate suggests an allergy or a viral infection. A preauricular adenopathy suggests an adenovirus infection. Meibomianitis and chronic blepharitis with an associated conjunctivitis are common.

Clinical examination requires good illumination and magnification. Attention should be directed to the presence or absence of preauricular adenopathy, involvement of the eyelid margins, patency of the lacrimal system, severity and nature of the conjunctival injection, follicle formation or papillary hypertrophy, and the nature of the secretion (Table 9-1).

Staining and culture. Initial treatment is based on Gram staining of smears of the conjunctival exudate. Intraepithelial gram-negative diplococci of gonorrhea ophthalmia may be demonstrated by Gram stain 48 hours before their demonstration in culture. Exudate for culture is collected with a calcium alginate swab moistened with sterile saline or broth. The material is collected from the lower con-

small follicles that are smaller and paler than papillae and lack the central core of blood vessels. Basically it is a lymphoid hyperplasia and occurs in some normal children, chlamydial infections, and T cell mediated reactions (type IV hypersensitivity).

Mucopurulent conjunctivitis. Bacterial organisms causing mucopurulent conjunctivitis in the United States include gram-positive cocci (*Staphylococcus aureus, Staphylococcus epidermidis, Streptococcus pyogenes,* and *Streptococcus pneumoniae*), gram-negative cocci (*Neisseria meningitidis, Moraxella lacunata* [of Morax-Axenfeld]), and gram-negative rods (genus *Haemophilus,* family Enterobacteriaceae [genera *Proteus* and *Klebsiella*]). Almost any bacteria may be involved. Additionally, the causative organism may be one of a number of bacteria or fungi intermediate between saprophytes and pathogens. They may be recovered in culture or found in epithelial scrapings that are Gram stained.

The onset is acute, and both eyes are involved with a mucopurulent exudate. Drying of inspissated pus during sleep may cause the eyelids to be agglutinated on awaking.

Physicians must wash their hands thoroughly and use eyedrops in individual containers to avoid transmitting infection. If ocular tension is measured, the tonometer must be sterilized after use. The patient should use only his own towels. Corticosteroids should not be used. The eye should not be patched.

Most bacterial inflammations of the conjunctiva are self-limited. However, treatment with topical sulfacetamide, sulfisoxazole, or antimicrobials may be helpful. Initial treatment should consist of hourly topical instillation of sulfonamides, erythromycin, or gentamicin. A poor clinical response after 48 to 72 hours indicates that insensitive bacteria are the cause or that the cause is not bacterial. Further therapy should be based on the results of culture. Conjunctivitis caused by gonococci, *Chlamydia trachomatis,* or *Pseudomonas* organisms may require systematic as well as topical treatment.

Purulent conjunctivitis. This is a severe, acute, purulent conjunctivitis caused by *Neisseria gonorrhea.* It has an incubation period of 2 to 5 days. It occurs in newborn infants who are infected during passage through the birth canal, and in older individuals as a result of contamination from acute gonorrheal urethritis. The occurrence of any discharge in the newborn is suspicious because tears are generally absent in newborns.

The inflammation may have a relatively mild onset but progresses rapidly. Marked swelling and redness of the eyelids and severe chemosis of the conjunctiva occur. The exudate is first serous and then purulent. The disease is well established after 2 days, reaches its height in 4 or 5 days, and then regresses over a 4- to 6-week period. Inflammation of the central cornea is common, and perforation may occur. The gram-negative intracellular organism may be demonstrated in conjunctival scrapings at the time of onset of the disease and in the exudate 48 hours later.

Infants with purulent conjunctivitis or complicated (disseminated) gonococcal infection should be hospitalized in isolation and managed with wound and skin precautions for 24 hours after initiation of treatment with crystalline penicillin G. Two doses of 25,000 units/kg of body weight should be given intravenously each day for 7 days. The eyes should be irrigated with saline. Many ophthalmologists use topical (not systemic) tetracycline rather than saline.

Full-term infants born to mothers with clinically apparent gonorrhea should receive a single intramuscular dose of 50,000 units of penicillin G. Low birth weight infants should receive 20,000 units. Infants with ophthalmia or disseminated gonococcal infection should be hospitalized under isolation with wound, skin, and secretion precautions. They should be treated with intravenous aqueous crystalline penicillin G, 25,000 units/kg of body weight, twice daily intravenously for 7 days. The eyes are irrigated with sterile saline.

Gonococcal urethritis is sometimes complicated by a bacteremia that causes an acute migratory polyarthritis or a tenosynovitis. A sterile catarrhal conjunctivitis occurs in about 10% of those affected. The condition must be differentiated from Reiter syndrome, which causes a sterile urethritis, arthritis, and iridocyclitis.

Ophthalmia neonatorum. Ophthalmia neonatorum is a conjunctivitis that occurs within the first 10 days of life. In most states it is a reportable infectious disease. The most serious cause is *Neisseria gonorrhoeae.* More common causes today are inclusion body conjunctivitis (*Chlamydia trachomatis*) and bacteria, mainly *Staphylococcus* species and *Streptococcus pneumoniae*. Diagnosis is based on epithelial scrapings stained with Gram stain, on fluorescent antibody staining, on culture, and on cytology of the exudate. Treatment with systemic and local antibiotics is effective in bacterial disease. Chlamydial conjunctivitis in the newborn must be treated by means of systemic and topical erythromycin (see below).

Credé prophylaxis. Credé prophylaxis for gonorrheal ophthalmia is the instillation of one drop of 1% silver nitrate solution into the lower conjunctival cul-de-sac of each eye immediately after birth. Only a single-dose ampule should be used. Alternatively an ophthalmic ointment containing 1% tetracycline or 0.5% erythromycin from single-use tubes may be used in each eye within 1 hour after birth. The agent should not be flushed from the eyes. Infants born by cesarean section should also be treated. Prophylaxis with erythromycin ointment prevents chlamydial infection, which is not prevented with either silver nitrate or tetracycline.

Trachoma and inclusion conjunctivitis (TRIC). The genus *Chlamydia* contains two species, *Chlamydia trachomatis* and *Chlamydia psittaci*. *Chlamydia trachomatis* is parasitic principally in humans and causes a variety of oculourogenital diseases: trachoma, inclusion conjunctivitis, lymphogranuloma venereum, urethritis, and proctitis. Pneumonitis occurs in the newborn. *Chlamydia psittaci* is an intraocular parasite of vertebrates and causes a variety of nonocular disorders in birds and mammals; parakeets occasionally transmit a chronic chlamydial conjunctivitis.

Inclusion conjunctivitis. Inclusion conjunctivitis is an acute ocular inflammation caused by *Chlamydia trachomatis*. Newborns are infected in the birth canal (inclusion blennorrhea) and develop an acute mucopurulent conjunctivitis after an incubation period of 5 to 14 days. Adult inclusion conjunctivitis is transmitted venereally and by contaminated eye cosmetics. About 90% of adult women who have chlamydial eye infection have an associated chlamydial genital infection.

Inclusion conjunctivitis is one cause of ophthalmia neonatorum. After a variable period of 5 to 14 days, an acute conjunctivitis occurs with profuse discharge. Because the newborn does not have conjunctival lymphoid tissue until 4 to 6 weeks of age, there is no follicular reaction. Epithelial scrapings stained with Giemsa stain show many basophilic inclusion bodies combined with initial and elementary bodies. Immunofluorescent staining using monoclonal or polyclonal antibodies is more sensitive. If not treated, the acute phase lasts 10 to 20 days and then subsides into a gradually diminishing chronic follicular conjunctivitis that persists 3 to 12 months. Infants should be treated daily for 21 days with both systemic erythromycin (30 mg/kg) and topical tetracycline ointment. Systemic tetracyclines are contraindicated in pregnant women and infants because of yellowing of permanent teeth. Both parents should be examined and treated.

Gonorrheal conjunctivitis may be differentiated by a shorter incubation period (1 to 3 days), by involvement of both the superior and inferior fornices, and by cytology and demonstration of the causative organism.

Adult inclusion conjunctivitis begins as an acute follicular conjunctivitis that persists 3 to 4 months. There may be an associated preauricular adenopathy, epithelial keratitis, and sometimes peripheral corneal focal infiltrates. There is follicular and papillary hypertrophy. The disease may be distinguished from adenovirus infections by the polymorphonuclear cytologic response and the basophilic intracytoplasmic inclusion bodies, in contrast to the mononuclear response seen in adenoviral infections. Other venereal diseases must be excluded; luetic serology should be routine. Patients and their sexual partners should be treated with systemic tetracycline (500 mg orally every 6 hours for at least 7 days) and topical tetracycline ointment. Infants, children, pregnant women, and nursing mothers should be treated with oral erythromycin rather than tetracycline, but topical tetracycline should be used. Adults should receive 500 mg orally every 6 hours on an empty stomach for at least 7 days; pediatric patients should receive oral erythromycin syrup, 50 mg/kg/day, in four divided doses for at least 2 weeks.

Trachoma. Trachoma is a chronic, bilateral, cicatrizing conjunctivitis caused by *Chlamydia trachomatis*. There are at least eight strains, and the disease varies considerably in severity. It is endemic, often associated with conjunctivitis, and is the chief cause of blindness in the world (20 million people are blind from trachoma). Basophilic inclusion bodies may be found, particularly in the acute stage, in epithelial scrapings stained with Giemsa stain. Antibodies to *Chlamydia* may be present both in eye secretions and in the serum. The severity of the disease varies markedly, and there are unexplained regional differences; in the United States, it is largely confined to American Indians in the Southwest. Entire populations in regions of poverty, flies, dryness, and poor hygiene may be infected. Scarring of the tarsal conjunctiva leads to entropion and trichiasis. The scarring occludes the orifices of goblet cells and accessory and main lacrimal glands with mucous deficiency and ocular drying. Corneal vascularization with superimposed infection with *Neisseria gonorrhoeae* or *Haemophilus aegyptius* (Koch-Weeks) further complicates the disease.

Chlamydia organisms are sensitive to sulfonamides, tetracyclines, and erythromycin. The compounds are preferably administered systemically. In adults, tetracycline and sulfadiazine (2 to 4 g daily for 14 days) are the preferred agents. Entire communities may be treated prophylactically. Flies must be eliminated and cleanliness improved, a major problem in regions without plumbing or running water. Active immunization by inoculation is complicated by the several strains, poor cross-immunity, and weak antigenicity. Surgery is commonly required for cicatricial distortion of the eyelids.

Virus inflammations. Invasions of the conjunctiva by a variety of viruses (See Chapter 23) can cause conjunctivitis. Many mild nonincapacitating conjunctival inflammations in which microorganisms are not demonstrated are probably caused by viruses. Conjunctival involvement may be part of a systemic infection, or the disease may be limited to the epithelium of the cornea (Chapter 10) and conjunctiva.

Adenovirus. This group of at least 31 human and 17 animal serotypes causes upper respiratory tract infection primarily in infants, children, and military recruits. Some strains cause conjunctivitis and preauricular adenopathy together with fever and pharyngitis (acute phar-yngoconjunctival fever), and other cause keratoconjunctivitis.

Acute pharyngoconjunctival fever. This is one of a spectrum of infections caused by the adenoviruses and is characterized by fever, pharyngitis, cervical adenopathy, and acute follicular conjunctivitis. The conjunctivitis is bilateral, often with intense hyperemia, particularly in the lower cul-de-sac, a scanty secretion, and often pseudomembranes. Adenovirus types 3 and 7 are particularly implicated in infections with severe conjunctival inflammation.

The parents of children with acute pharyngoconjunctival fever may develop a monocular conjunctivitis with follicle formation, preauricular adenopathy, and fever.

Acute hemorrhagic conjunctivitis. This is a specific violent inflammatory conjunctivitis caused by a picornavirus type 70 (see Chapter 23). The disorder is endemic but appears to be self-limited without sequelae. It was first seen in Africa in 1969, has appeared in west and north Africa, the Orient, Latin America, and Florida. There is an explosive onset of conjunctivitis with eyelid edema, tearing, serous discharge, and conjunctival hemorrhages. Conjunctival follicles and enlarged preauricular lymph nodes occur. Reticulomyelitis has been reported. Acute and convalescent serums indicate increasing titers of picornavirus type 70 antibodies, but the virus is seldom recovered from the eye.

Acute bacterial conjunctivitis caused by *Streptococcus pneumoniae*, other bacterial pathogens, or adenovirus infections may produce conjunctival hemorrhages without follicular reaction. By contrast, acute hemorrhagic conjunctivitis is explosive at onset, bilateral, and chracterized by eyelid edema, chemosis, follicles, and hemorrhages; the signs peak at 48 hours and clear rapidly thereafter.

Lacrimal conjunctivitis. Lacrimal conjunctivitis is a monocular conjunctivitis secondary to infections caused by microorganisms in the lacrimal sac in which drainage into the nose is blocked. The inflammation persists until lacrimal drainage is established. Usually dacryocystitis does not involve the conjunctiva. Pneumococcus infection of the lacrimal sac causes keratitis. Fungus occlusion of the canaliculi can sometimes be recognized by a scraping sound when the lacrimal system is probed.

Parinaud oculoglandular syndrome. This is a traditional ophthalmic eponym, but the condition is rarely seen. It consists of a monocular, granulomatous, necrotic conjunctival lesion associated with a suppurative preauricular adenopathy. The name must be differentiated from Parinaud sign, which is the inability to rotate the eyes upward because of a midbrain neoplasm, principally pinealoma. The chief causes of Parinaud oculoglandular syndrome include chancre, tuberculosis, lymphogranuloma venereum, oculoglandular tularemia, infectious mononucleosis, cat-scratch disease, and fungal infections.

Mycotic inflammations. Fungus inflammations of the conjunctiva are uncommon. They may be primary in the conjunctival sac, secondary to mycotic obstructions of the lacrimal system, or contiguous to adjacent inflammation. Treatment is that described for fungal keratitis.

Atopic conjunctivitis. Immediate hypersensitivity states (types I hypersensitivity reaction [anaphylaxis]) are characterized by rapidity of onset when an allergic individual is exposed to an antigen to which there is sensitivity. Contact with the antigen triggers an enzyme reaction in mast cells and basophils with the release of histamine and eosinophil chemotactic factor of anaphylaxis. A number of reactors are also released: (1) slow-reacting substance of anaphylaxis, (2) heparin, (3) prostaglandins, and (4) the platelet activating factor. The specific ocular diseases in which this mechanism plays a role include allergic rhinitis (hay fever), atopic keratoconjunctivitis, giant papillary conjunctivitis, vernal conjunctivitis, and insect bites and stings.

Allergic rhinitis (hay fever). This is a recurrent, seasonal hypersensitivity characterized by sneezing, rhinorrhea, obstruction of the nasal passages, and conjunctival and pharyngeal itching. The conjunctiva is milky or pale pink in color and edematous as are the eyelids. A clear, watery exudate in the acute phase becomes whitish, thick, and stringy in the chronic phase. Vasoconstrictive eyedrops, crushed ice compresses, and oral antihistamines provide symptomatic relief.

Atopic keratoconjunctivitis. Male teenagers with a history of childhood atopic dermatitis (often before the age of 2 years) may develop a bilateral conjunctival inflammation that resembles vernal conjunctivitis but is not seasonal. The conjunctiva is pale, and there are papillary hypertrophy, corneal pannus, keratoconus, punctate epithlial keratitis, and sometimes cataract. Itching, burning, tearing, and a watery discharge also occur. The personal and family history of atopic dermatitis, the wheal-and-flare reaction to many common antigens, help differentiate the condition from vernal conjunctivitis.

Giant papillary conjunctivitis. Hard and soft (rarely) contact lenses, an ocular prosthesis (artificial eye), or a buried suture may sometimes stimulate giant papillae on the upper tarsal conjunctiva. The papillae are similar to those of vernal conjunctivitis, but itching is less. There is increased mucus production. When contact lenses are the cause, wearing time is reduced and there is eventual intolerance. More thorough cleaning of contact lenses, a lens of different polymer, a switch from hard to soft lenses (or vice versa), or a different contact lens cleaning solution may be helpful. A new ocular prosthesis may be helpful. Irritating sutures must be removed. All symptoms and signs stop if the exciting agent is removed.

Insect bites and stings. These cause both a toxic inflammatory response and an immunologic IgE-mediated response. Hypersensitivity reactions vary from simple urticaria to anaphylactic shock. Mild symptoms of pruritis and urticaria can be controlled by administration of 0.2 to 0.5 ml of 1:1000 epinephrine subcutaneously. Severe symptoms require intravenous infusions, tracheostomy, and early supportive management to prevent death.

Vernal conjunctivitis. Vernal conjunctivitis is a bilateral recurrent hypersensitivity reaction that occurs during the warm months of the year, particularly in hot climates. It is a localized form of anaphylaxis (type I hypersensitivity) combined with a cell-mediated response (type IV hypersensitivity). Boys are more commonly affected until puberty; thereafter both sexes are affected equally. Three forms occur: (1) palpebral (Fig. 9-1), which involves the tarsal conjunctiva of the upper eyelid with the formation of typical thickened gelatinous vegetations; (2) limbal, the most common form in blacks, associated with the formation of a gelatinous, elevated area about 4 mm wide at the corneoscleral limbus, and (3) mixed.

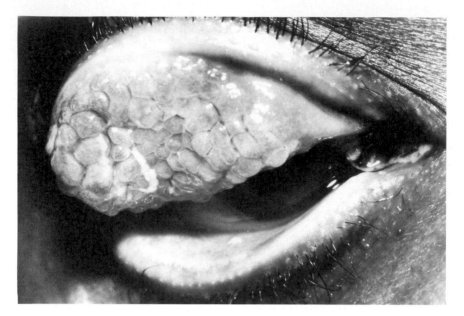

Fig. 9-1. Palpebral form of vernal conjunctivitis with marked papillary proliferation of the conjunctiva.

The principal symptom is itching, which may be nearly intolerable. It is aggravated by sweating, ocular irritation, and rubbing the eyes. Papillary hyperplasia of the upper tarsal conjunctiva appears as large, grayish pink, vegetating masses. Limbal nodules appear as small, semi-transparent elevations. There is a thin, ropy, white secretion. Conjunctival scrapings contain numerous eosinophils. Tear IgG and histamine levels are elevated.

The disorder gradually subsides over a 4- to 6-year period. Moving to a cool climate and air conditioning of the bedroom may be helpful. Removal of the thick ropy secretion with a 10% solution of acetylcysteine may be helpful. Topical corticosteroids, topical 2% cromolyn sodium are used. Radiation therapy is contraindicated.

Cell-mediated immune reactions. Type IV hypersensitivity reactions are caused by T lymphocyte sensitization to antigens fixed in the tissues. It is the usual type in microbial infections, in tissue rejection in transplants, in neoplasms, and in reactions to simple chemicals that are bound to a cell. The specific conjunctival disorders in which this mechanism plays a role include phlyctenulosis and contact conjunctivitis.

Phlyctenulosis. This is a monocular, localized, cell-mediated type (type IV) of conjunctival hypersensitivity. Hypersensitivity to tuberculoprotein and staphylococcal antigen are common causes. *Candida albicans, Coccidioides immitis, Leishmania* species, and the agent of lymphogranuloma venereum are also causes. Phlyctenulosis is most common during the first two decades of life, when there is a particularly high degree of responsiveness to cell-mediated hypersensitivity. Usually the bulbar conjunctiva is affected with a nodule 0.5 to 3 mm in size that follows a 10-day course of elevation, infiltration, ulceration, and resolution. There is severe photophobia if the cornea is involved, but otherwise symptoms are minimal. Corneal phlyctenules attract a stalk of new blood vessels from the corneoscleral limbus and may cause loss of vision, requiring keratoplasty. Phlyctenules caused by tuberculoprotein hypersensitivity respond quickly to topical corticosteroids. The *Staphylococcus* type requires treatment of the blepharitis.

Contact conjunctivitis. This occurs in one of two forms: (1) irritant (the most common), and (2) hypersensitive. Hypersensitive contact conjunctivitis (and dermatitis) is nearly always caused by tissue sensitization as the result of topical administration of ophthalmic drugs. Those most likely to induce sensitization are neomycin, atropine, idoxuridine, gentamicin, and thimerosal. Other medications include chloramphenicol, penicillin, topical anesthetics, antihistamines, homatropine, scopolamine, benzalkonium, and silver and zinc salts. Other substances include mascara, eye shadow, eyebrow pencil, soap, hair dye, nail polish, perfumes, cosmetics, shampoo, hair spray, eye makeup, and eyeglass cleaning fluid. The pattern of an eyelid reaction may be diagnostically helpful: adhesive tape and nickel (eyeglass nasal pad) cause sharply demarcated lesions; linear streaks are caused by plants; spreading lesions may be caused by cosmetics, poison oak, or poison ivy; and monocular lesions are caused by eyedrops. The condition is marked by itching, chemosis of the conjunctiva, and eosinophils in the scrapings.

Primary irritant contact conjunctivitis is a follicular type of conjunctivitis that is particularly marked in the lower cul-de-sac. Symptoms are minimal, and the disease is often listed as a chronic conjunctivitis. Eosinophils are not present in conjunctival scrapings. Almost any compound used in the treatment of ocular disease may be a source of such irritation. The conjunctivitis disappears when the compound is discontinued, and once it has improved, the drugs may be reinstituted without recurrence. The irritation may constitute an untoward reaction to the vehicle or a preservative rather than the active principle of the drug.

Contact with the offending agent must be eliminated. Corticosteroids may aggravate the condition, and the preservative in corticosteroid drugs may cause the condition.

Chronic conjunctivitis. Chronic conjunctivitis is a general term applied to persistent conjunctival inflammation characterized by injection, scanty exudation, and periodic exacerbations and remissions. It may be caused by many agents. Symptoms vary from mild grittiness or foreign body sensation, with heaviness of the eyelids, to burning, photophobia, and irritation. The symptoms may be severe enough to handicap the patient and are often disproportionately severe for the clinical signs of disease. Examination indicates hyperemia, microscopic papillae, thickening of the con-

junctiva in the fornices, mucous secretion, and sometimes epithelial keratitis. Causes include:

1. *Staphylococcus aureus* infection is usually associated with a chronic blepharitis and an epithelial keratitis involving the lower half of the cornea. Both *Moraxella* species and *Staphylococcus aureus* may cause inflammation of the temporal conjunctiva (angular). There may be a follicular reaction in patients with *Moraxella* infections.

2. A variety of microorganisms often considered nonpathogenic, such as demodex mites, have been implicated. These organisms often reside on body surfaces but may be found in almost pure culture. Presumably, when appropriate predisposing conditions are present, they may produce inflammation.

3. Molluscum contagiosum skin nodules and verruca vulgaris (warts) (see Chapter 23) of the eyelid margin may cause a chronic conjunctivitis with epithelial keratitis. Molluscum contagiosum nodules must be removed to relieve the conjunctivitis; excision of warts may lead to seeding. Cryotherapy is effective.

4. Chemical and physical irritants and unsuspected foreign bodies may be a cause. The use of sun lamps without ocular protection may give rise to an actinic keratoconjunctivitis. Chemical irritation from the chlorine in swimming pools is an obvious cause. Drugs used to treat ocular disease may cause irritant or contact conjunctivitis (see Chapter 8).

5. Excessive meibomian secretion is characterized by a frothy secretion at the angles and may either cause or complicate chronic conjunctivitis.

6. Acne rosacea may have conjunctival involvement that precedes rosacea corneal vascularization.

Treatment of chronic conjunctivitis is difficult. Careful diagnosis is essential, and the cause must be eliminated if possible. Lesions of the eyelids and eyelid margins, such as cysts, warts, and nodules of molluscum contagiosum, must be eliminated. Keratoconjunctivitis sicca must be excluded, and the tear ducts must be tested for patency. Allergy and irritations caused by chemicals, smoke, and cosmetics must be minimized. Many of the same symptoms result from abnormalities of the precorneal tear film.

OTHER CONJUNCTIVAL DISORDERS
Ocular cicatricial pemphigoid

Ocular cicatricial pemphigoid (benign mucous membrane pemphigoid, chronic cicatricial conjunctivitis, essential shrinkage of the conjunctiva) is a chronic, progressive bullous disorder of mucous membranes that particularly affects women over 60 years of age. Subepithelial fibrosis involves the conjunctiva and oral mucosa particularly, sometimes the oral, esophageal, pharyngeal, and nasal mucous membranes, and less frequently vaginal and anal mucosa. Initially there is a conjunctival inflammation with a mucoid discharge and loss of epithelial cells so that the conjunctiva stains with rose bengal and there is an associated subconjunctival fibrosis. The conjunctiva shrinks with obliteration of the fornices, ectropion, and trichiasis. Destruction of the goblet cells with loss of mucin leads to dryness of the eye with keratinization of the conjunctiva and cornea. The progressive scarring may obliterate the conjunctival fornices, fuse the eyelids together, and cover the cornea with a leathery membrane. Immunofluorescent studies show deposition of immunoglobulins, including IgG, IgA, and IgM, and complement 3 in the conjunctival basement membrane zone and in the conjunctival epithelium. There is circulating antibody to ocular surface epithelium in serum. There is an association with HLA-B12.

Treatment is often unsatisfactory. Artificial tears, all-trans retinoic acid ointment, and emollients are used for lubrication. Topical corticosteroid and antibacterial therapy may be necessary. Local instillation of 10% acetylcysteine solution may reduce ocular mucus. Contact lenses may protect the cornea. Early use of systemic corticosteroids and immunosuppressant drugs, particularly cyclophosphamide, may help, but one third of the patients are blinded by the disease. In some patients vision may be restored with a plastic cornea (keratoprosthesis).

Symblepharon

Symblepharon is a condition in which there are adhesions between the palpebral and bulbar conjunctivae (Fig. 9-2). It may obliterate conjunctival cul-de-sacs or form bands of scar tissue. Scarring results from conditions in which apposed areas of the conjunctiva lose their epithelial coverings. The chief causes are chemical burns (particularly caustics), trachoma, erythema multiforme (Stevens-Johnson syndrome), ocular cicatricial pemphigoid, and membranous conjunctivitis. The adhesions cause a mechanical defect, since the eyelids are adherent to the eyeball, and desiccation of the cornea and keratitis occur because of exposure, loss of conjunctival goblet cells, and atresia of the orifices of accessory and main lacrimal

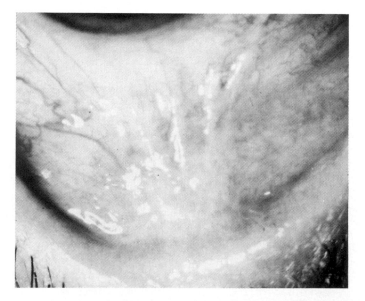

Fig. 9-2. Symblepharon after alkali burn of the bulbar and palpebral conjunctiva.

gland ducts. Treatment frequently is ineffective and disappointing. In the early stages it is directed toward periodic lysis of the adhesions with a glass rod (such as a clinical thermometer) and protection of the cornea with a soft contact lens. Replacement of the scarred conjunctiva with a buccal mucous membrane graft or conjunctiva from the fellow normal eye may be necessary.

Pterygium

A pterygium is a wing-shaped fibrovascular connective tissue overgrowth encroaching on the cornea from the conjunctiva in the interpalpebral fissure (Fig. 9-3). It usually advances from the nasal side and only rarely from the temporal side of the cornea. The cause is not known, but conjunctival irritations from sun and wind in individuals who spend much time outdoors are implicated. Histologically, there is elastotic degeneration (basophilic degeneration) caused by degeneration of subepithelial collagen and replacement with an abnormal material that stains for elastin but is not digested by elastase. There is dissolution of Bowman zone of the cornea and dyskeratotic epithelial cells overlying the pterygium. The stroma of the pterygium contains lymphocytes and plasma cells and immunofluorescent staining shows IgG and IgE immunoglobulins.

Initially there may be signs of chronic conjunctivitis, thickening of the conjunctiva, and symptoms of a mild conjunctivitis. The cosmetic appearance is often the only complaint.

In the temperate zone of the United States, pterygia seldom progress rapidly and usually require no treatment, but they respond well to any surgical procedure. In tropical areas pterygia progress rapidly, are commonly thick and vascular, and have a pronounced tendency to recur, irrespective of the type of surgery.

Every effort must be made to maintain a smooth corneal contour and avoid depressed areas of cornea that will create breaks in the precorneal tear film. Beta and grenz rays have been widely used to prevent recurrence. Beta-ray sources applied to the corneoscleral limbus may cause a sectorial radiation cataract caused by damage to cells in the replicative zone of the equatorial portion of the lens. Preoperatively and postoperatively, individuals with pterygia should be protected from ultraviolet light and irritation from wind or dust.

A pseudopterygium is an inflammatory adhesion of the conjunctiva to damaged cornea that occurs after corneal trauma or inflammation. It may occur at any point around the corneoscleral limbus and is not progressive. The pseudopterygium often bridges the corneoscleral limbus so that in this region a probe may be passed between it and the sclera.

Pinguecula

A pinguecula is a benign degenerative tumor of the bulbar conjunctiva that appears as a yellowish white, slightly elevated, oval-shaped tissue mass on either side of the cornea in the palpebral fissure. The lesions are usually bilateral and located nasally. They become more common with advancing age. They cause a cosmetic defect and in some instances appear to precede a pterygium. Treatment is usually unnecessary, but excision is simple. A pinguecula has the same histologic structure as a pterygium but is limited to the conjunctiva.

Lymphangiectasis

The lymphatic channels of the conjunctiva may become dilated and cause clear, serous conjunctival cysts. These appear on the bulbar conjunctiva as minute tubules filled with clear fluid. Symptoms are minimal. There is no effective treatment. (Note: There are no lymphatic channels within the orbit proper.)

Lithiasis

Degenerations of the conjunctival epithelium in the elderly or prolonged conjunctivitis may cause yellowish to white concretions in the ep-

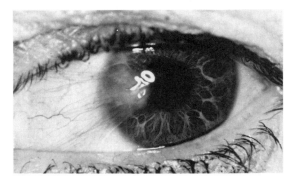

Fig. 9-3. Pterygium extending over the nasal portion of the cornea.

ithelium. The deposits may be seen in the tarsal conjunctiva or the inferior fornix. Rarely, there is dehiscence of the overlying epithelium, causing exposure of the concretion along with foreign body symptoms. The area stains with Bengal rose. The deposits may be removed easily with a sharp needle-knife after the instillation of a conjunctival anesthetic.

Granuloma

A granuloma may result from faulty closure of a conjunctival incision. It occurs particularly after retinal detachment and strabismus surgery. There is a large, fungating, reddish mass that bleeds readily. Usually simple excision is all that is required. Retained foreign bodies may also cause a granuloma.

Tumors, cysts, and neoplasms

Choristomas. Choristomas are congenital tumors composed of tissues not normally found in the region. Dermoid cysts of the conjunctiva may be cystic or solid and contain stratified squamous epithelium, hair follicles, sebaceous glands, hair shafts, brown tissue, teeth, and debris. An epidermal cyst contains stratified squamous epithelium only. A dermatolipoma occurs usually at the superior temporal corneoscleral limbus and appears as a sharply circumscribed, round, slightly yellowish, elevated mass involving the cornea and the sclera. It occurs frequently in mandibulofacial dysostosis. Hamartomas are congenital tumors composed of tissues normally found in the region.

Lymphomas. Lymphomatous disease (reactive lymphoid hyperplasia, lymphosarcoma, and reticulum cell sarcoma) may be manifest in the adenoid layer of the conjunctiva. A smooth elevated tumor mass, which may be widespread, develops, and there is protrusion of the conjunctiva. Retrobulbar extension may cause proptosis. The condition may be benign (80%) or malignant and associated with systemic lymphoma. The lesion must be studied histologically for diagnosis. The conjunctival lesion is extremely sensitive to roentgen-ray therapy.

Telangiectasis. Telangiectasis of the conjunctiva occurs in all cases of ataxia telangiectasia (Louis-Bar syndrome). There is nystagmus, progressive, cerebellar ataxia, deficiency in IgA, and impaired lymphocyte transformation.

Carcinoma of the conjunctiva. This may appear as an exposure keratosis, as an inflammatory lesion, or as a leukoplakia with a white shining lesion caused by keratinization of the conjunctival epithelium.

Conjunctival intraepithelial neoplasia (carcinoma in situ). This is a slow-growing, dysplastic, squamous cell tumor that usually involves the bulbar conjunctiva in the interpalpebral space in men (75%). The lesion is usually solitary and consists of a wide-demarcated, slightly elevated, reddish-gray gelatinous mass that may develop a dense white appearance secondary to surface keratosis (leukoplakia). Papanicolaou staining of scrapings may indicate abnormal cells. Complete excision is combined with radiation to prevent recurrence. The tumor cells may remain precancerous or undergo malignant transformation to squamous cell carcinoma, which may metastasize.

Squamous cell carcinoma. Squamous cell carcinoma (Fig. 9-4) may be confined to the superficial tissues, or it may invade the adjacent tissues, such as the eye or orbit. The tumor is extremely sensitive to radiation, which should be used if excisional biopsy fails. Basal cell carcinoma rarely occurs.

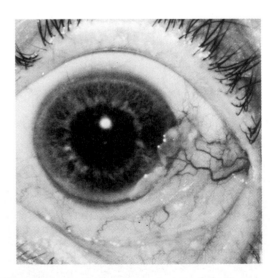

Fig. 9-4. Squamous cell carcinoma of the conjunctiva at the corneoscleral limbus. These tumors occur particularly in compromised hosts, and this 76-year-old patient had a pulmonary mass that could not be diagnosed.

Pigmented lesions of the conjunctiva

Benign melanosis. Benign melanosis consists of flat, brown patches of melanin granules produced by normal melanocytes. They occur most commonly in black patients (rarely in white patients) near the corneoscleral limbus in the interpalpebral space.

Nevi. Nevi occur commonly, often near the corneoscleral limbus, but may involve the conjunctiva anywhere. They appear as yellowish-red areas or deeply pigmented masses and occur usually before age 20. Sometimes nonpigmented nevi cause alarm when they become deeply pigmented, usually at puberty. Benign nevi are usually not excised unless cosmetically undesirable or if they enlarge enough to irritate the eye or suggest malignant degeneration.

Benign acquired melanosis. These are flat, acquired, pigmented blemishes of the conjunctiva. They originate from melanocytes that have migrated from the neural crest to the basal layer of the conjunctiva where they persist in the superficial or deep epithelium. The superficial layer contains dendritic melanocytes and nevocytic melanocytes, while the deep epidermis or subepithelium contains fusiform melanocytes. Dendritic melanocytes cause racial pigmentation, suntan, freckles, benign epithelial melanosis, and acquired melanosis. Nevocyte melanocytes form nevi. Fusiform melanocytes cause the nevus of Ota, melanosis oculi, and blue nevus. All three may cause benign acquired conjunctival melanosis, and all three, particularly dendritic melanocytes, have the potential for conversion to malignant melanoma.

Clinically, there are two types of conjunctival melanoma: (1) focal nodular melanoma that appears as an isolated elevated lesion, and (2) diffuse melanoma that extends radially. When there is involvement of the skin of the eyelids, it may be recognized as lentigo maligna melanoma (Hutchinson's melanotic freckle), but when limited to the conjunctiva this distinction is not possible.

All lesions of benign acquired melanosis should be completely excised. The specimen should be examined to determine the presence or absence of atypical cell structure. Hyperpigmentation of the conjunctival epithelium without melanocytic hyperplasia or melanocytic hyperplasia without atypical cells do not progress to malignancy. Lesions that involve the cornea or are imcompletely excised tend to recur. If atypical melanocytes are not arranged along the junction of the epithelium and substantia propria, progression to malignant melanoma is common (90%). When atypical melanocytes are combined with epithelial cells, progression is likely (75%). The problem is difficult inasmuch as skilled pathologists may disagree concerning the nature of the tumor. Often recurrent malignant melanoma of the conjunctiva requires exenteration of the orbit to prevent death from metastatic disease.

BIBLIOGRAPHY
General

Easty, D.L., and Smolin, G.: External eye disease, London, 1985, Butterworths.

Fedukowicz, H.B., and Stenson, S.: External infections of the eye, Norwalk, Conn., 1985, Appleton-Century-Crofts.

Ladas, I.D.: Histocompatibility (HLA) antigens and eye diseases other than uveitis, Surv. Ophthalmol. 27:233, 1983.

O'Connor, G.R., editor: Immunologic diseases of the mucous membranes: pathology, diagnosis, and treatment, New York, 1980, Masson Publishing USA.

Smolin, G., and O'Connor, G.R.: Ocular immunology, Philadelphia, 1981, Lea & Febiger.

Smolin, G., Tabbara, K., and Whitcher, J.: Infectious diseases of the eye, Baltimore, 1984, The William & Wilkins Co.

Conjunctivitis

American Academy of Pediatrics: Prophylaxis and treatment of neonatal gonococcal infections, Pediatrics 65:1047, 1980.

Browning, D.J.: Tear studies in ocular rosacea, Am. J. Ophthalmol. 99:530, 1985.

Donshik, P.C., and Ballow, M.: Tear immunoglobulins in giant papillary conjunctivitis induced by contact lenses, Am. J. Ophthalmol. 96:460, 1983.

Friendly, D.S.: Ophthalmia neonatorum, Pediatr. Clin. North Am. 30:1033, 1983.

Lemp, M.A., Mahmood, M.A., and Weiler, H.H.: Association of rosacea and keratoconjunctivitis sicca, Arch. Ophthalmol. 102:556, 1984.

Meisler, D.M., Berzins, U.J., Krachmer, J.H., and Stock, E.L.: Cromolyn treatment of giant papillary conjunctivitis, Arch. Ophthalmol. 100:1608, 1982.

Patriarca, P.A., Onorato, I.M., Sklar, V.E.F., Schonberger, L.B., Kaminski, R.M., Hatch, M.H., Morens, D.M., and Forster, D.K.: Acute hemorrhagic conjunctivitis, J.A.M.A. 249:1283, 1983.

Pemphigoid

Foster, C.S., Wilson, L.A., and Ekins, M.B.: Immunosuppressive therapy for progressive ocular cicatricial pemphigoid, Ophthalmology **89**:340, 1982.

Mondino, B.J., and Brown, S.I.: Immunosuppressive therapy in ocular cicatricial pemphigoid, Am. J. Ophthalmol. **96**:453, 1983.

Proia, A.D., Foulks, G.N., and Sanfilippo, F.P.: Ocular cicatricial pemphigoid with granular IgA and complement deposition, Arch. Ophthalmol. **103**:1669, 1985.

Thoft, R.A., Friend, J., Kinoshita, S., Nikolić, L., and Foster, C.S.: Ocular cicatricial pemphigoid association with hyperproliferation of the conjunctival epithelium, Am. J. Ophthalmol. **98**:37, 1984.

Lacrimal gland

Tseng, S.C.G., Hirst, L.W., Maumenee, A.E., Kenyon, K.R., Sun, T.T., and Green, W.R.: Possible mechanisms for the loss of goblet cells in mucin-deficient disorders, Ophthalmology **91**:545, 1984.

Pterygium

Pinkerton, O.D., Hokama, Y., Shigemura, L.A.: Immunologic basis for the pathogenesis of pterygium, Am. J. Ophthalmol. **98**:225, 1984.

Melanosis

Folberg, R., McLean, I.W., and Zimmerman, L.E.: Conjunctival melanosis and melanoma, Ophthalmology **91**:673, 1984.

10

THE CORNEA

The cornea is the transparent, avascular structure that forms the anterior one sixth of the globe through which the iris pattern and black pupil normally are clearly visible. Its most anterior layer, the precorneal tear film, covers a constantly renewed epithelium whose basement membrane is attached to the corneal stroma. The stroma constitutes 90% of the cornea; its anterior condensation, to which the basement membrane of the epithelium attaches, is the Bowman zone. The cornea is lined by a single endothelial cell layer adjacent to the aqueous humor of the anterior chamber. Descemet membrane, the basement membrane of the endothelium, separates the endothelium from the corneal stroma. The central cornea requires atmospheric oxygen for its aerobic metabolism; the peripheral cornea is nurtured by the superficial and deep corneal plexuses derived from the anterior ciliary arteries. The cornea is innervated by nonmedullated sensory fibers that pass to the long and short ciliary nerves of the ophthalmic division of the trigeminal nerve. The inferior cornea sensory innervation is by axons passing to the infraorbital branch of the trigeminal nerve.

The cornea, with its 42-diopter refractive power, is the principal refractive tissue of the eye because it separates air with an index of refraction of 1.0 and aqueous humor with an index of refraction of 1.34. The regular arrangement of the 200 corneal lamellae, the scarcity of keratocytes, the absence of blood vessels, and deturgescence (dehydration) make the cornea transparent. Corneal transparency requires integrity of both the epithelium and the endothelium.

The endothelium provides a mechanism that pumps fluid from the stroma into the aqueous humor. Failure of the endothelial pump causes a generalized corneal edema; the failure is sometimes called endothelial decompensation. Damage to the corneal epithelium causes a subepithelial edema, but the anterior condensation of the corneal stroma (Bowman zone) prevents stromal swelling. When a contact lens that is not permeable to oxygen is worn for a long period, subepithelial corneal edema develops (Sattler veil). The edema disappears spontaneously when the cornea comes in contact with the atmosphere.

The corneal epithelium, which is five to six layers thick, is continuous with the outer layers of the conjunctival epithelium; thus inflammatory diseases of the conjunctiva extend easily to the corneal epithelium. The basement membrane of the corneal epithelium must be adherent to the underlying condensation of the stroma (Bowman zone), or epithelial cells may be easily flicked away by blinking. Abnormalities of the eyelids or conjunctiva or a deficiency in the precorneal tear film results in localized areas of corneal drying.

SYMPTOMS AND SIGNS OF CORNEAL DISEASE

The three main symptoms of corneal disease are (1) iridescent vision (halos), (2) reduced visual acuity, and (3) pain. Iridescent vision results from epithelial and subepithelial edema, which divides white light into its component parts with blue in the center and red on the outside. The edema combined with the round pupil cause a halo effect in which lights are surrounded by a shimmering rainbow. Interference with the visual axis by scars, blood vessels, stromal edema, leukocytes, or other opacities reduces visual acuity.

The corneal epithelium is amply innervated by sensory nerves that do not have Schwann sheaths. Epithelial defects cause discomfort that may be described as a foreign body sensation, burning of the eyes, or pain so severe that it incapacitates the patient. Reflex lacrimation may occur.

The exposed position of the cornea and the lamination of the tissue allow easy observation and precise localization of corneal defects. Inspection through a +20 diopter condensing lens combined with penlight illumination often provides adequate magnification. Attention is directed to the diameter of the cornea, its shape, and the presence or absence of opacities in the normally transparent tissue. The normal cornea reflects a clear image of the examining light. In the region of disease, the light is distorted and dull. Corneal opacities or aqueous humor opacities may obscure the pattern of the iris and prevent observation of the normally black pupil. Fluorescein strips or solutions (2% sterile) stain areas of absent corneal epithelium bright green. Corneal sensation is measured by touching the cornea with a wisp of cotton and observing the eyelid closure reflex. Many conjunctival abnormalities, lacrimal disorders, and eyelid disorders may result in corneal disease.

OPACITIES

Opacities in the cornea may be central or peripheral. When located in the visual axis they may impair vision. A minor scar may severely distort vision because it disturbs the smooth curvature of the corneal refractive surface (irregular astigmatism). Three types of opacities involve the cornea:

1. Leukoma, in which the involved portion of the cornea is totally opaque. Localized leukoma appears as a whitish scar surrounded by normal cornea. In generalized leukoma the entire cornea is white, often with conspicuous blood vessels coursing across its surface.
2. Macula, in which the opacity is more transparent than in leukoma.
3. Nebula, which is a mild loss of corneal transparency.

Epithelial defects heal without scarring, in contrast to defects of the Bowman zone and the remaining stroma, which heal with permanent opacification. The human endothelium does not replicate, and if there are too few endothelial cells to cover a defect, stromal edema occurs. A corneal scar to which the iris is adherent is called an adherent leukoma.

Congenital leukomas (opacities). Embryologically the cornea has a complex origin. The epithelium is derived from surface ectoderm. The keratocytes of the stroma, Descemet membrane, and the endothelium are derived from neural crest cells (mesenchyme). (Most of the periocular mesenchyme is of neural crest origin as there are no mesodermal somites in the head and neck region.) Opacification of the cornea may be the result of several mechanisms, either singly or in combination: (1) the lens vesicle may not fully separate from the surface ectoderm; (2) endothelium may fail to form; (3) cornea and sclera may not differentiate (sclerocornea); or (4) the corneal stroma may be thinned. Embryogenesis of the cornea and anterior chamber angle are closely related. Corneal opacities thus often have associated abnormalities of the iris and iridocorneal angle.

Neurocristopathies. Neural crest cells that cap the primitive neural tube (see Chapter 1) migrate and differentiate to evolve into many structures. Neural crest cells either form or contribute to the formation of pigment cells (except those of the optic cup), parasympathetic and sympathetic ganglia, oligodentroglia, Schwann sheath cells, cranial nerves, membranous bones of the head, vascular pericytes, sclera, corneal stroma and endothelium, and the anterior chamber recess. A number of developmental abnormalities of neural crest origin (neurocristopathies) involve either the head or eye (Table 10-1) or other systems. Many are described elsewhere in this text.

Anterior segment mesenchymal dysgenesis (Peters anomaly) varies in severity from a focal thinning of the stroma (posterior keratoconus)

Table 10-1. Some disorders of neural crest origin

Deficient neural crest formation
  Brain-face-eye malformations: cyclopia, facial hemiatro-
    phy
Abnormal crest cell migration
  Congenital glaucoma, posterior embryotoxin, Axenfeld
    anomaly
  Riegers anomaly, sclerocornea
  Treacher Collins syndrome
Abnormal crest cell proliferation
  Iridocorneal-endothelial syndromes
  Waardenburg syndrome
Abnormal crest cell terminal differentiation
  Hereditary endothelial dystrophy
  Posterior polymorphous dystrophy
  Fuchs endothelial dystrophy
Generalized neurocristopathies with ocular signs
  Pheochromocytoma
  Neuroblastoma
  Medullary carcinoma of the thyroid
  Hirschsprung disease (heterochromia iridis)
  Von Recklinghausen disease
  Multiple endocrine neoplasia type IIb (III)
  Neurocutaneous melanomas

to a completely opacified cornea lined with uveal tissue that bulges forward (corneal staphyloma). In intermediate types, strands of iris attach to the margin of the corneal opacity or the anterior lens is adherent.

Sclerocornea is an abnormality in which the peripheral cornea blends with the sclera and the transition at the normal corneoscleral limbus is lost. It may be an isolated abnormality or part of Peters anomaly (above). In Reiger syndrome there is thickening of Schwalbe line (the termination of continuous corneal endothelium), with iris strands adherent to it, and hypoplastic iris stroma.

Corneal dystrophies (p. 242) that cause opacification, which is evident at birth, include endothelial dystrophy and posterior polymorphous dystrophy.

A dermoid (a choristoma containing histologically normal tissue foreign to its location) affects only the anterior corneal segment.

Corneal vascularization

The central cornea has no blood vessels but depends on atmospheric oxygen for its aerobic metabolism. The peripheral cornea is nurtured by superficial and deep arteries at the corneo-

scleral limbus. The superficial corneal vascular plexus is the source of subepithelial neovascularization. Interstitial (anterior stromal) neovascularization originates from the deep corneal plexus; apposition of the major arterial circle of the iris or radial vessels of the iris to the cornea results in posterior stromal neovascularization. Blood vessels may extend from the entire corneal circumference or radially from a portion of the corneal margin (fascicular). Subepithelial neovascularization combined with fibroblastic proliferation is called *pannus;* it usually involves the superior portion of the cornea.

In the acute stage of corneal neovascularization, new blood vessels are easily visible. There is an associated ciliary injection and a varying degree of corneal clouding. After the condition causing neovascularization subsides, these vessels may appear in a relatively clear cornea as a bloodless network (ghost vessels). Corneal neovascularization is part of the normal inflammatory response. Many corneal inflammations and infections resolve quickly after vascularization. The most serious consequence of corneal vascularization is the loss of corneal transparency combined with a biochemical modification of the corneal tissue that changes it from an avascular tissue not participating fully in the body's tissue immunity to one requiring a direct blood supply that partakes of antigen-antibody reactions.

Corneal edema

The integrity of both the epithelium and endothelium is necessary to maintain the cornea in its relatively deturgesced state. The desmosomes of the epithelial cells provide a barrier to external aqueous fluids, and the endothelium removes fluid from the corneal stroma. Damage to either of these structures may result in corneal edema. (A drug must be lipid soluble to pentrate the epithelium and aqueous soluble to penetrate the stroma and endothelium.)

If the corneal epithelium is deprived of atmospheric oxygen, as for example with a hard contact lens, or if the intraocular pressure rapidly increases to more than 50 mm Hg, an epithelial and a subepithelial edema develops. This edema is prevented from spreading deep into the stroma by the compactness of the Bowman zone. The cornea looks dull, uneven, and hazy. The patient has decreased visual acuity and iridescent vision. The edema rapidly disappears when the cause is removed.

Stromal edema indicates the failure of the corneal endothelium to pump an adequate amount of fluid from the stroma into the aqueous humor. In minor involvement, the cornea is thickened and has a dull appearance. In severe cases, the epithelium may be edematous; the condition is called bullous keratopathy. Vision is severely depressed. Endothelial dystrophy is the chief spontaneous cause. Iatrogenic pseudophakic bullous keratopathy mainly develops after cataract extraction with an intraocular lens implantation. The use of posterior chamber lenses with extracapsular cataract extraction reduces the incidence. A bullous keratopathy may develop months or years after insertion of an iris-supported intraocular lens.

Pigmentation

A brownish subepithelial line occurs in normal eyes (Hudson-Stähli line: horizontal), at the base of the cone in keratoconus (Fleischer ring: circular), at the head of a pterygium (Stocker line: verticle arc), immediately anterior to a filtering bleb (Ferry line: horizontal), and after any disturbance of the corneal epithelium. Pigmented subepithelial scars occur in about 10% of patients who have a radial keratotomy (see refractive surgery). Pigment lines are composed of ferritin deposited in widened intracellular spaces and within intracytoplasmic vacuoles of the corneal epithelium. Ferritin has a protein shell (apoferritin) and a core of ferric hydroxide. The mechanism of its deposition in the cornea is not known.

In Wilson hepatolenticular degeneration deposition of a copper-containing material in the inner layers of the cornea extends as far as the trabecular meshwork of the anterior chamber recess (Kayser-Fleischer ring). It ends abruptly at the posterior edge of the meshwork. The ring is often incomplete—it may be concealed in its early stages by the corneoscleral limbus and can be seen only by using a gonioscope.

The Krukenberg spindle is a vertical pigment deposit on the endothelial surface of the cornea, probably derived from uveal pigment. It is deposited by convection currents in the anterior chamber and is usually arranged in an approximately triangular pattern with the apex near the center of the cornea and the base in the 6 o'clock meridian. In the pigment dispersion syndrome patchy areas of iris depigmentation appear as defects by iris transillumination combined with pigment accumulation in the anterior chamber angle recess. Glaucoma may occur.

Keratic precipitates, which are inflammatory cells adherent to the endothelium in inflammations of the anterior ocular segment, may occasionally become pigmented.

Blood staining of the cornea usually follows injuries in which there has been blood in the anterior chamber followed by an increase in intraocular pressure. The anterior layers of the cornea are transparent, but the endothelium becomes glazed with a brownish tan pigment, which may obscure the iris entirely. If the cornea is incised for a third or more of its circumference, as is done in cataract extraction, blood staining may occur without increased intraocular pressure, although blood must be present in the anterior chamber.

Heavy metals such as silver (argyria), iron (siderosis), gold (chrysiasis), copper (chalcosis), and mercury may be deposited in the stroma adjacent to the Descemet membrane. Metals are introduced by local medication (silver), intraocular foreign bodies (iron or copper), intraocular blood (iron), systemic therapy (gold), toxic vapors (mercury), or a disordered metabolism (copper in hepatolenticular degeneration).

Superficial corneal lines

Microscopically thin parallel lines arranged in whorls and other concentric patterns originate in the epithelium and subepithelial tissue. The most common type, called fingerprint lines, may be associated with recurrent corneal erosion. When they are bilateral, they may constitute a type of superficial corneal dystrophy.

ABNORMAL DEPOSITS IN SYSTEMIC DISEASE

The cornea is frequently the site of deposition of abnormal metabolic products circulating in the blood. Often the deposition is not grossly evident and may be overlooked if special magnification is not used.

In corneal arcus (arcus senilis, gerontoxon), there is an extracellular lipid infiltration (neutral fats, phospholipids, and sterols) at the corneal periphery. It first appears inferiorly, then superiorly, and eventually circles the entire cornea, although it may often involve only a sector of the cornea. It appears as a grayish-white infiltrate separated from the white sclera by a clear interval of 1 mm. It occurs almost universally in humans over 60 years of age.

Corneal arcus tends to develop more commonly and earlier in life in blacks than in whites. Both races show a tendency to develop the lesion with increasing age. Myocardial infarction is twice as likely to occur in an individual 39 to 49 years of age who has corneal arcus than in one who does not. Additionally, young patients with corneal arcus are more likely to have higher serum cholesterol levels and to be smokers. It does not occur invariably in familial hypercholesterolemia, and there is no relationship between corneal arcus and secondary types of hypercholesterolemia that occur in diabetes mellitus, lipoid nephrosis, and myxedema.

Previous vascularization of the cornea leads to the deposition of lipid adjacent to the blood vessel in some patients with hypercholesterolemia and may occur in association with megalocornea. The optical zone of the cornea is not involved, there are no symtoms, and treatment of the cornea is not indicated.

Posterior embryotoxon (thickened Schwalbe line) with strands of iris attached (Axenfeld anomaly) is similar to corneal arcus, but the opacity is located on the inner surface of the cornea. Posterior embryotoxon is also seen in arteriohepatic dysplasia, an autosomal dominant failure of the hepatocyte to secrete bile, in which strabismus and retinal pigmentary degeneration may also occur.

Jet-black patches of adrenochrome may be seen in the cornea and conjunctiva after long-term use of epinephrine salts in the treatment of glaucomas. In blacks an irregular melanosis is often present in the superficial layers of the peripheral cornea. These appear as extensions of conjunctival pigmentation and are irregularly arranged peninsulas of pigment.

Calcium is deposited in the cornea in two forms: (1) diffuse subepithelial deposition of crystals, and (2) band keratopathy in which horizontal grayish band is interspersed with round dark areas that appear as "holes." The first type of deposition is seen in the milk-alkali syndrome (ingestion of milk and calcium carbonate) and is associated with glistening crystals deposited in the diffusely hyperemic conjunctiva. In hypophosphatemia, in which the tissues are unable to metabolize calcium because of a deficiency in the parathyroid hormone, the cornea, but not the conjunctiva, contains calcium crystals.

Band keratopathy results from the deposition of noncrystalline phosphate and carbonate calcium salts in the epithelium, in the subepithelial tissue, and between the stromal lamellae. In juvenile rheumatoid arthritis (Still disease), band keratopathy may complicate an indolent chronic iridocyclitis. Other causes include hyperparathyroidism, vitamin D poisoning, sarcoidosis, multiple myeloma, renal disorders, and keratoconjunctivitis sicca. It occurs in diseases associated with hypercalcemia, in association with ocular inflammation, and after repeated topical instillation of drugs that have calcium in the vehicle.

The calcium may be removed by first removing the corneal epithelium and then applying a chelating agent, usually sodium EDTA (ethylenediaminetetraacetic acid). Visual improvement is often temporary because additional calcium is deposited.

In some lysosomal storage diseases, the cornea, among other tissues accumulates an abnormal amount of the storage substances. The cornea is cloudy, not unlike its appearance in corneal edema, and the iris is difficult to see.

In cystine storage disease, cystine crystals in the conjunctiva and cornea appear as tinsellike, fine refractile crystals uniformly scattered throughout the tissue.

In dysproteinemias, particularly multiple myeloma, iridescent crystals may be scattered throughout the cornea and conjunctiva. Deep deposits similar to those in corneal dystrophy may be present in cryoglobulinemia.

Multiple endocrine neoplasia, type IIb (III) (a neurocristopathy) is characterized by the association of medullary thyroid carcinoma, multiple mucosa neuromas, pheochromocytoma, marfanoid habitus, characteristic facies with large lips, intestinal ganglioneuromatosis, and skeletal anomalies. Prominent corneal nerves occur in a clear corneal stroma. Additionally, conjunctival and eyelid neuromas are present, combined with keratoconjunctivitis sicca. Prompt identification of affected individuals facilitates early treatment of associated medullary carcinoma of the thyroid and pheochromocytoma.

ABNORMALITIES OF SIZE
Microcornea

In microcornea the cornea has a diameter of less than 10 mm as well as a decreased radius of curvature (Fig. 10-1). The majority of these eyes are hyperopic, and the development of glaucoma in later years is common. The term is reserved for eyes in which the small corneal diameter is the sole abnormality. When the entire eye is small, the condition is called microphthalmia. Vision is reduced, and ocular nystagmus and strabismus may occur. Usually there are numerous associated developmental abnormalities, and sometimes only cystic remnants of the eye are present (anophthalmos).

Megalocornea

Megalocornea (anterior megalophthalmos) is a bilateral abnormality in which each cornea has a diameter of more than 14 mm (Fig. 10-2). Glaucoma is not present, but many authorities believe that the corneal enlargment is sec-

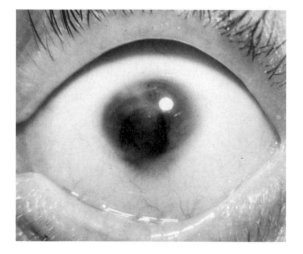

Fig. 10-1. Microcornea in which there is also a corneal nebula (opacity) and an iris coloboma. Vision was 3/200.

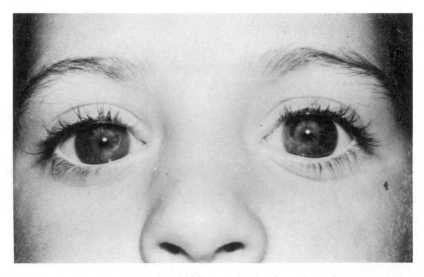

Fig. 10-2. Megalocornea in an 11-year-old boy. Despite the enlarged cornea, ocular tension and the optic nerves remain normal.

ondary to an arrested congenital glaucoma. The anterior chamber is deep, the iris stroma atrophic, and the iris tremulous. Posterior subcapsular cataract occurs with aging. Megalocornea must be differentiated from congenital glaucoma. Measurement of the intraocular pressure and study of the anterior chamber angle by means of a prism (gonioscopy) are essential in the differential diagnosis.

Staphyloma

An anterior staphyloma is an ectasia or bulging of the cornea that is lined with uveal tissue. It occurs most commonly in degenerated eyes after perforation of a corneal ulcer and is combined with iris prolapse. The anterior chamber is obliterated, and a secondary glaucoma is present. Often enucleation is required.

KERATITIS

Inflammation of the cornea may be caused by microbes, hypersensitivity, ischemia, nutritional deficiency, anesthesia from interruption of the sensory nerve supply, exposure, defects in the tear flow, and trauma. Ulcerative lesions involve the epithelium, stroma, or both in a progressive necrosis with loss of tissue that may affect the peripheral or central cornea. Corneal necrosis adjacent to the corneoscleral limbus stimulates early neovascularization from the corneal vascular arcade that results in rapid repair. Ulcerative lesions central to this area may have severe tissue destruction from a collagenase, possibly stimulated or provided by polymorphonuclear leukocytes.

Nonulcerative keratitis predominantly involves the subepithelium and stroma in lymphocytic infiltration, which may be generalized or nodular. There is no necrosis, but vision may be impaired by corneal opacification or neovascularization.

The periodic closure of the eyelids, Bell phenomenon, in which the eyes turn up and out in closure, the sensory innervation, the flow of tears, their antimicrobial action, and the tight junctions of the corneal epithelium protect the external eye. The general and local immune systems provide additional protection. The many nonpathogenic microorganisms normally present in the external eye may suppress the growth of pathogenic bacteria.

When inflammation interrupts the corneal epithelium, the defect stains with fluorescein.

Discomfort varies from a foreign body sensation to severe pain. The grossly transparent cornea becomes infiltrated with inflammatory cells, and blood vessels may invade the avascular stroma. The anterior ciliary arteries become injected. Peripheral corneal ulcers (marginal ulcers) often complicate staphylococcal conjunctivitis and reflect an antigen-antibody reaction to staphylococcal antigens or exotoxins. The immune complex binds complement, which attracts neutrophils that infiltrate the corneoscleral limbus.

Central ulcerative keratitis

These corneal inflammations are the most severe and most damaging. There is an outpouring of polymorphonuclear leukocytes into the cornea with a purulent infiltrate often combined with extensive stromal destruction. The leukocytes and the cornea itself produce collagenases that degrade corneal collagen. When severe, the cornea may perforate. The herpes simplex virus causes an epithelial inflammation that may extend to the corneal stroma as a disciform keratitis.

Except for *Neisseria gonorrheae*, all bacterial and fungal central ulceration requires a break in the epithelium. The organisms (Table 10-2) may be inoculated by a corneal foreign body; may be present in the lacrimal system, conjunctiva, or eyelids; or may be introduced into a damaged cornea by contamination. The herpes simplex virus requires intracellular activation after primary infection.

The major bacterial families that cause keratitis are: (1) Micrococcaccac (*Staphylococcus aureus*, *Staphylococcus epidermis*, and *Micrococcus*), (2) Streptococcaceae (hemolytic *Streptococcus* species and *Streptococcus pneumoniae*), (3) Pseudomonadaceae (*Pseudomonas aeruginosa*), and (4) Enterobacteriaceae. Less common bacterial causes include *Moraxella* species and *Serrata marcescens*.

Many "nonpathogenic" fungi cause keratitis, particularly in eyes treated with corticosteroids and after immune suppression. The most common fungi that cause corneal ulcers are *Aspergillus fumigatus*, *Candida albicans*, *Fusarium solani*, and *Curvularia*.

Management of central ulcerative keratitis requires preliminary identification of the likely organism followed by specific identification after appropriate microbial studies. Often treat-

Table 10-2. Microbial inflammation (keratitis)

Bacterial	
Keratoconjunctivitis	Extension of conjunctivitis to corneal margin, staphylococci, streptococci
Keratitis	Enterobacteriaceae, fecal contamination
Necrotizing keratitis	*Pseudomonas aeruginosa* and trauma, contaminated solutions
Acute hypopyon ulcer (pus in anterior chamber)	Trauma combined with *Streptococcus pneumoniae* or hemolytic streptococci
Indolent ulcer	*Haemophilus, Moraxella liquefaciens*
Pannus (vascularized scar)	*Chlamydia trachomatis*
Interstitial keratitis	Spirochaetaceae, *Treponema*, congenital syphilis (rare in acquired)
Fungal	
Keratomycosis	Injury by plant material, prolonged topical antibiotics and corticosteroids, compromised host
Viral	
Dendritic keratitis epithelitis	Herpes simplex (*Herpesvirus hominis* type 1)
Adenovirus keratitis	Any adenovirus
Epidemic keratoconjunctivitis	Adenovirus 8 or 19
Zoster keratitis; epithelitis (early); mucous plaques (late)	Varicella virus involving the ophthalmic branch of trigeminal nerve (N V)
Keratitis vaccinia or variola	Vaccination or smallpox

Table 10-3. Initial treatment of corneal ulcer before examination of scrapings

	Topical	Subconjunctival
Cefazolin	50 mg/ml	100 mg
Tobramycin	11 mg/ml	40 mg
Bacitracin	10,000 units/ml	
Gentamicin	15 mg/ml	40 mg
Methicillin		100 mg

ment is started empirically, and appropriate diagnostic steps are initiated only after the ulcer has progressed. Identification of the microbial cause may then be impossible.

The first step in management is to collect material by scraping the ulcer with a platinum spatula under magnification. Scraped material should be stained (Gram) for bacteria and fungi, Giemsa for cytology, and Grocott methenamine silver stain for fungi. The limulus lysate assay detects gram-negative endotoxin. Scrapings are plated on the following media: rabbit blood agar at 37° C; sheep blood agar at 25° C; chocolate blood agar at 37° C under increased CO_2 tension; Sabouraud's dextrose-peptone agar with yeast extract and 50 μg/ml of gentamicin, maintained on a rotary shaker at 25° C; and thioglycolate broth at 37° C. Usually virus infections are not cultured unless a superinfec-

tion is suspected; however, blood is drawn for measurement of antibodies.

Initial treatment with concentrated eyedrops is based on the results of the Gram stain (Table 10-3). The specific selection of an antibiotic agent is determined by local experience. After isolation of the organism, its antibiotic sensitivity may indicate specific therapy (Table 10-4).

Patients with ulcers less than 2 mm in size that involve the anterior one third of the cornea may be given ambulatory treatment; larger and deeper ulcers should be treated in a hospital. A 1% atropine solution is instilled two or three times daily. If there is severe corneal necrosis, a temporary bandage contact lens may be used.

Inflammations of the peripheral cornea are often associated with conjunctivitis. Initially there is a marginal corneal infiltrate that has a clear interval between the infiltrate and the corneoscleral limbus. Patients complain of tearing, redness, and photophobia. There is marked ciliary and conjunctival vascular congestion in the affected quadrant. The infiltration extends to form an elongated ulcer with its long axis parallel to the corneal margin. The most common cause is hypersensitivity to *Staphylococcus* exotoxin or antigen in blepharitis or conjunctivitis. Such ulcers respond favorably to corticosteroids and erythromycin or bacitracin ointments. An associated acne rosa-

Table 10-4. Treatment of microbial corneal ulcers based on Gram stain

Gram stain	Topical	Subconjunctival if central or peripheral more than 5 mm in diameter	Systemic if perforation threatened
Gram-positive cocci *Micrococcaceae,* *Streptococceae,* *Sarcina*	Cefazolin, 50 mg/ml, and tobra-mycin, 11 mg/ml	Cefazolin, 100 mg, and tobra-mycin, 40 mg	Methicillin, 200 mg/kg/day
Gram-positive rods *Corynebacterium,* Bacillaceae, *Pro-* *pionibacterium*	Penicillin G,* 100,000 units/ml; or gentamicin, 14 mg/ml; or tobramycin, 11 mg/ml, and cefazolin, 50 mg/ml	Penicillin G,* 500,000 units; gentamicin, 20-40 mg	Penicillin G,* 2-6 kg/4 hr; gentamicin, 5 mg/kg/day
Gram-negative cocci *Moraxella, Neisseria* (diplococci)	Penicillin G,* 100,000 units/ml	Penicillin G,* 500,000 units/ml	Penicillin G, 2-6 g/kg/4 hr
Gram-negative rods Pseudomonadaceae, Enterobacteriaceae (E coli, Proteus, Klebsiella pneumo- niae)	Tobramycin, 11 mg/ml, and car-benicillin 4 mg/ml	Tobramycin, 40 mg, and car-benicillin, 25 mg	Carbenicillin, 4-6 kg/4 hr
No organisms stained	Tobramycin, 11 mg/ml, and ce-fazolin, 50 mg/ml	Cefazolin, 100 mg, and tobra-mycin, 40 mg	Methicillin
Possible fungi	Natamycin, 50 mg/ml; or micon-azole, 10 mg/ml; or amphoter-icin B, 2.5-10 mg/ml Nystatin ointment, 100,000 units	Amphotericin 750 mcg	Amphotericin Ketoconazole, 200-400 mg/day Flucytosine, 150 mg/day

*If sensitive to penicillin, use topical gentamicin, tetracycline, or erythromycin.

cea requires the addition of tetracycline systemically.

Peripheral ulcers as a result of bacterial invasion may extend centrally and require the same treatment as central ulcerative keratitis.

Microbial keratitis

Acute hypopyon ulcer. An acute hypopyon ulcer (sometimes considered the classical central ulcerative keratitis) is a severe bacterial inflammation of the cornea associated with pus in the anterior chamber (hypopyon) and a severe iridocyclitis (Fig. 10-3). *Streptococcus pneumoniae* (pneumococcus) is the usual cause; the organism often has a focus in the lacrimal system. Other bacterial causes are S. *aureus* and *Moraxella* (in derelicts). Often the keratitis is preceded by mild trauma and loss of corneal epithelium, which allows entry of the organism. The ulcer is a dirty gray color, with overhanging margins. The cornea is thinned and the conjunctiva is violently injected. If untreated, the cornea may perforate and the eye may be lost because of purulent inflammation.

The bacteria are sensitive to many antibiotics, and the ulcer responds quickly to treatment. A concurrent pneumococcal dacryocystitis may necessitate dacryocystorhinostomy or occulusion of the canaliculi.

Pseudomonas aeruginosa central ulcer. *Pseudomonas aeruginosa* ulcer is caused by a common gram-negative aerobic bacillus found in the normal skin and intestinal tracts of humans. The organism produces an extracellular protease that enzymatically degrades corneal proteoglycans. Additionally, the invading polymorphonuclear leukocytes and the cornea itself produce collagenases that degrade corneal collagen.

Pseudomonas keratitis is more common in men than in women. A history of corneal trauma, current contact lens wear, previous inflammatory eye disease, or concurrent serious systemic disease is common. The ulcer (Fig. 10-4) usually begins centrally. It quickly broadens and deepens and has a fulminating course. The cornea may perforate within 48 hours of onset. Treatment is by subconjunctival injection of tobramycin or carbenicillin, and instillation of concentrated tobramycin and carbinicillin eyedrops every 30 minutes (Table 10-4).

Protozoan Infections

Acanthamoeba keratitis. A severe persistent keratitis, difficult to distinguish clinically from a stromal herpes infection, may be caused by members of the genus *Acanthamoeba*. These are small, ubiquitous, free-living protozoa that feed on bacteria and are found in contaminated water and material. The organisms may be introduced into the cornea by minor trauma; soft contact lenses may be a cause. The inflammation is resistant to medical treatment, and keratoplasty is required to remove the infected tis-

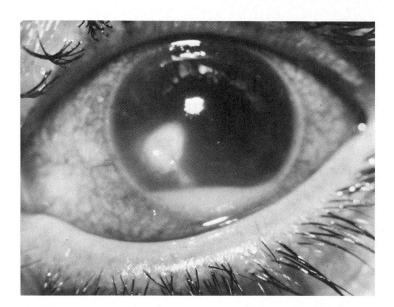

Fig. 10-3. Central ulcerative keratitis caused by a *Streptococcus* infection in a 69-year-old patient with facial nerve paralysis that prevented adequate closure of the eyelid.

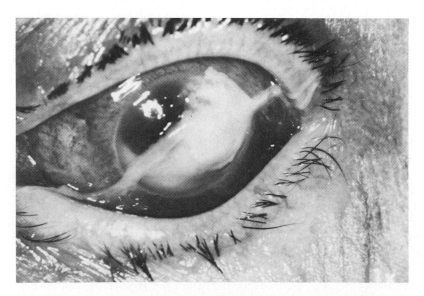

Fig. 10-4. *Pseudomonas aeruginosa* infection of 3 days' duration that developed during the topical treatment of uveitis with atropine and prednisolone.

sue. The epithelium is often intact, and there are small, white, round lesions in the corneal stroma. Keratitic precipitates are associated with a mild uveitis. Diagnosis is often made by histologic examination of the corneal button removed at the time of keratoplasty.

Fungal infections

Infection of the cornea by fungi has increased fifteenfold since the introduction of topical administration of corticosteroids and antibiotics. The disorder is common in subtropical climates during dry, windy months. Except for *Candida* infections, which often occur (55%) in women who have severe medical disease, most fungal infections occur in otherwise healthy men. There may be a history of topical therapy with corticosteroids and antibiotics.

Clinically, the fungus ulcer (Fig. 10-5) appears as a fluffy, white elevation surrounded by a shallow crater, which is surrounded by a grayish, sharply demarcated halo that persists for months. The central lesion may have satellite lesions of pseudopods. Corneal vascularization is minimal and hypoyon is frequent. The ciliary injection may be disproportionately severe for the amount of keratitis present.

The mycotic ulcer resembles those caused by bacteria. It has a rapid onset. A specimen obtained by scraping the base and edges of the ulcer is essential to the diagnosis. Treatment is difficult because many of the antifungal agents do not penetrate the cornea well (pimaricin and amphotericin B), are toxic both topically and systemically (amphotericin B), or have a limited antifungal range (flucytosine). Preferred therapies include topical atropine solution, topical (10 mg/ml) and subconjunctival (10 mg) miconazole, and oral ketoconazole (200 to 400 mg daily) (Chapter 3). These imidazole compounds have a broad antifungal spectrum and penetrate the cornea and ocular tissues well. Ocular preparations are not available and must be prepared from intravenous preparations. These agents are not effective against *Fusarium* sp., which require pimaricin.

Many eyes do not heal until a conjunctival flap is drawn over the cornea surgically. Mechanical removal of the fungi by curettage may be beneficial. Rapidly progressive deep ulcers with descemetocele or perforation require a penetrating transplant with a diameter that encompasses all of the pseudopods to remove as much of the fungi as possible. A lamellar corneal transplant may not be satisfactory because of failure to remove enough fungi.

Viral infections

Herpesvirus hominis infections of the cornea (Table 10-5) are initially limited to the epithelium but, with recurrence, involve the corneal stroma (disciform keratitis) in a central ulcerative keratitis. Conjunctival scrapings generally show a mononuclear leukocyte response; the virus may be isolated in tissue culture. Fluorescent antibody staining of corneal scrapings are generally more reliable and rapid than cultivation.

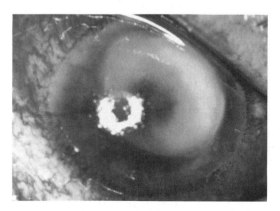

Fig. 10-5. Fungus ulcer of cornea with deep infiltrate and severe ciliary injection. There is no corneal vascularization.

Table 10-5. *Herpesvirus hominis* disease

Type 1: Lips, skin, eye, and genitalia
Type 2: Genitalia and lips, skin, eye
Primary herpes infection
Recurrent herpes infection
  Epithelial infectious keratitis
    Dendritic
    Geographic
Herpes-induced ocular abnormalities (noninfectious)
  Viral interstitial keratitis (antigen-antibody response to live virus)
  Disciform keratitis (T lymphocyte–mediated response to HSV antigens fixed to epithelial cells)
  Epithelial trophic keratitis (metaherpetica; secondary basement membrane defects)
  Sterile stromal ulceration (failure of corneal collagen synthesis, secondary to persistent absence of epithelium)
Iridocyclitis

There are two types of *Herpesvirus hominis:* type 1, the usual cause of facial, oral, or ocular lesions; and type 2, associated mainly with genital infections. Herpes simplex type 1 is becoming nearly as common a cause of genital infection as type 2.

Primary infection now affects about 30% of the population, predominately lower socioeconomic groups. Clinical signs occur in less than 10% of those with primary infection, but all become carriers and are subject to recurrent infections. Primary infection is usually transmitted by an individual with an acute recurrent inflammation of the lips or mouth. After primary infection, the virus persists in a latent form in ganglia. Replication of the virus may be triggered in some persons by fever, ultraviolet light, immunosuppression, trauma, stress, or menstruation. Most individuals have no specific initiating factor.

If primary infection causes clinical signs (10%), there may be vesiculation of the lips, mouth, genitalia, skin, or a severe systemic disorder (0.1%). Primary herpes infection of the eye is rare. Initial herpes vesicles of the eyelids are followed by unilateral, ulcerated blepharitis with preauricular adenopathy. Follicular or pseudomembranous conjunctivitis may occur with preauricular lymphadenopathy. The rare corneal involvement resembles small phlyctenular spicules.

Neonatal infection may follow prolonged labor or premature rupture of the membranes in mothers with genital lesions. Babies may also be infected from maternal nongenital lesions, from other infants in the nursery, and by professional staff. Neonatal ocular infection with herpes virus type 1 or type 2 causes a severe inflammation with conjunctivitis, keratitis, cataract, necrotizing retinitis, optic neuritis, and encephalitis.

After primary herpes infection, recurrent active inflammation occurs throughout life in an infected individual. Most individuals have no specific initiating factor; but in some persons, fever, ultraviolet light, immunosuppression, trauma, stress, or menstruation may trigger replication of the virus. The most common clinical sign of type 1 infection is vesiculation of the lips or mouth. A few individuals have recurrent keratitis.

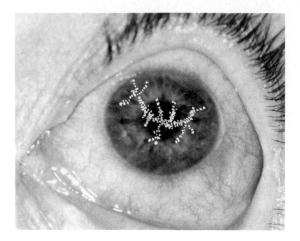

Fig. 10-6. The branching pattern of dendritic keratitis.

Dendritic keratitis. Dendritic keratitis (Gr. *dendron,* tree) is an acute and chronic corneal inflammation that occurs in an individual who has had a primary infection with *Herpesvirus hominis* type 1. The latent virus (or the virus genome) persists in the trigeminal ganglion. Thereafter, the same factors that precipitate recurrent active inflammation elsewhere may trigger keratitis.

Epithelial keratitis (Fig. 10-6) begins as punctate epithelial opacities that become vesicular and coalesce in a branching linear pattern that stains with fluorescein. Corneal sensitivity is markedly diminished. The epithelium between the dendrites is lost; the result is a sharply demarcated, irregularly shaped geographic (amoeboid) ulcer. Both eyes are infected in less than 10% of patients and rarely simultaneously. Symptoms include foreign body sensation, lacrimation, and reduction of vision if the optical area of the cornea is involved. After frequent attacks, the patient is aware of recurrence even before signs of inflammation are present.

Initial treatment consists of mechanical debridement of virus-laden epithelial cells by means of a moist cotton-tipped applicator, spatula, or scalpel blade; the basement membrane must not be damaged. If only dendritic lesions are present, an antiviral compound (see Chapter 3) may be instilled every 2 hours and at bedtime. Geographic lesions (see Table 10-5) require hourly instillation together with topical atropine solution (0.5%). Treatment should be continued for at least 1 week after the lesions heal. Corticosteroid preparations should never be used.

Stromal involvement occurs in several forms. The most common, disciform keratitis, consists of a disk-shaped grayish area of stromal edema, with localized keratitic precipitates. The edema may be limited to the stroma adjacent to the epithelium or involve the full thickness of the cornea. Disciform keratitis is presumably a T lymphocyte-mediated reaction (type IV hypersensitivity) against herpes virus antigens fixed to the corneal endothelium. The lesion may heal without residue or may cause severe corneal scarring. Treatment is individualized, depending on involvement of the visual axis and severity of the disease. Ophthalmic ointments prevent epithelial disruption, and cycloplegics combat the iritis. If the inflammation progresses or the visual axis is affected, prednisolone acetate 1% may be instilled every 2 to 4 hours, tapering the instillation to 0.125% daily. Antivirals must be instilled prophylactically at full dosage whenever the corticosteroid dosage exceeds one drop of 1% prednisolone daily. Patients readily become dependent on the relief of corticosteroids, and the corneal stroma may slowly dissolve with eventual corneal perforation.

Viral interstitial keratitis is probably an antigen-antibody reaction (type II hypersensitivity) to the live virus. There is necrosis of the corneal stroma with a white infiltrate, and a localized vasculitis at the corneoscleral limbus. If the visual axis is not involved, treatment consists of antivirals, cycloplegics, and artificial tears. If the disease is exceptionally severe, or if the visual axis is threatened, corticosteroids may be used cautiously as described above. The inflammation is protracted, and corticosteroid treatment, if used, must be gradually decreased over many months.

Trophic keratitis (metaherpetica) occurs because of damage to the epithelial basement membrane caused by previous infection and stromal scarring. Trophic defects have a smooth palisading arrangement of heaped-up epithelium at their margins. The treatment is the same as that for recurrent corneal erosion.

Sterile stromal keratitis (melting) is a sequela of a persistent epithelial defect. Every effort must be made to restore the integrity of the epithelial covering through the use of a soft contact lens, ocular ointments, and artificial tears. Medroxyprogesterone eyedrops, 1%, may be useful.

Peripheral ulcerative keratitis

The peripheral cornea is nurtured by the corneal capillary arcade so that this portion of the cornea is less vulnerable to progressive infection than the central cornea. Additionally, any opacities are not in the visual axis. Progressive necrosis, loss of tissue, and inflammation of the peripheral cornea occur less commonly than central ulcerative keratitis. The inflammation may be secondary to systemic disease, infection, bacterial hypersensitivity, or phlyctenular keratoconjunctivitis.

Ring-ulcer. A ring-ulcer begins at the corneoscleral limbus and extends to include almost the entire peripheral cornea in a mucopurulent inflammation. It may occur in acute leukemia, brucellosis, bacillary dysentery, dengue fever, gonococcal arthritis, hookworm infestation, influenza, lupus erythematosus, periarteritis nodosa, porphyria, rheumatoid arthritis, scleroderma, Sjögren syndrome, and Wegener granulomatosis. A ring-abscess starts as a minute, infected, purulent infiltrate about 1 mm within the corneoscleral limbus. It then circles the entire cornea. The subsequent central cornea sloughing results in panophthalmitis. Bacteria or fungi is the usual cause of the abscess.

Marginal catarrhal ulcers. Marginal catarrhal ulcers (Fig. 10-7) are an antigen-antibody reaction to either antigens or exotoxins of *Staphylococcus aureus* and other substances. The immune complex binds complement, which then attracts polymorphonuclear leukocytes to the site. There may be an associated conjunctivitis or blepharitis. The inflammation responds to the topical instillation of corticosteroids, but the source of the sensitizing material must be removed.

Mooren ulcer. This is a chronic, painful, progressive, nonpurulent, superficial ulceration that originates in the anterior layers of the peripheral cornea of elderly people. It may be bi-

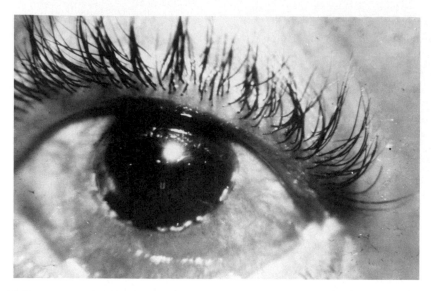

Fig. 10-7. Acute *Staphylococcus aureus* conjunctivitis with marginal corneal infiltrates caused by sensitivity to the exotoxin of the bacteria.

Table 10-6. Noninfectious corneal inflammation

Immunologic abnormalities
    Anaphylactic: Vernal keratoconjunctivitis
    Cytotoxic: Mooren ulcer
    Immune complex: Marginal ulcer
    Cell mediated: Phlyctenular keratitis
Vascular disease
    Arteritis: Interstitial keratitis and N VIII (Cogan)
    Ischemia: Surgical, systemic disease; collagen disease
Nutritional deficiency
    Vitamin A and protein: Keratomalacia
    Acne rosacea?
Innervational
    Neurotropic keratitis (section N V and N VIII)
Tear film abnormality
    Keratoconjunctivitis sicca
        Loss aqueous portion: Sjögren
        Loss mucin: Erythema multiforme, ocular cicatricial
            pemphigoid
        Local drying (delle, *pl.* dellen)
        Superior limbic (failure to wet epithelium)
Eyelid abnormalities
    Entropion or ectropion
    Trichiasis and eyelid margin abnormalities
    Corneal exposure: Lagophthalmos, exophthalmos
    Faulty blinking
Trauma
    Radiation: ultraviolet exposure, "snow blindness," laser
    Mechanical
    Chemical
    Climatic droplet keratopathy, spheroid degeneration
        (wind, sand, snow)

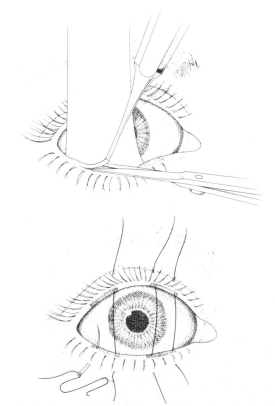

Fig. 10-8. Temporary tarsorrhaphy in which posterior portions of the upper and lower eyelid margin are denuded and brought together with sutures to prevent exposure of the cornea.

lateral (35%). The ulcer has a gray, overhanging margin that may be elevated. It extends circumlimbally or centrally and may cover the entire cornea with scar tissue. The ulceration may be caused by an autoimmune response of the corneal stroma to normal cornea or conjunctival epithelium.

Bilateral keratitis is less responsive to treatment than monocular ulcers. Initial treatment consists of 1% topical corticosteroids as often as every 30 minutes, day and night, as long as epithelial healing progresses. The corneal epithelium may be removed or the conjunctiva adjacent to the ulcer excised. Collagenase inhibitors may be effective. A soft contact lens relieves pain but has no effect on progression. Cyclophosphamide may be used for immunosuppression.

Phlyctenular keratoconjunctivitis. This is a cell-mediated immune response of the cornea and conjunctiva. It is a common cause of decreased vision among Eskimos, presumably because of their sensitivity to tuberculosis.

Noninfectious central ulcerative keratitis

Anesthesia of the cornea, failure of the eyelids to cover the eye, continued corneal irritation by the eyelashes or eyelid, dryness of the eye, or vitamin A deficiency may lead to a central ulcerative keratitis (Table 10-6).

Neurotropic keratitis. This is a corneal inflammation that results from anesthesia of the cornea, which permits trauma and desiccation of the corneal epithelium without reflex protection. Additionally, the trigeminal nerve may play a role in the metabolism of the cornea. Because the cornea is anesthetic, there is no pain, but the conjunctiva is injected, and there may be loss of vision. The lesion begins inferiorly with exfoliation and ulceration, and it may progress until there is loss of the globe. Suturing the upper to the lower eyelid (tarsorrhaphy, Fig. 10-8) is the usual method of treatment. If it is probable that both the trigeminal and facial nerves will be severed in a neurosurgical procedure, for example, in the removal of a cerebellar angle tumor, the keratitis should be anticipated and tarsorrhaphy should be performed before the cornea ulcerates.

Exposure keratitis. Exposure keratitis, sometimes called keratitis e lagophthalmos, is an inflammation caused by the failure of the eyelids to cover the globe. There is exfoliation of the corneal epithelium followed by secondary infection. The condition is most commonly associated with facial nerve disorders in which the orbicularis oculi muscle is paralyzed. The cornea may be similarly exposed after blepharoptosis surgery or in severe proptosis.

Keratitis e lagophthalmos causes pain and ciliary injection. It is evident on examination that the cornea is not protected by closure of the eyelids. Treatment is directed toward prevention of corneal drying. In mild cases, the instillation of an ointment at bedtime and protection of the globe are all that is required. In facial nerve paralysis, a temporary blepharoplasty may be carried out. Soft contact lenses may be effective. If the paralysis is permanent and there is no likelihood of restoration of the facial nerve function, a permanent type of blepharoplasty is done. Proptosis with exposure keratitis requires a central tarsorrhaphy.

Keratomalacia. Softening of the cornea results from vitamin A deficiency, which causes desiccation and necrosis of the cornea and the conjunctiva. Vitamin A is a fat-soluble vitamin derived either from conversion of carotene or from preformed vitamin in the diet. Carotene is present in many plants, particularly leafy greens and yellow vegetables. Preformed vitamin A is derived from butterfat, cheese, and liver. Failure to ingest adequate vitamin A or its precursors is commonly associated with other dietary deficiencies, notably inadequate protein. Secondary deficiency occurs because of inadequate saponification of vitamin A in the gut. The deficiency is observed in sprue, in celiac disease, after extensive resection of the small intestine, and in cystic fibrosis of the pancreas. Failure to store vitamin A occurs in cirrhosis of the liver.

Vitamin A deficiency in the retina has been studied carefully, particularly in animals in whom nutrition can be supported by administration of vitamin A acid, which is not converted to retinal. In humans, vitamin A deficiency causes blindness by (1) destruction of the cornea in xerophthalmia (dry eye) and keratomalacia (corneal softening), (2) loss of retinal in the photopigments of the retina, (3) faulty growth of bone causing optic nerve compression in the optic canal, and (4) faulty fetal development in a vitamin-deficient mother.

In children with acute but not chronic deficiency, dryness of the conjunctiva (xerosis conjunctivae) is the initial external sign of the deficiency. It is paralleled by night blindness, which may not be noticed. Bitot spot is present, particularly in boys. It occurs on the exposed bulbar conjunctiva, usually in the palpebral fissure on the temporal side. It appears as a highly refractile mass with a silvery gray hue and a foamy surface. It is superficial, and the foam may be rubbed off, leaving a roughened conjunctival surface that fills with foam again in several days.

The keratomalacia, or softening of the cornea, may be generalized or localized. It may lead to destruction of the eye if infection occurs. It is particularly common with an associated protein deficiency. Generally, it occurs in infants and not in adults.

Mild vitamin A deficiency caused by improper nutrition may be reversed by a diet that contains protein and carotene. Severe disease requires supplemental vitamin A.

Nonulcerative keratitis

Nonulcerative keratitis is a corneal inflammation that may be acute or chronic, progressive or stationary. Unlike ulcerative keratitis, it is not associated with tissue loss or tissue necrosis. It may involve the corneal epithelium, the subepithelium, or the corneal stroma. Epithelial keratitis occurs in conditions in which basal corneal cells are separated from their basement membrane, causing either punctate defects in the epithelium or large erosions. Subepithelial keratitis involves both the epithelium and basement membrane in a punctate inflammation, which is caused by trauma, ultraviolet burns, and adenovirus infection, but may also occur with spheroidal degeneration, acne rosacea, and onchocerciasis. Stromal keratitis or inflammation, particularly of the deeper layer of the cornea, is seen in syphilis, onchocerciasis, sarcoidosis, and tuberculosis, and with vestibuloauditory symptoms (of Cogan).

Epithelial keratitis. In epithelial keratitis, basal cells separate from the underlying basement membrane. In punctate keratitis, the cornea is studded with minute epithelial defects that stain with fluorescein solution. Patients complain of intermittent burning, irritation, tearing, and blurred vision. It may be traumatic, toxic, or inflammatory. It may occur in inherited lattice or Reis-Bückler corneal dystrophy. Treatment depends on the cause.

Superficial punctate keratitis. Superficial punctate keratitis (Thygeson) is a chronic, bilateral, possibly viral, disorder, in which numerous, irregular, randomly distributed, epithelial corneal opacities occur intermittently over a 3- or 4-year period. The lesions stain variably with fluorescein. Topical corticosteroids relieve the irritative symptoms and often resolve the epithelial lesions. Extended-wear contact lenses provide relief. If contact lens wear is discontinued for more than 48 hours, the lesions often recur.

There are numerous remissions and exacerbations and eventual healing without scars. Patients complain of intermittent burning, irritation, tearing, and blurred vision. Under magnification, from 1 to 50 (usually about 20) minute, oval, corneal opacities are visible. They are composed of a conglomeration of minute dots. New lesions appear as old ones heal so that their distribution varies from examination to examination. Hyperemia of the conjunctiva is present in the 12 o'clock meridian.

Superior limbic keratoconjunctivitis. This is a bilateral chronic keratinization of the superior bulbar conjunctiva, which results in a papillary reaction in the tarsal conjunctiva and punctate staining of the superior cornea sometimes (25%) with filaments. It occurs more often in women than in men. About 25% of the affected patients have signs of current or previous hyperthyroidism. The symptoms, which seem to originate from inadequate wetting of the superior cornea, may be treated with artificial tears, a soft contact lens, and, if necessary, resection of the superior conjunctiva so the cornea will be moistened by the tears.

Viral keratitis. Corneal inflammation occurs in many viral diseases (see Chapter 23) and may or may not be associated with systemic abnormalities that dominate the clinical picture. Many of the adenoviruses cause corneal inflammation. Zoster ophthalmicus caused by *Herpesvirus varicella* may cause severe anterior uveitis and keratitis. The photophobia observed in measles is caused by a keratoconjunctivitis that is frequently unobserved. Mumps may cause a transient corneal edema. Mononucleosis may be associated with deep corneal infiltrates.

Molluscum contagiosum. This is a mildly contagious skin disease caused by a virus of the pox group that is characterized by the occurence of smooth, waxy, umbilicated papules. When they occur on the eyelids, a follicular conjunctivitis and eptihelial keratitis may occur. Effective treatment requires removal of the papule, usually by lightly freezing it and removing its core with a curette.

Verruca. Verrucae of the eyelid margin or surface of the eye caused by the human papilloma (wart virus) usually disappear spontaneously and are usually not treated. Shedding of the virus into the conjunctival sac may cause inflammation that requires excision of the wart. Excision of warts may cause seeding; cryotherapy may be used.

Adenovirus infection. Subepithelial nonulcerative keratitis is associated with conjunctivitis (keratoconjunctivitis) and is most commonly caused by adenoviruses. Epidemic keratoconjunctivitis (EKC) is caused by adenovirus types 8 and 19. The disease is spread by eye to eye transmission.

Upper respiratory tract infection caused by adenovirus (pharyngoconjunctival fever) is a common disease that is especially widespread among children. Transmission from the respiratory tract to the eye is responsible for most instances of sporadic keratoconjunctivitis.

Adults between 20 and 40 years of age are most frequently affected, and the disease is more common in men than women (2:1). The incubation period ranges between 2 and 14 days, usually 7 to 9 days. The infection starts unilaterally as conjunctivitis with preauricular adenopathy. In most cases, keratitis develops 2 to 7 days later.

The initial symptoms are foreign body sensation, photophobia, lacrimation, discharge, and swelling. On examination, the bulbar conjunctiva is hyperemic, sometimes with severe chemosis. Conjunctival hemorrhages may occur with adenovirus types 8 and 19. Hyperemia is moderately severe, and diffuse infiltration and papillary and follicular hypertrophy are present. Papillary hypertrophy is more severe in the upper tarsal conjunctiva and may persist for 2 to 4 weeks. Follicular hypertrophy is

moderately severe and present mainly in the upper and lower fornices. Pseudomembranes may occur in severe cases of adenoconjunctivitis 8 and 19. Preauricular adenopathy is present.

Mild to moderate epithelial punctate keratitis with small corneal infiltrations may develop in the early stages. The duration of sporadic keratoconjunctivitis is less than 3 weeks, but epidemic keratoconjunctivitis lasts weeks longer. Subepithelial punctate keratitis with large, dense, well-marked corneal opacities in the subepithelial area of the cornea may develop in association with adenoviruses in both types of conjunctivitis. Generally, these opacities resolve within 3 months in all cases. Those caused by adenoviruses 8 and 19 may persist for several years.

Epidemic keratoconjunctivitis may occur in hospitals, outpatient departments, schools, and swimming pools. Institutional transmission may result from contaminated eye solutions, instruments, and contaminated fingers of doctors and nurses.

The differential diagnosis involves herpetic keratoconjunctivitis and chlamydial and bacterial conjunctivitis. Although the adenovirus has some in vitro sensitivity to idoxuridine and trifluorothymidine, no effective treatment is available. Frequent topical applications of antimicrobial drops may soothe the eye and prevent secondary bacterial infection.

Stromal nonulcerative keratitis. This disease particularly involves the deeper layers of the corneal stroma with infiltration of the edematous tissue by lymphocytes and plasma cells. There is often a severe associated iritis. In congenital syphilis, there is marked corneal vascularization deep in the stroma (interstitial keratitis). Superficial punctate and sclerosing keratitis occurs in onchocerciasis. In the late stages, a foreign body granuloma may cause complete opacification of the cornea.

Degenerations

Degenerative conditions that may affect the cornea are keratoconjunctivitis sicca, spheroid keratitis, corneal arcus, pterygium, gutter degeneration, band keratopathy, amyloidosis, and dellen. Persistent epithelial defects may develop in an eye that has a pre-existing abnormality of the ocular surface. Herpes keratitis, atrophy, ocular cicatricial pemphigoid, radiation keratitis, or chemical injury may result in chronic epithelial defects of the central stroma. Soft contact lenses, patching, and tarsorrhaphy may be helpful, but recurrence is common.

Spheroid keratitis (climatic droplet keratitis [Labrador keratitis]). This acquired degenerative corneal disease occurs mainly in elderly patients as subepithelial, spherical, golden, droplet-shaped opacities of various sizes in the superficial corneal stroma. It results from exposure to extreme heat or cold, dust, snow, ice particles, and ultraviolet radiation. The material is deposited in a horizontal fashion in the exposed portion of the conjunctiva and cornea that corresponds to the palpebral aperture with an appearance that resembles band keratopathy.

Marginal ectasia (Terrien). This is a slow, progressive, thinning of the peripheral cornea that results in ectasia and severe astigmatism. Rupture may occur with minor trauma. Excision of the ectatic corneal stroma and suturing the normal thickness stroma together alleviates the astigmatism.

CORNEAL DYSTROPHIES

Corneal dystrophies (Table 10-7) are bilateral hereditary disorders. They are occasionally present at birth but more frequently develop during adolescence and progress slowly throughout life. They are often described on the basis of their appearance or the layer of the cornea involved. Many do not interfere with vision but create interesting patterns in the normally transparent cornea. Most are transmitted as autosomal dominant disorders, but central macular dystrophy (Groenouw type II) is transmitted as an autosomal recessive defect.

Epithelial dystrophies

The juvenile epithelial dystrophy (of Meesmann) is a rare disorder that consists of clear dots or cysts in the corneal epithelium that occasionally rupture and stain. They are aggregates of an amorphous electron-dense material and marked irregularities in the architecture of the epithelium. Treatment is solely symptomatic.

Recurrent corneal erosion occurs after an uncomplicated corneal abrasion where regenerated epithelium does not adhere to the underlying basement membrane. About half of all patients have dystrophies of the epithelial basement membrane. In such an instance the patient, on awakening in the morning and opening or rubbing his eyes, will remove the epithelium. There is sudden onset of a foreign body sensation and lacrimation. Examination with high magnification between attacks shows a minute opacification in the subepithelial area. This area stains with fluorescein when the epithelium is removed. The disorder is disabling because of recurrent pain, but it causes no visual disability. Treatment is difficult. Recurrent corneal erosion is treated by removal of the abnormal epithelium and pressure dressing in the hope that the epithelium will attach itself normally to the underlying tissue. Removal of all epithelium as far as the corneoscleral limbus may be necessary. In some cases corticosteroids are used locally after removal of the epithelium. Often several treatments are required. The instillation of petrolatum lubricating or 5% sodium chloride ointment at bedtime may prevent the eyelid from adhering to the loose epithelium and may prevent flicking the epithelium off when the eyes are opened. A soft contact lens sometimes successfully prevents loss of epithelium.

A variety of epithelial basement membrane dystrophies (map-dot-fingerprint, bleb-like, microcytic) result from misdirected basal cells that generate excessive basement membrane, which triggers faulty epithelial desquamation,

Table 10-7. Corneal dystrophies

Epithelium: juvenile epithelial (Meesmann), recurrent erosions, map-dot-fingerprint, bleb-like, microcytic (Cogan)

Stroma:

  Bowman zone: Reis-Bücklers, anterior membrane, honeycomb, hereditary band keratopathy, anterior crocodile shagreen and mosaic pattern.

  Central: granular (Groenouw type I), macular (Groenouw type II), fleck, crystalline (central or marginal), cloudy, parenchymatous, posterior amorphous, hemochromatosis

  Pre-Descemet: farinata, primary, secondary

Endothelium: guttata, Fuchs, congenital hereditary endothelial, congenital hereditary stromal, posterior polymorphous

Ectatic: anterior keratoconus, keratoglobus, posterior keratoconus, Terrien marginal

intraepithelial microcysts, and poor epithelial adherence to the basement membrane. The condition is bilateral and usually occurs after age 40. There are no symptoms unless the epithelium erodes, causing a foreign body sensation. Deposits in the visual axis impair vision. Surgical removal of all corneal epithelium and use of a corneal contact bandage lens may provide significant improvement without recurrence.

Stromal dystrophies

Granular dystrophy (Groenouw type I) appears as irregularly shaped white spots surrounded by clear cornea in stroma underlying the Bowman zone. The disease begins in childhood and slowly progresses by late middle age, rarely resulting in loss of useful vision. Corneal transplantation may be performed, if necessary, to restore useful vision.

Central macular dystrophy of the cornea (Groenouw type II) begins in childhood as a diffuse clouding and progresses until, by middle age, the entire thickness of the cornea contains gray confluent spots. Mature keratan sulfate is absent from the cornea and blood stream.

Lattice dystrophy becomes evident in young adults; their anterior corneal stroma contains lines in irregular patterns made up of amyloid that has been locally synthesized by the cornea. The amyloid is composed of protein AA that occurs in secondary amyloidosis, combined with a structural protein AP (P for plasma). Protein AA does not occur in primary familial amyloidosis of the cornea. Painful epithelial erosions occur in early life, and early lamellar keratoplasty may be indicated.

Endothelial dystrophy

Human corneal endothelium does not regenerate, but when cells are lost, the adjoining cells spread out to cover the defect. If the defect is not covered, Descemet membrane develops round, wartlike excrescences that dip into the anterior chamber. These normally occur as a degenerative change with aging, are located at the periphery of the cornea, and are called Hassall-Henle bodies. They are of no clinical significance except as an indication of aging.

A similar loss of endothelium of the central cornea causes an endothelial dystrophy (Fuchs dystrophy, or cornea guttata). The condition is bilateral, but one eye is more extensively involved than the other. Biomicroscopically, minute spheres appear imbedded on the posterior cornea. They may vary from a few to so many that vision is impaired. The deposits may act as a diffraction grating and may cause iridescent vision. When the deposits are extensive, the deturgescent action of the endothelium is lost, and the cornea becomes edematous. This may occur spontaneously or may follow cataract surgery, corneal trauma, prolonged wearing of contact lenses, or tonography. The substantia propria is thickened and opaque, and epithelial edema is followed by erosion and bullae (bullous keratopathy or combined epithelial-endothelial dystrophy). Vision is markedly reduced. The bullae may rupture and expose corneal nerve endings, resulting in severe pain. Soft contact lenses relieve discomfort. Hypertonic saline or glucose solutions dehydrate the edematous cornea and may improve vision. Early endothelial and epithelial dystrophy responds well to penetrating transplant, provided all of the diseased tissue is removed.

Keratoconus

Keratoconus (conical cornea) is an abnormality in which the symmetric curvature of the cornea is distorted by an abnormal thinning and forward bulging of the central portion of the cornea (ectasia) (Fig. 10-9). The condition is usually bilateral, but one eye may be in-

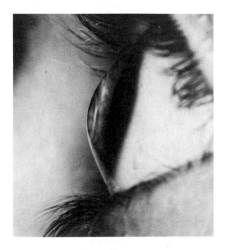

Fig. 10-9. Abnormal corneal profile in keratoconus.

volved long before its fellow. Onset is usually at the time of puberty. Women are affected more frequently than men. Keratoconus progresses slowly over many years but may become stationary at any time. The chief symptom is decreased visual acuity for far and near because of severe astigmatism, which, as the disease progresses, becomes irregular and cannot be improved with spectacles. Contact lenses provide a regular anterior curvature and usually provide visual improvement.

Diagnosis may be difficult in the early stages. Viewing the cornea from above by looking down from behind the patient and over the brow, as is done in the diagnosis of proptosis (see Chapter 6), may indicate the corneal cone (Munson sign). The corneal cone distorts the pattern of the Placido disk, a flat disk that has concentric black and white circles and a central opening to observe their corneal reflection. The light reflex in retinoscopy is irregular. The epithelium at the base of the cone may be infiltrated with a ferritin pigment, causing a Fleisher ring. Breaks in Descemet membrane allow aqueous humor to enter the stroma and cause a severe corneal edema, hydrops of the cornea, which is a common complication of Down syndrome.

Vision is usually maintained at a useful level by using hard contact lenses. If these cannot be used, a penetrating corneal transplant restores useful vision with a 95% success rate.

Keratoconus may be associated with a variety of other ocular disorders such as retinitis pigmentosa, retrolental fibroplasia, ectopia lentis, congenital cataract, microcornea, blue sclera, and vernal catarrh. Systemic disorders associated with ocular disorders include the following syndromes: osteogenesis imperfecta, Down, Marfan, Ehlers-Danlos, Crouzon, Laurence-Moon-Biedl, and van der Hoeve.

Therapeutic soft contact lenses

Soft contact lenses are hemispherical shells that cover the cornea and a portion of the adjacent sclera. When hydrated the lens is soft and pliable, and when dry it is hard and brittle. A dry lens requires about 2 hours of soaking in normal saline solution to become completely hydrated. Soft contact lenses are usually better tolerated than hard contact lenses, although visual improvement may not be as good. Soft

contact lenses have been useful in the treatment of bullous keratopathy, recurrent corneal erosion, and corneal ulcerations. They may protect the cornea in trichiasis. In dry eye syndromes such as Sjögren disease, ocular pemphigoid, erythema multiforme, and other conditions in which there is inadequate tearing, the lens is often not effective.

KERATOPLASTY

Corneal transplant, or keratoplasty, is the excision of corneal tissue and its replacement by a cornea from a human donor. One of two techniques is used: (1) the penetrating graft (Fig. 10-10), in which the entire thickness of cornea is removed and replaced by transparent corneal tissue, and (2) the nonpenetrating, or lamellar, keratoplasty, in which a superficial layer is removed and replaced without entry into the anterior chamber. The graft may vary in size from replacement of the entire cornea (total keratoplasty) to one in which a portion of the cornea is excised (partial). A diameter of 5 mm is the smallest size that will remain transparent in humans.

Because of improved surgery and better selection of donor material, the indications for transplant have been defined more in terms of the ocular disease necessitating the procedure than in the preoperative visual acuity. In diseases such as keratonconus, in which there is no corneal vascularization, the prognosis for improvement in vision is excellent. In corneal scars, such as those that occur after alkali burns, in which vascularization is superficial and deep, the graft is less likely to remain transparent. In every case, light perception and projection must be normal before surgery is considered. The prognosis in corneal dystrophies varies with the type and extent of the corneal abnormality. The dystrophy may recur in the donor graft.

The absence of blood vessels and lymphatics in the normal cornea prevents the donor cornea from sensitizing the recipient. Clear grafts follow transplants in minimally vascularized corneas but less frequently in severely vascularized corneas. Corneal graft rejection proceeds over a period of weeks and affects each layer separately.

Corneal graft reaction begins 3 or more weeks (sometimes years) after a technically suc-

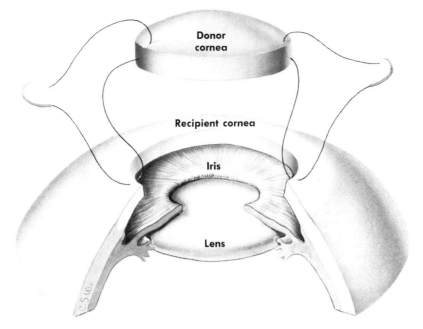

Fig. 10-10. The excised central portion of the cornea is being replaced with a clear donor cornea.

cessful clear transplant. The process begins with increased protein (flare) and cells in the anterior chamber. There is edema of the donor cornea. Keratitic precipitates accumulate on the endothelium and extend centrally to involve the entire graft. New blood vessels invade the graft, and the entire graft may become opaque. Removal of donor epithelium at the time of surgery reduces the antigenic level. A small graft, centrally placed, using nylon rather than silk sutures, minimizes reactions. Severely vascularized corneas are more likely to induce graft reaction. In grafts that were never clear after transplantation, it is difficult to determine whether subsequent inflammation is a graft reaction or complication of surgical technique. Treatment consists of frequent instillation of corticosteroids. Often the reaction disappears and the graft clears. The donor graft is never extruded but becomes opaque and often vascularized. Subsequent grafts may remain clear without a graft reaction developing, but the corneal blood vessels minimize the chances of a transparent graft.

Donor material is obtained from a noninfected adult, preferably between 25 and 35 years of age, who has died from an acute disease or from injury. Eyes from stillborn infants are less desirable, as are those patients who were ill for a long period before death. Eyes should not be used from patients who had terminal septicemia, Creutzfeldt-Jakob disease or other possible slow-virus disorders, AIDS, hepatitis, tumors of the anterior ocular segment, or leukemia. The donor ELISA titer for HLTV-III must be negative. The density of corneal endothelial cells decreases with aging and donor material from those aged more than 60 years is undesirable.

The donor eye should be enucleated within an hour after death by using sterile instruments and a sterile technique. If the eyelids are closed and a small icebag is placed over each eye, delays up to 5 hours are permissible. Many eye banks store donor corneal tissues as whole eyes in refrigerated, moist chambers for periods of 24 to 48 hours. Corneas may be stored for longer periods by carefully removing the cornea with a 3 mm rim of scleral tissue attached. The corneas must not be folded, because this damages the endothelium. The cornea may be stored in a modified tissue-culture medium (M-K medium) and stored at a temperature of 4° C.

Persons who wish to donate their eyes for use in keratoplasty should write to an eye bank that is a member of the Eye Bank Association of America.*

Penetrating keratoplasty

The excision of all layers of a central portion of the cornea (partial penetrating) and replacement with a clear donor cornea is the traditional type of keratoplasty. A penetrating transplant is complete when the entire cornea is excised and partial when it is not.

The operation is usually performed using topical and retrobulbar anesthesia and akinesia. The graft is removed from the donor eye with a trephine. The same trephine or a slightly larger one is used to remove the diseased area from the recipient eye. The donor cornea is then sutured into position.

To align the graft, temporary preplaced sutures may be inserted equidistantly in the four principal meridians of the donor button. Monofilament nylon (10-0) is used as either a continuous or an interrupted suture.

Lamellar keratoplasty

Since all layers of the cornea are not removed in nonpenetrating, or lamellar keratoplasty, it has a more limited application than the penetrating type. Conversely, the procedure is associated with fewer postoperative complications than penetrating keratoplasty, may be repeated with a good likelihood of success even after earlier failures, and does not complicate a subsequent penetrating graft.

Keratoprosthesis

Corneal implants (keratoprostheses) made of nonreactive plastic are used in individuals in whom corneal transplantation was previously contraindicated or foredoomed to failure because of excessive scarring or neovascularization. In densely scarred corneas, a central optical cylinder of plastic supported by a cuff of plastic or dentin from a tooth extracted from the patient may occasionally provide a marked improvement in vision.

Keratorefractive surgery

The cornea is the major refractive surface of the eye because it separates air from fluid (the

aqueous humor). A change in its curvature will therefore either decrease or increase its refractive power. Increased curvature will provide increased refractive power and will decrease the amount of hyperopia. A decreased curvature will decrease the amount of myopia. A number of procedures have been developed to correct refractive errors through modification of the corneal curvature: radial keratotomy, keratomileusis, keratophakia, epikeratophakia. Radial keratotomy is used to neutralize myopia with best results obtained in patients with refractive errors of less than 4 diopters. The other procedures require a lamellar-type keratoplasty and may correct from 12 to 20 diopters of refractive error. They are mainly used to correct hypertropia after cataract removal.

Radial keratotomy is the most widely performed procedure. It aims at reducing moderate degrees of myopia (1 diopter to 4 diopters) so that spectacles or contact lenses are not required for distance vision. A central optical zone 3 or 4 mm in diameter is untouched. A

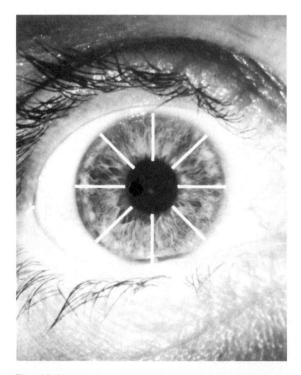

Fig. 10-11. The location of the incisions in radial keratotomy. The central 3 to 4 mm optical zone of the cornea is not incised, and the incisions do not extend beyond the corneoscleral limbus. Four, eight, or sixteen radial incisions are made.

*Eye Bank Association of America, 1511 K Street, N.W., Suite 830, Washington, DC 20005-1401, telephone (202) 628-4280.

series of equally spaced radial incisions then extend through most of the corneal thickness from the edge of the optical zone to, but not beyond, the corneoscleral limbus (Fig. 10-11). The intraocular pressure then pushes the weakened peripheral cornea forward and flattens the central optical zone, thus reducing its refractive power and the degree of myopia.

A central optical zone 3 mm in diameter provides a greater correction than one 4 mm in diameter. Four to sixteen radial incisions are used; eight is the usual number. The effect is proportionate to the depth of the incision, particularly near the central optical zone. Minute perforations into the anterior chamber heal without problems; if the anterior chamber is lost, the remaining incisions must be delayed until the cornea heals, usually about 1 month. Vision fluctuates with the level of the intraocular pressure during healing. In about 10% of the patients, there is microscopic pigmentation of the incision, which appears 6 to 12 months after the procedure. Generally about 3 to 4 diopters of correction is obtained. Most suitably selected patients have postoperative vision better than 20/40 without spectacles.

In keratomileusis (Fig. 10-12) the refractive power of the eye is increased by increasing the radius of curvature of the anterior surface of the cornea and thus neutralize or decrease hypermetropia, particularly that which follows cataract extraction. A disk of tissue 8.5 to 9.0 mm in diameter is resected from the patient's anterior corneal stroma, frozen, and reshaped on a computer-assisted lathe. The tissue is then reinserted in the cornea to provide an increased radius of curvature. The procedure is the most technically difficult of all the refractive surgical procedures.

Rather than using the corneal tissue of the patient, donor cornea may be reshaped and transplanted to the patient's anterior cornea (keratophakia). Intraocular lenses inserted at the time of cataract extraction, implantation of an intraocular lens sometime after cataract extraction (secondary implant), and the use of contact lenses reduce the need for keratomileusis. In addition to correction of hypermetropia, it may be useful in some patients with myopia of 6 to 18 diopters.

Epikeratophakia (see Fig. 10-12) is similar to keratophakia except that no corneal stroma is

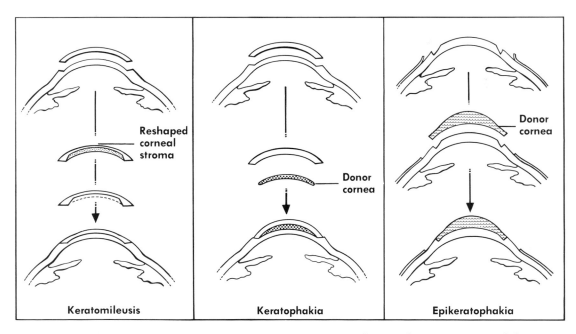

Fig. 10-12. Various types of corneal refractive surgery. In *keratomileusis*, a portion of the patient's cornea is reshaped to provide a different curvature; in *keratophakia*, donor cornea or a synthetic lens material is used; in *epikeratophakia*, the donor cornea is placed over the patient's cornea from which the epithelium has been removed.

removed from the patient. A thin disk of donor corneal stroma is sutured to the patient's cornea from which the epithelium has been removed. In 4 to 10 days the recipient's epithelium covers the tissue, and in 1 to 2 months the recipient's keratocytes repopulate the donor tissue. The donor tissue is easily removed if necessary.

Keratoepithelioplasty (see Fig. 10-12) is used for the treatment of persistent corneal epithelium defects in which the fellow eye is too impaired to provide donor material for a conjunctival transplant. Corneal epithelium with a thin layer of stroma as a carrier is obtained from a fresh cadaver eye and is transplanted to the sclera adjacent to the corneoscleral limbus of the recipient eye, which has had a superficial keratectomy. The donor epithelium covers the defect and replaces the damaged epithelium.

INJURIES

Foreign bodies of the cornea constitute about 25% of all significant eye injuries.

Abrasions

Removal of the corneal epithelium by an abrasion or ultraviolet light causes considerable pain and lacrimation, but the lesion heals quickly and is of little clinical importance unless infection occurs. The abraded area stains with fluorescein. The eye is usually more comfortable if tightly patched, and the majority of corneal abrasions heal with no treatment other than patching. Local anesthetics are contraindicated because they may delay epithelization. If infection is feared, it is better to use sulfacetamide solution locally than to use a broad-spectrum antibiotic.

Lacerations

Corneal lacerations are particularly serious, because the interior of the eye is opened to infection and there is the likelihood of additional injury to intraocular structures. Treatment is directed toward prevention of infection by administration of an antibiotic, avoidance of prolapse of intraocular contents that may occur with repeated examinations, and closure of the laceration with sutures after excision of prolapsed intraocular tissue. If the lens is lacerated, it is removed at the time the corneal laceration is repaired.

BIBLIOGRAPHY
General

Barraquer, J., and Rutlan, J.: Microsurgery of the cornea: an atlas and textbook, Barcelona, 1984, Ediciones Scriba, S.A.

Brown, S.I., and Mondino, B.J.: Therapy of Mooren's ulcer, Am. J. Ophthalmol. **98**:1, 1984.

Caldwell, D.R., Insler, M.S., Boutros, G., and Hawk, T.: Primary surgical repair of severe peripheral marginal ectasia in Terrien's marginal degeneration, Am. J. Ophthalmol. **97**:332, 1984.

Casey, T., and Daniel, M.: Corneal grafting, Philadelphia, 1984, W.B. Saunders Co.

Fedukowicz, H.B., and Stenson, S.: External infections of the eye, Norwalk, Conn., 1985, Appleton-Century-Crofts.

Grayson, M.: Diseases of the cornea, ed. 2, St. Louis, 1983, The C.V. Mosby Co.

Koch, D.D., Parke, D.W., and Paton, D.: Current management in ophthalmology, New York, 1983, Churchill Livingstone.

Leibowitz, H.M.: Corneal disorders: clinical diagnosis and management, Philadelphia, 1984, W.B. Saunders Co.

Lemp, M.A., Gold, J.B., Wong, S., Mahmood, M., and Guimaraes, R.: An in vivo study of corneal surface morphologic features in patients with keratoconjunctivitis sicca, Am. J. Ophthalmol. **98**:426, 1984.

Smolin, G., Tabbara, K., and Waitcher, J.: Infectious diseases of the eye, Baltimore, 1984, Williams & Wilkins Co.

Smolin, G., and Thoft, R.A.: The cornea: scientific foundations and clinical practice, Boston, 1983, Little, Brown, and Co.

Taylor, D.M., Atlas, B.F., Romanchuk, K.G., and Stern, A.L.: Pseudophakic bullous keratopathy, Ophthalmology **90**:19, 1983.

Developmental

Bahn, C.F., Falls, H.F., Varley, G.A., Meyer, R.F., Edelhauser, H.F., and Bourne, W.M.: Classification of corneal endothelial disorders based on neural crest origin, Ophthalmology **91**:448, 1984.

Beauchamp, G.R., and Knepper, P.A.: Role of the neural crest in anterior segment development and disease, J. Pediatr. Ophthalmol. Strabismus **21**:209, 1984.

Bolande, R.P.: The neurocristopathies: a unifying concept of disease arising in neural crest maldevelopment, Hum. Pathol. **5**:409, 1974.

Buxton, J.N., and Lash, R.S.: Results of penetrating keratoplasty in the iridocorneal endothelial syndrome, Am. J. Ophthalmol. **98**:297, 1984.

Kupfer, C., Kaiser-Kupfer, M.I., Datiles, M., and McCain, L.: The contralateral eye in the iridocorneal endothelial (ICE) syndrome, Ophthalmology **90:**1343, 1983.

Steinberg, E.B., Wilson, L.A., Waring, G.O. III, Lynn, M.J., and Coles, W.H.: Stellate iron lines in the corneal epithelium after radial keratotomy, Am. J. Ophthalmol. **98: 416–421, 1984.**

Keratitis

Boisjoly, H.M., Pavan-Langston, D., Kenyon, K.R., and Baker, A.S.: Superinfections in herpes simplex keratitis, Am. J. Ophthalmol. **96:**354, 1983.

Brown, S.I., and Mondino, B.J.: Therapy of Mooren's ulcer, Am. J. Ophthalmol. **98:**1-6, 1984.

Cohen, E.J., Buchanan, H.W., Laughrea, P.A., Adams, C.P., Galentine, P.G., Visvesvara, G.S., Folberg, R., Arentsen, J.J., and Laibson, P.R.: Diagnosis and management of *Acanthamoeba* keratitis, Am. J. Ophthalmol. **100:**389, 1985.

Ishibashi, Y., Matsumoto, Y., and Takei, K.: The effects of intravenous miconazole on fungal keratitis, Am. J. Ophthalmol. **98:**433, 1984.

Moore, M.B., McCulley, J.P., Luckenbach, M., Gelender, H., Newton, C., McDonald, M.B., and Visvesvara, G.S.: *Acanthamoeba* keratitis associated with soft contact lenses, Am. J. Ophthalmol. **100:**396, 1985.

Nesburn, A.B., Lowe, G.H. III, Lepoff, N.J., and Maguen, E.: Effect of topical trifluidine on Thygeson's superficial punctate keratitis, Ophthalmology **91:**1188, 1984.

Cornea

Parlato, C.J., Cohen, E.J., Sakauye, C.M., Dreizen, N.G., Galentine, P.G., and Laibson, P.R.: Role of debridement and trifluridine (trifluorothymidine) in herpes simplex dendritic keratitis, Arch. Ophthalmol. **103:**673, 1985.

Sanitato, J.J., Kelley, C.G., and Kaufman, H.E.: Surgical management of peripheral fungal keratitis (keratomycosis). Arch. Ophthalmol. **102:**1506, 1984.

Dystrophies

Krachmer, J.H., Feder, R.S., and Belin, M.W.: Keratoconus and related noninflammatory corneal thinning disorders, Surg. Ophthalmol. **28:**293, 1984.

Meisler, D.M., Langston, R.H.S., Naab, T.J., Aaby, A.A., McMahon, J.T., and Tubbs, R.R.: Infectious crystalline keratopathy, Am. J. Ophthalmol. **97:**337, 1984.

Surgery

Arentsen, J.J.: Corneal transplant allograft reaction, Trans. Am. Ophthalmol. Soc. **81:**361, 1983.

Arrowsmith, P.N., and Marks, R.G.: Visual, refractive, and keratometric results of radial keratotomy, Arch. Ophthalmol. **102:**1612, 1984.

Deitz, M.R., and Sanders, D.R.: Progressive hyperopia with long-term follow-up of radial keratotomy, Arch. Ophthalmol. **103:**782, 1985.

Friedlander, M.H., Safir, A., McDonald, M.B., Kaufman, H.E., and Granet, N.: Update on keratophakia, Ophthalmology **90:**365, 1983.

Ingraham, H.J., Guber, D., and Green, W.R.: Radial keratotomy, Arch. Ophthalmol. **103:**683, 1985.

MacRae, S.M., Matsuda, M., and Rich, L.F.: The effect of radial keratotomy on the corneal endothelium, Am. J. Ophthalmol. **100:**538, 1985.

Powers, M.K., Meyerowitz, B.E., Arrowsmith, P.N., and Marks, R.G.: Psychosocial findings in radial keratotomy patients two years after surgery, Ophthalmology **91:**1193, 1984.

Sanders, D.R., editor: Radial keratotomy, Thorofare, N.J., 1984, Slack, Inc.

Schanzlin, D.J., Robin, J.P., Gomez, D.S., Gindi, J.J., and Smith, R.E.: Results of penetrating keratoplasty for aphakic and pseudophakic bullous keratopathy, Am. J. Ophthalmol. **98:**320, 1984.

Thoft, R.A.: Keratoepithelioplasty, Am. J. Ophthalmol. **97:**1, 1984.

11

THE SCLERA

The sclera is a dense, connective tissue structure composed of collagen bundles of varying diameters. It constitutes the posterior five sixths of the globe. Its anterior portion is visible beneath the transparent conjunctiva as the white of the eye, but careful examination shows a fine network of blood vessels that make up the richly vascularized episclera located mainly in the anterior segment of the globe between the conjunctiva and sclera proper. Inflammations, often associated with connective tissue disorders, are the main disorders of the sclera. The tissue, however, undergoes changes in shape, size, and translucency that play an important role in the pathogenesis of other ocular disorders.

SYMPTOMS AND SIGNS OF SCLERAL DISEASE

Because of its rich sensory nerve innervation, inflammations of the sclera may cause severe or dull pain that is aggravated by contraction of an ocular muscle if the sclera is inflamed near its insertion. No signs may be apparent in inflammations of the posterior sclera, but pain on ocular movement suggests the cause. Unless the inflammation causes cataract, keratitis, uveitis, retinitis or detached retina, there is no loss of vision, which distinguishes the pain from that which occurs in retrobulbar neuritis.

Inflammation of the anterior portion of the sclera causes generalized or localized areas of deep reddish injection of the episcleral tissues. These areas may be painful on palpation. In thinning or necrosis of the sclera, the bluish-black choroidal pigment may be exposed.

Pigmentation of the sclera

The sclera is normally white. It appears blue in young children and sometimes in osteogenesis imperfecta, Ehlers-Danlos syndrome, pseudoxanthoma elasticum, and keratoconus.

Localized discolorations of the sclera occur in intrascleral nerve loops, in alkaptonuria and hyaline plaques (Fig. 11-1). A blue nevus may be associated with an underlying choroidal nevus or a melanocytoma with an underlying melanocytosis. The most serious abnormality is extension of a choroidal malignant melanoma through the sclera, often at the site of one of the small openings for the transmission of nerves or blood vessels. The differential diagnosis of a black elevated mass in the sclera includes staphyloma with an extremely thin sclera or extraocular extension of an intraocular malignant melanoma.

The sclera is not pigmented in jaundice. The yellowish appearance of the globe is caused by bilirubin in the conjunctiva.

INTRASCLERAL NERVE LOOP

An intrascleral nerve loop (of Axenfeld) is an anatomic variation in which an anomalous loop of a long ciliary nerve partially or completely perforates the sclera and then returns to the inner surface of the sclera, often accompanied by a blood vessel. It appears as a 1- to 2-mm black dot on the sclera, mainly in the lower half

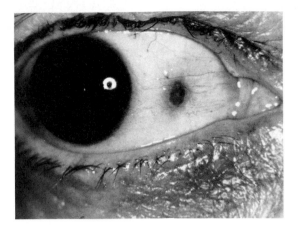

Fig. 11-1. Senile hyaline plaque located immediately in front of the insertion of the lateral rectus muscle in a 65-year-old man. The plaque shells out of the sclera easily and contains calcium sulfate (gypsum).

of the eye, some 2 to 4 mm from the corneoscleral limbus. Its unchanging appearance and location indicate its nature. Treatment is not indicated.

SENILE HYALINE PLAQUE

Senile hyaline plaque (Fig. 11-1) is the term mistakenly applied to a darkish deposition located immediately anterior to the insertion of the medial or lateral rectus muscle in the sclera. It occurs only in individuals over 50 years of age. It appears as an area of translucency in the sclera. It was formerly thought to be caused by thinning of the sclera because of traction of the recti muscles. The plaque may be easily shelled out of the slightly thinned sclera and histologically may contain calcium sulfate (gypsum).

STAPHYLOMA AND ECTASIA

Staphylomas and ectasias are bulgings or enlargements of the sclera secondary to embryologic defects of the sclera, localized areas of degeneration, or increased intraocular pressure. If only the sclera bulges, the condition is called an ectasia, whereas if the uvea lines the bulging sclera it is called a staphyloma.

Ectasias are usually associated with abnormalities in closure of the optic vesicle; thus, concurrent colobomas of the uveal tract and retina are common. Failure of the scleral mesoderm to form the lamina cribrosa gives the appearance of an enormous but normal optic disk at the bottom of a deep pit. In myopia a localized bulging of sclera may develop between the insertions of the recti muscles, and this bulging may be associated with a retinal separation. In adult glaucoma, the sclera propria (and cornea) is resistant to the increased intraocular pressure, but a partial ectasia forms at the lamina cribrosa along with the characteristic glaucomatous excavation (cupping) of the optic disk.

Staphylomas may be total or partial. In congenital glaucoma, uniform stretching of the sclera occurs before the scleral and corneal collagen fibers have matured. The result is the total staphyloma of buphthalmos (ox eye).

Localized staphylomas are dividied into anterior and posterior types. Anterior staphylomas occur anterior to the equator (calary), ciliary staphylomas over the ciliary body, and intercalary staphylomas between the ciliary body and the corneoscleral limbus. These bulgings most often follow inflammation of the anterior uveal tract or laceration of the sclera combined with constantly increased intraocular pressure. The involved area appears as a region of scleral thinning lined with the dark pigment of the uveal tract.

Posterior staphylomas occur in Marfan and Ehler-Danlos syndromes, and in pathologic myopia in which there is thinning and stretching of the posterior pole as the axial length of the globe increases. Vision is decreased. Ophthalmoscopic examination often shows central retinal degeneration. Indirect ophthalmoscopic examination shows a sharp, well-defined edge of posterior scleral outpouching.

Equatorial staphylomas and ectasias involve the areas near the points of exit of the four vortex veins from the eye. The localized bulging of the sclera may be a factor in retinal separation, though often it is not detected until the area is exposed surgically.

SCLERAL THINNING

In long-standing scleral or uveal inflammation, Marfan syndrome, myopia, aging, rheumatoid arthritis, and osteogenesis imperfecta, the underlying uveal pigment is visible because of scleral thinning. The sclera appears more blue than white. This coloration may be vivid in osteogenesis imperfecta.

INFLAMMATIONS

The sclera proper has a poor blood supply and an inactive metabolism, but the episclera has a rich vascular network. Scleral inflammations (Table 11-1) tend to be torpid and unresponsive to treatment. There is often an associated rheumatoid arthritis or other connective tissue disorder. The cause is obscure but may be the result of local tissue ischemia or an immune-complex-mediated hypersensitivity (type III).

EPISCLERITIS

Episcleritis (Fig. 11-2) is an inflammation of the episcleral tissue in the region between the insertion of the recti muscles and the corneoscleral limbus. There are two types: nodular and diffuse. It affects women twice as frequently as men and has its peak incidence between 30 and 40 years of age. The onset is sudden with intense redness, usually involving only one quadrant of the globe but sometimes all, and a sharpness or pricking discomfort. The affected episclera is edematous, and the blood vessels are engorged. The condition tends to spontaneous remission, sometimes within a few hours or days. There is a marked tendency for recurrence, sometimes cyclic, over a period of years.

Nodular episcleritis is similar to simple episcleritis but is associated with a tender, subconjunctival nodule 2 to 3 mm in size. There may be deep, boring pain, most severe at night, but the inflammation generally disappears spontaneously after 4 to 5 weeks, sometimes leaving a residue of a faintly pigmented patch to which the conjunctiva is adherent.

Scleritis

Scleritis is a more serious disease than episcleritis and is associated with more intense pain. Scleritis is more likely to be bilateral than episcleritis. Like episcleritis, it tends to recur.

Diffuse anterior scleritis has an insidious onset with generalized orbital aching. The blood vessels are intensely injected and appear as deep-seated, small numerous radial vessels surrounded by capillaries.

Posterior scleritis is a rare, unilateral inflammation, usually associated with anterior scleritis. It occurs more commonly in women than men in the fourth through sixth decades of life. Choroiditis, retinal detachment, macular edema, retinal folds, choroidal folds, and papilledema may occur. Retinal detachment with choroidal elevation and posterior uveitis may simulate a choroidal malignant melanoma.

Nodular scleritis is intensely painful with an extremely tender, firm, immobile nodule completely separated from the overlying congested episcleral tissues. The nodules may be multiple. Avascularity or progressive increase in size of the nodule indicates scleral necrosis.

There are two types of necrotizing anterior scleritis. In one a severe inflammation causes much pain and many ocular complications. It is often associated with severe systemic disorders such as systemic lupus erythematosus or Wegener granulomatosis. In the second, joint involvement or rheumatoid arthritis is prominent and ocular inflammation and symptoms are minimal as rheumatoid granulomas form in the sclera (scleromalacia perforans). The necrosis may follow an anterior scleritis. Avascular

Table 11-1. Inflammation of the sclera

Episcleritis
Diffuse
Nodular
Anterior scleritis
Diffuse
Brawny
Sclerokeratitis
Nodular
Necrotizing
With uveitis
Without inflammation (scleromalacia perforans)
Posterior scleritis

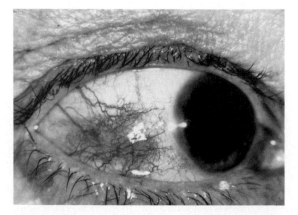

Fig. 11-2. Localized area of acute episcleritis on the temporal side of the sclera in a 35-year-old woman.

patches may perforate suddenly. The noninflammatory type may cause painless, large scleral defects through which the choroid bulges, usually without perforation, a disaster that may be precipitated by subconjunctival corticosteroid injection.

Treatment is difficult. Episcleritis improves spontaneously, although recovery may be hastened by administration of noncorticosteroidal anti-inflammatory drugs. Large doses of corticosteroids may be used, but the dangers of cataract and glaucoma must be appreciated. In severe necrotizing disease corticosteroids as well as immunosuppressive therapy and other compounds used in the treatment of connective tissue disease may be necessary.

INJURIES

Laceration of the sclera invariably involves the underlying uveal coat and is serious. Blunt trauma to the globe may rupture the posterior sclera as the result of contrecoup phenomenon. The history of blunt trauma associated with severe subconjunctival hemorrhage and a persistently soft globe suggests a posterior rupture of the globe. Usually an associated rupture of the retina and choroid occurs along with vitreous hemorrhage obscuring the tissues.

BIBLIOGRAPHY

Berger, B., and Reese, F.: Retinal pigment epithelial detachments in posterior scleritis, Am. J. Ophthalmol. **90:**604, 1980.

Cobo, M.: Inflammation of the sclera, Int. Ophthalmol. Clin. **23:**159, 1983.

Foster, C.S., Forstot, S.L., and Wilson, L.A.: Mortality rate in rheumatoid arthritis patients developing necrotizing scleritis or peripheral ulcerative keratitis: effect on systemic immunosuppression, Ophthalmology **91:**1253, 1984.

Watson, P.G., and Bovey, E.: Anterior segment fluorescein angiography in the diagnosis of scleral inflammation, Ophthalmology **92:**1, 1985.

Watson, P.G., and Hazelman, B.L.: Major problems in ophthalmology. Vol. 2: The sclera and systemic disorders, Philadelphia, 1976, W.B. Saunders Co.

Wilhelmus, K.R., Grierson, I., and Watson, P.G.: Histopathologic and clinical association of scleritis and glaucoma, Am. J. Ophthalmol. **91:**697, 1981.

Young, R.D., and Watson, P.G.: Microscopical studies of necrotising scleritis. I. Cellular aspects, Br. J. Ophthalmol. **68:**770, 1984.

Young, R.D., and Watson, P.G.: Microscopical studies of necrotising scleritis. II. Collagen degradation in the scleral stroma, Br. J. Ophthalmol. **68:**781, 1984.

12

THE LACRIMAL APPARATUS

The lacrimal system consists of a secretory and a drainage portion. The secretory portion comprises the lacrimal gland, which is divided into palpebral and orbital lobes, and basic secretors located in the margin of the eyelids and scattered throughout the conjunctiva. These are the meibomian glands, the sebaceous glands of Zeis, and the sweat glands of Moll that provide an oily secretion which minimizes tear evaporation. The lacrimal gland provides both aqueous and mucous components, and the accessory lacrimal glands of Krause and Wolfring contribute to the aqueous portion of tears. The conjunctival goblet cells, glands of Manz, and crypts of Henle secrete mucin that wets the hydrophobic epithelium.

The drainage portion consists of epithelium-lined tubes leading from the two openings on the eyelid margins (the puncta) through the canaliculi to the lacrimal sac, which lies in the lacrimal fossa. The lacrimal sac opens into the inferior nasal meatus by its inferior continuation, the nasolacrimal duct, which lies in the bony nasolacrimal canal.

The tears consist of a relatively stagnant layer, the precorneal tear film, that overlies the cornea and a fluid layer that flows in the lower fornix to the inferior punctum. The precorneal film provides the smooth and regular anterior refracting surface of the eye. It has three layers: (1) a superficial oily layer that prevents evaporation, (2) a middle aqueous layer, and (3) an inner mucin layer immediately adjacent to the corneal epithelium. The orbital and palpebral portions of the lacrimal gland provide reflex secretion controlled by the nervous system in response to changes in the surface of the eye. The remaining tear secretions produce their contribution to the tears at a steady and constant rate and are not controlled by the nervous system.

SYMPTOMS AND SIGNS OF LACRIMAL APPARATUS DISEASE

Diseases of the lacrimal system are divided into those involving abnormalities of the lacrimal glands and those involving defects in the drainage system. Excessive tear secretion usually occurs because of reflex stimulation of the gland, whereas decreased tear formation occurs because of either atrophy of glandular tissue or conjunctival scarring that occludes the orifices of the accessory and main lacrimal glands. Neoplasms and inflammatory diseases of the lacrimal gland cause a characteristic swelling and S-shaped curve of the upper eyelid.

Diseases of the lacrimal drainage apparatus obstruct the passages and cause tearing. The obstructed lacrimal sac may become acutely or chronically inflamed. Acute inflammation causes a generalized cellulitis of the sac and surrounding structures. Chronic inflammation is associated with few signs other than painless swelling of the lacrimal sac region and pus flowing from the puncta when pressure is applied to the sac.

The main symptoms of diseases of the lacrimal system are usually related to an excess or

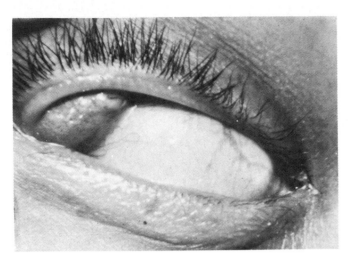

Fig. 12-1. Chronic dacryoadenitis in a 23-year-old man with sarcoidosis.

a deficiency of tears or to swelling of the lacrimal gland or lacrimal sac. Excessive tear formation or poor drainage is a nuisance, since vision is blurred by tears that overflow onto the face. Deficient tear secretion, however, may cause loss of the eye and may be associated with keratinization of the conjunctiva and cornea. It may cause nearly intolerable symptoms of burning and dryness of the eyes.

DISEASES OF THE LACRIMAL GLANDS

The lacrimal glands are tubuloracemose, similar in structure to the salivary glands. In general, they are subject to the same inflammations, diseases, and tumors. The two groups of glands are often involved in the same inflammatory and degenerative diseases.

Inflammation

Acute dacryoadenitis. Acute dacryoadenitis is an uncommon inflammation of the lacrimal gland that usually accompanies systemic diseases. Mumps and infectious mononucleosis are the usual systemic causes of an acute inflammation. A purulent infection may be secondary to extension of inflammation from the eyelids or the conjunctiva.

Pain and discomfort in the upper outer portion of the orbit are the chief symptoms. Swelling and redness of the lacrimal gland cause a mechanical blepharoptosis of the upper eyelid and an S-shaped curve of the eyelid margin. Other causes of cellulitis of the skin and orbit must be considered in the differential diagnosis. Eversion of the upper eyelid indicates a swollen, reddened gland.

Treatment is directed to the cause. If a purulent infection is present, antibiotics and local hot compresses, possibly combined with incision and drainage, are indicated. Dacryoadenitis is usually self-limited, and therapy is directed toward preventing the extension of any infection.

Chronic dacryoadenitis. Chronic dacryoadenitis is a proliferative inflammation of the lacrimal gland that occurs in a variety of disorders: sarcoidosis, Sjögren syndrome, leukemia, lymphoma, amyloidosis, tuberculosis, syphilis, posttraumatic and eosinophilic granuloma, and foreign body granuloma. Clinically it is characterized by painless enlargement of the lacrimal glands (Fig. 12-1), most evident when the upper eyelid is everted. Treatment must be directed toward the cause.

Sarcoidosis may cause chronic dacryoadenitis without enlargement of the gland. Dry eyes are the only symptom, but the gland accumulates radioactive gallium and has the histologic changes of sarcoid.

Mikulicz syndrome is the term applied to chronic bilateral swelling of the lacrimal and salivary glands. It may occur in reticuloendothelial disease, leukemias, Hodgkin disease, and sarcoidosis. It is not a specific entity.

TEARING AND DRY EYES

Excessive tear formation (lacrimation) or defective drainage of tears (epiphora) is associated

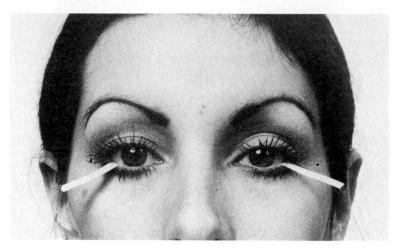

Fig. 12-2. Measurement of the quantity of tears using strips of filter paper hooked over the lateral portion of the lower eyelid.

with blurring of vision and constant discomfort caused by tears running down the cheek. In all instances it is necessary to learn whether there is excessive production or defective drainage of tears.

Measurements of quantity of tears

Tears are measured clinically (Table 12-1) using a 35 × 5.0 mm strip of Whatman 41 filter paper (available commercially as Iso-Sol strips) that is folded 5 mm from one end. The folded end is hooked over the lateral portion of the lower eyelid (Fig. 12-2). The extent to which the filter paper beyond the fold is wet by tears is measured after 5 minutes. The test is conducted in a dimly lit room with the patient facing away from bright light to diminish reflex stimulation.

Measurements of reflex tearing from the orbital and palpebral portion of the lacrimal gland are made without topical anesthesia (Schirmer I). Reflex tear formation is considered normal if 10 mm or more of the paper from the fold is moistened. In the absence of psychic tearing and excessive ocular irritation (the filter paper itself causes some irritation), more than 25 mm of wetting indicates excessive tear formation.

Basic tear secretion from the accessory lacrimal glands of Krause and Wolfring, and from the glands of Manz, Zeis, Moll, tarsal (meibomian), and goblet cells occurs at a constant rate and is not controlled by the nervous system. It is the sole supply of tears during sleep and in the newborn. Basic tear secretion is measured

with filter paper in the same way as reflex secretion, but the conjunctiva and cornea are first anesthetized with a topical anesthetic solution. Basic secretion is considered normal if 8 to 15 mm of the filter paper measured from the fold is moistened.

If the basic test is combined with irritation of the nasal mucosa with a cotton-tipped applicator to stimulate reflex tearing, both basic and reflex reaction is measured (Schirmer II). Less than 15 mm of wetting of the filter paper 2 minutes after hooking over the eyelid indicates failure of reflex tearing.

A drop of 1% bengal rose dye in the conjunctival sac stains dead or damaged conjunctival and corneal cells. Patients with a deficiency of the aqueous portion of tears have punctate staining of the lower two thirds of the cornea and the bulbar conjunctiva stains bright red in the area corresponding to the palpebral apertures.

Lacrimation

Lacrimation, or the overproduction of tears, results from emotional or reflex stimulation of the lacrimal gland, irritation or drying of the cornea and conjunctiva, or stimulation of the retina by excess light (Table 12-2). Excessive tearing may exhaust the lacrimal gland so that the tear tests show normal or decreased tear formation. Abnormal regeneration of the seventh cranial nerve after facial nerve paralysis may result in tearing and salivation during eating (crocodile tears). Hyperthyroidism, tic dou-

Table 12-1. Tests for tear secretion and patency of lacrimal drainage system

Type of test	Procedure
Tear secretion	
Schirmer I	Wetting of Whatman No. 41 filter paper
Basic secretion	Wetting of filter paper after topical anesthesia of eye
Schirmer II	Basic secretion combined with irritation of nasal mucosa membrane
Norn	Fluorescein dilution in cul-de-sac
Lacrimal system abnormality	
Jones I	Appearance of fluorescein* in the nose after its conjunctival instillation
Jones II	Appearance of fluorescein* in the nose after its lacrimal sac irrigation
Dye disappearance	Fluorescein disappearance from cul-de-sac (normal 1 minute)
Dacryocystography	Roentgenography after injection of radiopaque medium into lacrimal sac
Dacryoscintography	Gamma camera tracing of technetium (^{99m}Tc) instilled into cul-de-sac
Saccharine or quinine	Sweet or bitter taste after instillation of solution in conjunctival sac

*Use of cobalt light to excite fluorescence.

Table 12-2. Causes of excessive tear production (lacrimation)

A. Psychic stimulation
B. Parasympathetic stimulation
  1. Cholinergic drugs
  2. Anticholinesterase drugs
C. Lacrimal gland inflammations and neoplasms
D. Trigeminal irritation
  1. Lesions of the eyelids, conjunctiva, cornea, iris
  2. Glaucoma
E. Retinal stimulation by glare and excessive light
F. Facial nerve
  1. Sphenopalatine ganglion stimulation by inflammation and neoplasms
  2. Misdirected regeneration following seventh nerve paralysis (crocodile tears)

Table 12-3. Causes of defective tear drainage (epiphora)

A. Abnomalities of puncta
  1. Ectropion, orbicularis oculi muscle weakness, cicatrization, occlusion, congential absence
B. Lacrimal obstruction
  1. Canaliculi: inflammation, cicatrix, fungi impaction
  2. Lacrimal sac and duct: Congenital abnormalities, inflammation, neoplasms
  3. Meatus: Congenital or acquired stenosis, local nasal disease

loureux, pseudobulbar palsy, and cholinergic stimulation by either parasympathomimetic drugs or anticholinesterases may lead to a pharmacologic type of lacrimation. Often the cause of lacrimation can be easily identified and corrected.

Epiphora

Epiphora is that condition in which drainage of tears through the lacrimal passages is faulty (Table 12-3). It has a variety of causes: entropion or ectropion with faulty apposition of the lacrimal puncta to the lacrimal lake; scarring and occlusion of the puncta; paresis or paralysis of the orbicularis oculi muscle, which eliminates the pumping action of the canaliculi; foreign bodies in the canaliculi; occlusion of the canaliculi; and obstructions in the lacrimal sac and the nasolacrimal duct. The accumulation of tears at the inner canthus causes irritation, which reflexly stimulates additional tear formation.

The adequacy and patency of the lacrimal system may be demonstrated in several ways (Table 12-3). Simple inspection of the eyelids indicates whether the puncta are in contact with the lacrimal lake. Normally, when the eye is rotated upward, the inferior punctum is not visible unless the eyelid is everted. Forcible closure of the eyelids indicates the adequacy of the function of the orbicularis oculi muscle.

Fluorescein tests. Fluorescein solution (2%) instilled in the conjunctival sac is diluted and normally disappears within 1 minute. If the fluorescein can then be demonstrated in the nose or pharynx, the lacrimal passages are patent (Jones test I). A cobalt filter used to excite fluorescence of the fluorescein may enhance the accuracy. Sodium saccharide (10%) instilled in the conjunctival sac may be recognized by its sweet taste if it passes into the posterior pharynx.

If 2% fluorescein instilled in the conjunctival sac cannot be demonstrated in the nose or pharynx, the residual fluorescein is irrigated from the conjunctiva and the lacrimal system is irrigated with normal saline solution. Fluorescein found in the nasopharynx is evidence that it has reached the lacrimal sac and that the obstruction is in the nasolacrimal duct (Jones test II). If fluorescein cannot be demonstrated in the nose or pharynx by irrigation, the functional block is most likely in the canaliculi.

Sodium pertechnetate (^{99m}Tc) in dilute solution may be instilled in each conjunctival sac; a scintigram taken with a gamma camera will indicate its passage through the lacrimal drainage system (Fig. 12-3). This is a physiologic method of demonstrating obstruction, particularly minor blockage by folds of mucous membrane within the lacrimal sac and duct. Injection of a radiopaque compound such as iophendylate (Pantopaque) through the punctum and canaliculus and subsequent roentgenographic study demonstrate the lacrimal system less physiologically than instillation of a radioactive isotope.

Irrigation of the lacrimal system through the punctum demonstrates severe obstructions. If a fold of mucous membrane is the cause of obstruction, the force of irrigation may indicate a lacrimal sac to be patent.

Irrigation of the lacrimal system through the punctum demonstrates severe obstructions. However, when a fold of mucous membrane obstructs, the force of irrigation may indicate a lacrimal sac to be patent.

The management of epiphora depends on its cause. Surgery of the eyelid is indicated when the punctum is not in contact with the lacrimal lake. Obstruction in the lacrimal sac may require repeated probing with successively larger probes or a dacryocystorhinostomy. Atresia of the canaliculi may be difficult to correct. If the lacrimal sac has been obliterated, a glass tube extending from the conjunctival cul-de-sac into the nose or maxillary sinus will provide drainage.

Dry eye

Although a tearing eye may be a nuisance to the patient, it never causes permananet loss of vision. Absence of tears causes keratinization of the corneal and conjunctival epithelium and can result in blindness (Table 12-4). Removal of the lacrimal gland is not associated with drying of the eye, although reflex and psychic tearing is lost. The accessory lacrimal glands maintain normal moistening of the globe in most but not every individual.

Decreased tear secretion is particularly associated with conjunctival scarring that occludes the orifices of the glands that moisten the eye. Decreased tear secretion occurs predominantly in keratoconjunctivitis sicca and may occur in Sjögren syndrome, amyotrophic sclerosis, and some bulbar palsies. There is less than 10 mm of wetting of filter paper (Schirmer I test, see Fig. 12-2) in a 5-minute period even after stimulation of the nasal mucosa. The eyes burn, feel dry, and have a constant foreign body sensation. Symptoms are aggravated by warmth and conditions that cause rapid evaporation of tears. There may be punctate epithelial erosions of the cornea and the conjunctiva, which stain with rose bengal.

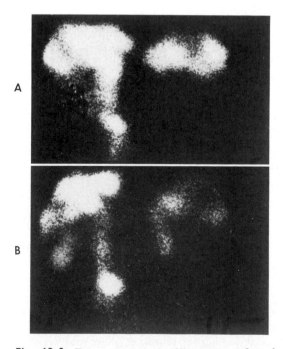

Fig. 12-3. Dacryoscintogram 15 minutes after the instillation of ^{99m}Tc in each cul-de-sac in a 72-year-old man who complained of tearing. **A,** Radioactive marker fills the entire nasal lacrimal excretory system on one side and remains largely in the conjunctival sac and canaliculus on the opposite side. **B,** After 45 minutes, a complete obstruction is demonstrated at about the level of the entrance of the sac to the nasal lacrimal canal. (Courtesy Malcolm Cooper, The University of Chicago.)

Conditions associated with conjunctival scarring include (1) erythema multiforme in its various ocular manifestations of Stevens-Johnson syndrome (Chapter 29), (2) trachoma, (3) ocular cicatricial pemphgoid, and (4) chemical and radiation burns of the conjunctiva. Sjögren syndrome (Chapter 29) is a systemic disease with widespread manifestations, mainly of keratoconjunctivitis sicca, xerostoma, and arthritis with laboratory signs of a severe inflammation.

Deficiency of the mucin layer of tears secreted by goblet cells is measured by the tear film breakup time. A small amount of fluorescein covers the cornea, and the patient is instructed not to blink as the cornea is studied by using a cobalt blue filter with the biomicroscope. In normal eyes, a dry spot appears within 15 to 34 seconds. In mucin-deficient eyes, dry spots appear in less than 10 seconds. Corneal filaments may be present together with cellular debris in the tear film.

The treatment of dry eyes is often unsatisfactory. Patients experiment until they find a method that provides relief. Artificial tears and long-acting inserts are commercially available, and frequent instillation may be required. Obstruction of the superior and inferior puncta to conserve moisture is often effective if tears are entirely absent. Avoidance of hot and dry atmospheres, which encourage tear evaporation, is helpful. Airtight covering of the eyes with

Table 12-4. Dry eyes (keratoconjunctivitis sicca)

I. Conjunctival cicatrization with loss of goblet cells and accessory lacrimal glands
   A. Erythema multiforme (Stevens-Johnson syndrome)
   B. Trachoma
   C. Ocular cicatricial pemphigoid
   D. Cicatricial
   E. Thermal, chemical, and radiation burns
II. Sjögren syndrome
III. Lagophthalmos
IV. Riley-Day syndrome
V. Absence of lacrimal gland
VI. Paralytic
   A. Facial nerve (between facial lacrimal nucleus and geniculate ganglion), greater superficial petrosal nerve, sphenopalatine ganglion
   B. Trigeminal nerve (decrease in reflex lacrimation)
VII. Toxic
   A. Cholinergic blockade (atropine-like drugs)
   B. Deep anesthesia
   C. Debilitating disease

---

diving goggles may help. If parotid gland secretion is not impaired, transplantation of the Stensen duct into the conjunctival sac may provide a generous salivary secretion.

Keratoconjunctivitis sicca. Keratoconjunctivitis sicca is a common symptom complex secondary to an abnormal precorneal tear film. Patients complain of gritty, sandy, foreign body sensations in the eye or irritation and itching, all of which are worsened by a hot, dry atmosphere and tobacco smoke. Symptoms may be aggravated by reading or by infrequent or incomplete blinking. The cornea loses its usual glossy appearance, and mucus floats as strands, sheets, or blobs in the tear film. Filamentary strands of epithelium may adhere to the cornea. The superficial conjunctiva and cornea stain with a 1% bengal rose solution.

When the eye is open some of the tear film evaporates, but in the normal eye blinking causes an exchange in the tear film spread over the exposed cornea and conjunctiva. In keratoconjunctivitis the stability of the precorneal tear film is disturbed, and dry spots form on the corneal epithelium. Mucous plaque may adhere to the corneal epithelium, and filaments may be present. *Staphylococcus* conjunctivitis and blepharitis are common. Four types occur.

1. In the fluid deficiency type, there has been atrophy of the main or accessory lacrimal glands, and the aqueous portion of the tear film is thinned and deficient. This is the classical type seen in Sjögren syndrome. A decreased amount of lacrimal gland tissue occurs in collagen diseases. In the Riley-Day syndrome, there is deficient lacrimal gland innervation that may be pharmacologically induced by ganglionic blockade.

2. Mucin deficiency occurs in conjunctival diseases such as ocular erythema multiforme (Stevens-Johnson syndrome) and ocular cicatricial pemphigoid (Chapter 9). These diseases also cause an eventual loss of the lacrimal aqueous phase as a result of scarring of the secretory ducts. Vitamin A deficiency and chemical burns also cause a loss of mucin. The mucin is secreted by goblet cells and is necessary to wet the hydrophobic corneal epithelium.

3. Elevated lesions of the cornea or conjunctiva may cause the tear film to break up at the apex of the lesion. This may occur in trachoma, herpes simplex, or other diseases

in which the corneal surface is irregular. A similar mechanism may cause the relatively depressed area adjacent to the elevated area to become dry with failure of corneal stroma renewal and the creation of a pit (Ger. *dellen,* pits or depressions).
4. Failure of blinking or infrequent or incomplete blinking may cause inadequate spread of tears with normal components. This occurs in neuroparalytic keratitis, dellen, and pterygium.

DISEASES OF THE LACRIMAL PASSAGES
Canaliculitis

Canaliculitis is an inflammation of the canaliculi that occurs because of infection. Most attention has been directed to inflammation associated with obstruction by *Actinomyces (Streptothrix).* Canaliculitis causes tearing and inflammation of the adjacent conjunctiva. Recovery of the organism from the canaliculus and a gritty foreign body sensation during probing in the canaliculus establish the diagnosis.

Dacryocystitis

Dacryocystitis is an acute or chronic inflammation of the lacrimal sac. The cause is obstruction of the lacrimal sac or the nasolacrimal duct followed by microbial infection.

Acute dacryocystitis. Acute dacryocystitis is a suppurative inflammation of the lacrimal sac with an associated cellulitis of the overlying tissues (Fig. 12-4). The onset is acute, and there are major symptoms of a suppurative infection at the inner canthus. Painful swelling occurs in

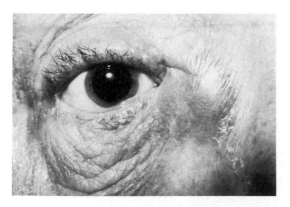

Fig. 12-4. Acute dacryocystitis in a 71-year-old woman.

the tissues overlying the lacrimal sac. Exquisite tenderness in the region is often combined with widespread cellulitis and associated constitutional symptoms. The main differential diagnosis involves other causes of acute suppurative inflammation in the area. Local hot compresses and systemic antibiotics are used in treatment. Incision and drainage are indicated if there is abscess formation.

Chronic dacryocystitis. Chronic dacryocystitis occurs because of obstruction of the nasolacrimal duct, and it is seen most frequently in the newborn period and in middle life. The chief symptoms are epiphora and regurgitation of pus through the puncta when the lacrimal sac is massaged.

Infantile stenosis. Dacryocystitis in infants occurs because of failure of the nasolacrimal duct to open into the inferior meatus, as normally occurs about the third week of life. The initial symptom is constant tearing of one eye. The tearing is distinguished from that in congenital glaucoma by the clear and transparent cornea and the absence of blepharospasm. Tearing is followed by regurgitation of pus through the puncta. Acute dacryocystitis is exceptional.

There is a strong tendency toward spontaneous patency with spontaneous drainage and disappearance of the condition by 6 months of age. Often a topical medication such as sulfacetamide is instilled topically to prevent lacrimal conjunctivitis. While awaiting spontaneous correction, the parents are instructed to massage the lacrimal sac daily to keep it empty of pus.

If the obstruction persists after 6 months of age, lacrimal probing is indicated. The patient is mummified in a blanket, and a local anesthetic is instilled into the conjunctival sac. General anesthesia may be used. A lacrimal probe is inserted into the upper punctum, directed medially and into the lacrimal sac, and then turned at right angles into the nasolacrimal canal and the inferior meatus. The nose is inspected to be certain that the tip of the probe is not covered by mucous membrane. Rarely, more than one probing must be done. In exceptional instances the nasolacrimal duct fails to canalize, and a dacryocystorhinostomy is necessary. Such surgery is wisely deferred until the child is 3 or 4 years of age. Because of the softness of the bone, it is an uncomplicated procedure in the very young.

Adult chronic dacryocystitis. Adult chronic dacryocystitis results from occlusion of the lacrimal sac, which may occur spontaneously or after injury or nasal disease in this region. Spontaneous atresia is more common in women in middle life. An annoying epiphora occurs initially, and, as the occlusion continues, pus regurgitates from the lacrimal sac. If neglected, marked dilation and thinning of its walls occur; this condition is known as mucocele or hydrops of the lacrimal sac. Acute suppuration is unusual. Differential diagnosis involves mainly the various causes of tearing and granulomatous infections of the lacrimal sac.

Surgery is the only satisfactory treatment. When not severe, instillation of zinc and epinephrine collyria may be helpful in the elderly. Probing of the lacrimal passages with probes of successively greater size may be useful, but for the most part relief is transient and the procedure is painful.

The surgical procedure of choice if the canaliculi are patent is a dacryocystorhinostomy, in which a connection is established between the lacrimal sac and the nose. Many procedures has been recommended. If the bony opening into the nose is large enough, most patients improve. Preoperative dacryoscintography is helpful to outline the lacrimal sac and localize the obstruction and rule out the rare neoplasm. Extirpation of the sac (dacryocystectomy) should not be carried out. In elderly patients who require intraocular surgery, the lacrimal sac is removed to eliminate the regurgitation of pus into the conjunctival sac.

Tumors

Tumors of the lacrimal gland may be benign, as occurs in benign lymphoid hyperplasia, chronic dacryoadenitis, and benign mixed cell tumor; or malignant, as in malignant lymphoma, adenoid cystic carcinoma, adenocarcinoma, and malignant degeneration of mixed cell tumor. Rarely, squamous cell carcinoma and its variant, mucoepidermoid carcinoma, occur. Additionally, neoplasms may metastasize to the lacrimal gland or extend to the gland from contiguous structures.

The tumor mass may cause a fullness of the upper outer portion of the eyelid that may simulate the appearance of a blepharoptosis. There may be proptosis with displacement of the eye downward and nasally with diplopia. Eversion of the eyelid may disclose the tumor mass.

Inflammatory, malignant, and lymphomatous tumors usually cause symptoms within 6 months of their onset, whereas benign mixed cell tumors grow slowly and may cause marked displacement of the globe with such gradual (painless) growth that the diplopia is not noted. Inflammatory and lymphomatous tumors do not cause erosion of the bone, whereas malignant tumors cause erosion relatively early and benign mixed cell tumors relatively late or not at all. The benign mixed cell tumor has an onset at about 35 years of age; other tumors have an onset after 50 years of age. An exception is Burkitt's lymphomatous tumor, which affects the orbit in childhood. All of the above mentioned tumors except the benign mixed cell tumor may cause pain.

About one fourth of all lacrimal gland tumors are malignant lymphomas. About 75% of the affected patients have systemic lymphoma, a disease that must be excluded in all patients with lacrimal gland lymphoma. The lacrimal gland tumor is sensitive to radiation, and of those treated, one fourth do not have and never develop systemic lymphoma.

Tumors of the lacrimal gland may be classified as follows:

Benign
    Mixed tumor, 50%
Malignant
    Adenoid cystic carcinoma (cylindroma) de nova, 27%
    Adenoid cystic carcinoma from benign mixed tumor, 3%
    Adenocarcinoma from benign mixed tumor, 9%
    Adenocarcinoma de novo, 7%
    Mucoepidermoid carcinoma, 2%
    Miscellaneous carcinoma, 2%

Benign mixed cell tumor (pleomorphic adenoma) is the most common epithelial tumor of the lacrimal gland. It contains mesenchymal elements (myxoid, chondroid, and osteoid) and doublelayered, tubular epithelial units. It is slowly progressive, predominantly involves men (1.5:1), and begins at a median age of 35 years. There is often a long history (1 to 4 years) of painless fullness of the upper, outer orbit and moderate proptosis with displacement of the globe downward and inward. There may be roentgen-ray evidence of erosion of the bone of the lacrimal fossa. The tumor should be removed through a lateral orbitotomy within its capsule. If there is bony involvement, the bone should be resected. Incisional biopsy results in recurrence.

A malignant mixed cell tumor originates as a benign mixed cell tumor but through seeding at the time of removal or nontreatment undergoes malignant degeneration into an adenocarcinoma or adenoid cystic carcinoma. It has no sex predilection and occurs most commonly after 50 years of age. There is sudden onset of pain, with rapid tumor growth, in a patient with a history of a recurrent benign mixed cell tumor or in a patient with a lacrimal mass present for several years. Erosion of the lacrimal fossa may occur.

The adenoid cystic carcinoma (cylindroma) is the most common malignant epithelial tumor of the lacrimal gland. It is notorious for slow, relentless spread, despite multiple radical excisions. It has the most unfavorable prognosis of all lacrimal gland malignancies. The most common symptom is proptosis with pain, diplopia, decreased visual acuity, blepharoptosis, and lacrimation. Histologically it is composed of aggregates of small undifferentiated neoplastic cells separated by small and large cystoid spaces containing mucosubstance ("Swiss cheese"). The onset is relatively rapid—always less than a year. Unlike patients with benign mixed cell tumor, patients have pain and diplopia. Roentgen-ray studies may show bone erosion.

Adenocarcinoma occurs slightly later in life than other lacrimal tumors, is more prevalent in men, and has a longer duration of symptoms than adenoid cystic carcinoma. It is more likely to metastasize than adenoid cystic carcinoma.

Older patients may develop squamous cell carcinomas, undifferentiated carcinomas, or mucoepidermoid carcinomas. These patients are from 50 to 70 years of age and have histories of recent onset and possible bone destruction. They should be treated as described for lacrimal gland mass of short duration.

Management of tumors of the lacrimal gland is not standardized. Possibly half the tumors are inflammatory or lymphomatous and responsive to corticosteroids or radiation. These tumors do not cause bone erosion. Thus, biopsy to obtain tissue for diagnosis is tempting. Biopsy, though, is associated with a high recurrence rate in benign mixed cell tumors and a low survival rate in malignant tumors. A 2-week trial of corticosteroids may cause 50% or more regressions of a benign lymphomatous hyperplasia and have far less effect on other tumors.

Removal through the intracranial approach is contraindicated because of possible direct seeding of the brain. An en bloc resection including the bony wall of the lacrimal gland fossa unnecessarily disfigures those patients with lymphoid tumors but may decrease the number of recurrences and deaths in those with epithelial tumors.

Tumors of the lacrimal sac are rare and involve its lining, the pseudostratified columnar epithelium. Most neoplasms are squamous cell carcinomas, transitional cell carcinomas, and adenocarcinomas. The initial symptom is tearing, which may be followed by the signs of chronic dacryocystitis with regurgitation of pus and mucus through the punctum. Regurgitation of blood is nearly always caused by a malignant tumor of the lacrimal sac. A painless, nonreducible swelling then occurs in the region of the sac, and eventually there is extension of the tumor outside the lacrimal fossa. Tumors can be demonstrated roentgenographically after injection of contrast media into the lacrimal passages. Squamous cell tumors must be completely excised.

BIBLIOGRAPHY

Benger, R.S., and Frueh, B.R.: Lacrimal drainage obstruction from lacrimal sac infiltration by lymphocytic neoplasia, Am. J. Ophthalmol. **101:**242, 1986.

Lee, D.A., Campbell, R.J., Waller, R.R., and Ilstrup, D.M.: A clinicopathologic study of primary adenoid cystic carcinoma of the lacrimal gland, Ophthalmology **92:**128, 1985.

Lemp, M.A., and Weiler, H.H.: How do tears exit? Invest. Ophthalmol. Vis. Sci. **24:**619, 1983.

Nik, N.A., Hurwitz, J.J., and Sang, H.C.: Mechanism of tear flow after dacryocystorhinostomy and Jones' tube surgery, Arch. Ophthalmol. **102:**1643, 1984.

13

THE ORBIT

The orbit is a pear-shaped cavity with a medial wall that extends directly anterior from its stem, or apex, and a lateral wall that diverges about 45%. The stem contains the annulus of Zinn, which is the circular fibrous origin of the recti muscles. It provides a passage for the blood vessels and nerves. The orbital apex is located almost directly posterior to the medial canthus (not directly posterior to the fovea centralis). The middle portion is expanded to contain the eye. The base forms the thick orbital margins for protection of the eye. Adjacent to the inferior wall of the orbit is the maxillary sinus. Adjacent to the medial wall is the ethmoid sinus. Laterally the temporalis muscle fossa is located anteriorly, whereas the temporal lobe of the brain is adjacent to the posterior part. Superiorly the frontal sinus is located anteriorly, and the frontal lobe of the brain is located posteriorly (Fig. 13-1). The junction of the anterior and middle cranial fossae is located at the apex of the orbits.

Affections of the orbit are a heterogeneous group of abnormalities that originate with a bony cavity, which provides expansion only anteriorly. The orbit contains tissue of neural crest, ectodermal, and mesodermal origin that may be primarily or secondarily affected. Moreover, tissues and tumors from the intracranial cavity or sinuses may herniate through bony defects into the orbit and cause displacement of the eye and impair its motor nerves. The venous drainage of the orbit is into the cavernous sinus, and rupture of an internal carotid artery aneurysm into the cavernous sinus may cause a pulsating protrusion of the globe.

SYMPTOMS AND SIGNS OF ORBITAL DISEASE

Diseases of the orbit often manifest themselves by displacement of the globe, sometimes associated with local pain, redness, and swelling. Proptosis often refers to unilateral displacement of an eye, exophthalmos, and bilateral protrusion of the eyes. Abnormalities at the apex of the orbit may paralyze structures innervated by the motor nerves of the eyes, affect their sensory nerve supply, or cause optic atrophy.

In proptosis or exophthalmos, the palpebral fissure widens, and a rim of sclera is often visible above and below the cornea. In thyroid disease, retraction of the upper eyelid accentuates this appearance. In enophthalmos, the palpebral aperture is more narrow, and a blepharoptosis may seem to be present.

Proptosis of an eye is detected by viewing the eyes over the brow of the patient from above and behind (see Fig. 6-2). Many devices are available to measure the distance between the anterior surface of the cornea and the zygomatic arch on the lateral margin of the orbit (Figs. 13-2 and 13-3). The measurements with the usual exophthalmometers are accurate to within 1 to 2 mm. An exophthalmometer may be improvised by holding a ruler against the zygoma of the maxilla to view the front surface of the cornea.

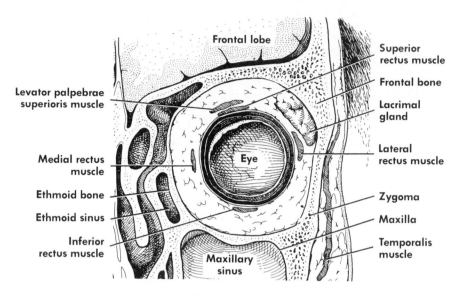

Fig. 13-1. Coronal section of the left orbit about 15 mm from the corneal apex. The frontal sinus is adjacent to the orbit in its anterior portion, whereas the frontal lobe is adjacent to the orbit posteriorly. Laterally the temporalis muscle is adjacent to the orbit anteriorly, whereas the temporal lobe of the brain is located posteriorly. The ethmoid sinus is located medially and the maxillary sinus inferiorly.

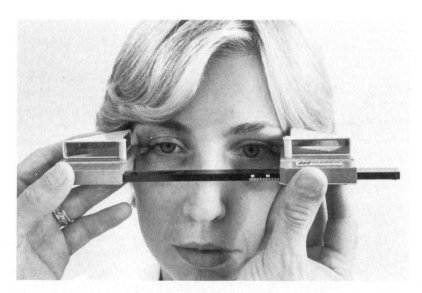

Fig. 13-2. Measurement of exophthalmos using a modified Hertel exophthalmometer. The observer views the position of the eyes in the mirrors. The numbers on the rule refer to the distance separating the two eyepieces and must be the same with repeated measurement.

Orbitonometry measures the backward displacement of the globe under different pressures. This may be estimated by means of palpation or measured by determining how much displacement of the globe occurs when a measured force is applied with a Copper orbitotonometer.

The direction of displacement of the eye may suggest the most likely cause. Exophthalmos of thyroid disease is often symmetrical unless muscle contracture occurs. Tumors within the muscle cone cause a symmetric proptosis in contrast to those outside the muscle cone, which cause the eye to be deviated up or down, in or out, in addition to forward.

Displacement of the globe is often complicated by visual abnormalities, congestion and edema of the eyelids and conjunctiva, occasionally by a bruit in the head, optic disk swelling, visual failure, choroidal folds, and venous congestion.

Displacement of the globe. A relatively small mass in the muscle cone causes early forward displacement of the globe. The nerve supply to the extraocular muscles may be affected, causing a paralytic strabismus (Chapter 21). Masses outside the muscle cone must be larger to displace the globe, and the proptosis is asymmetric. Tumors of the lacrimal gland may not cause proptosis, or they may displace the globe down and in. The lacrimal gland itself may be proptosed when there is a marked increase in the volume of the orbital contents.

Visual abnormalities. Diplopia is often an early sign of proptosis and may occur before development of gross displacement of the globe. Decrease of vision is generally a late sign. It may indicate corneal clouding from exposure, retinal edema, or optic nerve impairment.

Congestion and edema of the eyelids and conjunctiva. Marked congestion of the vessels of the globe suggests an infection, a thyroid abnormality with rapid progression of exophthalmos, or a carotid-cavernous sinus fistula.

Bruit in the head. An abnormal blowing sound heard on auscultation of the head is a classic sign of carotid-cavernous sinus fistula. The patient usually hears noises in the head, such as the sound of running water or the swishing of water. It may be most marked on the side of a carotid-cavernous sinus fistula. The bruit is synchronous with the heart and may disappear when pressure is applied to the carotid artery in the neck. Bruits occur with some orbital and intracranial tumors, and they may be present in normal infants.

Palpable tumors. Tumors located in the anterior half of the orbit may be palpated through the eyelids. Often a lateral canthotomy or a conjunctival incision in the lower outer canthus will permit the surgeon to palpate deep in the orbit. Such an incision should never be used in the upper eyelid because of possible damage to the levator palpebrae superioris muscle, causing blepharoptosis. The tendon of the superior oblique muscle, localized fat in the eyelids, and indurated orbital inflammatory tissue all yield the tactile sensation of a tumor.

Choroidal folds. Orbital tumors, hyperopia, Graves disease, and hypotony may cause folds or striae in the posterior fundus (Fig. 13-4). These appear as alternating bright and dark lines with the peaks being bright and the valleys a darker shade of red. They are more common temporally than nasally and may be associated with congestion of the optic disk. Fluorescein angiography causes the peaks to fluoresce brightly, creating a pattern of alternate bright and dark lines. Vision is unaffected, although there may be a shift of refraction toward hyperopia because the posterior pole of

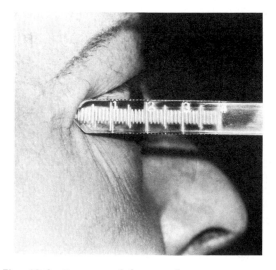

Fig. 13-3. Estimate of degree of proptosis using a transparent exophthalmometer (Luedde). Here the anterior surface of the cornea is 19 mm from the zygoma.

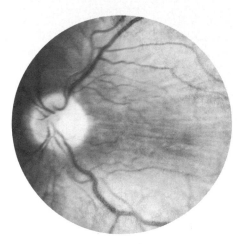

Fig. 13-4. Choroidal folds in a 53-year-old man with a long-standing hemangioma of the orbit.

the eye is displaced forward. With time, the slopes of the folds become pigmented.

Miscellaneous signs. Interference with the venous drainage of the optic nerve may cause a papilledema that may be followed by optic atrophy. Marked congestion of the orbit may severely restrict ocular movements. Prominence of the globe causes increased exposure of the cornea; lacrimation, photophobia, and exposure keratitis may develop.

DIAGNOSIS

An initial decision must be made as to whether ocular proptosis is actually present or whether the appearance is simulated by another condition. Retraction of the upper eyelid causes the eye to appear more prominent, although it is not displaced. Eyelid retraction is a common sign of thyroid disease. A slight blepharoptosis, as occurs in Horner syndrome, may simulate an ocular proptosis of the opposite side. Abnormalities of orbital structure that cause a shallow orbit, as in Crouzon disease, simulate proptosis. Marked enlargement of the eye such as occurs in congenital glaucoma or unilateral severe myopia makes the eye more prominent without displacement.

Physical examination should be directed to possible neoplasms in areas adjacent to the orbit, notably the nasopharynx and the intracranial cavity. Thyroid disease, lymphomatous disease, chronic inflammation of orbital muscles, and benign lymphoid hyperplasia must always

be excluded. A chest roentgenogram is desirable to exclude metastatic malignancy, although a normal chest x-ray does not exclude this possibility. Blood tests should exclude hematopoietic disease and syphilis, and attention should be directed to the causes of chronic granulomas. Removal of a portion or all of a tumor may provide both cure and a diagnosis. Following excisional biopsy, it is desirable to base the decision concerning further therapy on the best possible histologic sections and not on frozen sections. Lacrimal gland tumors (Chapter 12) must be completely resected to avoid seeding.

Computed tomography. Computed tomography has virtually replaced conventional roentgenography in the diagnosis of orbital abnormalities. Better spatial resolution and decreased scanning time of modern equipment make it possible to demonstrate muscle origin and insertions, fascial planes, large blood vessels, and bone detail. The computed tomography image distinguishes fat from solid tissues, and provides visualization of the location of the eye and intraocular portions in relation to other orbital structures.

The breakdown of the blood-tissue barriers makes possible contrast-enhancement, in which neoplastic and inflammatory tissue become more evident after the intravenous injection of an iodine-containing contrast medium.

Roentgenography. Roentgenography sometimes supplements computed tomography. The standard frontal projection allows a composite view of the bones of the orbit to permit comparison of the dimensions and density of the two orbits. The Water position is used for detailed study of the roof of the orbit. Separate oblique views are required for examination of the inner and outer walls. The Caldwell position is used for demonstration of the superior orbital (sphenoidal) fissure. Visualization of the inferior orbital (sphenomaxillary) fissure requires a special posteroanterior projection. This view demonstrates fractures of the floor of the orbit. Polytomography is used to study details too small to be visible on conventional roentgenographic examination and to visualize orbital structures without superimposition of surrounding structures.

Ultrasonography. Sound waves with frequencies of 5,000 to 20,000 kiloherz provide an

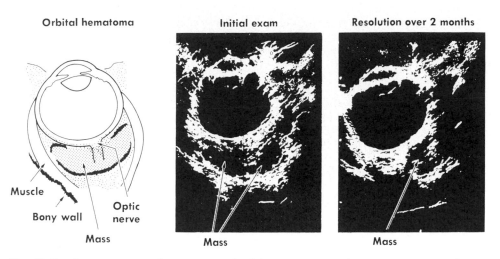

Fig. 13-5. Ultrasonograms of a compact orbital hematoma. By ultrasonic criteria the lesion appears to have many characteristics of a solid tumor. Repeat ultrasonography (right) 2 months after the original shows partial resolution of the lesion. Later it resolved completely without sequelae. More usual ultrasonic findings of orbital hemorrhage resemble those of orbital inflammation and are not confused with tumors. (From Dallow, R.L.: Ultrasonography in the diagnosis of orbital disease. In Brockhurst, R.J., Boruchoff, S.A., Hutchinson, B.T., and Lessell, S., editors: Controversy in ophthalmology, Philadelphia, 1977, W.B. Saunders Co.)

imaging technique used in the diagnosis of both intraocular and orbital tumors. High-frequency sound energy is projected through soft tissue of the orbit, and the sound waves are partially reflected at tissue interfaces of anatomic boundaries. The reflected sound waves (echos) are converted into an electric potential by a piezoelectric crystal and displayed on a cathode ray oscillograph as either spikes (A-scan ultrasonography) or dots (B-scan ultrasonography). Sometimes these systems are displayed simultaneously (Fig. 13-5).

B-scan dots provide a two-dimensional image that demonstrates globe contours, optic nerve, extraocular muscle, and retrobulbar fat. Tumors, swollen muscles, and inflamed tissue are similarly visualized. A-scan ultrasonography provides a spike that corresponds to the position of actual tissue. The amplitude of the echo spikes corresponds to the density of the surface of any reflecting tissues. The grouping of the spikes and their decreasing amplitude as they pass through a tissue mass permits differentiation of tissue into cystic, solid, angiomatous, and infiltrative.

Fine needle aspiration biopsy. Fine needle aspiration biopsy is most useful in establishing the diagnosis in orbital tumors, particularly malignancies. The tip of the aspirating needle may be observed using B-scan ultrasonic imaging as it advances and enters the tumor. A 22- or 23-gauge, 3.8 cm, thin-wall disposable needle is used, attached to a 20 ml syringe, which in turn is attached to a pistol-type syringe holder. After the needle enters the mass, aspiration pressure is applied and the needle angled to different positions in the tumor. Aspirate remaining in the needle may be used for preparation of a paraffin block while the aspirate in the syringe is prepared for microscopic study on slides.

DEVELOPMENTAL ABNORMALITIES

The orbit and its contents may be affected by a number of congenital abnormalities that involve the bones of the orbit, skull, or face (Table 13-1). Often the skull has a characteristic shape or the facial features are typical of the abnormality. There may be an associated exophthalmos from shallow orbits, optic atrophy, papilledema, and strabismus. Exotropia occurs with the orbits widely separated. Esotropia is often associated with poor vision. The neural crest contributes to the brachial arches, and abnormalities occur with a wide variety of hered-

Table 13-1. Developmental anomalies of the skull, face, and orbit

Dysostosis of the skull
  Craniosynostosis
    Oxycephaly (tower skull): Premature union of coronal suture, often with high forehead (dolichocephaly)
    Scaphocephaly (boat skull; long, narrow skull): Premature union of sagittal suture
    Trigonocephaly (egg-shaped skull): Premature closure of frontal suture
    Brachycephaly (short skull, cloverleaf skull): Premature union of all cranial sutures
  Upper face and skull
    Acrocephalosyndactyly (Apert)
    Crouzon
    Hypertelorism (Greig)
Mandibulofacial dysostosis
  First brachial arch
    Maxillary
      Palpebral fissures slant downward and outward
      Malar bone hypoplasia with sunken upper face
    Mandibular
      Receding chin
  Second brachial arch
    N VII
    Middle ear
    Posterior neck musculature
Developmental tumors
  Hemangiomas
  Lymphangiomas
  Dermoid cysts
  Lipomas
  Choristomas
Defects of orbital walls
  Mucocele
  Meningocele
  Encephalocele

itary, chromosomal, and congenital defects. The first brachial arch subdivides into maxillary and mandibular portions. Abnormalities of the maxillary portion result in down and outward-slanting palpebral fissures (antimongoloid) and a sunken upper face with depressed cheek bones. Abnormalities of the mandibular portion result in a receding chin. Abnormalities of the second brachial arch may cause nerve deafness and pterygium colli (a congenital web of skin of the neck).

Craniosynostosis. Craniosynostosis follows premature union of one or more cranial sutures. The closure causes a complete arrest of bone growth at right angles to the closed suture. Compensatory growth of the skull in other diameters causes anomalies in the shape of the skull. The deformity progresses until the brain ceases to grow at about 8 years of age.

Increased cerebrospinal fluid pressure is common and may cause secondary optic atrophy. Primary optic atrophy may occur because of pressure on the optic nerve by downward displacement of the base of the brain or because of compression of the nerve in the optic foramen. The orbit may be unusually shallow because of an abnormal growth of the lesser wing of the sphenoid bone and vertical inclination of the orbital root. Exotropia, or less commonly esotropia, may occur. The strabismus may be secondary to optic atrophy or may be the result of anatomic changes in the orbit.

Increased cerebrospinal fluid pressure, papilledema, and optic atrophy require cranial surgery. Some physicians advocate craniectomy in the early months of life in all instances of craniosynostosis to prevent mental retardation and the cosmetic defect. Others believe that the procedure should be individualized, that a cosmetic defect is not constantly produced, and that mental retardation is not caused by the bony abnormality.

Dysostosis of the upper face and skull

Dysostosis of the upper face and skull often involves widely spaced orbits (hypertelorism) with a resultant increase in interpupillary distance so that convergence is impaired. Most are associated with widespread abnormalities.

Acrocephalosyndactyly (Apert). This is an autosomal dominant disorder. The skull is tall (oxycephaly) and the occiput flat. The eyes are protruberant and widely spaced with the palpebral fissures slanting downward and outward. The maxilla and nasal bridge are underdeveloped. The cerebroventricles are dilated. In type I there is complete syndactyly of the fingers and toes ("mitten hands," "sock feet"); in type II the syndactyly is incomplete.

Medial cleft facial syndrome (hypertelorism of Greig). This is an autosomal dominant disorder characterized by widely spaced eyes, cleft tip of nose and premaxilla, V-shaped frontal hairline, primary telecanthus, and cranion bifidum occultum. There may be associated eyelid defects including epicanthal folds, accessory nasal tissue medially with displacement of the inferior puncti, colobomas of the eyelid, epibulbar dermoid tumors, unilateral microphthalmos, and hereditary vitreoretinal degeneration with retinal separation.

Craniofacial dysostosis (Crouzon). Craniofacial dysostosis is an autosomal dominant condition in which brachycephaly (widened skull) is combined with hypoplasia of the maxillary bones. The forehead is broad, and there is prominence of the anterior forehead region. The eyes are widely separated, and the shallow orbits make them prominent. The nose is broad and hooked, the upper dentition irregular, and the palate high. The earlobes are often large, and atresia of the external auditory canal is common. Optic atrophy may occur. Exposure keratitis may necessitate a lateral blepharoplasty.

Mandibulofacial dysostosis

Mandibulofacial dysostosis abnormalities affect the first and eventually the second brachial arch (see Table 13-1).

Collins-Franceschetti-Klein syndrome. This is an irregular autosomal dominant abnormality of the facial bones with hypoplasia of the zygomas and mandible. The palpebral fissure slants outward and downward. There may be colobomas of the lower eyelids, absence of eyelashes on the inner one third of the lower eyelid, and absence of lower lacrimal puncta. The external ears may be abnormally small (microtia), and there may be atresia of the external auditory canal. Atrophy of the mandible causes a prognathism of the upper jaw and an open bite. Associated skeletal abnormalities are common, and dermolipomas of the conjunctiva occur.

Dyscephalic syndrome (Hallerman-Streiff-François). This is a congenital disorder (probably) in which a large nose that resembles a parrot beak is combined with a receding chin to give a "bird face." Teeth are absent or malformed. Stature is small. Bilateral cataract and microphthalmia are present. The palpebral fissures slant downward and outward, and neural crest anomalies of the anterior ocular segment may be present (Chapter 10).

ORBITAL INFLAMMATION
Acute inflammation

Acute orbital inflammation (Table 13-2) is most commonly caused by direct bacterial spread from the ethmoid or maxillary sinus, by

Table 13-2. Orbital tumors

A. Primary
 1. Bone
   a. Chondrosarcoma
   b. Osteosarcoma
 2. Muscle
   a. Rhabdomyosarcoma
 3. Optic nerve
   a. Meningioma
   b. Glioma
 4. Lacrimal gland
   a. Benign: mixed, adenoma, cyst
   b. Malignant: mixed, adenocarcinoma, mucoepidermoid, squamous cell
 5. Connective tissue
   a. Fibroma
   b. Neurofibromatosis
B. Direct extension
 1. Eyelids
   a. Squamous cell, basal cell
 2. Eye
   a. Malignant melanoma
   b. Retinoblastoma
 3. Intracranial cavity
   a. Meningioma
 4. Nasal accessory sinuses
   a. Osteoma
   b. Chondrosarcoma
   c. Malignancies
C. Metastatic
 1. Sympathicoblastoma (neuroblastoma)
 2. Chloroma (in myeloblastic leukemia)
 3. Lymphoma (in lymphatic leukemia)
 4. Nephroblastoma
 5. Carcinoma: breast, uterus, thyroid, prostate, lung
D. Inflammatory: walls or contents
 1. Cellulitis: anterior; posterior
 2. Abscess
 3. Periostitis
 4. Chronic granuloma (pseudotumor)
 5. Gumma
 6. Tuberculoma
 7. Sarcoid granuloma

pyogenic thrombophlebitis from a focus in the skin of the eyelids in regions drained by orbital veins, or by a penetrating orbital trauma. The orbital septum, the dense fascia that separates the anterior eyelids from the orbital contents, prevents anterior inflammations, mainly periorbital cellulitis, from extending into the orbit proper. Acute intraorbital inflammations are far more serious than preseptal periorbital cellulitis and may involve both the anterior and posterior orbital contents.

Preseptal cellulitis has a sudden onset with swelling, redness, and increased warmth of the eyelids. There is conjunctival edema, leukocytosis, and sometimes fever. A fluctant mass signifies abscess formation. Preseptal inflammations are most common in patients less than 5 years of age.

Orbital cellulitis may have the same signs and symptoms as preseptal cellulitis, but they are more severe. Additionally, proptosis, anesthesia of the area innervated by the ophthalmic and maxillary branches of the trigeminal nerve, impaired ocular rotations, ocular pain aggravated by ocular rotation, and increased intraocular pressure occur. Increased severity of signs and symptoms, decreased visual acuity, afferent pupillary defect, venous congestion, and papilledema indicate abscess formation. Orbital cellulitis is dangerous to life, particularly in boys' second decade of life.

Management of both preseptal and orbital cellulitis requires a complete general and ocular examination. A complete and differential blood cell count as well as Gram stain and culture of secretions from the conjunctiva, nasopharynx, and any lacerations, abscesses, or fistulas are indicated. If meningeal signs are present, the cerebrospinal fluid is cultured. Initial treatment consists of appropriate intravenous antibiotics based on the results of Gram stain and culture. Abscess drainage with sinus drainage, sinus drainage solely, or incision and drainage of eyelid abscesses may be necessary. Cavernous sinus thrombosis, meningitis, brain abscess, optic nerve atrophy, and death may occur in neglected cases.

Cavernous sinus thrombosis. This is an acute thrombophlebitis that originates from a purulent infection of the face, sinus, ear, or other area that drains through veins to the cavernous sinus. Ophthalmoplegia occurs; the lateral rectus muscle is usually the first muscle involved. Involvement of the ophthalmic division of the trigeminal nerve causes severe pain. There may be papilledema, visual failure, and other signs of involvement of the nerves passing through the optic foramen and superior orbital fissure. The disease requires intensive antibiotic chemotherapy combined with anticoagulation.

Idiopathic orbital inflammation (pseudotumor)

This acute, nonmicrobial inflammation affects middle-aged men predominantly. The onset is acute, and there is a rapid development of proptosis, extraocular muscle weakness, decreased vision, pain, and erythema and swelling of the eyelids. At times the inflammatory signs may be sufficiently prominent to suggest an orbital cellulitis. Computed tomography demonstrates inflammation of extraocular muscles, orbital fat, and perineural connective tissue. Most pseudotumors are nonspecific reactions composed of perivascular lymphocytes, plasma cells, and some polymorphonuclear leukocytes. In children there may be a large eosinophilic component often correlated with a peripheral blood eosinophilia. In long-term cases, collagen is deposited in the orbital fat, within the extraocular muscles around the optic nerve, and within the lacrimal gland.

The main treatment consists of systemic administration of corticosteroids, often combined with retrobulbar corticosteroids. Resolution is often prompt, but proptosis persists in nonresponsive patients. The treatment is unsatisfactory, but often there is spontaneous remission. Excision is always incomplete and is usually followed by recurrence. A variety of surgical procedures may be used to protect the cornea from exposure, thus preventing keratitis e lagophthalmos. The fellow orbit becomes involved in about 25% of the cases.

Reactive lymphoid hyperplasia (pseudolymphoma) causes a slowly progressive, painless tumor of the orbit, lacrimal gland, conjunctiva, and rarely, the uvea. Histologically, mature lymphocytes arranged in accumulations of sheaths are found. Subconjunctival tumors occur in the fornices and are a salmon color. Orbital involvement occurs in middle-aged persons and causes a progressive proptosis. The majority of cells are T lymphocytes and the remainder polyclonal B lymphocytes. Malignant lymphomas are composed predominantly of monoclonal B lymphocytes. Radiotherapy is the preferred therapy for reactive lymphoid hyperplasia.

Burkitt lymphoma is the only lymphosarcoma that affects children. It probably originates in the abdomen and metastasizes to the facial bones and then encroaches on the orbit. Hepatosplenomegaly and central nervous system involvement occur. Chemotherapy is curative if done before central nervous system involvement.

TUMORS AND RELATED CONDITIONS

A large variety of new growths, inflammations, congenital abnormalities, and systemic diseases may reflect themselves by orbital involvement. Diagnosis is complicated by the frequency with which ocular manifestations of thyroid gland abnormalities and idiopathic orbital inflammation exhibit similar symptoms and signs. The medical history is helpful. A sudden onset and a rapid progression suggest an inflammatory process rather than a neoplasm. Orbital pain results commonly from inflammation. A history of hyperthyroidism suggests a thyroid abnormality even though the patient may be euthyroid or hypothyroid. A complaint of noise in the head is suggestive of a carotid-cavernous sinus fistula. Intermittent proptosis may be caused by varices of the orbit, and congestion is aggravated by increased venous pressure brought about by coughing or bending over.

The most common causes of proptosis of the adult orbit are thyroid disease, lymphomatous disease, idiopathic orbital inflammation, hemangioma, and mucocele of the frontal sinus (Table 13-3). There is considerable variation in the orbital diseases encountered in different institutions; this most likely reflects the interests of the staff and the type of patient referred for care.

Neuroblastomas in infants and children metastasize (20%) to the orbit. They sometimes occur together with periorbital ecchymosis. Neuroblastoma may also cause Horner syndrome. There may be opsoclonus-myoclonus ("dancing eyes").

Gliomas of the optic nerve may occur as an isolated tumor or in association with neurofibromatosis. Rhabdomyosarcoma occurs more frequently in the orbit than elsewhere in the body and is the most common primary orbital malignancy in children.

Superior orbital fissure syndrome. The superior orbital fissure syndrome is characterized by local pain, proptosis, and paralysis of cranial nerves III, IV, and VI. Usually there is loss of sensation in the area of distribution of only the ophthalmic division of the trigeminal nerve (N V). Proptosis and loss of corneal sensation distinguish the syndrome from cavernous sinus tumor. Blepharoptosis is present, and the eye is usually turned down and out. The most com-

Table 13-3. Systemic disorders affecting the orbit

A. Thyroid disease
B. Osteitis deformans (Paget disease), osteosarcoma following osteitis deformans
C. Histiocytosis
   1. Juvenile xanthogranuloma
   2. Eosinophilic granuloma
   3. Hand-Schüller-Christian disease
   4. Letterer-Siwe disease
D. Hematopoietic system
   1. Lymphoma
      a. Malignant lymphoma, lymphocytic type (nodular or diffuse)
         (1) Well differentiated
         (2) Poorly differentiated
      b. Malignant lymphoma, histiocytic type (diffuse)
      c. Malignant lymphoma, mixed (nodular)
      d. Hodgkin type
   2. Plasma cell
      a. Primary
      b. Metastatic
   3. Granulocytic sarcoma (chloroma)
E. Vascular abnormalities
   1. Carotid-cavernous sinus fistula
   2. Cavernous sinus thrombosis
   3. Orbital aneurysm
   4. Hemorrhage
   5. Angioneurotic edema

mon cause is a neoplasm that involves the apex of the orbit, but in many instances a pseudotumor may be responsible.

INJURIES

Blunt trauma to the orbit may cause severe intraorbital hemorrhage that suffuses readily beneath the conjunctiva and under the eyelids and may limit ocular movements markedly. Severe hemorrhage may also be a sign of fracture of the wall of the orbit and may be associated with serious brain damage. Penetrating injuries of the orbit may perforate its thin posterior walls to enter the brain or the sinuses. The most common fracture of the orbit is the result of a marked increase in intraorbital pressure that causes a blowout of the floor (see Chapter 7). The most common fracture of the orbital rim involves its medial margin and the nose and is particularly likely to occur as a result of automobile accidents. Fractures of the superior margin of the orbit may damage the trochlea and may cause the symptoms of a superior oblique muscle paralysis. Fractures of the lateral margin are fairly common and result in loss of the cheekbone. Early elevation of the zygomatic arch can prevent the need for much corrective surgery. Fractures of the inferior margin are frequently comminuted and associated with fractures of other facial bones. The medial wall of the orbit may be ruptured, and emphysema of the orbital or eyelid tissues occurs. This may be recognized by the peculiar crepitation with palpation.

SURGERY OF THE ORBIT

Procedures involving the orbit include decompression to permit expansion of orbital contents that cannot be removed, excision of orbital tumors, exenteration of all orbital contents, enucleation of the eye, and correction of bony defects.

Orbital decompression is mainly indicated in thyroid disease in which expansion of the orbital contents causes so much proptosis that the cornea is no longer protected by the eyelids. Provision of an additional opening allows the orbital contents to expand without pushing the eye forward. Decompression is often combined with procedures designed to decrease the width of the palpebral fissure by suturing the tissues of the upper eyelid to the lower eyelid (lateral blepharoplasty).

Tumors of the orbit may be approached from the orbit's anterior margin or its lateral or superior wall. The anterior approach is made through an eyebrow incision and is used solely for palpable tumors. The lateral approach is used for benign tumors of the posterior orbit. A combined anterior-lateral approach is used for malignant lacrimal gland tumors. The superior approach requires a craniotomy and is indicated mainly in tumors such as meningioma or glioma that involve both the orbital and cranial cavities. In desperate situations the cornea may be protected by adhesions between the upper and lower eyelids (blepharoplasty) or protected with a conjunctival flap.

Exenteration of the orbital contents is a mutilating procedure indicated mainly for malignancies of the lacrimal gland, for extension of eyelid malignancies into the orbit, for malignant melanoma of the conjunctiva, for malignant melanoma or retinoblastoma that has burst through the globe and caused marked orbital involvement, and for primary intraorbital malignancies such as rhabdomyosarcoma. The procedure may be lifesaving in lacrimal gland tumors in which areas of bony involvement must be removed. This usually necessitates exposing the dura mater. In malignancies that have extended into adjacent nasal sinuses and the intracranial cavity, the procedure is mainly palliative.

Removal of the eye. Enucleation of the eye is indicated in a blind and painful eye, in malignancies of the eye, in severe injuries of the globe when restoration of a functional eye is not possible, and in early sympathetic ophthalmia. The conjunctiva is opened as close to the corneoscleral limbus as possible and each muscle separated from the globe at its insertion. The optic nerve is then severed as far behind the globe as possible.

A number of ingenious procedures have been proposed to provide motility to the ocular prosthesis after enucleation. In general, however, they do not work well. Nonetheless, with careful matching of the normal eye the cosmetic defect is minimal. The artificial eye should be removed only once or twice a month, and every precaution should be taken to prevent contamination.

Loss of an eye does not cause a 50% loss of visual efficiency (one may estimate the loss by covering one's own eye) but may be accompanied by severe emotional problems.

Bony defects of the orbit. These may be repaired by means of Silastic implants or bone taken from the iliac ridge. Commonly the surgery is indicated because of incarceration of an ocular muscle in an orbital fracture and considerable judgment is essential so as not to overcorrect the defect.

BIBLIOGRAPHY
General

Gorman, C.A., Dyer, J.A., and Waller, R.R.: The eye and orbit in thyroid disease, New York, 1984, Raven Press.

Diagnosis

Augsburger, J.J., Shields, J.A., Folberg, R., Lang, W., O'Hara, B.J., and Claricci, J.D.: Fine needle aspiration biopsy in the diagnosis of intraocular cancer, Ophthalmology **92:**39, 1985.

Byrne, S.F.: Standardized echography in the differentiation or orbital lesions, Surv. Ophthalmol. **29:**226, 1984.

Kennerdell, J.S., Slamovits, T.L., Dekker, A., and Johnson, B.L.: Orbital fine-needle aspiration biopsy, Am. J. Ophthalmol. **99**:547, 1985.

Kincaid, M.C., and Green, W.R.: Diagnostic methods in orbital diseases, Ophthalmology **91**:719, 1984.

Newell, F.W.: Fundus changes in persistent and recurrent choroidal folds, Br. J. Ophthalmol. **68**:32, 1984.

Norris, J.L., and Stewart, W.B.: Bimanual endoscopic orbital biopsy: an emerging technique, Ophthalmology **92**:34, 1985.

Yeo, J.H., Jakobiec, F.A., Abbott, G.F., and Trokel, S.L.: Combined clinical and computed tomographic diagnosis of orbital lymphoid tumors, Am. J. Ophthalmol. **94**:235, 1982.

Developmental

Diamond, G.R., Katowitz, J.A., Whitaker, L.A., Quinn, G.E., and Schaffer, D.B.: Variations in extraocular muscle number and structure in craniofacial dysostosis, Am. J. Ophthalmol. **90**:416, 1980.

Judisch, G.F., Kraft, S.P., Barley, J.A., and Jacoby, C.G.: Orbital hypotelorism, Arch. Ophthalmol. **102**:995, 1984.

Inflammation

Newell, F.W., and Leveille, A.S.: Management and complications of bacterial periorbital and orbital cellulitis, Metab. Pediatr. Syst. Ophthalmol. **6**:209, 1982.

Rootman, J., and Nugent, R.: The classification and management of acute orbital pseudotumors, Ophthalmology **89**:1040, 1982.

Tumors

Henderson, J.W.: Orbital tumors, ed. 2, Philadelphia, 1973, W.B. Saunders Co.

Hornblass, A.: Tumors of the ocular adnexa and orbit, St. Louis, 1979, The C.V. Mosby Co.

Musarella, M.A., Chan, H.S.L., DeBoer, G., and Gallie, B.L.: Ocular involvement in neuroblastoma: prognostic implications, Ophthalmology **91**:936, 1984.

Seeger, R.C., Brodeur, G.M., Sather, H., Dalton, A., Siegel, S.E., Wong, K.Y., and Hammond, D.: Association of multiple copies of the N-*myc* oncogene with rapid progression of neuroblastomas, N. Engl. J. Med. **313**:1111, 1985.

Surgery

McCord, C.D., Jr.: Current trends in orbital decompression, Ophthalmology **92**:21, 1985.

Soll, D.B.: The anophthalmic socket, Ophthalmology **89**:407, 1982.

14

THE PUPIL

The pupil is the central opening of the iris. It regulates the amount of light entering the eye by constricting (miosis) in bright illumination and dilating (mydriasis) in the dark. Pupillary size is controlled by the opposed actions of two nonstriated muscles, both derived from the neuroectoderm of the secondary optic vesicle: the sphincter pupillae (N III parasympathetics) and the dilatator pupillae (sympathetics). The two layers of secondary optic vesicle fuse to form the pigment layer of the iris, and its most anterior portion at the pupillary margin may form a pigmented pupillary frill, conspicuous in ectropion uveae.

Normal pupils are round, regular in shape, and nearly equal in size. There may rarely be a physiologic difference in pupil size (physiologic anisocoria). Each pupil is located with its center a little below and slightly to the nasal side of the cornea. The pupils are constricted in infancy and in old age and are at their maximal size during childhood and adolescence.

The pupils are dilated (mydriasis) in excitement and in the dark. They are constricted (miosis) in sleep, in light, and with ocular convergence (not accommodation). Pupils are constricted in neonates, reach their maximal diameter at about 21 years of age, and constrict thereafter to become small in old age (involutional miosis). Pupils are considered miotic if they are less than 2 mm in diameter and mydriatic if they are more than 6 mm in diameter.

The sphincter pupillae muscle is a typical annular sphincter muscle located next to the pu-

pillary margin deep in the iris stroma. It is innervated by efferent visceral fibers that originate in the Edinger-Westphal portion of the oculomotor nucleus (N III). Preganglionic fibers enter the orbit with the inferior branch of the oculomotor nerve. A short motor branch is sent to the ciliary ganglion, where synapse is made with postganglionic fibers. Three to six postganglionic nerves extend forward from the ganglion. They divide into 6 to 20 short ciliary nerves that penetrate the sclera around the optic nerve and pass forward in the suprachoroidal space; about 97% of the fibers are distributed to the ciliary muscle (accommodation) and the remainder to the sphincter pupillae muscle (miosis).

The dilatator pupillae muscle is arranged radially deep in the iris stroma. It extends from the outer edge of the sphincter muscle to the root of the iris and contains pigment. It is innervated by sympathetic fibers that originate in the hypothalamus. From here the fibers descend in the lateral columns of the cervical cord and emerge with the eighth cervical and first thoracic ventral nerve roots. The fibers then ascend the sympathetic chain to the superior cervical ganglion, where they synapse. Postganglionic fibers extend cranially along the internal carotid artery and reach the dilator pupillae muscle mainly with the two long ciliary nerve branches of the nasociliary branch of the fifth (trigeminal) cranial nerve. Some sympathetic fibers that pass through but do not synapse in the ciliary ganglion are mainly va-

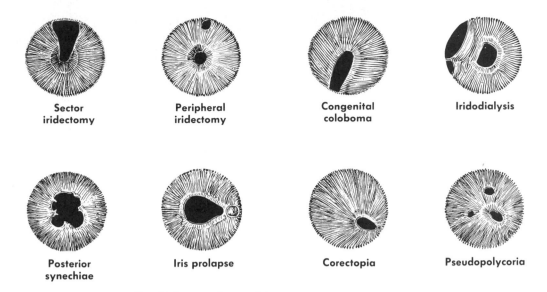

Sector
iridectomy

Peripheral
iridectomy

Congenital
coloboma

Iridodialysis

Posterior
synechiae

Iris prolapse

Corectopia

Pseudopolycoria

Fig. 14-1. Irregularity of the pupil in various disorders.

somotor to choroidal arterioles and do not innervate the dilatator pupillae muscle.

Since the sphincter pupillae muscle and the dilatator pupillae muscle are integral parts of the iris, their function may be altered in iris inflammations, degenerations, and congenital abnormalities. Additionally, the pupil provides passage between the posterior and anterior chambers for aqueous humor. If the aqueous humor is prevented from passing through the pupil (pupillary block or iris bombé), glaucoma occurs.

Abnormalities of the pupil may be the result of local disease or injury to the iris, or reflect an abnormality of the afferent or efferent innervation. Dyscoria refers to abnormalities in the shape of the pupil. Corectopia refers to displacement of the pupil from its normal position. Polycoria describes additional openings in the iris (Fig. 14-1). Miosis is the condition of excessive constriction of the pupil, generally to a diameter of less than 2 mm. Mydriasis is the condition of excessive dilation of the pupil, generally to a diameter of more than 6 mm. In anisocoria the pupils are of different size. Usually if the anisocoria is most marked in bright light, the size of the larger pupil is abnormal. If the inequality is most marked in dim illumination, the size of the smaller pupil is abnormal. Iridoplegia is failure of the pupil to constrict to light or to a near stimulus.

SYMPTOMS OF PUPILLARY ABNORMALITIES

The chief symptoms resulting from abnormalities of the pupil relate to its function as a diaphragm in controlling the amount of light that enters the eye. When the pupil is dilated, approximately 50 times as much energy enters the eye as when it is constricted. Dilation and constriction occur constantly in the normal eye in response to the amount of light stimulating the retina.

A convex lens provides magnification to observe minimal pupillary reflexes, which may be difficult to evaluate when the pupils are constricted.

A dilated pupil causes more chromatic and spherical aberration and less depth of focus, as is true of a camera with the diaphragm opened widely (The normal eye is about f 5.6.)

A marked constriction of the pupil interferes with vision in dim illumination because of failure of the pupil to dilate in response to the reduced lighting. The visual loss caused by minor opacities of the lens may be severely aggravated by pupillary constriction, which is often a serious problem in the treatment of glaucoma.

Openings in the iris in addition to the pupil may cause monocular double vision (diplopia). Surgical iridectomies are usually located near the 12 o'clock meridian; they are covered by the upper eyelid and cause no symptoms. In conditions such as polycoria (multiple pupils) or iridodialysis, which is a separation of the base of the iris from the ciliary body (see Fig. 14-1), diplopia may be an annoying symptom.

PUPILLARY REFLEXES

Pupils should be examined in a dimly illuminated room that is bright enough to observe the pupils. Attention should be directed to any difference in size (anisocoria), shape (dyscoria), or position (corectopia) of the pupils.

To test the pupillary reflexes a flashlight with fresh batteries should be used. The patient is directed to look in the distance to avoid near stimulation. The light is directed into the eye from below to avoid corneal reflections and the shadow of the nose. Each eye should be stimulated for an equal period of time. Attention is directed to the initial constriction of the pupil and to any dilation of the pupil that is not present in the fellow eye as the light stimulus continues. When initial constriction is the end point, each eye should be stimulated for about 1 second. When pupillary dilation with continued light stimulation is the end point, each eye should be stimulated for 3 seconds with nearly instantaneous alternation between the two eyes. An asymmetry of the pupillary response provides significant information that may be approximately quantitated by the use of a 0.3 log neutral density filter to reduce the intensity of the light stimulus.

When light is directed into one eye, the pupil constricts (direct light reflex), and normally the opposite pupil simultaneously constricts a similar amount (consensual light reflex). The receptors for the light reflex are the retinal rods and cones. The afferent axons responsible for conduction of the impulse are separate from the visual fibers but follow the same course in the optic nerve and chiasm; they separate from visual fibers at the level of the lateral geniculate body and do not synapse but pass through the brachium of the superior colliculus and synapse in the pretectal region. Here the fibers pass with partial decussation to the Edinger-Westphal portion of the oculomotor nucleus (N III). Visceral motor efferent fibers pass from the nucleus in the oculomotor nerve to synapse in the ciliary ganglion. Postganglionic fibers reach the sphincter pupillae muscle by the short ciliary nerves (see Fig. 2-24).

Synkinetic, or associated, constriction of the pupil occurs with convergence (not accommodation). It is not a reflex but an associated reaction that occurs because of the common innervation of the medial rectus muscle active in convergence and the sphincter pupillae muscle. A less commonly observed synkinetic reaction is the pupillary constriction that may follow contraction of the orbicularis oculi muscle innervated by nerve VII.

Hippus, a rhythmic dilation and contraction of the pupils (physiologic pupillary unrest), cannot be reliably associated with any nervous disorder.

In unilateral defects of the afferent branch of the light reflex arc, the pupils are of the same size because of the consensual reflex originating from the normal fellow eye. In unilateral defects of the parasympathetic efferent arc, the affected pupil is larger than the normal fellow eye. In unilateral defects of the sympathetic arc, the affected pupil is smaller than the normal fellow eye.

In patients who have a hemianopsia caused by lesions in nerve fibers posterior to the lateral geniculate body, the pupillary reaction to light is intact, since the afferent pupillary fibers are not affected. Thus a patient may be blind from lesions posterior to the lateral geniculate body and the pupillary reactions will be normal.

In patients who have a hemianopsia caused by an optic tract lesion, light stimulation of the portion of the retina corresponding to field defect causes a diminished or absent direct light reflex. This is called the hemianopic pupillary reflex. Detection requires a small bundle of light rays so that the uninvolved side is not stimulated by scattered light within the eye. Mainly retinal lesions affect the pupillary response only when extensive. Optic nerve disease causes an afferent pupillary defect (Chapter 18).

CONGENITAL ABNORMALITIES

Since the pupil is an opening in the iris, it is evident that developmental pupillary abnormalities result because of abnormalities of the iris or the innervation of its muscles. The most striking change, however, may be the alteration in the appearance of the pupil. In aniridia (Chapter 15) the iris is rudimentary and the eye appears to be jet black with no iris present.

A coloboma of the iris (see Figs. 14-1 and 15-3) may be associated with faulty closure of the retinal fissure and typical defects in the optic nerve and choroid. More common is simple coloboma of the iris, in which one or more layers of the iris are absent in a localized area, either extending as far as the ciliary body (total) or involving only a portion of a sector (partial). The pupil is pear shaped because of the absence of iris, but the usual layers are retained in the normal sector, and thus the iris shows normal reflexes. Colobomas may be completely surrounded by iris tissue (Fig. 14-1) and appear as additional pupils (pseudopolycoria). True polycoria, with multiple pupils each having a sphincter muscle, is extremely rare. The condition of multiple pupils is called pseudopolycoria. The openings lack a sphincter and do not react to light. Conspicuous displacement of the pupil from its normal position is corectopia, or ectopic pupil. Relatively minor displacement is common and causes no symptoms. When severe, the eyes are generally myopic and vision is poor. Severe displacement is often accompanied by subluxation of the lens in the direction opposite the corectopia. Severe corectopia is often an autosomal dominant defect. Rarely, a congenital absence of the dilatator pupillae muscle causes a miosis as a result of unopposed action of the sphincter pupillae muscle.

Small clusters of black pigment may occur at the pupillary margin. They originate from the pigment epithelium of the iris and may be caused by instillation of miotics in children who have accommodative esotropia.

Persistent pupillary fibers. The anterior portion of the tunica vasculosa lentis, which nourishes the lens during embryonic life, is derived from anterior ciliary vessels. These nutritional vessels atrophy about the eighth month and recede to the collarette of the pupil. Occasionally, delicate strands of fibers remain and extend from the collarette to the anterior lens capsule. Rarely they are sturdy and pigmented, but they do not interfere with vision.

MIOSIS AND MYDRIASIS
Miosis

Constriction of the pupil to less than 2.0 mm is called miosis. The pupil is abnormal if it does not dilate in darkness. The most common cause of the condition is the instillation of cholinergic-stimulating drugs, which contract the sphincter pupillae muscle, in the treatment of glaucoma. Accidental or systemic administration of these compounds may cause miosis, depending on the dose. Morphine causes extreme constriction of the pupil. During sleep the pupils constrict, and the miosis may distinguish true sleep from simulated sleep (as does involuntary fluttering of the eyelids in simulated sleep). With aging, the pupils become smaller (involutional miosis), but normal reflexes are retained. Bilateral adhesion of the iris to the lens (posterior synechiae) may cause small, irregular pupils. Congenital absence of the dilatator pupillae muscle results in miosis because of unopposed action of the sphincter pupillae muscle.

Irritation of the conjunctiva, cornea, or iris may cause miosis. Irritative lesions of the efferent parasympathetic pathway, as in meningitis, encephalitis, cavernous sinus thrombosis, lesions within the superior orbital fissure or orbit, may result in miosis.

Mydriasis

Dilation of both pupils to more than 6.0 mm combined with failure to constrict when stimulated with light occurs after local instillation of drugs that paralyze the sphincter pupillae muscle (Table 14-1). Pupils dilated with drugs such as atropine do not constrict promptly when 1% pilocarpine solution is instilled. Pupils that are dilated as a result of interference with the nerves involved in the reflex arc constrict promptly after instillation of pilocarpine. Usually, systemic administration of cholinergic blocking compounds has a minimal pupillary effect. In bilateral blindness caused by lesions anterior to the lateral geniculate body, the pupils are dilated and do not constrict when stimulated with light.

In their course from the Edinger-Westphal nuclei in the midbrain to the eye, paralytic lesions of the parasympathetic efferent pathway of pupillary motor fibers may result in mydriasis. Blunt ocular trauma may rupture the sphincter pupillae muscle causing mydriasis (traumatic iridoplegia). Increased cerebrospinal pressure, intracranial neoplasms, and aneurysms each may cause mydriasis.

During general anesthesia, the pupils are usually dilated in stages I and II because of excitement, alarm, or adrenergic stimuli. During stage III, the pupils reflect the miosis of coma.

Table 14-1. Possible causes of a dilated pupil that does not constrict to light

I. Iris involvement*
  A. Inflammatory disease, posterior synechiae
  B. Ischemic sphincter muscle with acute increase in intraocular pressure
  C. Contusion injury to sphincter (traumatic iridoplegia)
  D. Cholinergic blockage of sphincter (atropine and related compounds)
II. Ciliary ganglion or short ciliary nerves†
  A. Adie syndrome
  B. Ciliary ganglion inflammation (zoster, viral ganglionitis)
  C. Orbital or choroidal trauma or tumor
III. Preganglionic N III†
  A. Aneurysm of circle of Willis
  B. Herniation of the uncus of the temporal lobe
  C. Parasellar tumors (pituitary adenoma, meningioma, craniopharyngioma, nasopharyngeal carcinoma)
  D. Parasellar inflammation (Tolosa-Hunt syndrome, zoster, giant cell arteritis)
IV. Edinger-Westphal nucleus†
  A. Dorsal: uncommon, bilateral, near-vision reaction retained, supranuclear vertical gaze palsy present
  B. Ventral: associated neurologic defects (Nothnagel, Benedikt, Weber syndromes) and paralysis of ocular muscles, innervated N III

*Pupil does not constrict with topical 1% pilocarpine.
†Pupil constricts with topical 1% pilocarpine.

Table 14-2. Some causes of inequality of pupil size (anisocoria)

I. Local ocular causes
  A. Drugs topically instilled: mydriasis or miosis
  B. Injury
    1. Rupture of iris sphincter with contusion (traumatic iridoplegia)
    2. Adhesions between iris and cornea following laceration (adherent leukoma or anterior synechiae)
  C. Inflammation
    1. Keratitis (miosis)
    2. Acute iridocyclitis (middilation)
    3. Adhesions between iris and lens (posterior synechiae)
  D. Closed-angle glaucoma (middilation)
  E. Ischemia of iris
    1. Ocular surgery
    2. Internal carotid artery insufficiency (dilation)
  F. Diseases of iris
    1. Iridocorneal syndromes
    2. Aniridia
    3. Congenital variation
II. Paralysis of sphincter pupillae muscle (pupil dilated)
  A. Intracranial disease
    1. Neoplasm, aneurysm, degeneration
    2. Infection: syphilis, herpes zoster ophthalmicus, meningitis, encephalitis, botulism, diphtheria, tuberculous meningitis (pupil dilated, fixed)
    3. Vascular disease: cavernous sinus thrombosis, hemorrhage
  B. Toxic polyneuritis (alcohol, lead, arsenic, carbon dioxide)
  C. Diabetes mellitus (pupil spared in 75% of cases of diabetic ophthalmoplegia)
III. Paralysis of dilatator pupillae muscle (pupil constricted)
  A. Horner syndrome
IV. Lesions of intercalated neuron
  A. Argyll Robertson pupil (tabes dorsalis, pupil constricted)

In stage IV, hypoxia of the midbrain and the Edinger-Westphal nuclei causes pupillary dilation. Surprise, fear, and pain cause dilation of the pupil, as does any strong emotion, pleasant or unpleasant, or vestibular stimulation.

The pupil may be dilated in carotid artery aneurysm and in orbital or intracranial trauma caused by injury to pupillary fibers in the oculomotor nerve (N III). In acute closed-angle glaucoma, the pupil may be middilated because of sphincter hypoxia and may be fixed. In Adie syndrome, the pupil reacts slowly to light and is larger initially than the fellow pupil.

Irregularity

Irregularly shaped pupils occur in a variety of disorders (see Fig. 14-1). After a corneal laceration, the iris prolapses into the wound, causing a tear-drop-shaped pupil. After blunt trauma to the eye, the iris may be torn from its insertion at the scleral spur, causing an iridodialysis. The sector of the pupil corresponding to the iridodialysis is flattened and becomes a chord of the circular pupil.

In uveitis the iris may be bound to the lens by posterior synechiae. These may be evident only when the pupil is dilated, but if they

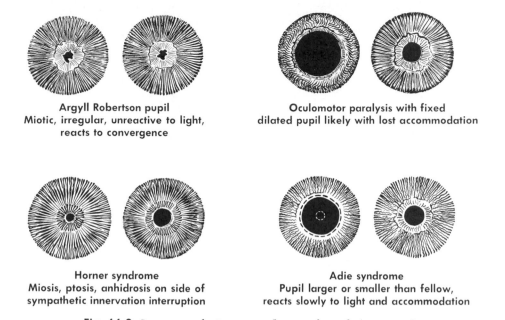

Argyll Robertson pupil
Miotic, irregular, unreactive to light,
reacts to convergence

Oculomotor paralysis with fixed
dilated pupil likely with lost accommodation

Horner syndrome
Miosis, ptosis, anhidrosis on side of
sympathetic innervation interruption

Adie syndrome
Pupil larger or smaller than fellow,
reacts slowly to light and accommodation

Fig. 14-2. Some neurologic causes of unequal pupils (anisocoria).

formed when the pupil was miotic, the irregularity of the pupillary margin will be marked.

Surgical excisions of part of the iris may be recognized by their usual location near the 12 o'clock meridian and by the deficiency of the iris pigment frill at the edges of the incision. A congenital coloboma involves the inferior nasal iris, and the frill of pupillary pigment lines the margins.

Anisocoria

Anisocoria (Fig. 14-2), or unequal size of the pupils, is a common variation. The normal difference in diameter, however, is less than 1 or 2 mm and often is not noted. About 20% of apparently normal individuals have a detectable difference in the size of the pupils, but the pupillary reflexes are normal. The cause is unknown but may be familial. The difference in size persists with variation in lighting, whereas pathologic anisocoria increases or decreases with changes in illumination (Table 14-2).

Inequality in size of the pupils or in a difference in their reflex reactions or responses to locally instilled drugs may indicate serious ocular or neurologic disease, which demands careful study. If the afferent pupillary fibers in one eye and the optic nerve are intact, the pupils or both eyes will remain equal in size even if there is a lesion of the optic nerve of the fellow

eye. This is because of the decussation of the efferent outflow so that the iris muscles of the involved eye are innervated normally. Anisocoria thus mainly reflects an abnormality involving the iris musculature of one eye, the eye itself, or the efferent parasympathetic or sympathetic motor innervation. The involved pupil may be either smaller or larger than the fellow. Irritative lesions of the parasympathetic pathway cause constriction, whereas paralytic lesions cause dilation. Irritative lesions of the sympathetic pathway cause dilation, whereas paralytic lesions cause constriction.

Anisocoria is studied in both a bright and a dim illumination. A flow chart (Fig. 14-3) simplifies the task. Often pupils are photographed in bright light and then in the dark by using a flash that photographs the pupils before they react. A variety of pharmacologic agents aid in the diagnosis (Table 14-3).

Afferent pupillary defect

The afferent pupillary defect (Robert Marcus Gunn) occurs in transmission defects of the optic nerve. It consists of a diminished amplitude of pupillary light reaction, a lengthened latent period, and pupillary dilation (escape) with continuous light stimulus. Patients with this disorder may note a decreased light sensitivity on the affected side, which is indicative of a

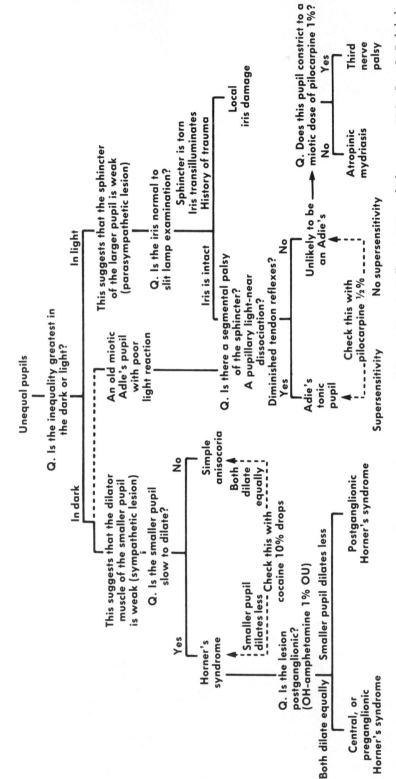

Fig. 14-3. A flow chart to assist in evaluation of anisocoria. (By permission of Czarnecki, J.S., Pilley, S.F.J., and Thompson, H.S.: Can. J. Ophthalmol. 14:297, 1979.)

Table 14-3. Pharmacologic response of unequal pupils

Compound	Normal pupil	Horner syndrome		Oculomotor nerve	
		Preganglionic lesion	Postganglionic lesion	Preganglionic lesion	Postganglionic* lesion
Epinephrine (0.1%)	0	0	Dilation	0	0
Hydroxyamphetamine (1%)	Dilation	Dilation	0	Dilation	Dilation
Cocaine (4%)	Dilation	0	0	Dilation	Dilation
Pilocarpine (0.125%)	0	0	0	?	Miosis
Pilocarpine (1%)	Constriction	Constriction	Constriction	Constriction	Constriction

*Excludes absent response in sphincter pupillae involvement in inflammation, posterior synechiae, cholinergic blockade (atropine).

conduction interference. The pupils are of equal size. The normally slow dilation of the pupil because of retinal adaptation as light continues to be directed into the eye must be distinguished from the more rapid dilation that occurs in afferent pupillary defects.

The afferent pupillary defect is most diagnostic in patients who have sudden decrease of vision in one eye without a conspicuous retinal lesion evident on ophthalmoscopy. In cystoid macular edema the pupils react normally. In optic neuritis an afferent pupillary defect is present. Patients with strabismus and amblyopia have normal pupillary reflexes. Patients with conversion reactions or simulated loss of vision have normal pupillary reactions.

Amaurotic pupil

The pupil of an eye that is blind as the result of local disease or optic nerve disease will not constrict when stimulated with light. The pupil of the normal fellow eye will not constrict. When the normal eye is stimulated with light, its pupil constricts promptly. The pupil in the blind eye constricts because its efferent innervation is intact.

Tonic pupil

Tonic pupil is a disorder in which the postganglionic parasympathetic innervation of the sphincter pupillae muscle, the ciliary muscle, or both, is impaired. There is supersensitivity of the cholinergic stimulation so that the pupil constricts or accommodation increases after the instillation of 0.125% pilocarpine, a concentration that does not affect the normal eye. Tonic pupil may occur with orbital tumors, zoster ophthalmicus, anesthesia, trauma, neuropathy

in diabetes mellitus or dysautonomia, idiopathically with reduced tendon reflexes (Adie syndrome), and after inferior oblique muscle surgery (injury to ciliary ganglia).

The Adie pupil (see Fig. 14-2) occurs more often in women than men and has its onset in one eye at about age 32. It is initially uniocular but involves the second eye at a rate of about 4% per year. Impairment of the iris sphincter causes a poor pupillary reaction to light that may involve the entire muscle or only a segment. Impairment of the ciliary muscle causes a weakness accommodation, induced lenticular astigmatism at near, and occasional cramps of the ciliary muscle with pain and delay in focusing.

The anisocoria causes photophobia, impaired dark adaptation, and a cosmetic defect in blue eyes. Ciliary muscle involvement causes headache and blurring of vision that diminish in severity within 2 years. There is decreased corneal sensitivity in affected eyes. Deep tendon reflexes are diminished or absent.

Initially the tonic pupil is large but it becomes smaller with time. When the patient converges, a slow and delayed pupillary constriction appears. This response may be marked and may exceed that of the normal pupil. After the pupil constricts for convergence, it slowly redilates but may remain smaller than the normal pupil for some time. Eventually the involved eye develops a permanently miotic pupil.

There is no effective treatment. Miotics reduce the anisocoria but may induce a spasm of the ciliary muscle. Spasms of the ciliary muscle are relieved by anticholinergic drugs, but these cause anisocoria.

Horner syndrome

Interruption of the sympathetic nerve supply to the dilatator pupillae muscle results in a constricted pupil and blepharoptosis. The miosis is not marked and is often not noticed. Interruption of the sympathetic nerves anywhere in their course from the hypothalamus to the orbit results in Horner (Johann F.) syndrome. In addition to the miosis and blepharoptosis, there is an anhidrosis, and, in experimental animals but not in humans, an enophthalamos.

The blepharoptosis is the result of loss of sympathetic nerve supply to the Müller smooth muscle of the upper eyelid, which provides its "tone." The eyelid droops only 1 or 2 mm. The anhidrosis follows loss of the sympathetic nerve fibers to the face and neck. The sweating fibers accompany the external carotid artery, and in lesions occurring between the bifurcation of the common carotid artery and the orbit, they are not affected. The enophthalmos is not present in humans but is simulated by the slight blepharoptosis. It is marked in animals that have much smooth muscle in the orbit.

Horner syndrome is usually caused by interruption of the cervical sympathetic trunk or the lower cervical and upper thoracic anterior spinal roots. The most common causes are mediastinal tumors, particularly bronchogenic carcinoma, Hodgkin disease, and metastatic tumors. Large adenomas of the thyroid gland and neurofibromatosis may be causes. Surgical and accidental traumas to the neck are the next most common causes. Diseases within the central nervous system that may cause this syndrome include occlusion of the posterior inferior cerebellar artery, multiple sclerosis or syringomyelia involving the reticular substance of the pons, and tumors of the cervical cord. Dissecting aneurysms of the internal carotid artery may cause pain in the ipsilateral forehead, eye, temple, cheek, teeth, and neck, combined with oculosympathetic palsy. A transient Horner syndrome may complicate an obstetrical epidural block. Its development signals close monitoring of the anesthesia. Insertion of a central venous catheter by means of percutaneous puncture of the internal jugular vein may produce a permanent Horner syndrome. Congenital and, occasionally, acquired Horner syndrome may be associated with less pigment in the iris on the affected side than there is in the fellow eye (heterochromia iridis).

The affected pupil does not dilate after instillation of 4% cocaine solution, but the normal pupil does. This occurs because cocaine dilates the pupil by preventing reuptake of norepinephrine at the postganglionic nerve terminal. Because of the absent norepinephrine in the affected eye, instillation of cocaine has little effect. Instillation of 1% hydroxyamphetamine is used to distinguish between preganglionic and postganglionic lesions causing Horner syndrome. In central and preganglionic lesions, the drug causes prompt dilation of the pupils of both eyes. In postganglionic lesions, the drug does not dilate the pupil on the affected side.

Argyll Robertson pupil

The Douglas M.C.L. Argyll Robertson pupil (see Fig. 14-2) is a bilateral abnormality characterized by failure of the pupils to constrict with light but retention of pupillary constriction with convergence. The entire syndrome includes miotic, irregular, and unequal pupils, the presence of some vision in each eye, failure of the pupils to dilate after local scopolamine instillation, and further miosis after eserine instillation. When all signs are present, they characterize tabes dorsalis of central nervous system syphilis. The lesion is thought to be in the pretectal region, where the afferent pupillary fibers synapse with nerve fibers going to the Edinger-Westphal nucleus. Hemorrhage and tumors involving the pretectal region may be associated with failure of the pupils to react to light and retention of the reaction to convergence; however, the pupils are not miotic, unequal, or irregular and are not typical of those described by Robertson.

BIBLIOGRAPHY

Burde, R.M., Savino, P.J., and Trobe, J.D.: Clinical decisions in neuro-ophthalmology, St. Louis, 1985, The C.V. Mosby Co.

Miller, N.R.: Walsh and Hoyt's clinical neuro-ophthalmology, ed. 4, Vol. 2, Baltimore, 1985, The Williams & Wilkins Co.

Thompson, H.S., Corbett, J.J., and Cox, T.A.: How to measure the relative afferent pupillary defect, Surv. Ophthalmol. 26:39, 1981.

Trobe, J.D.: Isolated pupil-sparing third nerve palsy, Ophthalmology **92:**58, 1985.

15

THE MIDDLE COAT: THE UVEA

The middle coat of the eye, the uvea (L. *uva*, grape), consists of the choroid, the ciliary body, and the iris. The choroid is the vascular layer of the posterior three fifths of the eye that nurtures the adjacent retinal pigment epithelium and the outer portion of the sensory retina. The ciliary body secretes aqueous humor and contains the smooth muscle (N III) that governs accommodation. The iris, a diaphragm that rests upon the lens, separates the anterior and posterior chambers of the eye. It contains a central opening, the pupil, through which aqueous humor passes from the posterior to the anterior chamber; it also contains two muscles, the sphincter pupillae (N III, parasympathetics) and the dilatator pupillae (sympathetics), which regulate the amount of light entering the eye.

The choroid extends from the margin of the optic nerve posteriorly to the ciliary body anteriorly. It consists of the choriocapillaris, an inner layer of specialized, large-diameter (21 μm), fenestrated capillaries (Fig. 15-1), which is separated from the retinal pigment epithelium by the lamina basalis choroideae (Bruch membrane). The outer layers of the choroid, which are closest to the sclera, consist of arteries and veins of successively larger diameter that empty into the vortex veins. The blood supply of the posterior half of the choroid is derived from 10 to 20 short posterior ciliary arteries, while that of the anterior half is derived from the long posterior and anterior ciliary arteries. The iris and ciliary body have the same blood supply as the anterior choroid.

The ciliary body is composed of a corona ciliaris (pars plicata), which contains ciliary processes, and an orbicularis ciliaris (pars plana), a transitional area with the choroid. The ciliary processes secrete the aqueous humor into the posterior chamber.

Located within the ciliary body is the ciliary muscle, divided into well-defined longitudinal and circular muscle fibers and poorly defined radial muscle fibers. Zonular fibers, which do not have contractile properties, connect the equatorial areas of the lens with the ciliary muscles. Contraction of the ciliary muscles re-

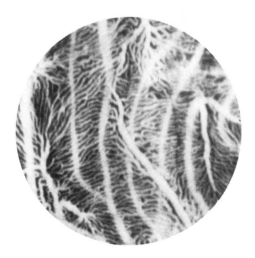

Fig. 15-1. Injected specimen of human choroid showing choriocapillaris and large collecting veins. The choriocapillaris is composed of such large vessels that it resembles vascular sinuses rather than the usual capillaries.

283

laxes the zonule so that the lens becomes more spherical (accommodation).

The iris contains a variable amount of pigment in its anterior stroma. The anterior stroma is absent in some areas, forming iris crypts. The stroma rests upon a layer of pigment epithelium continuous with that of the retina. The pigment epithelium contains the dilatator pupillae muscle on its anterior surface. The sphincter pupillae muscle is located near the pupil in the posterior iris stroma. Both muscles originate from neural ectoderm. The iris is divided by the collarette into a central pupillary zone (concentric with the pupil) and a peripheral ciliary zone. The collarette is the remnant of the minor vascular circle of the iris. The blood vessels of the iris are arranged in a radial pattern and have a thick adventitia. The blood vessels of the iris and ciliary body (and retina) are not permeable to large molecules (blood-aqueous barrier).

SYMPTOMS AND SIGNS OF UVEAL DISEASE

The symptoms and signs vary considerably with the portion of the uvea affected. Abnormalities of the iris may distort the shape of the pupil or may interfere with its dilation and constriction. Inflammations of the iris and the ciliary body cause a ciliary type of injection. Diseases of the ciliary body and the iris may be associated with severe, deep, boring, dull, aching pain within the eye. Inflammation of the posterior choroid occurs without ciliary injection or pain.

In most local diseases of the ciliary body, spasm of the ciliary muscle is painful and increases accommodation. Impairment of the oculomotor nerve supply causes pupillary dilation and loss of accommodation. Diseases of the choroid often extend to the overlying retina and reduce vision. Impairment of nutrition of the retina by the choriocapillaris results in abnormalities of visual acuity, visual field, or both. Inflammations of the choroid often extend into the adjacent retina, causing exudation of inflammatory cells and protein into the vitreous cavity and decreased vision. Ciliary body inflammations release cells and protein into both the vitreous cavity and anterior chamber, whereas inflammatory cells from the iris are confined to the anterior chamber.

The iris may be examined directly; the cornea provides magnification for study. The ciliary body can be seen with a gonioscope after maximal pupillary dilation or by using indirect ophthalmoscopy and scleral indentation.

Ophthalmoscopic visualization of choroidal details is usually obscured by the pigment epithelium of the retina, causing the fundus to appear reddish brown. Often a portion of the choroid is visible at the temporal side of the optic disk as a choroidal crescent. In blond individuals, the large choroidal veins may be seen. A white sclera may be observed between blood vessels that usually belong to the outer vessel layer of the choroid (Haller), which consists of veins that have a considerably larger diameter than the corresponding retinal arteries. Details of the choriocapillaris may be seen with fluorescein angiography, but ophthalmoscopically it consists of a thin sheet of blood that results in the red fundus reflex. In atrophy of the choriocapillaris, the choroidal veins may be seen as a dense network of white vessels (see Fig. 15-4).

The melanin of the choroid is browner than the jet-black retinal pigment. The choroidal pigment cells do not proliferate in inflammatory irritation as do the retinal pigment epithelium cells.

The lamina basalis choroideae (Bruch membrane) is composed of the basement membrane of the choriocapillaris endothelium, an elastic tissue layer sandwiched between two collagen layers, and the basement membrane of the retinal pigment epithelium. Deficiencies in the elastic layer cause a variety of fundus abnormalities, such as angioid streaks and rare hereditary diseases, and precede subretinal neovascularization, which complicates many retinal disorders.

CONGENITAL AND DEVELOPMENTAL ANOMALIES
Coloboma

Failure of the optic cup to close in the region of the retinal fissure results in a coloboma, an absence of uveal tissue in the region. Colobomas involve the inferior nasal quadrant and may extend from the optic nerve to the pupil. The retinal pigment epithelium is missing; the sensory retina is usually present but is transparent, and only its blood vessels can be seen with the ophthalmoscope. The CHARGE association is an acronym for an ill-defined group of developmental anomalies that include coloboma-ocular, heart disease, atresia choanae, retarded growth and development, genital malformations, and ear malformations. The cause is unknown.

The white sclera is seen ophthalmoscopically at the base of choroidal colobomas (Fig. 15-2). The sclera may bulge outward (ectasia). A coloboma of the ciliary body may be associated with a notching defect of the lens that corresponds to the deficient zonule in the area. The appearance of a choroidal coloboma may be simulated by prenatal retinochoroiditis caused by toxoplasmosis. These inflammatory lesions, however, do not usually occur in the inferior nasal quadrant, and there is proliferation of the retinal pigment epithelium.

Typical congenital colobomas of the iris involve the inferior nasal portion and cause a (key hole) defect in the shape of the pupil (Fig. 15-3). The margins of the coloboma show the pupillary frill with pigment epithelium, unlike surgical iridectomies.

Aniridia

Aniridia (absence of the iris) is a congenital, often hereditary, usually bilateral, failure of growth and differentiation of the anterior portion of the optic cup. The iris is not absent but is more or less rudimentary. When visible, its remnants can be seen by means of gonioscopy behind the corneoscleral limbus. Aniridia occurs mainly as an autosomal dominant (sometimes autosomal recessive) condition with almost complete penetrance. Rarely, it occurs in association with Wilms' tumor and deletion of band p 13 of chromosome 11 (11 p 13). Sporadic aniridia represents a new autosomal dominant condition.

Clinically, the corneal region appears black with no iris (or pupil) visible. Photophobia is often present and patients squeeze the eyelids almost closed and furrow the brow. Family members may have hypoplastic irides or iris colobomas. Visual acuity is about 20/100 or poorer, but in some kindred vision is good. Visual acuity may deteriorate because of glaucoma. In the usual phenotype, aniridia is associated with nystagmus, foveal and optic nerve hypoplasia, corneal pannus, cataract, secondary

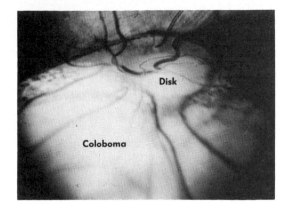

Fig. 15-2. Large coloboma of the inferior choroid. The retinal arteries and veins are present, but the large white area is sclera photographed through the transparent sensory retina, which lacks its normal blood supply from the choriocapillaris.

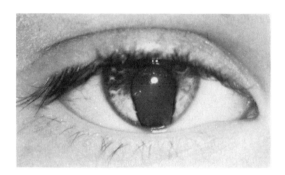

Fig. 15-3. Congenital coloboma of the iris in the characteristic down and slightly nasal position in the region of the site of closure of the fetal fissure.

glaucoma, and strabismus. Blood vessels may occur in the normal avascular foveal centralis.

Nonhereditary aniridia may be associated with a variety of systemic disorders: mental retardation, microcephaly, hemihypertrophy, horseshoe kidney, and genital abnormalities (cryptorchidism, hypospadias, and pseudohermaphrodism).

The gene for autosomal dominant aniridia has been mapped to chromosome 1 by linkage with the Rh, Duffy, and PGM loci and to chromosome 2 by linkage to acid phosphatase-1. All patients who have Wilms' tumor and 11 p 13 have aniridia, but not all patients with aniridia and 11 p 13 develop Wilms' tumor. Rhabdomyosarcoma, nephroblastoma, adrenal tumors, hepatoblastoma, and gonadoblastoma have also been described. As in retinoblastoma, the gene on one of the pair of chromosome 11 is deleted, and a second mutational event on the homologous chromosome results in tumor formation.

Provision of an artificial pupil by means of an iris painted on a contact lens reduces photophobia but does not improve vision. Glaucoma often develops in adolescence. The glaucoma responds poorly to surgery and medical treatment.

Atrophy of the choriocapillaris

Atrophy of the choriocapillaris occurs in two forms: (1) a benign type, depigmentation in situ, in which there is no functional impairment, and (2) a degenerative type, that may be either generalized or focal, in which functional impairment is severe. The sole pathologic change in the benign type is attenuated pigment in the retinal pigment epithelium. In the degenerative type, the choriocapillaris is absent, as are the retinal pigment epithelium and the outer layers of the sensory retina in the affected areas. Sclerosis of the choroidal vessels does not occur in either condition.

Depigmentation in situ is seen commonly in simple myopia and less frequently as a change with aging. The choroidal vasculature is conspicuous ophthalmoscopically. Vision and fluorescein angiography are normal.

Degenerative choriocapillary atrophy occurs in a generalized or diffuse form or in a focal form confined to the posterior pole of the eye. The generalized form occurs sporadically (Fig. 15-4) in X chromosome–linked choroideremia, gyrate atrophy, and hereditary and toxic retinal pigmentary degeneration. The focal type (also known as central areolar choroidal sclerosis, central progressive areolar choroidal dystrophy, or central choroidal sclerosis) occurs mainly as an autosomal disorder. Central vision is reduced in both types. In the generalized type there is night blindness, loss of the electroretinographic response to light, and a reduced electro-oculographic light-dark ratio.

Degenerative choroidal sclerosis begins in the retinal pigment epithelium and is followed shortly thereafter by impaired filling of the lobules of the choriocapillaris and then atrophy. With atrophy, the retinal pigment epithelium together with the adjacent outer retina degenerates, and the major arteries and veins of the choroid become visible. The precapillary arterioles and branches of the short posterior ciliary arteries also atrophy, but to a lesser extent than the choriocapillaris.

Choroideremia. Choroideremia is an X chromosome-linked choroidal atrophy with secondary atrophy of the retina, causing night blindness.

In the female carrier, the condition is asymp-

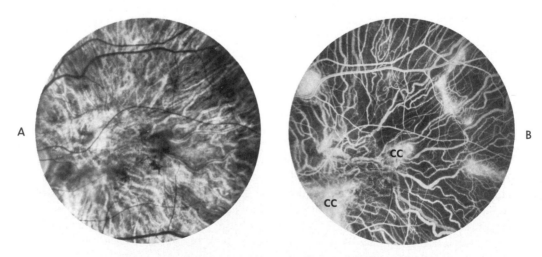

Fig. 15-4. A, Light ophthalmoscopy of choriocapillaris atrophy. The choroidal vessels appear as white lines through the atrophic pigment epithelium. **B,** Choroidal circulation in the late phase of fluorescein angiography. There is atrophy of the choriocapillaris, and the choroidal arteries and veins are clearly seen. Some islands of choriocapillaris (*CC*) remain.

tomatic and is associated with increased pigmentation and depigmentation of the fundus that is most marked in the equatorial region. The pigment granules have an irregular, square appearance similar to chunks of coal and are about 100 μm in diameter (the optic disk is 1,500 μm). Under or adjacent to the clumps of pigment are depigmented areas up to 0.5 disk diameter in size. They may appear paler than the rest of the fundus or have a bright yellow color.

Choroideremia in the hemizygous male usually has its onset between 10 and 13 years of age. Night blindness, which becomes complete in about 10 years, is the initial symptom. The peripheral field then begins to contract, and finally, after about 35 years, all vision is lost. The earliest fundus lesions resemble the pigmentary changes of the female carriers. Eventually atrophic changes dominate, and the white sclera becomes exposed in the equatorial region. At this time, night blindness occurs and an annular scotoma is present. The atrophy then spreads centrally and peripherally until all vision is lost. The retinal vessels are normal.

Gyrate atrophy of the choroid. This is a progressive autosomal recessive disorder with diffuse chorioretinal atrophy. Myopia occurs in the first decade, night blindness in the second, severe cataract in the third, and pigmentary changes of the macula with progressive vision loss in the fourth. The chorioretinal atrophy begins at the equator of the fundus with sharply punched-out oval areas of atrophy with scalloped borders, obliteration of the choriocapillaris, narrowing of the retinal vessels, and optic nerve atrophy. The chorioretinal atrophy slowly spreads toward the fovea centralis, which is preserved until adulthood. Clinically, the disorder resembles choroideremia, but is transmitted as an autosomal recessive disorder. In the late stages of gyrate atrophy, there is fine, velvety pigmentation with glittering crystals not seen in choroideremia. Additionally, the central retinal pigmentation conceals the choroid, which is exposed in choroideremia.

The plasma levels of the nonprotein amino acid ornithine are increased some twentyfold. There is a deficiency of the enzyme ornithine aminotransferase. Heterozygotes for the defect have intermediate levels of the enzyme and no ocular defects. Plasma levels of ammonia and its precursors, glutamine and glutamic acid, which are derived from ornithine, are low. Treatment with a low arginine diet (the precursor of ornithine in the urea cycle) restores normal plasma levels of ornithine, ammonia, glutamine, and glutamic acid.

Congenital ectropion uveae

The pigmented margin of the pupil marks the anterior border of the secondary optic cup. Rarely, flocculi or cystic dilations of the marginal sinus of the pupillary margin develop into dark brown bodies that may extend on the surface of the iris. They may occasionally break free to appear as movable pigment masses on the iris surface. They have no harmful effects.

Heterochromia iridis

In heterochromia iridis, the two irises differ in color (Table 15-1). In simple heterochromia iridis, there is relative hypoplasia of the lighter-colored iris combined with a relative hyperplasia of the iris architecture on the side of the darker-colored iris. The abnormality may be transmitted as an autosomal dominant trait. Displacement of the medial canthi, hypertrophy of the nasal bridge, white forelock, and deafness constitute the Waardenburg-Klein syndrome, an abnormality of neural crest cells.

In hypochromic heterochromia, the eye with the lighter-colored iris is abnormal. The difference between the two eyes may be extremely

Table 15-1. Heterochromia iridis

Lighter-colored iris abnormality
Simple heterochromia iridis
Arachnodactyly
Facial hemiatrophy
Mandibulo-oculofacial dyscephaly
Hallerman-Streiff syndrome
Waardenburg-Klein syndrome
Horner syndrome
Heterochromic cyclitis of Fuchs
Glaucomatocyclitic crisis
Amelanotic tumors
Cutaneous xanthomatosis
Reactive lymphoid hyperplasia of uvea
Darker-colored iris abnormality
Retention intraocular iron foreign body
Malignant melanoma of the iris
Ocular hemosiderosis
Trauma
Microcornea

slight when both irises are blue. The condition occurs in many different disorders. In Horner syndrome, there is paralysis of the dilatator muscle of the iris. In Fuchs heterochromic cyclitis there is a mild inflammation of the iris as well as the ciliary body, often complicated with cataract and sometimes with glaucoma. In glaucomatocyclitic crisis, there is diffuse iris atrophy secondary to inflammation, trauma, and ischemia of the iris. Infiltration of the iris by any nonpigmented tumor causes a hypochromic iris.

In hyperchromic iridis, the iris on the side of the anomaly or disease is darker than its fellow. The condition occurs with retention of an iron foreign body in the eye (siderosis), with malignant melanoma of the iris, in monocular melanosis in which there are excess chromatophores in the iris stroma, after anterior chamber hemorrhage from any cause, after perforating injuries or contusion of the globe before 10 years of age, and in association with microcornea.

Iris atrophy

Normally the pupillary zone of the iris is relatively flat because of an atrophy of the anterior leaf of the stroma. The gossamer appearance of the ciliary zone may be lost in conditions in which the blood vessels and fine collagen fibers atrophy and are replaced by a sclerosed network. Hypochromia iridis causes such an atrophy combined with a loss of chromatophores. If chromatophores are not lost, the iris looks dull and patternless and has the same color as its fellow. Such atrophy may be diffuse or localized. Minor degrees of iris atrophy occur with aging, and the atrophy may be severe after ocular inflammation, trauma, ischemia, and glaucoma. It may occur in tabes dorsalis without pupillary abnormalities.

Iridocorneal endothelial syndrome. Glaucoma, progressive iris atrophy, abnormal corneal endothelium, extensive peripheral anterior synechiae, multiple iris nodules, and a transparent membrane covering the anterior surface of the iris are seen in varying combinations in three conditions: (1) progressive essential iris atrophy, (2) iris atrophy with corneal edema and glaucoma (Chandler), and (3) iris-nevus syndrome (Cogan and Reese).

The disorders are slowly progressive over a period of 10 or more years. Women are more

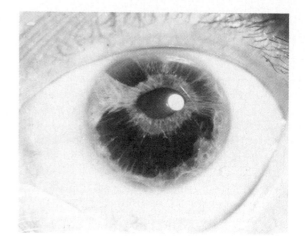

Fig. 15-5. Essential atrophy of the iris with loss of iris stroma below and an opening through all layers of the iris in a 33-year-old woman. Intraocular pressure is easily controlled by instillation of 2% pilocarpine, but when treatment is omitted, pressure rises precipitously, resulting in corneal edema and loss of vision.

commonly affected than men. After metaplasia, the corneal endothelium proliferates and is disrupted by loss of cells. Minor increases in intraocular pressure cause severe corneal edema, particularly in the Chandler syndrome. The iris stroma atrophies and develops a matted appearance caused by abnormalities of its basement membrane.

Essential iris atrophy (Fig. 15-5) is a rare, progressive, usually unilateral disease predominantly affecting women in their middle years (38.6 years). It is characterized by a distorted, displaced pupil, corneal endothelial degeneration, patchy atrophy of the iris with partial or complete hole formation, peripheral anterior synechiae, and secondary glaucoma. The onset is gradual, and the patient is aware only of a change in shape or position of the pupil. During the next several years, holes develop in the iris. Secondary glaucoma then ensues from peripheral anterior synechiae and damage to the trabecular meshwork from a cuticular membrane. Direct inspection of the iris indicates the loss of iris tissue and displacement of the pupil. Treatment is directed toward the secondary glaucoma and is often not effective. Visual loss results from either corneal edema or secondary glaucoma.

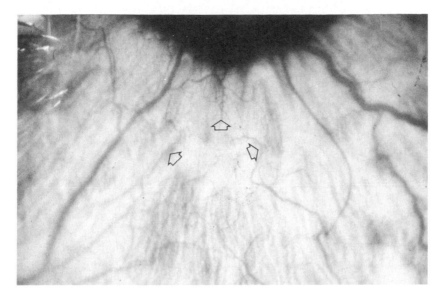

Fig. 15-6. New blood on surface of the iris (*arrows:* rubeosis iridis) in a 48-year-old diabetic patient.

A less severe form of iris atrophy (Chandler syndrome) is associated with an endothelial disturbance and corneal edema combined with multiple small nodules and an ectopic Descemet membrane on the iris surface. Glaucoma eventually may occur secondary to obstruction of outflow by peripheral anterior synechiae. Corneal edema occurs with minor increases in intraocular pressure.

The iris-nevus syndrome begins as a progressive iris atrophy, but after many years light tan, yellow, or dark brown nodules appear as little spheres of tissue in the iris stroma. Similar nodules may also be seen in the neurofibromatosis (Lish), in melanomas, in flocculus of the iris, and as inflammatory granulomas.

Secondary iris atrophy. Secondary iris atrophy does not cause the frank holes seen in the essential type. The atrophy may result from anterior uveitis, ocular trauma, or zoster ophthalmicus. The iris sphincer muscle may atrophy after an attack of closed-angle glaucoma. Iris atrophy may be caused by ischemia of the iris secondary to closure of the anterior ciliary arteries or long ciliary arteries that may follow carotid artery insufficiency or lupus erythematosus. Local interference with blood supply may follow retinal detachment operations, freezing or cauterizing of the corneoscleral limbus region, or detachment of three or four recti muscles.

Rubeosis of the iris (rubeosis iridis)

Neovascularization of the iris (Fig. 15-6) occurs as an irregularly distributed network of new vessels on the iris surface and stroma or as a fine, markedly tortuous, anastomosed, tightly meshed network on the surface and stroma of the entire iris. The new blood vessels and associated fibrous tissue may cover the trabecular meshwork and cause peripheral anterior synechiae that close the anterior chamber angle and cause an intractable neovascular glaucoma. Hemorrhage into the anterior chamber may occur.

Diabetes mellitus is a frequent cause of rubeosis iridis. The disorder often occurs after central vein closure and, more rarely, after central retinal artery closure. It occurs in many vascular abnormalities, such as aortic arch syndrome, carotid artery occlusive disease, carotid artery fistula, giant cell arteritis, anterior ocular segment ischemia, and intraocular tumors, and after ocular radiation and intraocular inflammation. It is the most common complication of vitrectomy, particularly if the lens is absent.

Neovascular glaucoma is difficult to relieve. Panretinal photocoagulation (ablation) of a neovascularized retina may be followed by involution of the iris vessels. Photocoagulation of the iris and anterior chamber angle causes a temporary ischemia that allows a filtering operation or implantation of a filtering valve. Cryotherapy of the ciliary body (cyclocryotherapy) may reduce the secretion of aqueous and possibly impair sensory innervation. Retrobulbar alcohol injection relieves pain for up to 3 months. Enucleation may be deferred if the eye is not too unsightly and if ultrasonography confirms the absence of an intraocular tumor.

INFLAMMATORY DISORDERS

Inflammations of the uveal tract may be divided as follows: suppurative or nonsuppurative; endogenous or exogenous (mainly trauma); anterior, intermediate, posterior; infectious or noninfectious. The suppurative types include panophthalmitis, in which the entire inner eye is inflamed, including the sclera, and endophthalmitis, in which not all layers of the globe are affected and the globe does not rupture.

Nonsuppurative inflammations may occur because of exogenous or endogenous causes. In exogenous disease the causative agent is introduced from the outside directly into the eye through an opening in the cornea or sclera. Endogenous inflammations result from systemic disease, from intraocular abnormalities such as hypermature cataract or uveal tissue necrosis, or because of an immunologic response of a previously sensitized tissue.

Inflammations have a variety of designations:

Inflammation of iris, ciliary body, and choroid: uveitis
Iris: iritis
Ciliary body: cyclitis
Iris and ciliary body: iridocyclitis
Anterior uveitis: iris and pars plicata
Intermediate uveitis: pars plana ciliaris and adjacent 1 mm of choroid
Posterior uveitis: choroid
Choroid: choroiditis

The iris, ciliary body, and anterior choroid share a common blood supply and tend to be involved to a greater or lesser extent in the same inflammatory processes. Inflammations of the posterior choroid, unless exceptionally severe, do not involve the anterior uveal tract.

Inflammations of the choroid often affect the overlying retina, resulting in a loss of vision. Inflammatory cells from the ciliary body may cloud the vitreous, enter the aqueous, and adhere to the cornea (keratic precipitates, KPs). Adhesions between the iris and lens (synechiae) may cause a pupillary block glaucoma (iris bombé). Inflammatory debris in the trabecular meshwork that prevents the outflow of aqueous causes an open-angle secondary glaucoma.

In the past, acute inflammation was classed as a nongranulomatous type of uveitis and chronic inflammation was classed as a granulomatous type of uveitis. Nongranulomatous inflammations were considered to be the result of previous systemic infection, particularly by streptococci. Granulomatous inflammations were thought to be caused by delayed hypersensitivity (T-cell mediated) such as that which occurs in tubercle infection in a previously infected patient. Granulomas, however, do not occur in most chronic inflammations, even those that have a prominent epithelioid cell reaction.

Endogenous uveitis may be caused by a variety of pathogens: (1) protozoa (*Toxoplasma, Trypanosoma*), amebae; (2) viruses (herpes, slow measles); (3) bacteria (tuberculosis, syphilis, leprosy, and leptospirosis); (4) fungi (*Candida, Coccidioides, Histoplasma, Sporotrichum, Cryptococcus,* and *Aspergillus*); and (5) parasitic worms (*Toxocara, Onchocerca, Cysticercus* [*Taenia*], and *Schistosoma*).

A variety of nonsuppurative inflammations are of immunologic origin: Behçet disease, Fuchs heterochromic iridocyclitis, serum sickness, acute multifocal posterior placoid epitheliopathy, and polyarteritis. Many of immunologic origin are associated with arthritis: rheumatoid arthritis, ankylosing spondylitis, Reiter syndrome, pauciarticular juvenile rheumatoid arthritis (Still), psoriasis, and ulcerative colitis (either with or without spondylitis).

Several types of uveitis are impossible to classify: sarcoid, Vogt-Koyangi, Harada syndrome, bird-shot retinochoroidopathy, uveal effusion syndrome, Posner-Schlossman syndrome, and pars planitis (peripheral uveitis or intermediate uveitis).

Table 15-2. Characteristics of acute and chronic uveitis

	Chronic	Acute
Anterior uvea		
Pain, photophobia	Minimal or absent	Severe
Vision	Gradual reduction	Abrupt reduction
Course	Protracted, remissions, and exacerbations	Self-limited (1-6 weeks), often recurrent
Keratic deposits	Heavy, coalescent, often "mutton fat," crenated margins, macrophages, phagocytized pigment	Pinpoint
Aqueous humor	Few cells, often large, variable aqueous flare	Many cells, intense aqueous flare, sometimes protein coagulation
Iris nodules and precipitates	Frequent	None
Posterior uvea		
Retinal and subretinal edema	Usually slight or moderate and localized around exudates	Marked and generalized, with blurring of neuroretinal margins and retinal vascular bed
Choroidal exudates	Heavy massive exudates with edges blurred by surrounding retinal and subretinal edema	No heavy massive exudates, occasionally localized areas of deeper infiltration
Secondary retinal involvement	Almost invariable, with retinal destruction	None or limited to pigment epithelium and rods and cones
Residual organic damage	Heavy glial scars with massive pigment surrounding the lesion	None or fine granular changes in pigment epithelium with damage to neuroepithelium and superficial gliosis
Anterior segment changes	Sometimes mutton-fat keratic deposits	Usually none
Vitreous changes	Usually heavy vitreous blurring; heavy, veillike opacities frequent	Slight to intense general blurring, fine, stringlike, fibrinous opacities

Acute uveitis

The nonsuppurative, self-limited, often recurrent inflammation of the uveal tract is characterized by edema, capillary dilation, and an exudation of polymorphonuclear leukocytes, which are quickly replaced by lymphocytes and plasma cells. Inflammation of the anterior segment is characterized by acute and severe inflammatory signs with a sudden onset, severe symptoms, and a tendency to spontaneous remission. The disease may recur or continue chronically (Table 15-2). Lesions in the choroid are rare and are associated with fine cells in the vitreous body and retinal edema without exudation.

The inflammation may be exogenous or endogenous (Table 15-3). Exogenous causes include ocular contusion, which often produces a transient anterior uveitis (traumatic iridocyclitis), alkali burns of the external eye, and a non-

Table 15-3. Acute, subacute, or chronic uveitis with predominately lymphocytic and plasma cell reaction

I. Exogenous
  A. Ocular contusion (traumatic iridocyclitis)
  B. Alkali burns
  C. Accidental and surgical penetrating injuries with noncontaminated foreign bodies, blood and its degradation products, necrotic intraocular tissue, intraocular lenses
II. Endogenous
  A. Without evident systemic disease: chronic idiopathic uveitis (the common type)
  B. With noninfectious systemic disease: rheumatoid arthritis, ankylosing spondylitis, Still disease, Reiter syndrome, Behçet disease, collagen disorders, regional enteritis, atopic disorders
  C. With infectious systemic disease: rubella, rubeola, mumps, herpes simplex, subacute sclerosing panencephalitis, Kawasaki syndrome
  D. Ocular syndromes: uveal effusion, glaucoma-cyclitis crisis, heterochromic cyclitis, pars planitis

infected foreign body. There are numerous endogenous causes, but idiopathic uveitis constitutes the most prevalent type of inflammation. Blood and its degradation products and necrotic intraocular tissue may produce a uveitis. In most instances, there is no obvious ocular or systemic cause. Noninfectious systemic disorders, ranging from arthritis to infectious diseases, may be associated with uveitis of varying degrees of severity. Uveitis is often not recognized although present in rubella, rubeola, mumps, or Kasaska syndrome.

Chronic uveitis

Chronic uveitis is a usually progressive inflammation of the uveal tract in which there is cellular infiltration, chiefly by mononuclear cells, macrophages, and epithelioid cells, with tissue necrosis and repair by fibrosis. Involvement of the anterior uvea in granulomatous inflammation is characterized by a torpid chronic course and minimal signs of inflammation. "Mutton fat" KPs form, and there is a mild aqueous flare with few cells in the aqueous humor. There is a marked tendency toward formation of posterior synechiae and decreased vision.

Chronic uveitis of the posterior eye clouds the vitreous with dense opacities. One or more choroidal exudative areas that involve the overlying pigment epithelium of the retina may be present.

The inflammation may be caused by microbes or parasites, or it may occur with a wide variety of noninfectious systemic diseases. There are a number of strictly ocular causes (Table 15-4).

Symptoms and signs of uveitis

The symptoms of nonsuppurative uveitis vary with the portion of the uveal tract involved. Visual loss is the main symptom of posterior inflammations, whereas anterior uveitis may initially cause pain, photophobia, and lacrimation. Pain is more common in acute iridocyclitis than in chronic iridocyclitis and is particularly severe when associated with keratitis. It centers in the periorbital and ocular region and is aggravated by exposure to light and by pressure on the eye. Photophobia varies in severity and may be so marked that the eyelids cannot be opened to examine the eye. Lacri-

Table 15-4. Chronic uveitis

I. Exogenous
 A. Foreign body granuloma
II. Endogenous
 A. With infectious systemic or local disease
  1. Bacterial: *Mycobacterium tuberculosis, M. leprae, Treponema, Francisella tularensis*
  2. Fungal: *Blastomyces dermatitidis, Cryptococcus neoformans, Coccidioides immitis, rhinosporidiosis*
  3. Viral: herpes simplex, herpes zoster, cytomegalic inclusion disease
  4. Parasitic: *Cysticerus cellulosae, Toxocara canis, Toxocara catis, Toxoplasma gondii, Trichinella spiralis, Echinococcus granulosus,* schistosomiasis, visceral larva migrans
 B. With noninfectious systemic disease: sarcoidosis, Vogt-Koyanagi-Harada syndrome, familial chronic granulomatous disease of childhood, Chédiak-Higashi syndrome, juvenile xanthogranuloma, relapsing febrile nodular nonsuppurative panniculitis
 C. Ocular syndromes: sympathetic ophthalmia, phacoanaphylactica, granulomatous scleritis

mation is usually proportionate to the degree of photophobia. Decreased vision occurs because of exudation of cells and protein-rich fluid and fibrin into either the anterior chamber or vitreous body. Inflammation of the choroid beneath the fovea centralis causes an early loss of visual acuity that is often disproportionately severe in comparison to the amount of choroidal involvement. Choroidal inflammation that is distant from the posterior pole, although damaging to the overlying retina, may cause only minimal changes in the peripheral visual field. Edema of the posterior pole of the eye, along with swelling of the optic disk (papillitis) and central cystoid edema, occurs with severe inflammations of both the anterior and posterior portions of the uvea and causes decreased vision.

Anterior uveitis. The signs of anterior uveitis include ciliary injection, exudation into the anterior chamber, iris and lens (posterior synechiae).

Ciliary injection. Dilation and congestion of the anterior ciliary arteries that nurture the iris and ciliary body are referred to as ciliary injection. This must be distinguished from conjunctival injection seen in conjunctivitis. The severity varies with the degree of inflammation. Little or none occurs in chronic iridocyclitis, whereas in severe acute inflammation there may be associated episcleral and conjunctival injection and conjunctival edema. In less acute inflammation there is a deep circumcorneal injection with a violet hue. The injection fades in the conjunctival fornix and does not blanch when 1:1,000 epinephrine is instilled (see Chapter 6).

Exudation into the anterior chamber. Inflammation of the iris and ciliary body releases prostaglandins, particularly from the anterior ciliary body, and breaks down the blood-aqueous barrier, so that increased protein, fibrin, and inflammatory cells are present in the aqueous humor. The protein causes a translucence of the aqueous humor, called aqueous flare, which can be seen with the biomicroscope. The cells are suspended in the aqueous humor and, because of thermal convection currents, rise when close to the iris and descend at the cooler cornea. Keratic precipitates (KPs) adhere to the corneal endothelial surface. Two main types of KPs occur: (1) large, heavy, greasy, fat KPs (mutton-fat KPs) composed of macrophages and phagocytized pigment, and (2) small, white, punctate accumulations composed of lymphocytes and plasma cells. Macrophages appear at the pupillary margin (Koeppe nodules), on the surface of the iris (floccules of Busacca), on the lens surface, and in the anterior chamber angle. Occasionally in severe acute iridocyclitis so many cells are present that a hypopyon forms, or, rarely, diapedesis of erythrocytes causes a hyphema.

Iris changes. In acute iridocyclitis, the pupil may be constricted or in middilation. The iris may be edematous with its pattern blurred ("muddy") and the capillaries engorged. In chronic iridocyclitis, nodules may originate from proliferation of the iris pigment epithelium or infiltration of the iris with round cells and macrophages. Typical granulomatous nodules such as tubercles or sarcoid nodules may be found. These may be followed by a patchy area of iris atrophy. Diffuse iris atrophy with loss of iris pattern follows prolonged iridocyclitis and may involve both the stroma (mesodermal) and pigment (ectodermal) layers.

Posterior synechiae. These adhesions bind the iris to the lens or to the anterior vitreous face, if the lens is absent. They cause a small, irregular pupil that does not constrict to light in the area of the adhesions. Sometimes small or large clumps of iris pigment remain on the anterior lens capsule, an indication of past or present iritis or ocular trauma. If posterior synechiae involve the entire pupillary margin, aqueous humor cannot flow from the posterior chamber into the anterior chamber, and the resultant iris bombé causes a secondary pupillary block glaucoma.

Posterior uveitis. The two most important signs of posterior uveitis are vitreous opacities and chorioretinitis (choroiditis).

Vitreous opacities. A variable degree of cloudiness of the vitreous occurs in posterior uveitis because of exudation of inflammatory cells and a protein-rich fluid combined with erythrocytes. Vitreous opacities consist of aggregates of cells, coagulated exudate and fibrin, and strands of degenerated vitreous body. Ophthalmoscopically, they appear as black dots against the red background of the fundus or may be so numerous that they obscure all fundus details. They are best studied by means of the biomicroscope combined with a concave lens to neutralize the refractive power of the cornea.

Choroiditis. Acute choroiditis appears ophthalmoscopically as an ill-defined grayish yellow or grayish white area surrounded by the normal colored fundus. The lesions may be single or multiple. The adjacent sensory retina becomes edematous and opaque and is so often inflamed that the lesion is described as chorioretinitis. Inflammatory cells and exudate may burst through the sensory retina to cloud the vitreous, which further obscures the ophthalmoscopic details of the lesion.

With healing, the margins of the lesion become more sharply defined and the vitreous clouding clears. If the choroid has been the main site of the lesion, it appears as a whitish yellow area stippled with pigment. When the retinal pigment epithelium has been destroyed, a patch of white scar appears that consists of either a fibrous replacement of retina and choroid or stark, white sclera over which both the retina and choroid have been destroyed. The retinal pigment epithelium proliferates, particularly at the margins of the lesions, and the final ophthalmoscopic appearance is often one of white sclera surrounded by black pigment. Pigment proliferation does not always occur following severe inflammation, presumably because of destruction of the retinal pigment epithelium.

Diagnosis and etiologic factors

Acute iridocyclitis has the signs and symptoms of the red eye, and closed-angle glaucoma, keratitis, or conjunctivitis is usually easily excluded. The diagnosis is confirmed by biomicroscopic examination and observation of keratic precipitates, aqueous flare, and cells. Clouding of the vitreous and ophthalmoscopic observation of a chorioretinal inflammatory lesion are diagnostic of posterior uveitis.

The endogenous etiologic factor may be immediately evident when associated with systemic disease, but in most instances it is impossible to demonstrate. The problem of diagnosis is complicated by the inability to secure uveal tissue for study, so that even after effective specific therapy, the cause remains presumptive. In many patients the etiologic factor is diagnosed only by exclusion of other possible causes; in other patients, such as those with arthritis or genitourinary tract disease, one knows only that the uveal tissue is inflamed, as are other organs. Moreover, the uveal inflammation may be caused by a different condition than a concurrent systemic disease, even if the disease is often associated with uveal inflammation.

Many patients in whom the cause of uveitis is not found have only a single attack; others are seen with chorioretinal scars or anterior segment lesions from asymptomatic inflammations that have occurred previously. In conditions such as heterochromic cyclitis and glaucomatocyclitic crises, no systemic abnormality has ever been found and etiologic studies are usually not useful.

Local ocular disease with uveitis. A variety of inflammations and diseases may be associated with uveitis:

1. Inflammation of adjacent tissues.
   a. Severe infection of the conjunctiva or cornea, which may involve the uvea by direct extension or by entry of the exotoxin into the eye (the infection may be bacterial, viral [often herpes simplex], or fungal). Herpes zoster ophthalmicus is associated with both uveitis and keratitis.
   b. Orbital abscess extending along the vortex veins.
   c. Meningitis extending along the sheaths of the optic nerve.
2. Disease of the lens.
   a. Hypermature cataract with release of toxic proteins within the eye causing a phacolytic uveitis. The prognosis is good if the lens is removed.
   b. Endophthalmitis phacoanaphylactica, an autoimmune process, in which the eye has become sensitive to its own lens protein. Usually, the sensitization occurs after extracapsular lens extraction. Retained lens protein stimulates B-lymphocytes to produce lens antibodies. After extracapsular extraction of the lens in the fellow eye, an antigen-antibody reaction occurs in the second eye. It is not a true anaphylactic reaction since IgE is not involved. Treatment consists of topical corticosteroids and removal of all retained lens material.
   c. Retention of the lens nucleus or particles after extracapsular lens extraction.
3. Trauma.
   a. Sympathetic ophthalmia is a rare, bilateral, diffuse, nonnecrotizing granulomatous uveitis that usually follows a laceration of one eye and prolapse of the iris or ciliary body. It is likely an autoimmune sensitization with T cell–mediated hypersensitivity (type IV). T lymphocytes are possibly directed at surface membrane antigens shared by photoreceptors, retinal pigment epithelial cells, and choroidal melanocytes.
   b. Retained intraocular foreign body.
   c. Contusion damage from blunt trauma.
   d. Chemical injury: (miosis, vascular dilation, and permeability are mediated by substance P and not prostaglandins).
   e. Blood within the eye after trauma or hemorrhagic intraocular disease.
   f. Perforation of the lens capsule.
4. Heterochromic cyllitis, a nongranulomatous iridocyclitis occurring in an eye lighter in color than the fellow eye.
5. Blind eyes with degenerative changes. Often these eyes have a chronic uveitis, and a decision must be made as to whether enucleation is preferable to continued discomfort.

6. Necrosis of intraocular tumor. In most instances the cause of the uveitis is obvious. Ultrasonography and computed tomography are valuable in demonstrating a tumor if the fundus cannot be seen.

The etiologic diagnosis of uveitis is often based on the following:

1. A uveitis of a type associated with a particular systemic disease.
2. Exclusion of all other likely causes of the uveitis.
3. Therapeutic improvement with specific medication. Many inflammations are self-limited, and a diagnosis based on improvement with specific medication may be erroneous.

The major conditions considered in the diagnosis of uveitis without obvious cause vary with time and locality. Attention is directed to sarcoidosis, arthritis, genitourinary tract disease, toxoplasmosis, histoplasmosis, and delineation of specific syndromes such as pars planitis.

Sarcoidosis. Sarcoidosis involves the uveal tract in about 50% of the cases. The disease may excite a minimal inflammatory reaction, and attention is not directed to the eyes. Anterior inflammation is associated with a granulomatous type of inflammation with numerous mutton-fat KPs and a few cells evident by means of biomicroscopy of the anterior chamber. Periphlebitis of veins in the peripheral fundus may occur with neovascularization. The choroidal lesion destroys the overlying retina, causing a severe inflammation with exudation of cells into the vitreous body and the formation of veils, "snowball" floaters, and membranes. The choroiditis often responds to corticosteroid therapy (see Chapter 23).

Arthritis. Patients with ankylosing spondylitis (Marie-Strümpell disease) develop an intermittent nongranulomatous anterior unveitis in 15% of the cases. The ocular disease is never particularly severe and responds readily to local medication. Ocular inflammation may precede joint disease. Young men are mainly affected; often there is a family history of ankylosing spondylitis or rheumatoid arthritis. The involvement of cervical vertebrae often makes it difficult for such a patient to place his head in position for biomicroscopy. The lumbosacral spine is initially affected, and the disease may easily escape diagnosis. The HLA-

B27 allele is present in more than 90% of affected individuals compared to 8% of the normal population (see Chapter 29).

Uveitis with pauciarticular juvenile rheumatoid arthritis (Still disease) is complicated by band keratopathy. The initial sign of the disease may be uveitis with minimal inflammatory signs. Many complications occur: cataract, glaucoma, and persistent uveitis.

Genitourinary tract disease. In the past, focal infection in the genitourinary tract was considered second to infections of the paranasal sinuses and nasopharynx as a cause of uveitis. Uveitis may complicate a metastatic gonorrhea in which there is an acute or chronic urethritis followed by arthralgia and ocular inflammation. Even before antibiotic treatment for gonorrhea, such instances were uncommon.

Uveitis occurs in two relatively uncommon multisystem disorders that have genitourinary tract symptoms often associated with arthritis: Behçet disease and Reiter disease.

Behçet disease. This rare (in the United States) chronic disease is classically associated with aphthous ulceration of the mouth (canker sores), genital ulcers, skin lesions, and ocular inflammation. It occurs in a chronic mucocutaneous form and in a neuro-ocular form that may cause blindness and death.

The mouth and genital region are ulcerated in the mucocutaneous form, and there is an associated conjunctivitis but no uveitis. Erythema nodosum, thrombophlebitis, cutaneous vasculitis, and papulopustular eruption in the extremities are seen.

The neuro-ocular form includes conjunctivitis, iritis, iridocyclitis (sometimes with hypopyon), keratitis, and retinal vasculitis. Meningoencephalitis with general or focal neurologic deficits occurs. The lesions of the mucocutaneous type are sometimes present.

Both types may have associated synovitis, superficial or deep thrombophlebitis, and gastrointestinal ulcerations mimicking ulcerative colitis. Natural killer-cell activity and serum interferon level are decreased during ocular exacerbations.

Reiter disease. Reiter disease comprises nongonococcal sterile urethritis, polyarthritis, and conjunctivitis or iritis. Genitourinary symptoms usually precede ocular or rheumatic features. The cause of the disease is not known, but bacillary dysentery has preceded the inflammation in some patients. Some 20% of individuals who have the HLA-B27 allele will develop Reiter syndrome after *Shigella* infections. HLA-B27 antigen is found in 92% of patients with the full syndrome. The conjunctivitis is usually mucorpurulent with preauricular adenopathy, chemosis, eyelid edema, and conjunctival hemorrhage. It resolves in 8 to 10 days. Anterior uveitis may be recurrent and is bilateral in recurrences although unilateral with first attacks. Scleritis, episcleritis, retinal edema, and optic neuritis have been described.

Histoplasmosis. Histoplasmosis is a fungus infection caused by *Histoplasma capsulatum* that is endemic in the Mississippi Valley. It occurs mainly as a subclinical disease demonstrable only by skin hypersensitivity and positive complement fixation. The organism has not been found in the eye except in endophthalmitis, but the positive lymphocyte transformation test suggests a cell-mediated abnormality.

Presumed ocular histoplasmosis is initially diagnosed because of loss of vision caused by a subretinal neovascular membrane. Recurrent hemorrhage beneath the retinal pigment epithelium is common. Blood sometimes seeps into the sensory retina, forming a dark lesion caused by the deeper blood and a bright red lesion caused by blood in the sensory retina. There are many small, discrete, atrophic areas of the choroid ("histo spots") of healed chorioretinitis at the equator and a healed chorioretinal inflammation at the optic disk margin resembling a choroidal crescent. The cellular reaction is minimal (see Chapter 23).

Pars planitis. Pars planitis (peripheral uveitis, chronic cyclitis) is a chorioretinitis that causes fibrovascular proliferation at the inferior ora serrata. There is cellular exudation into the overlying vitreous body. It is often bilateral and occurs in the first two decades of life. Periodic exacerbation and remission occur. After chronic progression, cystoid macular degeneration and cataract reduce vision. In unilateral cases, sub-Tenon injections of corticosteroids are used. In cases that do not respond to treatment, transscleral cryotherapy of the inflamed uvea may be helpful.

Reticulum cell sarcoma is a bilateral lymphoma that simulates diffuse uveitis. There are yellow-white chorioretinal infiltrates and vitreous exudates. The disease occurs after 50 years of age and is exacerbated by corticosteroids and cytoxic agents. Brain disease (microgliomatosis) causes generalized nonlocalizing neurologic signs and dementia.

Diffuse reactive lymphoid hyperplasia of the uvea may cause cells and flare in the anterior chamber and cells in the vitreous humor. Additionally, there may be heterochromia iridis, glaucoma, choroidal thickening, and retinal detachment. Ultrasonography of the eye aids in diagnosis. The lesion is sensitive to radiation. Systemic lymphosarcoma rarely causes intraocular lesions.

Immunogenic uveitis

The cornea and lens, because of their avascularity, and the retina, because of the blood-retinal barriers, partake minimally in antigen-antibody reactions. However, the choroid, with its fenestrated capillaries, and the highly vascular perilimbal conjunctiva are susceptible to deposition of immune complexes, so that once stimulated, these tissues are able to form antibody in a manner analogous to a regional lymph node. The type of subsequent inflammation depends on whether B-lymphocytes or T-lymphocytes are involved.

Immunogenic uveitis. Microbes are rarely found within the eye in endogenous, nonsuppurative uveitis. In many instances, it seems likely that an antigen stimulates immunologically competent lymphocytes within the uvea. Further exposure to the same antigen results in an immune complex or cell-mediated inflammatory reaction of the uvea.

Intravenous administration of lipopolysaccharides (endotoxin) induces an acute anterior uveitis in rats or rabbits. The inflammatory response is prevented by pretreatment with indomethacin, which suggests that prostaglandins are involved. In rabbits immunized with bovine serum albumin, uveitis may be induced with a challenge dose of intravitreal endotoxin. After the uveitis resolves, intravenous bovine serum albumin reactivates a uveitis in the eye that received the intravitreal endotoxin. Immune complexes are deposited in the uveal tract.

An ocular antigen-antibody reaction is easily produced in laboratory animals and is described as immunogenic uveitis. It either is induced by systemic or ocular hypersensitivity to an antigen. The antigen selected is usually an animal serum albumin, whole blood, egg albumin, antitoxin, or a similarly well-defined protein. If the animal is sensitized by means of a systemically administered antigen, subsequent injection of the same antigen into the vitreous body causes a severe self-limited uveitis.

If the antigen is injected initially into the vitreous body, there is an immediate inflammatory response, presumably to the trauma of injection, which persists for several days and then subsides. A uveitis of several days' duration occurs 7 to 14 days later. This delayed inflammation can be prevented by whole-body x-radiation, but it is not prevented by x-radiation of the eye only. The uveitis is likely caused by the reaction of antibody to antigen that is still retained within the eye. Once the eye is sensitized, ocular or systemic administration of the same protein elicits a violent uveitis.

Soluble retinal antigen (S-antigen), purified from photoreceptor outer segments, injected at a distant site in a dose as low as 5 μg will provoke a severe uveitis in most laboratory species. Some patients (about 25%) with choroiditis affecting the retina have lymphocytes with a positive memory response to human retinal antigen.

Diagnostic measures

Frequently the etiologic factor is not actively sought in self-limited acute inflammations, because they respond readily to corticosteroids. When such inflammations are recurrent, as they often are, attention is usually directed to systemic diseases such as rheumatoid arthritis or infections of the genitourinary tract.

In chronic inflammations, the etiologic diagnosis is based on the ophthalmoscopic appearance of lesions in the diagnosis of toxoplasmosis and histoplasmosis. Sarcoid is sought in black patients.

In many patients the following diagnostic procedures are carried out: (1) VDRL or serum fluorescent treponemal antibody absorption test for syphilis; (2) chest roentgenograms that direct particular attention to primary tuberculosis, sarcoid, and histoplasmosis; (3) leukocyte and eosinophil count and sedimentation rate; (4) profiles for immunologic abnormalities occurring in connective tissue disorders; (5) skin testing with tuberculin to detect delayed hypersensitivity; (6) complement-fixation test for histoplasmosis (prior histoplasmin skin testing may increase the complement-fixation titer); (7) angiotensin-converting enzyme and lysozyme tests for sarcoid; (8) HLA-B27 testing; and (9) lumbosacral roentgenograms for ankylosing spondylitis. The medical history and systemic physical examination are often noncontributory. Physical examination is directed particularly to cutaneous and mucous membrane lesions, involvement of joints in arthritic lesions, and genitourinary tract infection.

Treatment

If possible, specific treatment is carried out. For inflammation of unknown cause that is confined to the iris and the ciliary body, the pupil is dilated and accommodation paralyzed by topical instillation of 1% atropine solution. Full pupillary dilation is desired to prevent posterior synechiae. Corticosteroid preparations are instilled at frequent intervals. Subconjunctival injections may be used. Ocular pressure must be measured regularly, and any increase treated with carbonic anhydrase inhibitors and topical beta blockers.

Systemic corticosteroids are the main treatment for posterior uveitis. Retrobulbar or sub-Tenon injection of corticosteroids and, rarely, systemic cytotoxic anti-inflammatory agents may be used. Early syphilitic inflammations respond readily to antibiotics. Tuberculosis responds to ethambutol and similar agents, but there are few cases in which they are indicated. Antibiotics are not administered empirically.

Cytotoxic agents may be used in patients in whom corticosteroids have failed in the hope of modifying some immune process. Cyclosporin A inhibits the development of uveitis in rats administered retinal S antigen. It has been effective in some patients with uveitis but nephrotoxicity may restrict its usefulness. Chlorambucil has long been used with variable results. Evaluation of therapy is difficult.

Complications

The tendency for inflammation of the uveal tract to extend to adjacent tissues leads to many complications. Often the complications lead to marked loss of vision.

Keratitis and keratopathy. Corneal involvement may occur in several ways. The corneal and anterior uvea may be nearly simultaneously inflamed in herpes simplex keratitis, herpes zoster ophthalmicus, and syphilitic interstitial keratitis. Iridocyclitis, sometimes with hemorrhage, is a late complication of severe herpes simplex keratitis.

Prolonged iridocyclitis damages the corneal endothelium, causing folds in Descemet membrane, haziness, and stromal and epithelial edema. Continued edema is followed by vascularization of the cornea.

Band keratopathy, in which there is a progressive deposition of calcium in the Bowman zone in a horizontal band across the cornea, often complicates uveitis in young persons. It has been described principally in pauciarticular juvenile rheumatoid arthritis (Still disease), but it also occurs in older individuals after severe ocular uveitis. The calcium may be removed with chelating agents, but if the cause is not eliminated, it recurs.

Intraocular pressure. Uveitis causes a hyposecretion of aqueous humor; the intraocular pressure is usually low. Glaucoma may occur by one of several mechanisms. Topical instillation of corticosteroids in genetically susceptible individuals increases resistance to outflow from the anterior chamber, as happens in open-angle glaucoma. The trabecular meshwork may be inflamed or may be occluded with inflammatory cells and protein in severe acute iridocyclitis. Repeated or prolonged inflammation damages the trabecular meshwork and leads to a permanent glaucoma that is similar to open-angle glaucoma.

Pupillary block by posterior synechiae causes an angle-closure glaucoma by preventing the passage of the aqueous humor from the posterior to the anterior chamber (iris bombé). Peripheral anterior synechiae may form between the iris and the cornea because of a shallow anterior chamber, exudate between the two structures, or edema of the root of the iris or ciliary body.

The treatment of glaucoma complicating uveitis requires a balance between measures directed against the increased intraocular pressure and those used to treat the inflammation. If increased intraocular pressure is caused by corticosteroids, their use is reduced. The pupil is not constricted. Carbonic anhydrase inhibitors are used systemically and often combined with the local instillation of epinephrine and topical beta blockers. In iris bombé, the ballooning iris may be opened by a laser iridotomy. Ocular surgical procedures that are necessary because of peripheral anterior synechiae or damage to the trabecular meshwork should be postponed until cessation of the inflammation.

Cataract. Systemic or topical corticosteroid administration for a long period, particularly in patients with rheumatoid arthritis, may cause posterior subcapsular cataracts identical to those caused by uveitis. The typical cataract in uveitis (complicated cataract) occurs in long-standing cyclitis and involves the subcapsular region of the posterior pole in a lens opacity that has many colors (polychromatic). In particularly severe cyclitis, the cataract may involve both the anterior and posterior subcapsular regions.

Cystoid macular edema. In this abnormality (see Chapter 16) the capillaries of the central retina become abnormally permeable with edema of the posterior pole. Vision is markedly reduced. A uveitis in the region of the ora serrata (peripheral uveitis, pars planitis, or cyclitis) is only one of the numerous causes of this abnormality.

Retinal detachment. Fibrovascular proliferation after exudation into the vitreous may create vitreous traction bands that detach the sensory retina. Severe effusion from the uveal tract may elevate the retina in a uveal effusion.

Two syndromes with chronic bilateral exudative uveitis that occur mainly in middle-aged Orientals are associated with retinal separation. In Vogt-Koyanagi syndrome, predominantly anterior uveitis is associated with vitiligo, alopecia, localized whiteness of the hair (poliosis), and deafness. The visual prognosis is poor. In Harada syndrome, the uveitis is posterior, retinal separation is more common, and meningeal irritation with increased cerebrospinal fluid protein level and pleocytosis occurs. Hearing defects are common, but skin and hair changes are rare. Prognosis is better than in Vogt-Koyanagi syndrome, but the two diseases may be combined.

Chorioretinitis may cause a periphlebitis in the overlying retinal veins. Peripheral sea-fan-shaped neovascularization similar to that seen in sickle cell disease may occur and cause secondary traction or rhegmatogenous retinal detachment.

Suppurative uveitis

Suppurative uveitis is caused mainly by pyogenic (pus-producing) bacteria and rarely by fungi (Table 15-5). In exogenous infection the organisms are introduced into the eye after an accidental or surgical penetrating wound, after rupture of a corneal ulcer, or through a cystic filtering bleb after glaucoma surgery. Endogenous septic emboli may infect the eye in bacterial endocarditis or during the bacteremic stage of meningococcic meningitis. Septicemia may follow surgical procedures performed elsewhere in the body, particularly genitourinary tract operations in the elderly. Common organisms include *Staphylococcus aureus*, *Bacillus subtilis*, *Pseudomonas aeruginosa*, *Proteus*, coliform bacilli, and fungi. The purulent inflammation is classified as either a panophthalmitis involving the vitreous cavity and all coats of the eye, including the sclera, or an endophthalmitis limited to the intraocular contents.

Panophthalmitis. Panophthalmitis is an acute suppurative inflammation of the inner eye with necrosis of the sclera, and sometimes the cornea, and extension of the inflammation into the orbit. The causes are mainly bacterial. The incubation period is only a few hours, and the disease follows an acute course. The eyelids are red and swollen, and there is severe chemosis of the conjunctiva. Extension to the orbit may cause proptosis. The cornea is often a whitish mass of necrotic tissue, and if there has been a laceration or surgical incision, pus exudes from the wound. There may be severe ocular pain, and the globe may rupture. The signs gradually subside, and the eye becomes a shrunken mass of fibrous tissue (phthisis bulbi).

Although it is often not successful, treatment must be prompt and vigorous. Because the causative organism and its antibiotic sensitivity are not known until culture, broad-spectrum antibiotics to which penicillinase-producing staphylococci and gram-negative bacteria are sensitive are used systemically, topically, subconjunctivally, and intraocularly. The pus from the wound, the aqueous humor, and the vitreous humor are stained and cultured. Initial treatment is based on the findings of the Gram stain, but in about half the patients no organism is found. A vitrectomy to remove microbes and leukocytes and passage through a Millipore filter may concentrate the organism for staining

Table 15-5. Suppurative uveitis

I. Exogenous
  A. Intraocular infection with pus-producing bacteria after accidental or surgical penetrating wound, rupture of corneal ulcer, or microbial invasion of intraocular filtering bleb after glaucoma surgery
II. Endogenous
  A. Septic emboli in bacterial endocarditis, meningococcemia, bacteremia, viremia, and fungemia; septic emboli after urologic surgery
  B. Spread from adjacent structure: orbital abscess, pharyngeal phycomycosis

and culture. Initial antibiotic therapy is modified as necessary on the basis of the cultured characteristics and antibiotic sensitivity of the organism. Systemic corticosteroids may reduce the fibroblastic response to inflammation.

Endophthalmitis. Endophthalmitis is a suppurative inflammation of the intraocular contents in which not all layers of the globe are affected and in which the eye does not rupture. Endophthalmitis follows penetrating wounds of the eye (either surgical or accidental), metastatic infections, or intraocular foreign bodies. The onset is less violent than that of panophthalmitis; the inflammation gradually increases in severity. Fungi, necrosis of intraocular tumors, and retained intraocular foreign bodies often cause a purulent endophthalmitis. Leukocytes may accumulate in the anterior chamber (hypopyon), and the vitreous body may be filled with inflammatory cells. Treatment is the same as for panophthalmitis.

INJURIES
Contusions

Contusion to the eye may cause a variety of injuries to the uvea: (1) rupture of the sphincter pupillae muscle, with a sector of the pupil unresponsive (iridoplegia); (2) iridodialysis, in which the root of the iris is torn from its insertion, causing an additional opening at the periphery of the iris and the pupil in the sector of the defect to become a chord rather than an arc; (3) hemorrhage into the anterior chamber (hyphema), vitreous, or both; (4) glaucoma; (5) choroidal hemorrhage; and (6) choroidal tears.

The ciliary body is seldom visibly involved. However, many hyphemas probably originate from a tearing of the ciliary body from the scleral spur with bleeding from the major arterial circle of the iris. Gonioscopy indicates a localized deepening (recession) of the anterior chamber angle.

Hemorrhage into the choroid varies from a small intrachoroidal hemorrhage to massive bleeding. When located in the choroid, the hemorrhagic area is a dark brown elevation with pink to red edges evident in retroillumination. Hemorrhagic areas frequently absorb slowly and leave a residue of mottled pigment in the retinal pigment epithelium with areas of hypopigmentation and hyperpigmentation.

Choroidal tears (Fig. 15-7) are a common result of severe contusions to the anterior segment of the eyeball. They occur most frequently on the temporal side of the fundus, are concentric with the optic disk, and usually located between the disk and the fovea centralis or temporal to the fovea centralis. They may be single or multiple. They probably result from stretching of the posterior choroid caused by compression of the eye, the temporal side being more vulnerable because of its greater extent and the blow being more commonly directed from the less protected temporal side.

The tears are crescentic, vertical, and of variable length. Hemorrhage into the choroid, subretinal area, or retina frequently accompanies a disruption of the tissue. As hemorrhage and edema absorb, the yellowish gray lesions become well defined. When the tear is between the optic disk and the fovea centralis, vision is usually reduced and disruption of the overlying sensory retina causes a nerve fiber bundle visual field defect. Tears of the choroid lateral to the fovea centralis may affect vision minimally.

Choroidal effusion

Choroidal effusion (choroidal edema, combined retinal-choroidal detachment) occurs frequently after intraocular surgery. Five to 15 days after the procedure, folds develop in Descemet membrane and the choroidal detachment causes a low intraocular pressure. Occasionally, leakage of aqueous humor from the corneoscleral wound causes hypotony. Through a widely dilated pupil, the detachment of the choroid appears as a dark gray-brown mass. Ophthalmoscopically, the detachment is a smooth, round swelling, extending hemispher-

ically into the vitreous cavity. The detachment may be single or multiple and usually is located in the inferior fundus anterior to the equator. The borders are dark and well defined.

Trauma combined with decreased intraocular pressure (hypotony) is required to produce choroidal detachment. The normal pressure relationships within the choroid are disturbed, producing a transudation of fluid in the suprachoroidal space and resulting in choroidal edema. The serous choroidal detachment often slowly recedes after the wound heals, and the injury from the surgical manipulation subsides. This may occur within several days or, occasionally, months. A small wound fistula that permits loss of aqueous humor is a common cause of a persistent serous choroidal detachment. If this cause can be excluded, the persistence may be caused by hemorrhage. The latter complication may take months to resorb or may persist, owing to organization of blood in the suprachoroidal space.

Lacerations

A laceration of the cornea may be followed immediately by prolapse of the iris into the wound. If the wound is small, the pupil is distorted and has a teardrop shape. If extensive, the entire iris may be prolapsed.

Prolapse of the ciliary body through a scleral or corneal laceration is particularly serious be-

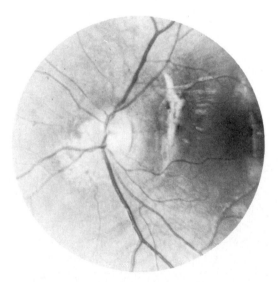

Fig. 15-7. Choroidal tears following blunt trauma to the anterior portion of the eye.

cause vitreous humor is lost and the zonule is damaged. Neglected prolapse of the ciliary body is more likely to cause a sympathetic ophthalmia than prolapse of other portions of the uveal tract.

TUMORS OF THE CHOROID
Malignant melanoma

The most common intraocular tumor is malignant melanoma of the choroid (Fig. 15-8). It usually occurs after puberty and increases in frequency between the ages of 30 and 70 years. Rare in blacks, it is slightly more common in women than men. Most eyes removed because of malignant melanoma contain benign nevi along the edges or within the tumor. These cells, however, may reflect the effects of tumor on the cells of the choroid. Most malignant melanomas of the uveal tract develop from preexisting benign melanomas commonly designated as nevi. Most benign melanomas never undergo malignant transformation. Malignant melanomas are found in approximately 10% of eyes blind from injury of inflammation, a finding that suggests that irritation may play a role in malignant transformation.

Malignant melanomas originate most frequently in the outer layers of the choroid and may spread carpetlike between the sclera and Bruch membrane. Tumors may remain quiescent for long periods and then without appar-ent reason suddenly begin rapid growth. With increase in size (Fig. 15-9), there may be globular growth inward. Eventually Bruch membrane perforates, and there is sudden growth of a mushroom or collar-button shape.

Symptoms and signs. The chief symptoms of malignant melanoma result from the nonrhegmatogenous retinal detachment caused by the increase in choroidal volume. Early metamorphopsia may be associated with macropsia or micropsia. This may be followed by a loss of visual field in the area corresponding to the area of the tumor. An overlying secondary serous retinal detachment causes more extensive visual field loss than would be anticipated from the size of the tumor. Glaucoma may occur late in the development of the tumor, but initially the tension is low because of decreased aqueous humor secretion. A malignant melanoma of the choroid must be considered as the cause of obscure intraocular inflammation, particularly when opaque media make it impossible to inspect the fundus. Ultrasonography and computed tomography aid in the diagnosis when the fundus cannot be seen.

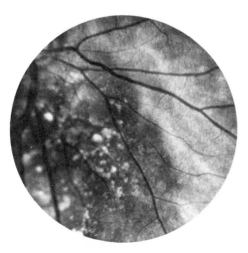

Fig. 15-8. Malignant melanoma of the choroid causing a solid retinal detachment. Numerous drusen are evident over the surface of the tumor.

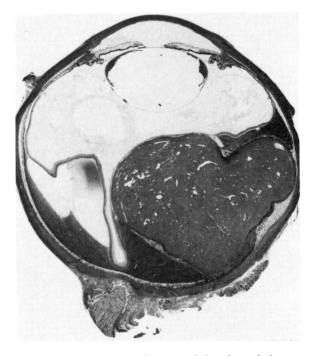

Fig. 15-9. Malignant melanoma of the choroid that has ruptured through the Bruch membrane into the eye. (Hematoxylin and eosin stain; ×5.)

Sudden loss of vision or rapid increase in the size of a mass over several days' time suggests that a lesion is not a malignant melanoma. A drawing of the tumor, with emphasis on its relationship to blood vessels, and photography with fluorescein angiography of the lesion may be helpful in making an exact diagnosis and in following slight increases in the size of the tumor. Physical examination, with particular attention to possible liver metastasis, should be done, although the presence of another malignancy does not exclude a primary ocular malignant melanoma. Neovascularization or vasodilation of episcleral vessels in the quadrant of involvement suggests a neoplasm, as does melanosis oculi. A vascularized mass on the sclera suggests an extraocular extension. Anesthesia of the cornea, partial paralysis of the iris, or dilated iris vessels occurring in the sector of tumor involvement and vitreous hemorrhage have been noted in some cases.

Ophthalmoscopy indicates a retinal detachment of grayish brown color. The pigmentation is distinctly lighter than the jet-black color seen in inflammatory retinal proliferation. Pigment spots of light orange pigmentation (lipofuscin) may occur over the detachment. Drusen may be scattered superficially. The retina is smoothly elevated, usually without a break, and has little tendency to form traction folds. There may be two areas of detachment, seemingly not connected. With increase in size a malignant melanoma becomes more distinct, but with inflammation the lesion becomes less distinct. Bed rest does not reduce the extent of the detachment in malignant melanoma.

Vessels on the retinal surface not associated with the retinal vasculature are suggestive of tumor. Hemorrhage is uncommon except when large necrotic tumors break through Bruch membrane.

Biomicroscopy of the fundus by using a Goldmann or Hruby lens with the pupil fully dilated provides retinal details. Cystoid degeneration of the overlying retina suggests a malignant melanoma. Cells in the vitreous body and an indistinct retina suggest an inflammatory lesion, unless a necrotic tumor has broken through Bruch membrane. Ophthalmoscopic study of the border of an elevated lesion may show a reddish or pink halo, indicating a hemorrhage rather than a tumor.

Visual field studies are valuable in differentiating between a benign and a malignant melanoma. Usually the choriocapillaris is intact when a benign melanoma is present; either there is no field defect or the defect is proportionate to the size of the lesion. In malignant melanoma, the defect is larger and progressive. A hemangioma causes a sector-shaped field defect.

After intravenous injection of sodium fluorescein, most malignant melanomas of the choroid begin to fluoresce slightly before or during the retinal arterial phase. Their fluorescence increases in intensity, and staining of the tumor may persist for 45 to 60 minutes after injection. Metastatic tumors of the choroid and hemangiomas may have a similar hyperfluorescence. Sometimes hemorrhage or pigment overlying a malignant melanoma will prevent visualization of the fluorescence.

Simultaneous A- and B-scan display (Fig. 15-10) is helpful in the diagnosis of choroidal neoplasms. When the A-scan ultrasonic beam strikes the tumor, high-amplitude echoes are reflected from the anterior boundary of the mass. As the beam traverses the tumor, there is a steep decay in the amplitude of the echo in malignant melanomas. The B-scan display shows a smooth convex tumor surface with an echo-free area appearing within the depth of the melanoma and a characteristic apparent excavation of the tumor and sclera posteriorly.

Measurement of the uptake of radioactive phosphorus may be helpful in the differential diagnosis of choroidal but not iris malignant melanomas. Usually measurements are made 48 hours after the administration of the isotope. The lesion is accurately localized and the probe placed directly over it by using a conjunctival incision if necessary. A difference of more than 100% in the number of counts over the tumor and over a normal area of the same eye is considered positive. The test is less helpful in differentiating small, malignant melanomas from nevi, melanocytomas, metastatic carcinomas, and uveal inflammation.

The eye should be evaluated by fundus photography, fluorescein angiography, A- and B-scan ultrsonography, ophthalmoloscopy, and perimetry.

The single most important clinical prognostic factor is the size of the tumor. If the largest

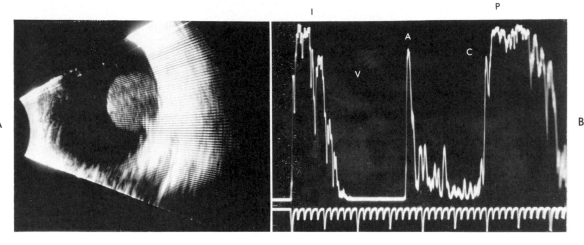

Fig. 15-10. A, B-scan echogram of a melanoma of the choroid. **B,** A-scan of the same melanoma. *I* is the initial spike that corresponds to the surface of the eye opposite the tumor; *V* corresponds to the vitreous; *A* indicates the anterior tumor surface; and *P* indicates the posterior surface on the inner surface of the sclera. The small spike at *C* is the interface between the tumor proper and the infiltrated cornea. (Courtesy Prof. Karl C. Ossoinig, M.D., The University of Iowa.)

tumor diameter in contact with the sclera is 10 mm or less (6⅔ disk diameters), the mortality is 13%, but if the size exceeds 12 mm, the mortality is 70%.

Patients with tumors composed of epithelioid cells, or epithelioid cells with spindle cell A or B, or with necrotic tumor have a grave prognosis. Such patients may benefit from nonspecific stimulation of the immune system by means of methanol extracted residue (MER) of BCG (bacillus Calmette-Guérin) or interferon. Spindle cell A tumors have the best prognosis.

Treatment. The appropriate treatment of malignant melanoma of the choroid is debated. The topic is complicated by inability to provide histologic diagnosis in eyes that are treated and not removed. Previously, survival studies were marred by an excessive loss to follow-up and inability to learn the immediate cause of death. Generally the size of the tumor, its location in the eye, and the absence of metastatic disease govern the type of treatment.

Small (up to 10 mm in diameter and 3 mm in height) tumors may be followed each 6 months for evidence of growth, using ultrasonography to measure the height of the tumor and fluorescein angiography to document its size. Most choroidal melanomas confined to the eye have little tendency to grow and no ten-

dency to metastasize. In the event of growth, a peripheral tumor may be treated by means of laser photocoagulation, by means of a radioactive plaque attached to the overlying sclera, or by using proton external beam radiation, or helium ion radiation. Tumors located in the anterior portion of the eye have less malignant potential than tumors located in the posterior portion of the eye. Some tumors of the anterior choroid may be removed by a resection of the sclera and the underlying tumor.

Eyes that contain large tumors or blind painful eyes require enucleation. Every effort must be made not to put pressure upon the eye during surgery. Once the ocular blood supply is isolated, the tumor is frozen through the sclera by means of liquid nitrogen, which is applied intermittently so as not to freeze the orbit, and the eye is removed.

The liver is usually the first and often the sole site of metastasis from uveal tract melanoma. Every patient in whom enucleation is contemplated should have radioactive isotope liver scanning and serum enzyme testing (alkaline phosphatase, lactate dehydrogenase, and gamma glutaryl transpeptidase) to exclude metastasis. Equivocal results may require hepatic arteriography or peritonoscopy and biopsy of suspicious nodules.

Choroidal nevi

Nevi of the choroid or ciliary body occur in about 30% of white individuals, are multiple in one eye in about 7%, and bilateral in about 4%. Often (55%) there are iris freckles or nevi in the same eye. Nevi are oval or circular in outline, vary from 0.5 to 4 disk diameters in size, and occur most commonly at the posterior half of the fundus. The lesion is sharply demarcated from the surrounding fundus, but the contrast between the melanoma and the adjacent choroid may be so slight that careful ophthalmoscopic examination is necessary for detection. The lesion usually becomes pigmented between 6 and 10 years of age.

The tumor varies in color from "slate gray" to "blue ointment." The choroidal pattern can easily be seen encircling the tumor. Since nevi do not involve the choriocapillaris layer, there is usually no visual field defect, as there is with malignant melanoma. Treatment is not indicated.

Hemangiomas

Hemangiomas (angiomas) of the choroid are rare and are associated in about one half of individuals affected with skin angioma (nevus flammeus), frequently in the region innervated by the first or second branch of the trigeminal nerve. The Stürge-Weber syndrome consists of intracranial angiomas, nevus flammeus, and glaucoma. A number of variants may occur. Glaucoma develops in some 30% of those affected. The glaucoma may develop before the age of 2 years (60%) with buphthalmos and a chamber angle malformation resembling that seen in congenital glaucoma. The glaucoma develops in the remaining patients (40%) in late childhood and early adulthood and resembles chronic open-angle glaucoma. Neurologic signs may occur occasionally; the hemangiomas are then a manifestation of the Sturge-Weber syndrome.

Choroidal hemangiomas vary in size from 2 to 17 mm in diameter and from 1 to 9 mm in thickness. They may increase slowly in thickness, causing a progressive hyperopia when the hemangioma involves the posterior pole. Rarely, both eyes may be involved in a similar process.

Metastatic carcinoma

The breast and lung in women and the lung in men are the most common primary sites of tumors that metastasize to the choroid. Other sites are uncommon in women. In men, tumors in the kidney, testicle, and prostate gland may metastasize to the choroid. Choroidal metastases are fairly common in the terminal stages of malignant disease; however, patients are so ill that the diagnosis is not made. Both eyes are affected with equal frequency. Involvement of the choroid in preference to the retina may reflect the larger number of blood vessels that go to the choroid from the ophthalmic artery.

Metastasis to the choroid leads to an overlying serous retinal detachment, which causes loss of vision in the area of involvement. The posterior segment is most often involved, and early loss of central vision occurs. The ophthalmoscopic appearance is characteristic. There is a yellow-orange elevation of the retinal pigment epithelium and an overlying serous retinal detachment with sharp delineation and no retinal breaks. There may be rapid growth of the tumor anteriorly, but usually there is a rim of undetached retina between the tumor and the periphery.

The diagnosis depends mainly upon an accurate history and careful physical examination. The primary malignancy may have been resected from months to years before the onset of symptoms. There may be no evidence of metastasis elsewhere in the body, but commonly osteolytic or pulmonary lesions can be demonstrated.

Treatment of a metastatic malignancy to the choroid must be directed to the primary disease. In tumors that are not hormone-dependent, the ocular treatment is related to the life expectancy and whether both eyes are involved. Enucleation is not indicated. Radiotherapy with a tumor dose of 2,500 to 3,500 r may be used, with appropriate precautions to protect the lens. The adult lens is so resistant to radiation that cataract formation will probably not be a problem because of the limited life expectancy of the patient. If the metastasis is binocular and the patient is not within the final weeks of life, radiotherapy may be carried out on both eyes.

CILIARY BODY TUMORS

Tumors of the ciliary body may involve the pigmented or nonpigmented epithelium or the stroma. The epithelium may be involved in a variety of uncommon types of hyperplasia or in a neoplastic process, medulloblastoma. The stromal tumors are essentially the same as those of the choroid, and malignant melanoma is the predominating type. A leiomyoma may originate from muscle cells.

Malignant melanomas

Malignant melanomas of the ciliary body (Fig. 15-11) are less frequent than malignant melanomas of the choroid. They tend to extend to the choroid, the iris, or both. They may follow the course of the major arterial circle of the iris and spread in a ring around the ciliary body. Because of their location, symptoms are minimal, and diagnosis may be delayed until the tumor causes a serous retinal detachment or extends to the anterior chamber. The mass may be seen by indirect ophthalmoscopy or gonioscopy.

Since melanomas of the ciliary body have a low degree of malignancy, resection rather than enucleation is often indicated.

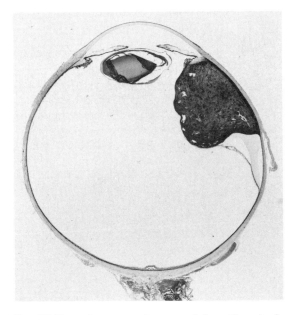

Fig. 15-11. Malignant melanoma of the ciliary body that has detached the peripheral retina. (Hematoxylin and eosin stain; ×4.)

Medulloepithelioma (diktyoma)

Intraocular medulloepitheliomas are embryonal neuroepithelial tumors that originate from the embryonic or developing nonpigmented epithelium of the ciliary body. They are divided into medulloepithelioma and teratoid medulloepithelioma (heteroplasia with hyaline cartilage, cerebral tissue, and skeletal muscle). They are further divided into benign and malignant forms. They are unilateral and nearly always occur in children. Enucleation is done at a median age of 5 years (range 1 to 43 years). There may be poor vision and pain. There may be a white pupil, a mass in the iris, anterior chamber, or ciliary body, glaucoma, cataract, iritis, and rubeosis iridis. Local excision is preferred, but commonly the tumor reaches large size before producing symptoms and requires enucleation.

Leiomyoma of the ciliary muscle

Leiomyoma of the ciliary muscle is an uncommon neoplasm that requires electron microscopy to differentiate it from an amelanotic spindle cell melanoma. It also may occur in the iris musculature.

Ciliary body cysts

Ciliary body cysts form in the nonpigmented epithelium of the pars plana and pars plicata. Those in the pars plicata contain proliferated nonpigmented epithelium and a watery substance. Cysts of the pars plicata contain hyaluronic acid. In multiple myeloma, cysts may occur in either location and contain IgG.

TUMORS OF THE IRIS

There is considerable variation in the amount of pigment in the anterior stroma of the iris. About half of all whites have pigment flecks on the surface of the iris that are of no pathologic significance. Histologically they occur because of increased pigmentation of melanocytes that do not proliferate.

An iris nevus consisting of a slightly elevated, localized, discrete, pigmented mass (Fig. 15-12) is composed of proliferated melanocytes. They may be associated with peripheral anterior synechiae in the iris-nevus syndrome. Iris nevi are associated with neurofibromatosis and malignant melanoma of the choroid and cil-

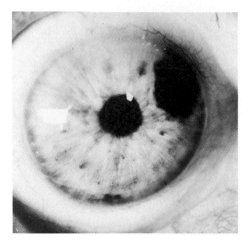

Fig. 15-12. Benign melanoma of the iris. There are freckles in the interior portion of the iris.

iary body. These nevi (benign melanomas) are not progressive and do not distort the pupil.

Malignant melanomas of the iris are predominantly spindle A type and do not metastasize. Mixed spindle cell and epithelial cell tumors metastasize, a complication favored by incomplete excision. A pigmented tumor that increases in size may be difficult to diagnose clinically. Inflammatory nodules, iris cysts, metastatic tumors, lymphoid tumors, and iris abscesses have all been mistaken for malignant melanoma. Fluorescein angiography of the iris defines the tumor limits for follow-up evaluation but is of uncertain value in differentiating malignant from benign lesions.

Juvenile xanthogranuloma is a skin disorder with yellowish-orange accumulations of histiocytes in the dermis layer. Infiltration of the iris causes a glaucoma and spontaneous bleeding into the anterior chamber (hyphema).

BIBLIOGRAPHY

Anirida

Nelson, L.B., Spaeth, G.L., Nowinski, T.S., Margo, C.E., and Jackson, L.: Aniridia: a review, Surv. Ophthalmol. **28**:621, 1984.

Solomon, E.: Recessive mutation in aetiology of Wilms' tumor, Nature **309**:111, 1984.

Coloboma

Pagon, R.A., Graham, J.M., Jr., Zonana, J., and Yong, S.-L.: Coloboma, congenital heart disease, and choanal atresia with multiple anomalies: CHARGE association, J. Pediatr. **99**:223, 1981.

Gyrate atrophy

Kaiser-Kupfer, M.I., Ludwig, I.H., de Monasterio, F.M., Valle, D., and Krieger, I.: Gyrate atrophy of the choroid and retina: early findings, Ophthalmology **92**:394, 1985.

Iridocorneal syndrome

Kupfer, C., Kaiser-Kupfer, M.I., Datiles, M., and McCain, L.: The contralateral eye in the iridocorneal endothelial (ICE) syndrome, Ophthalmology **90**:1343, 1983.

Rodrigues, M.M., Stulting, R.D., and Waring, G.O. III: Clinical, electron microscopic, and immunohistochemical study of the corneal endothelium and Descemet's membrane in the iridocorneal endothelial syndrome, Am. J. Ophthalmol. **101**:16, 1986.

Uveitis

Chan, C.-C., BenEzra, D., Hsu, S.-M., Palestine, A.G., and Nussenblatt, R.B.: Granulomas in sympathetic ophthalmia and sarcoidosis, Arch. Ophthalmol. **103**:198, 1985.

Jakobiec, F.A., Marboe, C.C., Knowles, D.M. II, Iwamoto, T., Harrison, W., Chang, S., and Coleman, D.J.: Human sympathetic ophthalmia: an analysis of the inflammatory infiltrate by hybridoma-monoclonal antibodies, immunochemistry, and correlative electron microscopy, Ophthalmology **90**:76, 1983.

Lyon, C.E., Grimson, B.S., Peiffer, R.L., Jr., and Merritt, J.C.: Clinicopathologic correlation of a solitary choroidal tuberculoma, Ophthalmology **92**:845, 1985.

Michaelson, J.B., Chisari, F.V., and Kansu, T.: Antibodies to oral mucosa in patients with ocular Behçet's disease, Ophthalmology **92**:1277, 1985.

Nussenblatt, R.B., Palestine, A.G., and Chan, C.-C.: Cyclosporin A therapy in the treatment of intraocular inflammatory disease resistant to systemic corticosteroids and cytotoxic agents, Am. J. Ophthalmol. **96**:275, 1983.

O'Connor, G.R.: Factors related to the initiation and recurrence of uveitis, Am. J. Ophthalmol. **96**:557, 1983.

Reynard, M., Riffenburg, R.S., and Maes, E.F.: Effect of corticosteroid treatment and enucleation on the visual prognosis of sympathetic ophthalmia, Am. J. Ophthalmol. **96**:96, 1983.

Uveal tumors

Brownstein, S., Barsoum-Homsy, M., Conway, V.H., Sales, C., and Condon, G.: Nonteratoid medulloepithelioma of the ciliary body, Ophthalmology **91**:1118, 1984.

Cantrill, H.L., Cameron, J.D., Ramsay, R.C., and

Knobloch, W.H.: Retinal vascular changes in malignant melanoma of the choroid, Am. J. Ophthalmol. **97**:411, 1984.

Coleman, D.J., and Lizzi, F.L.: Computerized ultrasonic tissue characterization of ocular tumors, Am. J. Ophthalmol. **96**:165, 1983.

Folberg, R., McLean, I.W., and Zimmerman, L.E.: Conjunctival melanosis and melanoma, Ophthalmology **91**:673, 1984.

Gamei, J.W., and McLean, I.W.: Modern developments in histopathologic assessment of uveal melanomas, Ophthalmology **91**:679, 1984.

Gass, D.M.: Comparison of prognosis after enucleation vs cobalt 60 irradiation of melanomas, Arch. Ophthalmol. **103**:6, 1985.

Gass, D.M.: Comparison of uveal melanoma growth rates with mitotic index and mortality, Arch. Ophthalmol. **103**:4, 1985.

Geisse, L.J., and Robertson, D.M.: Iris melanomas, Am. J. Ophthalmol. **99**:638, 1985.

McLean, I.W., Foster, W.D., and Zimmerman, L.E.: Modifications of Callender's classification of uveal melanoma at the Armed Forces Institute of Pathology, Am. J. Ophthalmol. **96**:502, 1983.

Seddon, J.M., Gragoudas, E.S., Albert, D.M., Hsieh, C.-C., Polivogianis, L., and Friedenberg, G.R.: Comparison of survival rates for patients with uveal melanoma after treatment with proton beam irradiation or enucleation, Am. J. Ophthalmol. **99**:282, 1985.

Shields, J.A.: Diagnosis and management of intraocular tumors, St. Louis, 1983, The C.V. Mosby Co.

Tse, D.T., Dutton, J.J., Weingeist, T.A., Hermsen, V.M., and Kersten, R.C.: Hematoporphyrin photoradiation therapy for intraocular and orbital melanoma, Arch. Ophthalmol. **102**:833, 1984.

16

THE RETINA

The invagination of the lateral optic vesicles in embryonic life forms the double-walled secondary optic vesicles, or optic cups. The inner wall forms the light-sensitive sensory retina. The outer wall thins to a single layer, the retinal pigment epithelium. The photosensitive pigment molecules located in the disks of the rod and cone outer segments absorb light that passes through the transparent inner portion of the sensory retina (*inner*, nearer the vitreous cavity; *outer*, nearer the choriocapillaris). The light converts 11-*cis*-retinal of the pigment molecule to an all-*trans* configuration. This process initiates a graded potential that is modulated and amplified in the retina and transmitted to the brain as spike discharges. Axons of the rods and cones synapse with bipolar and horizontal cells that have their cell bodies in the inner nuclear layer. Bipolar and amacrine cells synapse with each other and with ganglion cells. The axons of ganglion cells form the nerve fiber layer of the sensory retina and pass in the optic nerve to synapse in the lateral geniculate body (visual) or the pretectal region (pupil).

The retinal pigment epithelium lines the outer sensory retina. The outer segments are enmeshed in the pigment epithelium microvilli. The disks of the outer segments are continuously renewed by their cell bodies, and clumps of the oldest disks are phagocytized by the retinal pigment epithelium. If this phagocytosis stops, the sensory retina degenerates.

The sensory retina may be divided into a central portion (macula), which contains the fovea centralis that functions in photopic vision, and into four peripheral quadrants that function in spatial orientation and scotopic vision. The central retina, located between the superior and inferior temporal vessels, extends temporally from the optic disk to about 2 disk diameters lateral to the fovea centralis. It contains the fovea centralis, a pit in the retina in which the innermost layers of the sensory retina are displaced so that light falls directly upon the cone photoreceptors without transversing the inner retinal layers. The foveola at the center of the fovea centralis contains only cones. The clinical and anatomic names (Table 16-1) for these areas are sometimes used interchangeably. The fovea centralis functions in bright illumination (photopic vision), form vision, and color vision. Rod photoreceptors are most common in the peripheral quadrants and function in dim illumination (scotopic vision).

The blood supply to the retina in humans is derived from two sources: (1) the choriocapillaris, which nurtures the retinal pigment epithelium and the outer portion of the sensory retina adjacent to the choroid, and (2) the branches of the central retinal artery, which supply the inner half of the retina. Both systems are necessary for retinal function.

The central retinal artery is a medium-sized artery that branches from the ophthalmic artery immediately after its entry into the orbit; consequently, its intravascular pressure is high. The central retinal artery within the optic nerve has the usual three layers of intima, me-

Table 16-1. Clinical and anatomic terminology of the central retina

Anatomic terms	Clinical terms
Area centralis	Posterior pole, macula
Fovea centralis (1.5 mm)	Macula
Foveola (350 μm)	Fovea

dia, and adventitia, with well-developed elastic and muscular components. As the artery passes through the lamina cribrosa to enter the eye, the internal elastic lamina is reduced to a single layer and is entirely lost after the first or second bifurcation. Within the eye the muscle of the medial coat of the arterioles is markedly decreased, although contractile elements persist as far as the precapillary arterioles.

The arterioles and veins of the retina share a common adventitial sheath at their crossings. A similar anatomic arrangement is seen elsewhere only in the afferent and efferent arteries of the glomerulus. The common adventitial sheath anatomically causes some branch retinal vein occlusions and is the cause of venous sclerosis at arteriovenous crossings.

SYMPTOMS

The main symptom of retinal abnormalities is visual disturbance without pain. Disorders that predominantly affect peripheral (rod) function are associated with night blindness (impaired vision in reduced illumination) or impaired peripheral vision. Disorders of foveal (cone) function result in reduced visual acuity and impaired color vision. Opacities of the ocular media that impair image formation at the fovea centralis depress vision generally. Localized disturbances in the fovea centralis, such as hemorrhage, edema, deposits, or tumors, may cause a metamorphopsia, such as micropsia (small images) or macropsia (large images).

Traction on the retina may cause photopsia, which consists of sparks, rings, lightning flashes, or luminous bodies observed when the eyes are closed. Unlike visual hallucinations originating from lesions in the temporal or occipital lobes, photopsia does not involve both eyes simultaneously. Frequently the patient is unaware of retinal disease, and the abnormality is detected by means of functional testing or ophthalmoscopic examination.

FUNCTION

Five main factors determine the functions of the sensory retina: (1) visual acuity (the form sense), (2) dark adaptation, (3) color vision, (4) central and peripheral visual fields, and (5) electroretinography. The function of the retinal pigment epithelium is inferred from electro-oculography.

To exclude refractive errors as a cause of decreased vision, visual acuity must be measured while the patient is wearing appropriate lenses for the distance of vision being tested. Measurement of dark adaptation is a sensitive index of the synthesis of photopigments, particularly rhodopsin, in the rods. The common types of hereditary defects in color perception are transmitted as X chromosome-linked recessive defects, and affected individuals have good visual acuity. In most patients with acquired central retinal lesions, such as central retinal (macular) degeneration, the defect in color perception parallels the reduction in visual acuity. Some individuals may have marked impairment of color vision, decreased visual acuity, and nystagmus transmitted as an autosomal recessive condition (achromatopsia); others may be born with normal color vision but develop hereditary types of cone degenerations heralded by characteristic impairment in color perception and in the photopic electroretinogram. Parietal lobe disorders may impair color-naming ability and sometimes color perception.

Measurement of the central visual field tests the retinal function within 30° from the fixation point. Measurement of the peripheral field is less sensitive and determines the function of the entire retina. Since the optic nerve is composed of axons of the ganglion cells that form the nerve fiber layer of the retina, optic nerve disease may cause many of the same symptoms as retinal disease.

Electroretinography measures the action potential evoked by light stimulation of the retina. Because this is a mass response, it may be normal when retinal lesions are focal.

Electro-oculography measures the standing potential between the cornea and the retina. A decrease in the ratio between the response in the light- and dark-adapted retina indicates a disorder of the retinal pigment epithelium.

OPHTHALMOSCOPIC FINDINGS

The retina is examined with a direct or indirect ophthalmoscope or with a biomicroscope and a concave lens to neutralize corneal refraction. The main abnormalities of the fundus that are visible ophthalmoscopically include: (1) disturbances of the blood vessels, (2) opacities of the sensory retina, including hemorrhages, exudates, edema residues, cotton-wool patches, and vascular and glial tissue proliferation, (3) disturbances in the position of the sensory retina in rhegmatogenous (with hole formation) and nonrehegmatogenous (without hole formation) retinal detachment, (4) derangements of the retinal pigment epithelium, and (5) abnormalities of Bruch membrane and choroid.

Disturbances of blood vessels

The skilled observer constantly changes the focus of the direct ophthalmoscope to permit better definition of the size, shape, and depth of lesions. When viewed with an ophthalmoscope, the normal sensory retina is transparent, except for the blood vessels. The major retinal vessels are located in the nerve fiber layer, and the capillary plexuses are in this layer and the inner nuclear layer. Occlusive disease of the blood vessels affects mainly the inner layers of the retina. New blood vessels form on the inner (vitreal) surface of the retina, the surface of the optic nerve, and between the retinal pigment epithelium and the choroid.

The retinal blood vessels are normally transparent tubes through which the contained blood is visible with an ophthalmoscope. The oxygenated blood in the artery is brighter red than the blood in the veins, and the medial coat of the artery reflects light and causes a white reflex paralleling the axis of the vessel. Because retinal vessels lack direct nervous innervation, their constriction and dilation are based on autoregulation (intravascular resistance-pressure and PCO_2). The endothelial cells lining the retinal vessels are nonfenestrated and tightly joined. These vessels provide a portion of the blood-retina barrier that is similar to the blood-brain barrier. The retinal blood vessels are susceptible to the same diseases as blood vessels elsewhere in the body; but because their intravascular pressure must exceed the intraocular pressure to prevent collapse,

they form a highly specialized vascular bed without counterpart elsewhere.

Vascular pulsation. Visible pulsation of arteries or veins occurs when the intraocular pressure equals the pressure within the vessel. The normal pulsation of the central retinal vein is best seen on the surface of the optic disk. It is synchronous with the heart, and it comes from transmitted central retinal artery pulsation. If the venous pulsation cannot be detected, gentle pressure upon the globe will elicit it. Venous pulsation is absent and cannot be elicited in impending central vein closure; it usually cannot be elicited in papilledema.

Spontaneous arterial pulsation is always pathologic. It occurs when the intraocular pressure is equal to the diastolic blood pressure (in glaucoma) and in aortic regurgitation, in which there is a high pulse pressure. It may be elicited by pressure on the globe as is done diagnostically in ophthalmodynamometry.

Venous dilation. Increased venous pressure, markedly decreased intraocular pressure, or hyperviscosity of the blood causes dilated veins. Tortuosity increases because the vessel wall widens in three dimensions. Thus, dilated veins are visible in diabetes mellitus at any stage, in papilledema, in impending or partial closure of the central retinal vein, in vascular tumors of the retinal blood vessels, and in hyperviscosity blood syndromes.

Neovascularization. New blood vessels originating from retinal veins may carpet the inner (vitreal) surface of the sensory retina or optic disk or extend into the vitreous cavity. New blood vessels originating from the choriocapillaris may extend between the choriocapillaris and the retinal pigment epithelium and between the retinal pigment epithelium and the sensory retina.

Retinal neovascularization requires a diseased retina combined with a disturbed vascular bed; new vessels form predominantly from the venous side of circulation. The stimulus is presumably a diffusible factor because new vessels may be stimulated to form on the optic disk and iris. The vitreous humor also contains a factor that normally inhibits neovascularization. The new vessels consist of fenestrated endothelial tubes that leak protein and tend to bleed. Some new blood vessels on the iris, disk, and retina distant from sites of treatment may disappear after retinal photocoagulation, possibly because of removal of an angiogenic factor. Subretinal neovascularization originating from the choriocapillaris occurs after defects in Bruch membrane.

Neovascularization of the retina is seen in a variety of conditions in which the circulation is impaired: stasis caused by hyperviscosity of the blood or decreased flow, vascular occlusion (particularly venous closure), sickle cell trait (SC), inflammation, Eales disease, familial exudative vitreoretinopathy, talc emboli, sarcoidosis, diabetes mellitus, and retinopathy of prematurity. The first arteriovenous crossing in the superior temporal quadrant is the most vulnerable area, followed in turn by the inferior temporal quadrant, the superior nasal quadrant, and the inferior nasal quadrant. In conditions associated with retinal neovascularization, preexisting vascular channels located within the sensory retina may dilate, resulting in many more visible vascular channels. New blood vessels may extend along the inner surface of the retina. They may grow into the vitreous cavity as a network of endothelial channels (rete mirabile) with supporting tissue (proliferative retinopathy).

Subretinal neovascular membranes. New blood vessels originating in the choriocapillaris and developing between Bruch membrane and the retinal pigment epithelium and subsequently between the retinal pigment epithelium and the sensory retina cause visual loss in retinal drusen, disciform macular degeneration, angoid streaks, degenerative myopia, and presumed ocular histoplasmosis. These vascular membranes may occur in any part of the fundus, but are particularly common beneath the fovea centralis where a hemorrhage, which occurs in about two thirds of the cases, severely impairs vision.

The initial event is formation of a hole in Bruch membrane. Plasma from the choriocapillaris results in its separation from the retinal pigment epithelium. A capillary then extends from the choriocapillaris to the region between Bruch membrane and the retinal pigment epithelium. A defect in the retinal pigment epithelium permits the new blood vessels to proliferate between the pigment epithelium and

sensory retina. Hemorrhage into the sensory retina is followed by fibrous metaplasia of the retinal pigment epithelium. This obliterates the capillary network but causes the fibrous scar of disciform degeneration. If the fovea centralis is affected, final vision is 20/200 or less.

The membrane appears as a dark green circular or oval area. There may be a ring of pigment (Fig. 16-1, A). The overlying retina may be detached, infiltrated with hard yellow deposits, or swollen with cystoid edema. Blood in the sensory retina is bright red, crescent shaped, and located at the outer edge of the neovascular membrane. Fluorescein angiography demonstrates the network of new blood vessels derived from the choriocapillaris and not the retinal blood vessels (Fig. 16-1, B-D). Fluorescein leakage may be marked in the late phases of angiography.

Photocoagulation of the initial break and retinal pigment epithelium detachment may prevent neovascularization. The break must not be beneath the fovea centralis or photocoagulation will itself impair central vision. Once neovascularization starts, the entire membrane must be effectively photocoagulated because partial coagulation stimulates proliferation of additional blood vessels.

Hemorrhage. Hemorrhages within the retina assume different shapes, depending on the layer in which they occur. Preretinal hemorrhages (Fig. 16-2) occur between the retina and the vitreous body. They are characteristically large with a tendency to meniscus formation because the blood is not clotted and is only loosely restricted. Flame-shaped hemorrhages (Fig. 16-3) occur at the level of the nerve fiber layer and tend to parallel the course of the nerve fibers in the region of the retina where they occur. Round hemorrhages originate from the deep capillaries of the retina. They are confined by Müller cells to the outer nuclear layer and the fibers of the inner and outer plexiform layers. Hemorrhages in the sensory layer of the retina initially are a bright red and tend to become yellow as they slowly absorb. Hemorrhage between the choriocapillaris and retinal pigment epithelium is dark brown, well circumscribed, and sometimes elevated and may simulate a neoplasm. The blood may rupture into the sensory retina and appear as a bright red crescent at the margin of the subretinal neovascular membrane. Hemorrhage may occur in the retinal pigment epithelium and burst in the sensory retina, often with a bright red crescent-shaped hemorrhage at the edge of the lesion.

Retinal and subhyaloid (preretinal) hemorrhages occur in 15% of the adults and almost 70% of the young children with subarachnoid and subdural hemorrhage. The mortality in individuals with intraocular hemorrhages exceeds 50% in contrast to a mortality of about 20% in those without such hemorrhages. Mortality is higher in those with bilateral intraocular hemorrhages (58%) than in those with uniocular hemorrhage (48%). Usually the hemorrhages absorb without sequelae. However, when they break into the vitreous, they cause the same complications as other intravitreal bleeding.

Retinal hemorrhages occur because of an abnormality between the blood pressure within a vessel and the ocular pressure surrounding it, abnormalities of the blood vessel wall, retinal and subretinal neovascularization, diseases of

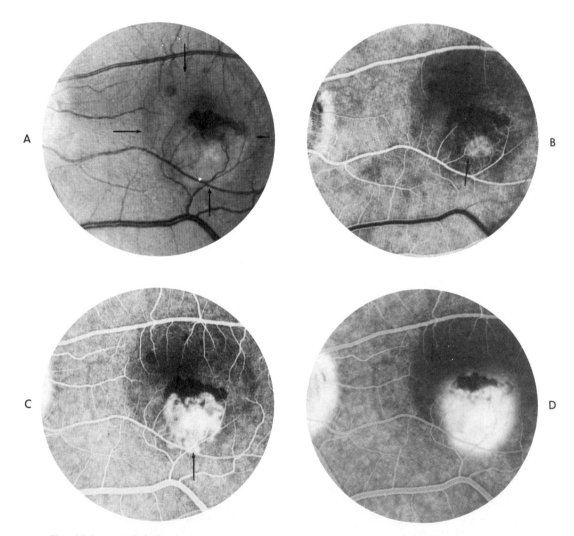

Fig. 16-1. A, Ophthalmoscopic appearance of subretinal neovascular membrane in presumed ocular histoplasmosis. There is hemorrhage into the sensory retina above the membrane and there is marked retinal edema *(arrows).* **B,** A fine tracery of choroidal blood vessels appears *(arrow)* beneath the sensory retina early in fluorescein angiography. **C,** The blood vessels of the network *(arrow)* are filled with fluorescein. **D,** At 90 seconds, the neovascular membrane leaks fluorescein.

the blood, or vitreous traction on the blood vessel. Ocular causes include trauma, vascular obstruction, and vasculitis. Systemic causes include diabetes mellitus, hypertension, and blood dyscrasias. A preretinal hemorrhage adjacent to the optic disk may be a sign of subarachnoid hemorrhage or glaucoma.

Microaneurysms. Microaneurysms are a common retinal abnormality. Large numbers form in diabetes mellitus, and these are char-

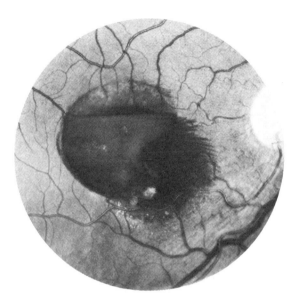

Fig. 16-2. Preretinal hemorrhage in macular region. A meniscus of blood forms when the head is erect.

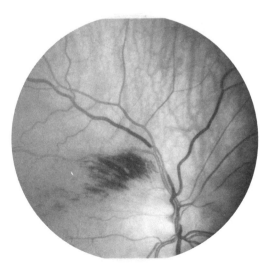

Fig. 16-3. Flame-shaped hemorrhage in the nerve fiber layer of the retina.

acteristically on the venous side of the capillary network (see Chapter 24). Microaneurysms may be seen in most of the conditions associated with retinal venous stasis—central or branch vein obstruction, Coats disease, periphlebitis, and hyperviscosity of the blood. Microaneurysms can be identified with certainty by fluorescein angiography or histologic examination. Ophthalmoscopically they appear as minute red dots of unchanging appearance that are unrelated to visible blood vessels. They remain unchanged for months but eventually become minute white dots or disappear. Small, deep, round hemorrhages with a similar appearance absorb more rapidly and disappear without leaving a residue. Microaneurysms leak plasma and are often surrounded by edema, which gives the retina a hazy appearance. Sometimes hard yellow deposits (edema residues) surround the microaneurysms. Although microaneurysms occur in many conditions, it is only in diabetes mellitus that large numbers occur predominantly at the posterior pole.

The resolving power of the direct ophthalmoscope is about 75 mμ. Most retinal microaneurysms are smaller than that and are invisible ophthalmoscopically, but they may be demonstrated by fluorescein angiography or histologically in flat preparations of the retina.

Capillary perfusion. Fluorescein angiography indicates that poor retinal function in vascular closure and diabetic retinopathy is secondary to inadequate perfusion of the retinal capillaries.

The various abnormalities causing decreased capillary perfusion are discussed in several different sections: carotid artery occlusive disease; ophthalmic artery occlusive disease; ischemic neuropathy of the optic nerve; vascular stasis in glaucoma; blood disorders such as leukemia, polycythemia, hemorrhage, hemoglobinopathies, and dysproteinemias; vascular inflammations; diabetes; and vascular hypertension.

Opacities of the sensory retina

The sensory retina is ophthalmoscopically transparent with a red-brown background caused by blood in the choriocapillaris and by the pigment in the retinal pigment epithelium. The normal red fundus reflex may be obscured by the following: (1) opacities of the media (cornea, lens, vitreous); (2) inflammatory exudates; (3) deposits (acute or chronic edema); (4) hemorrhages (preretinal, retinal, subretinal); (5) blood vessel malformation (neovascularization, aneurysms); (6) epiretinal membranes; and (7) detachment of the sensory retina from the underlying retinal pigment epithelium.

Inflammatory retinal exudates are opacities that result from inflammation of the retina or choroid. Often inflammatory cells in the vitreous obscure them. They appear as grayish-white areas with ill-defined margins. The underlying retinal pigment epithelium and choroid may be destroyed and the cells of the retinal pigment epithelium proliferate.

Retinal deposits (also called hard exudates, fatty exudates, chronic edema residues) originate from localized areas of retinal edema. They consist of fats and lipid-filled macrophages in the outer plexiform layer of the retina. They are distributed in the following patterns: (1) as a ring or partial ring in circinate retinopathy; (2) as a foveal star; or (3) as scattered irregular deposits in diffuse disorders such as diabetes mellitus or Coats retinal telangiectasis. They occur at the junction between leaking and competent retinal capillaries.

Retinal deposits at the posterior pole may have a circular or arcuate (circinate) pattern that surrounds an abnormally permeable blood vessel such as an aneurysm, shunt, or area of neovascularization (Fig. 16-4). A circinate pattern may be seen in diabetes mellitus, vascular hypertension, and other retinopathies. Deposits in the outer plexiform layer that surrounds the fovea centralis (Henle layer) result in a foveal star (Fig. 16-5), which appears as broken lines radiating from the fovea centralis but not reaching the outer plexiform layer. The pattern is visible in accelerated vascular hypertension, papilledema, and papillitis, and is caused by leakage from the capillaries of the optic disk. Diffuse lipid deposits (chronic edema residues) are similar to the deposits of circinate retinopathy but have no circular pattern and appear as scattered yellowish to white regions of varying size with sharply defined edges. In Coats disease there is a massive outpouring of lipids, mainly cholesterol, into and beneath the retina.

Cystoid central retinal edema results from a variety of conditions that cause abnormal permeability of the capillaries surrounding the fovea centralis. The retina appears slightly raised and white, with a cystoid pattern of edema that is visible ophthalmoscopically. The loss of vision directs most attention to the condition. However, fluorescein angiography pro-

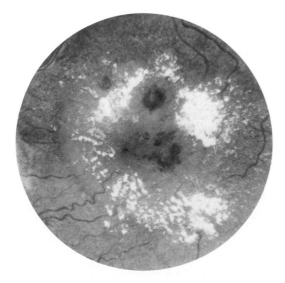

Fig. 16-4. Lipid deposits (edema residues) surrounding area of retinal microangiopathy in a patient with diabetes mellitus.

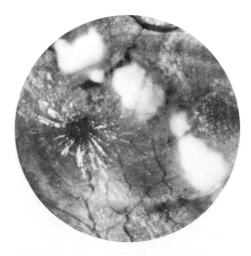

Fig. 16-5. Foveal star of edema in the outer plexiform layer of the retina (Henle layer), which surrounds the foveola. The cotton-wool patches are in the nerve fiber layer. These changes occurred in a 39-year-old man with accelerated vascular hypertension.

vides a typical picture with spokes radiating from the fovea centralis.

Cotton-wool patches (cytoid bodies). Cotton-wool patches appear ophthalmoscopically as indistinct, white retinal opacities with a hazy, irregular outline ("soft" exudates) (see Fig. 16-5). They are usually ovoid in shape, variable in size and number, and mainly seen in the posterior segment. They occur in the nerve fiber layer of the retina as a result of capillary infarction. Cotton-wool patches occur in the retina following retinal trauma and in severe arterial hypertension, severe anemia, papilledema, diabetic retinopathy, generalized carcinomatosis, acute systemic lupus erythematosus, and dermatomyositis, and the *acquired immune deficiency syndrome* (AIDS).

Microscopically, cotton-wool patches occur in axons in the nerve fiber layer of the retina. They consist of an accumulation of cell organelles and reflect obstruction of axonal flow in the nerve fiber layer. They do not contain infective particles.

Epiretinal membranes. Membranes on the vitreal surface of the retina result from proliferation of one or more of three retinal elements: (1) fibrous astrocytes, (2) fibrocytes, and (3) retinal pigment epithelial cells. Localized epiretinal membranes may occur at the posterior pole of the eye without clinical signs or may cause marked loss of vision as the result of covering, distorting, or detaching the fovea centralis. Epiretinal membranes may cause vascular leakage and secondary retinal edema. Some in younger individuals appear to be developmental in origin, while others are idiopathic and occur in otherwise normal eyes. The majority occur in association with retinal holes, ocular concussions, retinal inflammation, or after ocular surgery. A number of terms are applied: surface wrinkling retinopathy, when mild; macular pucker, when severe; and massive periretinal proliferation, when extensive. They may be removed by vitreous surgery when vision is impaired.

Disturbances in the position of the sensory retina

The sensory retina normally lines the globe smoothly without elevation or distortion. In senile retinoschisis the retina divides into two layers at the level of the inner plexiform layer.

In retinal detachment (separation), serous fluid or blood accumulates between the sensory retina and the retinal pigment epithelium. Vision is impaired because the outer layers of the sensory retina depend on the retinal pigment epithelium for nutrition, orientation, vitamin A, and phagocytosis. The entire sensory retina or a localized portion may be involved. The area of detachment loses the red reflex of the choroid and its sheen and appears gray.

Retinal detachment may be divided into rhegmatogenous (Gr. *rhegma:* breakage + *gen:* producing), in which a retinal hole is present, and nonrhegmatogenous or serous, in which there is no break in the continuity of the sensory retina.

Derangements of the retinal pigment epithelium

The retinal pigment epithelium obscures the view of the choriocapillaris, and the amount of melanin in its cells largely determines the degree of redness of the normal ocular fundus. A decrease in pigmentation occurs in aging, myopia, and atrophy of the choriocapillaris. The pigment (but not the pigment cell) is absent in albinism. The choroidal blood vessels are clearly visible, and if the choroid is lightly pigmented, the white sclera may be seen. In destructive inflammatory lesions involving both the choroid and the retina, all retinal and choroidal layers may be destroyed so that the white sclera is visible. Proliferation of the retinal pigment epithelium is stimulated in inflammatory processes, with resultant deep black pigmentation that commonly surrounds an area of chorioretinitis. In tapetoretinal degenerations, the pigment often has a central nucleus with dendrites (bone-corpuscle pigment) and is most marked at the equator.

In detachment of the retinal pigment epithelium, serous fluid or blood accumulates between the pigment epithelium and Bruch membrane, which elevates the sensory retina in the area.

Abnormalities of Bruch membrane (lamina basalis choroideae)

The main abnormalities recognized ophthalmoscopically are breaks in the elastic layer of Bruch membrane with replacement by fibrous tissue, which causes angioid streaks and drusen. Both conditions favor the formation of a subretinal neovascular membrane.

CONGENITAL AND DEVELOPMENTAL ABNORMALITIES

Myelinated nerve fibers. Myelination of the optic nerve is completed shortly after birth. Sometimes the process does not stop at the lamina cribrosa but extends a short distance over the retinal surface (see Fig. 16-5).

Additionally, the nerve fiber layer in the peripheral retina may be myelinated. The involved area is translucent, with the blood vessels visible beneath a thin, stark white opacity that is more dense nearer the disk and follows the distribution of the nerve fiber layer. The visual field is normal.

Melanosis of the retina. Melanosis of the retina, or grouped pigmentation, is a rare nonfamilial, nonprogressive retinal abnormality characterized by small grayish to black spots scattered throughout the fundus or limited to a single quadrant. They vary in size and sometimes are grouped aggregations that resemble animal footprints ("bear tracks") on the surface of the retina. They are composed of densely pigmented accumulations of cells from the retinal pigment epithelium that have migrated to the region normally occupied by photoreceptors that have failed to develop. There are no symptoms, although minute visual field defects may be demonstrated in these areas.

Retinal dysplasia. Retinal dysplasia is a congenital, sometimes hereditary, often bilateral retinal abnormality characterized by outer nuclear retinal cells at various stages of differentiation, arranged in a palisading or radiating pattern surrounding a central ocular space. The eye is often microphthalmic with a shallow anterior chamber. The retina forms tubes, and one-, two-, or three-layer rosettes form that are suggestive of a detached mature retina that has been thrown into folds.

The condition may occur because of separation of the sensory retina from the adjacent retinal pigment epithelium during a critical stage of its differentiation. Retinal dysplasia is associated with trisomy 13-15 and other chromosomal abnormalities, congenital retinal folds, Norrie disease, colobomas or cysts, and cyclopia. A small blind eye with a white mass in the pupil (leukocoria) characterizes the condition.

Pseudoglioma (pseudoretinoblastoma) is an obsolete term used to describe many conditions that cause a white pupillary reflex (leukocoria) or amaurotic "cat's eye reflex." It may be produced by persistent hyperplastic primary vitreous, retinal dysplasia, congenital retinal folds, Norrie disease, chromosome 13 trisomy, retrolental fibroplasia, Coats disease, larval granulomatosis, toxoplasmosis, retinoblastoma, incontinenti pigmenti, massive retinal fibrosis caused by organization of neonatal retinal hemorrhage, metastatic retinitis, secondary retinal detachment, juvenile retinoschisis, and embryonal medulloepithelium.

Phakomatoses. This is a group of conditions in which there are congenital, disseminated, usually benign tumors of blood vessels or neural tissues (disseminated hamartomas). There are often ocular, cutaneous, and intracranial tumors. A variety of conditions are included: (1) neurofibromatosis (von Recklinghausen), (2) tuberous sclerosis (Bourneville-Pringle), (3) encephalotrigeminal angiomatosis (Sturge-Weber-Dimitri), (4) angiomatosis retinae (von Hippel), (5) angiomatosis retinae with cerebellar hemangioblastoma (von Hippel-Lindau), (6) ataxia telangiectasia (Louis-Bar), and (7) encephalo-ocular arteriovenous shunts (Wynburn-Mason).

Neurofibromatosis is an autosomal dominant disorder of neural crest cells. There is wide variability but 100% penetrance, in which multiple tumors originate from astrocytes of the central nervous system and Schwann cells of peripheral nerves. Tumors of the Schwann cells of the nerves of the skin are associated with café au lait spots, axillary or other intertrigenous freckling, and cutaneous neurofibromas. Small, discrete, grayish neuromas of the iris (Lisch nodules) are diagnostic. Ocular changes include corneal nodules and corneal nerve enlargement, asymmetry of the orbital walls with bony defects, fibroma molluscum or plexiform neuromas causing thickness of the eyelids, and orbital tumors. There may be blepharoptosis, trichiasis, strabismus, proptosis (sometimes pulsating), visual failure, buphthalmos, glaucoma, and papilledema. Computed tomography of the orbit indicates glioma (astrocytoma) of the optic nerve and chiasm (some asymptomatic) in 15% of patients with neurofibromatosis. In patients without a family history of neurofibromatosis, the incidence is 60%. About 30% of all optic nerve gliomas occur in association with neurofibromatosis. Astrocytic hamartomas of the retina and optic disk appear as small hemispheres resting upon a refractile, white, slightly uneven base.

Tuberous ("potato-like") *sclerosis* is an irregular autosomal dominant and sporadic disorder with the diagnostic triad of mental deficiency, adenoma sebaceum (angiofibroma), and seizures. Symptoms begin during the first 3 years of life, and most patients die before the age of 21 years. Congenital patches of hypopigmented skin occur on the trunk and limbs. Peduncilated tumors may occur on the eyelids and palpebral conjunctiva. Astrocytic hamartomas of the retina appear initially on smooth, grayish white masses that develop into elevated, nodular tumors with a granular (mulberry-like) surface. Glial hamartomas of the optic disk ("giant drusen") tend to calcify. Astrocytic hamartomas of the brain, which account for the seizures and mental deficiency, tend to calcify ("brainstones") in more than half of the cases.

Encephalotrigeminal angiomatosis is a congenital, nonhereditary disorder in which there is a nevus flammeus (port-wine stain) along the distribution of the trigeminal nerve, a cavernous hemangioma of the choroid causing glaucoma, and hemangioma of the meninges on the same side often associated with intracranial calcification. Focal seizures and mental retardation are common.

Angiomatosis retinae is an autosomal dominant disorder with retinal hemangioblastoma involving one or both eyes. Ophthalmoscopic examination discloses a reddish, slightly elevated tumor about the size of the optic disk, or smaller, that is nourished by a large artery and vein. Coagulation of the tumor by means of photocoagulation or transscleral diathermy prevents hemorrhages, deposits, and secondary glaucoma. Similar angiomas may occur in the cerebellum and spinal cord. Cysts of the pancreas, kidneys, epididymus, liver, lung, adrenals, bone, omentum, and mesocolon may occur as well as renal carcinomas, pheochromocytomas, and meningiomas. Manifestations vary widely among kindreds.

Ataxia telangiectasia is an autosomal recessive neurocutaneous disorder that begins with the first decade of life. There are prominent telangiectatic lesions of the bulbar conjunctiva; the dilated blood vessels suggest conjunctivitis. There may be telangiectasis of the cheek bones, earlobes, and sometimes upper neck. There is a cerebellar ataxis and pendular nystagmus. IgA and IgE are absent or reduced. Translocation of chromosome 14 and broken chromosomes may be present. The alpha-fetoprotein of the serum, which usually reaches a peak concentration at about the thirteenth week of gestation, is increased. There are widespread immunologic defects related mainly to T-lymphocyte functions.

Encephalo-ocular arteriovenous shunts are a familial abnormality with an absence of capillaries between arteries and veins giving rise to aneurysms and angiomas in the retina, midbrain, and face. There may be ocular muscle paralysis, pulsating exophthalmos, and intracranial calcification.

Coats disease. This is a chronic, progressive, vascular abnormality in which telangiectatic retinal vessels leak fluid, which results in an exudative, bullous retinal detachment. It affects boys, predominantly between 18 months and 18 years of age, with peak incidence at about 10 years of age. It is usually unilateral, but when both eyes are involved, one is affected more seriously than the other.

The main symptom is a decrease in central or peripheral vision. In the very young, attention may be directed to the abnormality because of a white mass behind the lens, suggesting a retinoblastoma, which may lead to enucleation. Pathologically, there are telangiectatic retinal vessels, an eosinophilic transudate predominantly in the outer retinal layer, and a massive subretinal fluid containing foamy macrophages and cholesterol crystals.

Ophthalmoscopic examination discloses yellowish white exudative patches beneath telangiectatic retinal blood vessels. These wax and wane and may disappear in one area while occurring in another. Subretinal hemorrhages are frequent and are usually associated with numerous glistening cholesterol deposits. The retinal vessels may have a tortuous course, aneurysms, fusiform dilatations, and loops. Hemorrhage into the vitreous humor may occur with subsequent development of proliferative retinopathy. Eventually there may be detachment of the entire retina, iritis, cataract, and glaucoma.

Treatment is frequently ineffective, but early photocoagulation or cryotherapy may be helpful.

Retinopathy of prematurity. The retinopathy of prematurity (retrolental fibroplasia is the final cicatricial condition) is a bilateral (usually) vascular abnormality of the retina with neovascularization and its resultant sequelae. It occurs almost exclusively in premature infants with a birth weight of less than 1500 g. Before 1970 overuse of oxygen was probably the major, but not the only, cause; today, with meticulous oxygen monitoring, the prematurity itself may be responsible.

The human retina is avascular until the fourth gestational month when vessels begin to extend from the optic nerve to the ora serrata. The peripheral portion of the nasal retina is vascularized by the eighth month, but the process is completed in the temporal periphery only after full-term birth. Premature birth may impair the growth of retinal blood vessels from the normally vascularized retina into the yet avascular retina.

Normally the posterior pole of the fundus of a premature infant is lightly pigmented. The periphery is gray-white and avascular. The media are often hazy. The arteries and veins of the retina branch at angles of 30° and 60°, and there is an abrupt junction between the vascular and avascular retina, especially in the temporal fundus. At this junction there is an abundance of small, dilated blood vessels. The blood vessels gradually extend peripherally, and the retina is usually normally avascularized when the infant is 9 months postconception.

The retinopathy of prematury mainly affects the periphery of the temporal retina. The initial change (stage I) is a thin, flat, gray-white, tortuous demarcational line that separates the anterior avascular retina from the posterior vascular retina. Blood vessels that reach the demarcation line branch excessively. The demarcation line may extend in height and width to become a pink ridge (stage II). Retinal vessels leave the surface of the retina to enter the ridge, but there is no retinal detachment. There is neovascularization near its posterior edge, and the vitreous humor becomes increasingly hazy. Fibrovascular proliferation (stage

III) of varying severity may then extend into the vitreous from the ridge or may be seen adjacent to or attached to its posterior edge. Retinal detachment (stage IV) and cicatricial changes may follow as a result of subretinal effusion, traction on the retina, or both. Cicatricial changes vary from a small mass of opaque tissue in the retinal periphery, with or without a retinal detachment, to retrolental tissue occupying a part or all of the pupillary area. (Retinal vascular engorgement and tortuosity is recorded as a plus sign to the stages noted above.) At any stage of the disorder, the peripheral retinal vessels may become tortuous and dilated. The iris vessels may become engorged and the pupil rigid.

Screening for the retinopathy of prematurity is indicated in infants with a birth weight of less than 1700 g during the seventh to ninth week of life. The ocular fundi of premature infants may be studied with the indirect ophthalmoscope after topical application of 1% phenylephrine and 0.2% cyclopentolate (Cyclomydril). The eyelids are separated with a Saver or Cook infant speculum, and particular attention is directed to the temporal retinal periphery, using scleral depression if necessary.

The diagnosis of the fully developed retrolental fibroplasia is evident. The eyes are small and sunken with fetal grayish-blue irises. A white mass presses against the lens. Frequently glaucoma occurs accompanied by tearing and corneal edema, but without ocular enlargement. The infant often sits rocking back and forth grinding his eyes with his fists.

Early arrested stages of the retinopathy of prematurity may be associated with a variety of ocular abnormalities. Myopia is common. The blood vessels at the posterior pole may appear to be dragged temporally. The fovea centralis may be displaced temporally (ectopia maculae), causing a divergent strabismus. Minimal degenerative changes in the peripheral retina and abnormal vitreoretinal adhesions may result in a retinal detachment that requires surgical correction.

The idiopathic respiratory distress syndrome affects 10% of all infants weighing less than 2500 g at birth. High concentrations of oxygen are required for several days after birth. The cardiac and pulmonary deficiencies may disappear at any time, but the high oxygen concentration of the arterial blood may cause retinal damage.

The retinopathy of prematurity does not reflect poor, dangerous, or inept medical care. Rather, it reflects essential care for an often fatal condition. Pediatricians and parents must weigh the risk of treatment and ocular involvement.

The ocular status of the premature infant should be evaluated during the seventh to ninth week of life. The purpose of the ocular examination is to learn the presence or absence of ocular disease and to advise the parents. If there are signs of retinopathy, the infant should be reexamined at 3 months of age to learn if the disease has progressed. Thereafter the child should be examined every 3 months for the first 2 years, every 4 months for the next 2 years, every 6 months for the next 3 years, and then annually. In all infants, oxygen must be administered only when necessitated by hypoxia. The oxygen should be terminated, reduced, or used intermittently as early as the general condition permits.

Photocoagulation or cryotherapy for the active stage of the retinopathy of prematurity may be beneficial. Bilateral total traction retinal detachment may be treated with scleral buckling. Normal anatomical attachment of the retina may be brought about by vitrectomy with an approach through the pars plana. Administration of large doses (25 to 100 mg/kg of body weight) of oral vitamin E from birth is the subject of a long-term study.

Familial exudative vitreoretinopathy. This is an autosomal dominant disorder that occurs in individuals of normal birth weight, normal gestation, and an uneventful neonatal course. Most patients are asymptomatic, and peripheral incomplete retinal vascularization with abnormally straight blood vessels anastomosing along the avascular interface is detected only after the severe disorder in siblings prompts examination. The severe form has its onset between 3 months and 11 years of age. There is an accumulation of subretinal exudates, progressive traction on the central retina, cicatricial changes in the temporal retina, and peripheral vitreous hemorrhages. Temporal displacement of the fovea centralis causes a pseudostrabismus as the result of an abnormal angle kappa. The condition is distinguished from the retinopathy of prematurity by the normal birth weight, usual absence of myopia, and family studies.

VASCULAR DISORDERS

In humans, capillaries derived from branches of the central retinal artery nurture the inner layers of the sensory retina. There are capillaries at the level of the nerve fiber layer and in the inner nuclear layer. Interference with blood flow through these vessels results in decrease or failure of retinal perfusion and loss of function in the affected portion of the retina. Normal perfusion requires that the vascular pressure in the retinal arteries, capillaries, and veins exceed the intraocular pressure.

Retinal artery occlusion

Occlusions of the central retinal artery (Fig. 16-6) causes sudden, painless loss of vision. Occlusion of a branch causes a defect in the field of vision corresponding to the branch affected. The main causes of central retinal artery occlusion are emboli from carotid artery atherosclerotic plaques in older patients, emboli from cardiac valves in younger individuals, and thrombosis from arteriosclerosis (Table 16-2). Branch artery occlusions are usually caused by

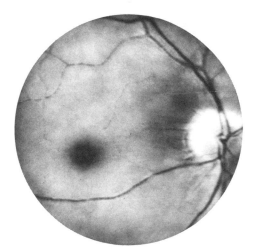

Fig. 16-6. Central retinal artery occlusion in a 19-year-old woman with mitral heart disease. Vision was suddenly lost 24 hours earlier. The sensory retina is edematous, but the normal red reflex is retained at the fovea centralis, causing a cherry-red spot. The blood column is segmented ("box cars") in the superior temporal artery.

Table 16-2. Some causes of retinal artery occlusion

I. Cardiac disease
   A. Valvular
      1. Mitral stenosis, regurgitation, or prolapse
      2. Aortic stenosis
   B. Atrial myxoma
II. Carotid artery disease
   A. Atherosclerosis
III. Systemic vascular disease
   A. Hypertension
   B. Atherosclerosis
   C. Giant cell arteritis
   D. Takayasu disease
   E. Collagen disease
   F. Wegener granulomatosis
   G. Pancreatitis (fat emboli)
   H. Midline granuloma
IV. Hyperviscosity of blood
   A. Dysproteinemia
V. Trauma
   A. Long bone fracture (fat emboli)
VI. Drug abuse
VII. Oral contraceptives
VIII. Systemic disease
   A. Diabetes mellitus
   B. Syphilis
   C. Sickle cell trait (SC)
   D. Thromboangiitis obliterans

emboli. Other conditions that cause arterial occlusion include atheroma formation complicated by subintimal hemorrhage, vascular spasm, and a dissecting aneurysm of the central retinal artery. Arterial emboli may develop in patients with chronic rheumatic heart disease (particularly mitral stenosis) and in myocardial infarction with mural thrombi. Vasospasm is secondary to arteritis in elderly persons or to vasomotor instability in younger individuals.

Occlusion by emboli may be preceded by episodes of flickering vision caused by minute emboli momentarily stopping blood flow in an arteriole but disintegrating and passing to the periphery. A large embolus may then cause a sudden loss of vision that is complete if the central artery is affected or involves a sector of the visual field if a branch is affected. Vasospastic disease is often preceded by repeated transient episodes of decreased vision or blindness in the affected eye (amaurosis fugax), and finally there is an attack in which vision does not return. The symptom of unilateral periodic blindness must be differentiated from the vas-

cular spasm of internal carotid-basilar occlusive disease, in which ophthalmodynamometry indicates a decreased pressure in the ophthalmic artery. Visual loss in carotid occlusive disease is seldom permanent or complete, even though the carotid artery is completely occluded, provided the central retinal artery is patent.

Ophthalmoscopic examination after central retinal artery occlusion reveals that the inner layers of the sensory retina are opaque and white because of edema. Because the inner layers are absent at the fovea centralis, it stands out conspicuously as a cherry-red spot. The retinal arteries appear as thin red threads. The blood column may be segmented so that there are segments with blood interspersed with empty segments. On fluorescein angiography, the artery fills with the dye after a delay, but the dye does not perfuse the retinal capillaries. After a week, the retina resumes its normal ophthalmoscopic appearance. The arteries, however, may remain as thin lines that, in time, may develop parallel sheathing and appear as white threads. The optic nerve becomes atrophic and appears deadwhite against the normally red fundus background.

Occlusion of the arterial blood supply causes a retinal ischemia with a coagulative necrosis of the inner layers of the retina. This is followed by autolysis and macrophages loaded with lipids. In the final stages, the outer half of the retina, which is nurtured by the choriocapillaris, is well preserved but the boundaries between the layers in the inner half are obliterated and are relatively acellular.

The prognosis is related to the cause, the degree of obstruction, and the length of time the occlusion has persisted. Relief within 1 hour may restore all vision, whereas relief within 3 or 4 hours may restore peripheral vision with a persistent defect of central vision. After this period has elapsed, or after development of a cherry-red spot, the visual defect is likely to be permanent.

Treatment is directed toward relief of vasospasm or an attempt to dislodge an embolus to a more peripheral and smaller vessel. Immediate intermittent massage of the globe is indicated. Moderate pressure is applied to the globe for a period of 5 seconds, then suddenly released for 5 seconds, and then repeated. Respiration of 5% carbon dioxide and 95% oxygen for 10 minutes each hour may be helpful. Stellate ganglion block with procaine or lidocaine (Xylocaine) may be helpful, as may retrobulbar injection with the same drugs or with acetylcholine, tolazoline, or papaverine. Immediate anticoagulation may be helpful prior to the development of a cherry-red spot.

Transient emboli of the retinal arteries may result from atherosclerotic occlusive disease of the carotid arteries or from diseased heart valves. The emboli are of two main types: cholesterol ester flakes from atheromatous ulcers in the carotid artery or platelet-fibrin aggregates from thrombi in the carotid artery or the heart. The embolus causes a transient loss of vision corresponding to the branch in which it lodges. Attacks caused by platelet emboli are brief and frequent and often involve the same vessel. There is no residual abnormality in the retinal blood vessel. Those caused by cholesterol emboli are more variable both in severity and frequency. They may be associated with a lasting visual field defect and visible emboli in the retinal blood vessels.

Patients with retinal artery occlusion require careful evaluation of the cardiovascular system, especially the carotid arteries (auscultation for bruits, palpation of facial pulses, ophthalmoscopy for emboli, ophthalmodynamometry, and angiography when suggested by previous findings). Systemic diseases include those associated with atherosclerotic cardiovascular disease and with hypertension. In addition to hematologic and systemic disease studies, patients less than 40 years of age require an echocardiogram or cardiac catheterization, or both, to screen for atrial myxoma or mitral valve prolpase (Fig. 16-7).

Retinal vein occlusion

Retinal vein occlusion may involve the central retinal vein, which causes immediate severe loss of vision, or a branch retinal vein, which results in partial loss of vision, depending on the region of the retina drained by the vein. Three basic mechanisms are involved in both types: (1) external compression of the vein, (2) venous stasis, and (3) degenerative disease of the venous endothelium.

External compression results from arteriosclerosis or arteriolosclerosis affecting the central retinal artery or its branches adjacent to

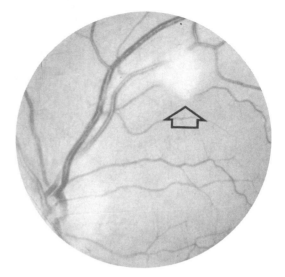

Fig. 16-7. Capillary occlusion by an embolus in a 32-year-old man with mitral valve prolapse. The cotton-wool patch was the sole evidence of the embolus. A permanent paracentral scotoma resulted.

the central retinal vein within the optic nerve or at arteriovenous crossings within the eye. Additionally, a connective tissue strand within the floor of the physiologic cup or from the cribriform plate may compress the central vein.

Venous stasis occurs with spasm in the corresponding retinal artery or arteriole, causing a low venous perfusion pressure that is often aggravated by retinal edema. Other causes include reduction in systemic blood pressure in cardiac decompensation, therapy for vascular hypertension, carotid occlusive disease, traumatic or surgical shock, dysproteinemias, and increased blood viscosity in obstructive pulmonary disease.

Degenerative disease of the venous endothelium causes intravascular detachment, proliferation, and hydrops. It occurs in severe systemic disease, such as arterial hypertension, cardiac decompensation, and diabetes mellitus. A similar mechanism may result from inflammation of the optic nerve or from systemic granulomatous disease. Additional factors include head trauma and oral contraceptives in women.

Central retinal vein closure is often preceded by episodes of transient decrease in vision. Visual loss does not occur within seconds, as in central retinal artery closure, but develops over several hours.

Ophthalmoscopic examination indicates engorgement of the venous tree (Fig. 16-8). Physiologic pulsation of the vein is absent and cannot be elicited by pressure on the eye. The involved retina has scattered, numerous, superficial, deep hemorrhages. The optic disk may be covered with hemorrhages, which may break into the vitreous humor. The veins are enlarged, engorged, tortuous, and dark blue. Segments may be hidden beneath edematous retina. Cotton-wool patches may be present, which indicates concomitant retinal ischemia. Fluorescein angiography shows marked leakage of the dye at the site of the occlusion.

The pathologic changes are dominated by hemorrhage, retinal edema, neovascularization, and glaucoma. There is secondary destruction of the retina, which is replaced with glial tissue. Hemosiderosis of the retina occurs with most hemosiderin located within macrophages. Some eyes develop neovascularization of the iris (rubeosis iridis), which may cause a painful hemorrhagic glaucoma.

Primary or secondary glaucoma is more likely to precede central vein closure than a branch vein closure. Additionally, about 20% of patients with central vein occlusion later develop rubeosis iridis and glaucoma.

Treatment of central vein occlusion is not satisfactory. Rubeosis iridis may be prevented by ablation of the retina with photocoagulation. Major attention should be directed to the prevention of a similar episode in the fellow eye. Glaucoma or ocular hypertension must be treated and intraocular pressure maintained at the lowest possible level. Anticoagulation is indicated if pulsation of the central retinal vein of the uninvolved eye cannot be induced with pressure upon the globe. Usually bishydroxycoumarin (Dicumarol) is used after initial anticoagulation with heparin. Patients and physicians must be on the alert for transient diminution of vision and signs of venous engorgement, after the fellow eye has been lost from a venous occlusion. Anticoagulation may have to be continued indefinitely. Venous occlusion during therapy suggests failure to maintain the prothrombin times in a therapeutic range.

Branch retinal vein occlusion may occur near

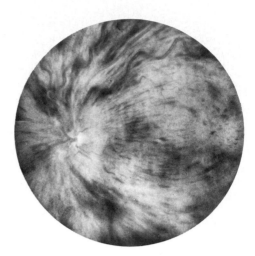

Fig. 16-8. Occlusion of the central vein of the retina. The old term "retinal apoplexy" is highly descriptive. The disk margins and the arteries are blurred by retinal edema. The veins are dilated. There are retinal hemorrhages that parallel the distribution of the nerve fiber layer of the retina in the central retinal area.

the optic disk and involve a major quadrant of the retina (Fig. 16-9), or it may occur at a peripheral crossing of an artery or vein. If a temporal branch is occluded, vision will be reduced if there is hemorrhage into or edema of the fovea centralis. Occlusion of a nasal branch or of a branch temporal to the fovea centralis may cause an inconspicuous loss of visual field that is not noticed by the patient.

The pathogenesis is complex. If capillary perfusion is not impaired, vision often returns to normal. If arteriolar perfusion is impaired, or if there is actual arteriolar insufficiency and retinal ischemia, permanent retinal changes occur. Ophthalmoscopically, retinal hemorrhages, retinal edema, and sometimes cotton-wool patches are visible. The affected vein is dilated and tortuous and may appear segmented. Fluorescein angiography may show diffuse staining and leakage from the involved venous and arterial trees. As the hemorrhage clears, dilated and tortuous collateral vessels may course across the central retina and the median raphe from normal to abnormal retina (Fig. 16-10). The capillaries are dilated and leak plasma. Surface neovascularization occurs, and there may be proliferative retinopathy and vitreous bleeding. The leakage of plasma from

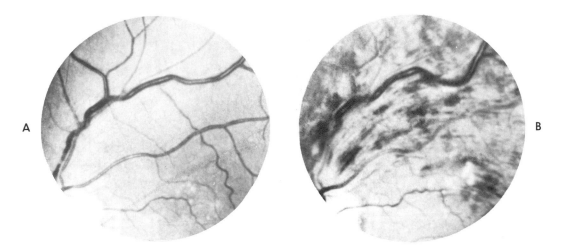

Fig. 16-9. Retinal branch vein closure in a 70-year-old woman. **A,** When the woman was 66 years of age the superior temporal vein was found to have multiple arteriovenous crossings with venous notching and peripheral dilation. There were a few drusen inferiorly. **B,** Four years later a branch vein occlusion occurred with flame-shaped hemorrhages and deposits; vision was reduced to 20/60.

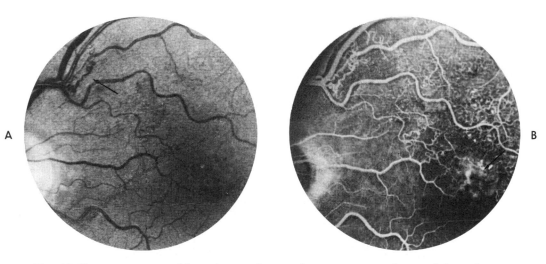

Fig. 16-10. A, Compensated branch vein closure of superior temporal vein of the right eye. New blood vessels direct blood around obstruction. **B,** Late venous angiogram of occlusion showing numerous dilated collateral vessels and many microaneurysms. There is plasma leakage above the fovea centralis that could cause loss of vision.

capillaries causes central retinal edema with reduced vision even after the absorption of the hemorrhage.

The main differential diagnosis includes those conditions that cause dilation and tortuosity of retinal veins in the prodromal stage and the same vascular signs associated with hemorrhage after frank occlusion has occurred.

Those conditions that may cause venous dilation include diabetes mellitus, blood dyscrasias (particularly those with associated increased blood viscosity), congenital tortuosity of retinal vessels, arteriovenous aneurysms of the retina, angiomas of the retina, papilledema, and congenital heart disease.

Treatment is directed to removal of the underlying cause if possible. Systemic corticosteroids may be used to minimize retinal edema and phlebitis. Anticoagulation may be used to open collateral venous channels. I sometimes prescribe 200 mg of aspirin every third day to inhibit thromboxane A synthesis and to inhibit prostaglandin synthesis by blood vessel walls. Higher doses of aspirin may inhibit prostacyclin synthesis by the blood vessel wall and cause vasoconstriction. Glaucoma, if present, must be vigorously treated. I sometimes prescribe topical timolol in the affected eye together with systemic acetazolamide. Controlled

studies have not been done. Venous stasis and signs of impending vein occlusion in the fellow eye require anticoagulation.

Retinal photocoagulation is indicated to prevent visual loss from macular edema, neovascularization, and vitreous hemorrhage from new blood vessels. Many patients do not develop these complications, and careful evaluation, including fluorescein angiography, is essential. Branch occlusions of nasal blood veins are usually minor and do not cause macular edema, although neovascularization occurs. Occlusion of the inferior temporal vein is less

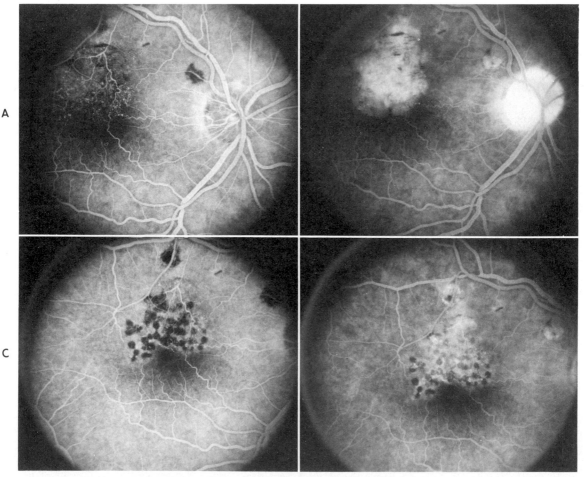

Fig. 16-11. A, Pretreatment fluorescein angiogram, transit phase, showing dilated retinal capillaries superior to the fovea centralis. **B,** Pretreatment fluorescein angiogram, late phase, showing leakage of fluorescein from dilated retinal capillaries. **C,** Posttreatment (6 weeks after argon laser photocoagulation) fluorescein angiogram, transit phase, showing pattern of photocoagulation to region of permeable capillaries. **D,** Posttreatment fluorescein angiogram, late phase, demonstrating decrease of edema. (From the Branch Vein Occlusion Study Group: Argon laser photocoagulation for macular edema in branch vein occlusion, Am. J. Ophthalmol. **98:**271, 1984.)

likely to cause macular edema than occlusion of the superior temporal vein. Occlusions of branches beyond the foveal region are unlikely to cause macular edema. Eyes with large areas (5 or more disk diameters in size) of capillary nonperfusion are most likely to develop neovascularization. Macular edema present within 3 months after branch vein occlusion should be treated with photocoagulation of the region of abnormally permeable blood vessels (Fig. 16-11). All areas of neovascularization should be treated. Treatment of areas of capillary nonperfusion in which there is no neovascularization is difficult to evaluate, since many of these eyes do poorly with or without treatment. Generally, too, the prognosis is poorer with eyes with large areas of capillary nonperfusion.

Hyperviscosity syndromes. Patients with extreme hyperviscosity of the blood ophthalmoscopically shows venous dilation and tortuosity, hemorrhages, microaneurysms, exudates, and papilledema. The condition resembles an impending venous closure and may cause frank occlusion. The blood serum causes include macroglobulinemia, hyperglobulinemia, and cryoglobulinemia, whereas the blood cell causes are leukemia and polycythemia. A similar pattern occurs in stasis retinopathy secondary to carotid artery occlusive disease.

Retinal vasculitis

Retinal vasculitis is primarily limited to veins. The most frequent cause is extension of an adjacent chorioretinitis. Other causes include necrotizing angiitis, multiple sclerosis, tuberculosis, sarcoidosis, syphilis, Behçet disease, and cytomegalic inclusion disease. The capillaries of the central retina may be inflamed in a number of conditions and cause a cystoid central retinal edema with the reduced vision.

Retinal arteriolitis may occur spontaneously or in cases of necrotizing angiitis. Inflammation of both arteries and veins leads to localized thrombus formation followed by neovascularization.

Retinal phlebitis. Phlebitis may rarely involve the central vein. Ophthalmoscopically, the disk is swollen as in papillitis, but vision is not reduced. Branch vein phlebitis appears as a branch vein closure, which clears spontaneously. Vaso-obliterative vasculitis may occur in peripheral retinal veins.

Eales disease is a nonspecific peripheral periphlebitis that mainly affects men between 15 and 30 years of age. It is characterized by recurrent retinal hemorrhage adjacent to the involved veins and by vitreous hemorrhage. Both eyes are involved in about half the cases. The cause is not known, but the condition may result from a T cell-mediated vascular hypersensitivity. The chief symptom is loss of vision caused by vitreous hemorrhage. Although this hemorrhage tends to absorb rapidly, repeated hemorrhages result in vascularization of the vitreous humor, chronic uveitis, and glaucoma.

Ophthalmoscopic examination indicates segmental, dilated, beaded, occluded veins, with sheathing or exudation, and blood in the vitreous body and the retina.

Occlusion of the affected vessels by means of photocoagulation is remarkably effective in preventing progression. Photocoagulation may have to be repeated.

Retinal edema

The nonfenestrated retinal blood vessels and the zonulae occludentes of the retinal pigment epithelium (blood-retina barrier) limit plasma from entering the sensory retina that has but a small extracellular space. Failure of this blood-retina barrier increases the extracellular fluid within the sensory retina. Excessive flow through the retinal pigment epithelium causes a central serous choroidopathy. Retinal branch vein occlusion or arterial macroaneurysms may cause diffuse retinal edema. Intrinsic capillary endothelial dysfunction in diabetes mellitus may result in edema that appears as "hard exudates." Retinal edema, particularly prominent in the central retina (cystoid macular edema), commonly occurs in chronic low-grade uveitis as in pars planitis, after cataract extraction, senile hyalitis, and retinitis pigmentosa.

Cystoid central retinal (macular) edema

This is a condition of the sensory retina in which the capillary bed in and surrounding the fovea centralis becomes abnormally permeable and leaks fluid into the retina. The fluid accumulates in the outer plexiform layer (which in this region courses tangentially from the fovea centralis) and causes edema and cysts. Visual

Table 16-3. Major causes of leakage of perifoveal capillary network resulting in cystoid macular edema

Retinal vascular disorders
  Diabetic retinopathy
  Central retinal vein occlusion
  Branch retinal vein occlusion
  Retinal telangiectasis (Coats)
Intraocular inflammation
  Pars planitis
  Retinal vasculitis (Eales, Behçet, sarcoidosis, necrotizing angiitis, multiple sclerosis, cytomegalic inclusion disease)
After ocular surgery
  Vitreous adherent to wound
  Intracapsular lens extraction with lens implantation
Retinal degenerations
  Preretinal fibrosis
  Retinitis pigmentosa
Drugs
  Topical epinephrine after lens extraction

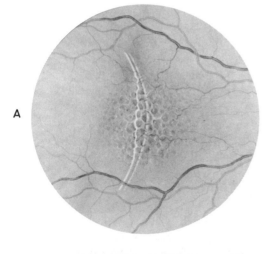

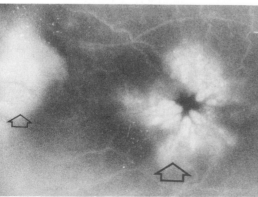

acuity is often reduced to 20/200, and ophthalmoscopic signs are minimal. Careful study indicates an irregularity and blurring of the foveal reflex. The retina is edematous and wrinkled, and cystic changes are sometimes present. Fluorescein angiography demonstrates leakage of the dye from the perifoveal capillaries and accumulation within the retina. In the late stages a spoke pattern develops in which the fluorescein surrounds the capillary-free area that marks the foveola where the inner plexiform layer is absent (Fig. 16-12).

There are many causes (Table 16-3). Originally the disorder was described as following cataract extraction (40% to 60%), particularly with vitreous adherent to the wound edges (Irvine-Gass syndrome). The lesion is nonspecific and occurs with a variety of retinal vascular abnormalities, degeneration, and intraocular inflammations as well as intraocular surgery.

The edema is usually self-limited and improvement is spontaneous. Systemic corticosteroids are often used in vascular and inflammatory disorders. Extracapsular cataract extraction with a posterior chamber intraocular lens is often substituted for intracapsular lens extraction to reduce the possibility of postoperative cystoid edema. In about one third of aphakic eyes, topical epinephrine causes retinal edema, which is reversible when the medication is stopped. Both systemic and topical forms of indomethacin have been used, but results are disappointing.

CENTRAL SEROUS CHORIORETINOPATHY

The choriocapillaris nurtures Bruch membrane, retinal pigment epithelium, and adjacent sensory retina. The numerous plasma infoldings at the base of the retinal pigment epithelium cells indicate an active fluid exchange. The tight junctions (zonulae occludentes) at the apices of the cell prevent fluid

Fig. 16-12. A, The biomicroscopic appearance of cystoid macular (central) edema. (Courtesy Henkind P.: Surv. Ophthalmol. **28** [suppl.]: cover, May 1984.) **B,** Late fluorescein angiogram of cystoid macular edema that occurred after cataract extraction in a 78-year-old man. Vision was reduced to 20/200 but later improved to 20/60.

from passing between the cells. Damage to the pigment epithelium permits fluid to pass between the cells and to accumulate between Bruch membrane and the sensory retina.

In central serous chorioretinopathy, a serous detachment of the retina occurs without obvious cause. Men are affected more than women, with the peak incidence about 55 years of age. Both eyes may be involved, but only one is usually affected at one time. When the fovea centralis is elevated, vision is reduced.

Ophthalmoscopically, the fundus lesion is characterized by one or more circumscribed el-

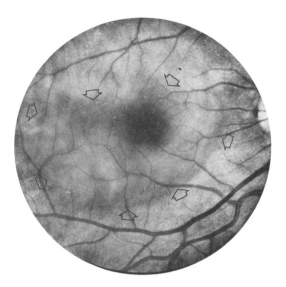

evations of the pigment epithelium or sensory retina at the posterior pole (Fig. 16-13). The lesions tend to remain unchanged for long periods but spontaneously resolve. Histologically, there is dilation and stasis in the orbital and vortex veins and their tributaries, and the lesion is suggestive of a systemic hemodynamic disturbance. There may be active proliferation of the pigment epithelium, producing elevated, pigmented lesions that suggest chorioretinitis. The lesions tend to disappear, leaving a residue of whitish-yellowish deposits deep to a sensory retina or areas of hypopigmentation and hyperpigmentation.

Fluorescein angiography indicates one or more areas of leakage in the choriocapillaris (Fig. 16-14). Photocoagulation of the area is followed by prompt resolution, but spontaneous, although delayed, resolution is usual. Often initial attacks are not photocoagulated, but recurrent attacks are promptly photocoagulated.

Fig. 16-13. Central serous chorioretinopathy of the right eye. There is elevation of the sensory retina in the region of the central retina. Arrows indicate lower border of the elevation. A fluid level is visible just above the foveal region. Small white dots adjacent to the superior blood vessels are residues of chronic edema.

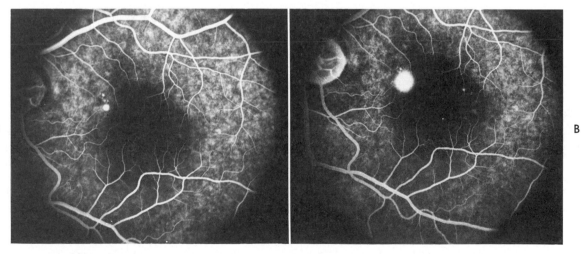

Fig. 16-14. Fluorescein angiograms of serous choroidopathy. **A,** Late phase showing leakage of fluorescein from choriocapillaris through retinal pigment epithelium and under sensory retina. **B,** Late phase (5 minutes) showing increased accumulation of fluorescein.

The cause of the reduced vision may be difficult to establish. If a small penlight is directed into the eye for 10 seconds, vision may be reduced one line or more in eyes with serous chorioretinopathy for more than 1 minute. Eyes with optic nerve disease recover within 30 seconds. Pupillary constriction to light stimulation is prompt in choroidopathy, whereas in optic nerve inflammation an afferent pupillary defect occurs.

Shunt vessels between choroidal and retinal vascular circulation

Anastomoses between the retinal and choroidal vascular beds are relatively common and consist mainly of capillaries. Large, anomalous shunt vessels that cause retinal blood to be drained into the choroidal circulation on the surface of the optic disk occur fairly commonly in occlusive retinal venous disease, glaucomatous optic atrophy, retinal proliferative vascular syndromes, and congenital diseases. When there is interference with the venous outflow in the optic nerve just behind the globe, convoluted dilated channels of preexisting capillaries develop on the surface of the disk. These occur with optic nerve gliomas, chronic atrophic papilledema, orbital cysts, and orbital meningiomas. The triad of shunt vessels, disk pallor, and loss of vision in middle-aged women suggests meningioma of the sheath of the optic nerve. The outlook for retained vision is poor.

RETINAL INFLAMMATIONS

The retina may be inflamed in exogenous and endogenous inflammations of the vitreous body, choroid, or retinal vessels. The main cause is an inflammatory lesion in the adjacent choroid causing a chorioretinitis. Inflammation of the sensory retina leads to an exudation of cells into the vitreous body, and if marked, this may cause diffraction of light and interference with vision. Inflammations affecting the posterior pole may disturb the fovea centralis and visual acuity. Ophthalmoscopically, in the acute stage the inflamed area appears yellowish white with ill-defined borders caused by edematous exudate.

A retinal inflammation may destroy the adjacent retinal pigment epithelium and expose the underlying choroidal vascular bed. Ophthalmoscopically, these regions appear to be a brighter red than the surrounding fundus and are crossed by relatively large choroidal veins. If the inflammation destroys both the choroid and retina, the white sclera is exposed. Alternatively, the retinal pigment epithelium may proliferate. (The choroidal melanocytes do not proliferate). After inflammation, particularly retinochoroiditis caused by congenital toxoplasmosis, the white sclera is surrounded by black areas of proliferated retinal pigment epithelium. Causes of primary retinal inflammation include toxoplasmosis, visceral larva migrans, rubella acquired in utero during the first trimester of pregnancy, syphilis, and sarcoid. Retinal infection may occur in the compromised host because of proliferation of viruses, particularly herpes simplex and cytomegalic virus, protozoa, and fungi not recognized previously as involving the retina. The inflammatory reponse varies with the degree of immunosuppression. The disease may terminate spontaneously, resulting in healing and pigment proliferation. The septicemia that causes the retinitis is often fatal.

Toxoplasmosis. Toxoplasmosis is caused by the obligate intracellular protozoa, *Toxoplasmosis gondii;* the cat is the definitive host. It occurs in a congenital form that is acquired transplacentally during the first 7 months of pregnancy and in an acquired form. Possibly all ocular inflammation is caused by the recurrence of the congenital type, although signs and symptoms may not be present at birth even though the infant is infected. Postnatally acquired clinical toxoplasmosis is usually associated with fever, lethargy, and malaise, sometimes with lymphadenopathy. It is diagnosed by assay of specific IgM by an enzyme-linked immunosorbent assay (ELISA).

The characteristic lesion of toxoplasmosis is a focal nectrotizing retinitis. The fovea centralis is commonly destroyed, causing loss of central vision. The lesion is sharply demarcated, with pigmented borders and atrophy of both the retina and the choroid, so that the white sclera is seen (Fig. 16-15). There may be satellite lesions. Usually the vitreous humor is clear, and there is no active inflammation. Because of the loss of central vision, there may be an associated esotropia, exotropia, or an ocular type of nystagmus. Children of subsequent pregnancies are not affected (see Chapter 23).

Congenitally infected individuals who are initally without visible retinal lesions may develop retinal inflammations 10 to 20 years later. A nonspecific local or generalized retinitis develops in either the anterior or posterior segment. Posterior retinitis causes vitreous exudates and veils, whereas anterior lesions cause mutton-fat keratic precipitates, aqueous flare, posterior synechiae, and complicated cataract.

Cytomegalovirus disease. Cytomegalovirus retinitis is a necrotizing inflammation of the sensory retina and choroid that occurs in immune-compromised individuals. The fundus shows scattered gray patches of necrotic retina with sheathing of adjacent retinal vessels (Fig. 16-16). Superficial and deep retinal hemorrhages are present. The vitreous contains inflammatory cells but disproportionately few for the severity of inflammation. There are large areas of chorioretinal atrophy with healing. The inflammation is aggravated by systemic corticosteroid therapy. Administration of investigational antivirals similar to acyclovir may result in disappearance of the virus from the blood

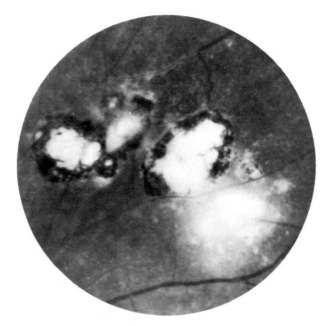

Fig. 16-15. Retinochoroiditis in an 18-year-old woman with toxoplasmosis. The multiple lesions of varying size with peripheral pigment proliferation and central destruction of the retina and choroid are characteristic of toxoplasmosis.

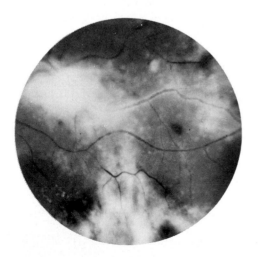

Fig. 16-16. Necrotizing cytomegalovirus retinopathy in a 25-year-old woman treated with chemotherapy for fulminating Hodgkin disease.

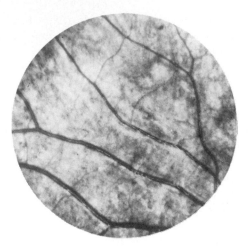

Fig. 16-17. Areas of pigmentation and depigmentation of the peripheral retina in fetal rubella.

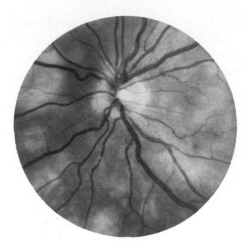

Fig. 16-18. Acute posterior multifocal placoid pigment epitheliopathy with multiple lesions deep to the sensory retina.

stream and resolution of the retinitis. There is relapse in patients with AIDS shortly after stopping therapy.

Acquired immune deficiency syndrome. Acquired immune deficiency syndrome (AIDS) is an abnormality in which previously healthy persons without other immunosuppressive disorders develop Kaposi sarcoma, opportunistic infections, or both (see Chapter 23). It is caused by a human T cell leukemia virus (LAV/HLTV-III). Patients at risk for the disorder include homosexual men, intravenous drug abusers, hemophiliacs and other recipients of blood products, and sexual contacts of individuals with the disorder.

Ocular lesions include Kaposi sarcoma of the eyelids, and noninfectious and infectious lesions. Noninfectious cotton-wool patches and retinal hemorrhages develop in up to 75% of the patients. They do not correlate with the clinical course of the disease.

Cytomegalic retinitis is the most common infectious ocular mainfestation. It appears as a hemorrhagic retinitis with granular areas of white retinal necrosis. There is a minimal cellular reaction in the vitreous. Treatment is not effective. *Pneumocystis carinii*, a common cause of pulmonary disease, has never been shown to cause retinal lesions. Curiously, the common opportunistic infections of the disorder, such as toxoplasmosis, fungi, and herpes, rarely involve the eye.

Toxocariasis. The larva of the common roundworm of the dog or cat may cause an eosinophilic granuloma of the retina. It appears as a whitish elevated area approximately the size of the optic disk. The dark-colored larva, which excites little cellular or pigmentary reaction, may sometimes be seen in the mass. Bands of retinal fibrosis radiate from the mass. Less common is a chronic endophthalmitis, which may lead to enucleation because of a diagnosis of retinoblastoma (see Chapter 23).

Rubella. Fetal rubella involves predominantly the retinal pigment epithelium and causes a slight disturbance in the melanin distribution. Ophthalmoscopically, there are discrete areas of pigmentation and depigmentation (Fig. 16-17). The electroretinogram is of limited value, since it may be normal, subnormal, or nonrecordable. The retinopathy does not progress, in contrast to primary retinal degenerations.

Acute posterior multifocal placoid pigment epitheliopathy. This inflammatory disease is characterized by the acute onset of multiple, flat or slightly elevated, yellow-white lesions of the posterior pole at the level of the retinal pigment epithelium (Fig. 16-18). These resolve spontaneously, leaving extensive degeneration of the pigment epithelium, as shown on fluorescein angiography, but with minimal alteration of the choroid or sensory retina. Lesions located in the central retinal area rapidly reduce visual acuity, which may improve spontaneously over several weeks. In the early stages, the inflammation blocks the transmission of choroidal fluorescence. Later the lesions gradually stain and fluoresce. Both eyes are usually affected, though not always simultaneously. After healing, there are extensive transmission defects in the pigment epithelium without late staining or leakage of dye.

The disease particulary affects young women who often have an upper repiratory tract illness 1 or 2 weeks earlier. There may be an associated mild uveitis with keratic precipitates and aqueous humor flare and cells in the vitreous. Erythema nodosum and episcleritis may occur. Rarely, headache and cells in the cerebrospinal fluid suggest a mild cerebral vasculitis. The cause is unknown, but the history of an earlier illness suggests a virus as the precipitating cause. Viral particles or antigens in the choriocapillaris may induce a localized obstruction as the result of immune complex deposition or as the result of an immune reaction.

Acute retinal pigment epitheliitis. This is a self-limited, benign condition in which tiny black spots surrounded by a yellow halo occur in the retinal pigment epithelium. The lesion may be single, but it more commonly occurs in clusters in the posterior pole. Vision may be blurred, but symptoms may not occur. Fluorescein angiography shows transmission defects in the retinal pigment epithelium that do not leak or change in size and shape. Men are affected in 75% of the cases. The median age is 45 years, and there is bilateral involvement in 38% of the patients.

Birdshot retinochoroidopathy. This is an inflammation of the retina, choroid, and their blood vessels. Numerous depigmented spots in the fundus, cystoid macular edema, disk edema, inflammatory cells in the vitreous, and retinal vascular leakage occur. Multiple spots in the choroid vary in size, shape, and color, Initially the spots are creamy-yellow in color but become white, atrophic, sharply circumscribed lesions. Some 80% of the patients have HLA-A29, compared to 7% of the control population. The cause is not known.

Acute retinal necrosis. One or both eyes of otherwise healthy patients of either sex or of any age may be affected in a severe destructive retinal inflammation. The disorder begins with a mild anterior and posterior granulomatous uveitis with pain disproportionately severe for the degree of inflammation. Secondary glaucoma may be present. Within days or weeks, multiple white patches develop in the peripheral retina with prominent arterial and venous vasculitis and occlusion. The vitreous becomes turbid, the optic disk and macular region are swollen. The condition may regress quickly with sharply delineated areas of pigmentary scarring, or progress with inflammatory tissue in the vitreous leading to traction and rhegmatogenous retinal detachment. Repair of the retinal detachment is complicated by optic atrophy, macular edema, and macular pucker. The differential diagnosis includes trauma, endophthalmitis, and retinitis seen in immune suppression. A herpesvirus group was found in one case.

RETINAL DEGENERATIONS

Genetic defects, inflammation, trauma, vascular disease, or aging cause either focal or generalized retinal degeneration. An accurate diagnosis often requires psychophysical and ophthalmic studies combined with fluorescein angiography of the patient and family members. Unfortunately, many of these disorders have not been studied histologically or they have been studied only in their end stages, when nonspecific changes predominated. Histologic and biochemical studies of human eyes in the early stages of disease are essential to provide more precise information.

Previously the retinal pigment epithelium was called the tapetum (Gr., *rug*). The term *tapetoretinal degeneration* describes hereditary disorders of the layer, although the primary site is not always in this layer. Sometimes phagocytosis of photoreceptor outer segments by the retinal pigment epithelium fails. In other individuals, atrophy of the choriocapillaris reduces the blood supply to the overlying pigment epithelium and sensory portion of the retina. Some disorders seem to affect the longevity of rods and cones, whereas others cause defects in lipid transport, defects in synthesis of rod membranes, or faulty or absent visual pigments. Subretinal neovascularization causes disciform degeneration of the retina in a variety of acquired and hereditary disorders. Many disorders once thought to involve the central retina predominantly are now recognized as involving the entire retina, with attention directed to the fovea centralis because of decreased visual acuity.

Retinal pigment epithelium. Most pigmentary degenerations of the retina involve predominantly the photoreceptors and the retinal pigment epithelium. Nutrition for the photoreceptor layer must pass through the retinal pigment epithelium and it provides phagocytosis and removal of the rod and cone outer segments. Failure of the lysosomal system of the pigment epithelium results in a failure to digest rod outer segments or in accumulation of cellular debris with degeneration of the overlying receptors.

Rod-cone dystrophy. This hereditary group of progressive disorders of vision is caused by different genes. The disorder is called by a variety of names: primary, hereditary, pigmentary retinopathy, retinitis pigmentosa, and tapetoretinal degeneration. Initially retinal rods or the retinal pigment epithelium are affected; eventually all visual cells are impaired. X chromosome–linked forms of the disease (mainly recessive) are rare and the most severe; autosomal dominant forms are the least severe; autosomal recessive forms are moderately severe. Most sporadic instances are autosomal recessive.

In adolescence, night blindness is the initial sign of the disorder. A ring scotoma develops and then extends peripherally and centrally until only a small contracted visual field remains (tubular vision). Eventually this too is lost. The scotopic electroretinogram is reduced in amplitude and becomes nonrecordable. The amplitude of the electro-oculogram does not increase in light. Eventually all vision is lost—earliest in the X chromosome–linked form and latest in the autosomal dominant form.

Ophthalmoscopic examination (Fig. 16-19) in advanced cases discloses a waxy-yellowish optic nerve, secondary to glial proliferation. The blood vessels are markedly attenuated. There is atrophy of the retinal pigment epithelium and later of the choriocapillaris. The retinal pigment epithelium may have a mottled gray appearance, and there are areas of hyperpigmentation and hypopigmentation. There are accumulations of pigment shaped as bone corpuscles. Pigment proliferation often begins in the midperiphery and then extends centrally and peripherally. With atrophy of the chorio-

capillaris, large vessels of the choroid are exposed and the fundus develops a whitish yellow appearance. A tapetoretinal reflex occurs at some time during the disorder in some patients. It has a metallic yellowish refractile appearance, affecting particularly the temporal retina.

Fluorescein angiography shows a mottled hyperfluorescence of the posterior fundus, sometimes with exposed large choroidal blood vessels. The retinal capillaries perfuse poorly, and there is often low perfusion pressure in the retinal, but not in the choroidal, blood vessels.

Myopia is common. A posterior subcapsular complicated cataract may reduce vision and require extraction. Cystoid macular degeneration occurs in young individuals. Some cases are associated with drusen of the optic disk or optic disk hamartomas.

Rod-cone dystrophy may occur solely with ocular changes or there may be metabolic, neurologic, or visceral abnormalities. The fundus appearance varies widely, but the night blindness, visual field constriction, and diminished retinal electrical responses occur in all.

There have been a number of different treatments suggested: vitamin A in high doses, cataract extraction, various subconjunctival injections, and the like. In 1916 Leber suggested that exposure to light accelerated the process and the degeneration of the retina. Animals de-

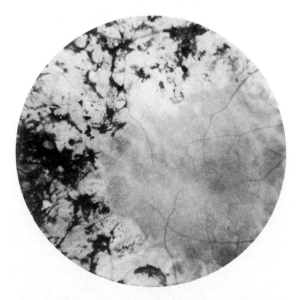

Fig. 16-19. Bone-corpuscle pigment proliferation and attenuated arterioles of primary pigmentary dystrophy of the retina (retinitis pigmentosa).

ficient in vitamin A develop retinal degeneration only when they are exposed to light. Thus the most recent trials aim to preserve vision in one eye by excluding it from light with an opaque shell. Evaluation of treatment requires exact diagnosis of the type of disease, knowledge of its hereditary pattern, long-term observation, and double-masked clinical trials. Inability to provide effective treatment has made the victims of the disease and their families easy prey from many nostrums.

I suggest the following regimen for patients afflicted with any form of retinitis pigmentosa:

1. Examination of the eyes annually to determine the progression of the disease.
2. Complete family history and examination to classify the disorder accurately. The possibility of affected children may be estimated through known family inheritance patterns.
3. Small doses of vitamins A and E, which may be helpful. The standard vitamin dosage should not be exceeded.

I believe it unwise for individuals with pigmentary degeneration to be exposed to bright sunlight. If such exposure is necessary, extremely dark sunglasses should be worn (lenses with less than 15% transmission). Additionally, pupillary constriction markedly limits the amount of light that can enter the eye. Cautious consideration may be given to the use of drugs that constrict the pupil, because these drugs may also cause minor opacities in the lens.

Secondary pigmentary retinopathy occurs in congenital and acquired syphilis and may be caused by retained intraocular iron or copper foreign bodies.

Leber congenital amaurosis. This is an autosomal recessively inherited, often consanguineous disorder in which there is either no light perception or near blindness from birth. The pupillary constriction to light is sluggish or absent. Pendular nystagmus and photophobia may be present. Initially the fundus may appear normal, but it subsequently shows areas of hyperpigmentation and hypopigmentation because of retinal pigmentary degeneration. The electroretinogram shows no response to light stimuli even when the retina appears normal. The ocular disorder may be associated with mental retardation and epilepsy as well as cataract and keratoconus. In ocular or oculocu-

taneous albinism and total loss of color vision (achromatopsia), visual acuity is somewhat better, although nystagmus is present. Congenital glaucoma with tearing, irritated eyes and subsequent ocular enlargement, congenital cataract, and various failures of development, such as microphthalmia, all manifest abnormalities on external examination. The absence of pupillary constriction to light in Leber disease distinguishes it from a rare disorder in which there is near blindness during the first year of life and eventual normal visual development. This disorder results presumably from delayed maturation of the visual system.

One type of Leber disease progresses to complete blindness; the other type appears stationary. Histologically the condition seems to occur because the sensory retina does not develop. There are oval-shaped, abnormal nuclei in the outer nuclear layer, abnormal fine structures of the inner segment, and a lack of basal foldings in the retinal pigment epithelium.

Vitelliform degeneration. Vitelliform degeneration (Best disease) is an autosomal dominant disorder with onset at birth or shortly thereafter. The central retinal region is occupied by a bright orange deposit that looks like the yolk of a "sunny-side up" fried egg (Fig. 16-20). The electro-oculogram is decreased, and there is a mild disturbance of dark adaptation. Tests indicate a generalized involvement of the retinal pigment epithelium, although the lesion appears to be confined to the central retinal region. Vision is normal as long as the "sunny-

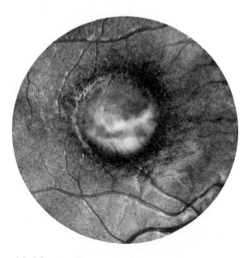

Fig. 16-20. Vitelliruptive degeneration in a 9-year-old girl with normal vision.

side up" appearance continues. Between 7 and 15 years of age, the material is dispersed ("scrambled") and scarring and pigmentary changes occur with loss of central vision. The fundus lesion may spare the fovea centralis, and in some family members there are no gross ocular lesions. Although the fundi may appear normal, all affected individuals have a decreased light-dark ratio with electro-oculography.

Drusen. Retinal drusen are localized deposits that lie between the basement membrane of the retinal pigment epithelium and the remainder of Bruch membrane. They may occur as an autosomal dominant disorder, secondary to a variety of ocular and systemic disorders, and with aging. They reflect an out-pouching of the basal cytoplasm and basement membrane of the retinal pigment epithelial cell into the Bruch membrane. The basement membrane subsequently degenerates and the cell fragments separate from the parent cell and in turn degenerate also. They are associated with serous detachment of the retinal pigment epithelium, subretinal choroidal neovascularization, and disciform scarring of the macula. (Drusen of the optic disk are a different and unrelated disorder.)

Drusen may be divided into nodular (hard) and granular (soft) types. Nodular drusen ophthalmoscopically appear as discrete, small, round, globular, golden masses, usually no larger than the diameter of a tertiary arteriole. Granular drusen are larger, amorphous, yellow deposits with indistinct margins, irregular shape, and varying size. They tend to change in shape and size and may even disappear. Both types may become calcified, and there are often small flecks of pigment surrounding them. Drusen cause "window defects" on fluorescein angiography (Fig. 16-21) in which the fluorescein in the choroidal vasculature is clearly seen. The drusen themselves stain but do not cause fluorescein leakage.

Drusen occur commonly as an aging change and occur in association with ocular diseases such as angioid streaks and systemic diseases such as recurrent polyserositis, scleroderma, and Rendu-Osler-Weber disease. They occur almost universally with aging, particularly in the peripheral fundi. Secondary drusen often, but not invariably, precede the subretinal neovascularization of disciform degenerations of the retina. Degenerative drusen occur in endophthalmitis and in eyes that are becoming phthisical. Secondary drusen may occur adjacent to areas of choroidal abnormality, such as

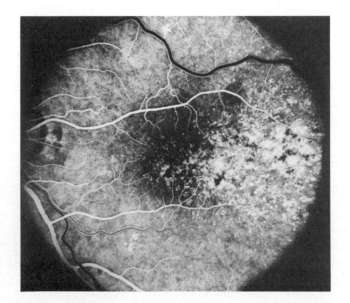

Fig. 16-21. Early venous angiogram of drusen. There is an absence of melanin in the retinal pigment epithelium overlying the summit of drusen that provides windows through which choroidal fluorescence is seen.

malignant melanoma. Senile drusen tend to involve the equatorial to peripheral retina, whereas familial drusen affect both the posterior pole and the periphery.

In some patients, mainly white, heavily pigmented women, drusen may be preceded by innumerable, small, discrete, round, yellow, subretinal deposits described as "stars in the sky." They are caused by focal nodular thickening of the basement membrane of the retinal pigment epithelium. These may cause a yellow subretinal exudate as well as initiate larger drusen.

Familial drusen occur as an autosomal dominant disorder. They are divided into three stages on the basis of their ophthalmoscopic appearance. During the first to third decades, they appear as small, discrete spots that are slightly pinker than the surrounding fundus. Eventually the dots become bright yellow, and larger ones tend to appear. Later, they tend to calcify and form minute pigment clumps. Eventually familial drusen become confluent and plaque formation occurs, particularly in the central retina.

The defects in the retinal pigment epithelium caused by drusen commonly lead to a subretinal fibrovascular membrane and retinal degeneration. Serous elevation of the central retina with hemorrhagic and edematous subretinal areas may be the first sign of neovascularization. If the initial neovascularization is not immediately beneath the fovea centralis, argon laser photocoagulation may be used to obliterate the new blood vessels.

Fundus flavimaculatus. Fundus flavimaculatus consists of multiple, round and linear, pisciform, yellow or yellow-white lesions, usually involving the posterior fundus (Fig. 16-22). The flecks vary in size, shape, outline, density, and apparent depth. The abnormality is transmitted as an autosomal recessive disorder and occasionally as an autosomal dominant one.

The disorder has its onset in the first or second decade and may take one of several courses: atrophy of the central retina with development of flecks, cone degeneration with severe color vision impairment, mild loss of visual acuity followed by flecks, or development of flecks without preceding macular involvement. Some of these patients lose vision because of a deposit of flecks beneath the fovea centralis, which causes secondary changes in the overlying cones.

The deposits usually first appear in the perimacular area and are isolated with fairly sharp borders and variable shapes, many of them linear and fishtaillike. Clusters of fresh lesions appear from time to time, and older lesions eventually disappear. The older lesions are less sharply demarcated, appear less dense, and show a greater tendency toward confluence.

Fluorescein angiography does not demonstrate the early lesions, since fresh lesions do not fluoresce. Hyperfluorescence is seen only at the sites of old lesions when choroidal fluorescence is viewed through abnormal retinal pigment epithelium. The fuzzy, irregular hyperfluorescent blotches at such sites are entirely different from the discrete, sharply outlined hyperfluorescent areas seen in drusen.

Fundus albipunctatus. Fundus albipunctatus is a rare autosomal recessive disorder characterized by yellowish-white dots of uniform size located in the retinal pigment epithelium and particularly concentrated at the midperiphery of the fundus. The deposits usually increase in number, but occasionally they may decrease or even disappear.

Progressive retinitis albipunctatus has a similar ophthalmoscopic picture at its onset. The electroretinogram is nonrecordable, and there is a markedly increased rod threshold with dark adaptation. Eventually bone spicule pigmenta-

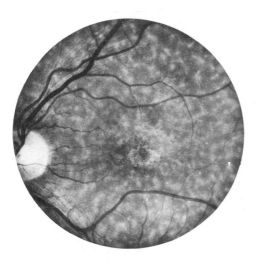

Fig. 16-22. Fundus flavimaculatus with central atrophic lesion (Stargardt disease).

tion, vascular attenuation, and optic atrophy develop as in rod-cone dystrophy.

Bruch membrane (lamina basalis choroideae). Bruch membrane separates the choriocapillaris from the retinal pigment epithelium. It consists of the basement membrane of the retinal pigment epithelium and the basement membrane of the endothelium of the choriocapillaris. It has inner and outer collagen layers that are separated by a layer of elastic tissue. It is freely permeable. Drusen of the retinal pigment epithelium rest on Bruch membrane and thus have been incorrectly designated as emerging from it. Ruptures of the elastic layer of Bruch membrane occur in angioid streaks, subretinal neovascularization, and pathologic myopia.

Angioid streaks. Angioid streaks consist of an irregular and jagged network of red to green striations, visible through an attenuated retinal pigment epithelium. They are produced by linear dehiscences developing as cracks in the collagenous and elastic portion of Bruch membrane. The condition is bilateral, but ocular involvement is not symmetrical. Both sexes are affected equally.

The optic disk is surrounded by one or more rings with offshoots extending toward the equator in a radial distribution (Fig. 16-23). In the early stages, the streaks are red but later become gray, brown, or black. The striations are flat, serrated, and may be several times wider

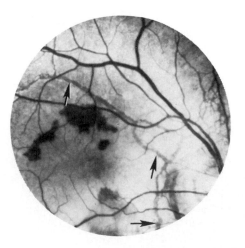

Fig. 16-23. Marked angioid streaks *(arrows)*. There has been subretinal neovascular membrane with bleeding and early development of disciform degeneration.

than retinal veins. They gradually taper off toward the periphery of the fundus, where they appear as thin lines. They do not branch dichotomously as do retinal vessels, and they give the appearance of cracks in dry mud.

Angioid streaks occur most commonly in pseudoxanthoma elasticum (of Grönblad and Strandberg) and fibrodysplasia hyperelastica (of Ehlers-Danlos). In these diseases there is a degeneration of the elastic tissue portion of the Bruch membrane, which ruptures and secondarily calcifies. Other causes include sickle cell anemia (5%), osteitis deformans (of Paget), and rarely, acromegaly, hypercalcemia, and lead poisoning. Those conditions with generalized elastic tissue disease may show concurrent vascular hypertension because of involvement of elastic tissue in the walls of arteries.

Ocular changes are asymptomatic unless a subretinal vascular membrane forms. This is often heralded by a retinal hemorrhage followed by a subretinal neovascular network.

Macular degenerations

The central retina (macula) is located temporal to the optic disk and surrounds the fovea centralis. The fovea centralis contains the cones mainly responsible for form vision and color vision. The area is involved in the same vascular, inflammatory, and degenerative diseases that affect the retina and underlying choroidal vasculature elsewhere. Several factors so modify disease in the central retina that its abnormalities are often considered apart from diseases of the remainder of the retina. A minute lesion that would not affect visual function if located peripherally may cause a severe loss of visual acuity. Additionally, the spreading of the inner layers of the retina to expose the cones in the fovea centralis is conducive to swelling of the outer plexiform layer of the retina (called the Henle layer in this region). This swelling is seen particularly in neuroretinitis with the formation of a circular area of deposits surrounding the fovea centralis (macular star). The optical system of the eye focuses light energy in this region, so that degeneration of the area may result from unwise exposure to the light of the sun, as occurs in eclipse retinopathy. Additionally, the central retinal area is involved preferentially in a variety of degenerative conditions.

Degeneration of the fovea centralis may be divided into primary and secondary types. The primary type results from a genetically transmitted defect, which is familial, bilateral, and progressive. It includes vitelliform degeneration, fundus flavimaculatus, autosomal dominant drusen, and typical achromatopsia.

Other primary types include abnormalities with central nervous system involvement. Central nervous system involvement occurs because the abnormalities, such as gangliosidosis and ceroid neuronal lipofucinosis (Batten), affect the ganglion cells of both the retina and the brain. Involvement of the central nervous system frequently leads to early death. Some cases are not accurately diagnosed because the fundi have not been examined.

Age-related macular degeneration. Age-related macular degeneration (senile macular degeneration) is the most common cause of legal blindness in the United States in persons older than 60 years. Its prevalence increases markedly after the age of 65 years, and it affects some 28% of individuals between the age of 75 and 85 years. It is more common in individuals of short stature and is associated with arteriosclerosis, stroke, and ischemic attacks. Possibly the degeneration is associated with chronic vascular hypertension.

Most age-related macular degeneration is preceded by retinal drusen that seem to predispose to degeneration. Two main types occur: areolar (geographic) atrophy of the retinal pigment epithelium and disciform macular scarring. A disciform scar is preceded by subretinal neovascularization that causes a serous or hemorrhagic detachment of the retinal pigment epithelium. About a quarter of individuals with areolar atrophy develop subretinal neovascularization and a disciform scar.

Areolar (geographic) atrophy of the retinal pigment epithelium is preceded by nodular (hard) drusen that sometimes become calcified. There is gradual diminution of central vision. Ophthalmoscopically, the foveal reflex is lost. There is depigmentation with baring of the choroidal vessels. There are small areas of mild pigment proliferation. The changes are subtle, and often the surrounding drusen are more conspicuous than the foveal lesion. In some patients several large confluent drusen coalesce and split Bruch membrane to cause a detachment of the retinal pigment epithelium, so-called exudative maculopathy.

Disciform scarring is the result of fibrous metaplasia of the retinal pigment epithelium. It is preceded by granular (soft) drusen that have indistinct borders and a tendency to confluence. There is a sudden onset of decreased vision and metamorphopsia with bending of straight lines or micropsia (objects appear smaller). A subretinal neovascular membrane appears as a greenish or green pigmentation deep to the retinal pigment epithelium. There may be retinal or subretinal blood or serous fluid. Hard deposits may be present in the retina. With progression, bright red blood is evident in the sensory retina followed by a white-gray area with scattered pigment that involves the entire fovea and adjacent tissue. Vision is often reduced to 3/200 or less.

Treatment of age-related macular degeneration is not satisfactory. I recommend that aged patients with drusen take 400 units of vitamin E twice daily. Each patient with drusen should check the central field of each eye daily, using an Amsler chart (Chapter 5) to detect metamorphopsia. Early detection of subretinal fluid secondary to subretinal neovascular membrane allows photocoagulation of the blood vessels, provided they are 200 μm or more from the center of the fovea. Photocoagulation of a membrane beneath the fovea centralis destroys the overlying sensory retina and causes a loss of vision similar to that caused by the disease.

Every patient with age-related macular degeneration should be assured that peripheral vision will be retained and that the loss of central vision will not cause loss in independence. Some patients obtain useful vision with telescopic lenses, special magnifying lenses, and similar optical aids. Although the proportion of patients who obtain satisfaction is disappointingly small, each patient should try these lenses before it is concluded that they are of no use. There are many devices and services of value that many with low vision find useful.

Secondary macular degeneration may follow trauma from mechanical or radiant energy injuries as well as from vascular, inflammatory, or degenerative disease. Secondary degeneration is commonly unilateral and frequently does not progress after the cause has been removed.

FLUID-SEPARATING RETINAL LAYERS

The smooth surface of the retina lining the globe may be disturbed by a number of abnormalities. Giant cysts in the outer plexiform layer of the sensory retina give rise to retinoschisis. Traction, holes, or exudation beneath the sensory retina may separate it from the pigment epithelium in retinal separation or detachment. Fluid between the Bruch membrane and the choriocapillaris may cause a detachment of the retinal pigment epithelium. Both the sensory retina and pigment epithelium may be elevated by tumors and fluid in the choroid—a combined detachment.

Retinoschisis

Retinoschisis (Gr. *schisis:* division). Splitting of the sensory retina occurs in two forms: (1) X chromosome–linked type that affects the central and peripheral retina, and (2) degenerative peripheral type that is not hereditary and does not involve the central retina. Rarely a peripheral type occurs in retrolental fibroplasia or diabetic retinopathy. Patients may complain of light flashes and floaters.

Degenerative retinoschisis. This usually occurs after 40 years of age. The retina splits into two layers at the level of the outer plexiform layer (rarely the inner plexiform layer). It begins as a cystic degeneration of the extreme retinal periphery, most commonly in the inferior temporal quadrant. The schisis cavity contains a glycosaminoglycan that is sensitive to hyaluronidase. The cavity may extend nasally to encompass the entire retinal periphery, and the cysts consolidate to form a huge elevation. Generally the condition is not progressive.

Patients may complain of light flashes and floaters. Ophthalmoscopically, there is a transparent elevation of the retina, which has a smooth, convex, sharply limited surface.

Usually no treatment is indicated. Annual ophthalmic and perimetric examinations are advised. Progression may be limited when necessary by photocoagulation, surface diathermy, or cryotherapy of the advancing edge of the retinoschisis. The development of a hole in the outer retina leads to a detachment of the sensory retina from the retinal pigment epithelium that must be treated.

X chromosome–linked juvenile retinoschisis. This is an X chromosome recessive disorder in which initially a cystlike structure involves the fovea centralis. It has a spoke pattern with the hub corresponding to the foveola. Later the radial folds disappear and are replaced by a nonspecific atrophic appearance. In about half the patients there is a peripheral retinoschisis, often in the inferior temporal region. there are silver-gray glistening spots scattered throughout the retina in all cases. The vitreous contains veils, most often in the periphery.

Vision may be normal in early childhood and may gradually deteriorate to about 20/200 at puberty. Strabismus and nystagmus may occur, but most commonly the condition is detected when the child fails to pass vision tests on entering school. The electroretinographic b-wave amplitude is reduced with a normal electrooculogram. There are no signs in carrier females.

Retinal detachment

The invagination of the primary optic vesicle forms two primitive retinal layers: the outer retinal pigment epithelium and an inner sensory retina. Traction on the inner sensory layer or an opening (hole, break, tear) in this layer permits the accumulation of fluid between the two layers of the primitive retina, causing a retinal detachment (separation). Retinal detachments with hole formation are called rhegmatogenous. Those without a break in the continuity of the inner retina are called nonrhegmatogenous or serous detachments.

Rhegmatogenous retinal detachment occurs secondary to the formation of breaks, tears, or holes in the continuity of the sensory layer of the retina (Fig. 16-24) or because of separation of this layer at the ora serrata. Retinal breaks result from vitreous traction on the sensory retina, because of retinal degeneration, and after laceration or contusion of the eye. Breaks caused by vitreous traction are either horseshoe-shaped or round. The vitreous remains attached to the flap (operculum) of a horseshoe-shaped tear and elevates the edges of the tear. Degeneration of the retina causes small round holes without opercula, a purely degenerative or atrophic process without traction. Detachment of the retina at the ora serrata, a retinal disinsertion, occurs mainly in young individuals as either a congenital or traumatic defect.

Lattice degeneration of the retina is present

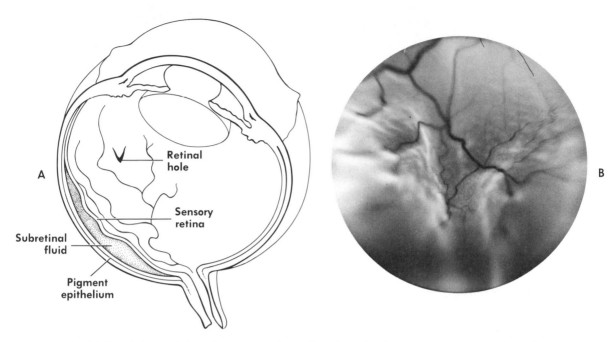

Fig. 16-24. A, Retinal detachment with horseshoe-shaped hole in superior temporal quadrant. **B,** Ophthalmoscopic appearance of a retinal detachment.

in about 30% of all rhegmatogenous separations and occurs far more frequently but without causing detachment. It is a sharply demarcated retinal thinning located at the ocular equator or anterior to it. Located within are a network of fine white lines that are continuous with blood vessels. Pigment accumulates along the white lines. Small white particles are on the surface of the lines and in the adjacent vitreous. There is liquefaction of the adjacent vitreous humor, but the vitreous strands may attach to the margins of the area of retinal thinning. Both tractional and nontractional tears may develop in this area of retinal thinning.

Retinal detachment occurs more commonly in men than in women, in eyes with degenerative myopia, in aging, and in aphakia. (The aphakic eye is 100 times more likely to develop a retinal detachment than an eye with the lens present.) Retinal detachment may occur after an uncomplicated cataract extraction, but it is seen more often if vitreous humor has been lost during surgery.

The detachment tends to be bilateral in about one third of the patients with degenerative retinal changes. The time interval between the detachment in the first and then the second eye may be as long as 10 years. The role of ocular trauma is obvious when there is a direct ocular contusion or a penetrating injury. Often, however, the history of trauma is obscure, and degenerative changes in each eye account for the separation.

Detachments tend to occur in youthful patients because of retinal dialysis or lattice degeneration. Retinal detachments occur in older patients because of tractional horseshoe-shaped tears, lattice degeneration, or aphakia.

In tractional detachments, the two main premonitory symptoms of retinal separation are (1) photopsia, or flashes of light without retinal stimulation by light caused by vitreous traction on the retina, and (2) a sudden shower of black dots in the peripheral visual field resulting from a minute vitreous hemorrhage at the point of a retinal break. Without traction, premonitory symptoms are absent and the first symptoms are decreased vision and a progressive defect in the visual field corresponding to the area of detachment.

The diagnosis of retinal detachment is based on the ophthalmoscopic appearance of the retina. Indirect ophthalmoscopy may be combined with scleral depression, and the examiner may study the retina from the optic disk to the ora serrata. Full pupillary dilation is required—2.5% phenylephrine combined with 1% tropicamide (Mydriacyl) are frequently used. The peripheral retina may be studied with a biomicroscope and a contact lens containing prisms that allow visualization of the periphery.

On ophthalmoscopic examination, the detached retina is gray or translucent and the normal choroidal pattern cannot be seen. The retina may be thrown into folds that change in location or shape with shifts in position of the eye or the head. The retinal vessels are dark red in the area of detachment and have an undulating course over its surface. The arteries and veins may appear to contain blood of the same color.

Retinal breaks are recognized by the bright red choroid shining through the grayish, opaque veil of detached retina. Additional holes may be found in areas of attached retina. Horseshoe-shaped tears with their base toward the ora serrata are common in the superior temporal quadrant anterior to the equator. Small round holes may be found anywhere and are frequently seen anterior to the equator. Retinal dialysis usually occurs in the inferior quadrants. It is most often single, semilunar, and at the extreme retinal periphery.

Retinal detachments with hole formation are usually readily diagnosed. Nonetheless, in rhegmatogenous retinal separation, holes are not found in 5% to 15% of the patients.

The most important differential point is the solid detachment caused by tumor, particularly malignant melanoma of the choroid. Failure of the detachment to regress with bed rest, the darker color, yellowish infiltrates, associated drusen, failure to transilluminate, and absence of hole formation suggest a tumor.

The treatment of rhegmatogenous retinal detachment is essentially surgical and directed toward closure of breaks in the retina. Once the diagnosis has been established, immediate treatment is indicated.

Retinal holes are closed by producing an area of chorioretinitis in the region of the defect so that adhesions between the edge of the hole and the retinal pigment epithelium will seal the opening. The chorioretinal reaction may be produced by cryosurgery with application of intense cold ($-80°$ C) or diathermy to the sclera in the region of the hole. Diathermy is used

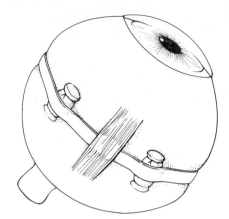

Fig. 16-25. Encircling rod (cerclage) with two radial sponges to indent the choroid to a retinal hole.

when the sclera is thin and the dark choroid gives a slate gray color, or after scleral dissection. Cryosurgery is used when the sclera is of normal white color and of unknown thickness. Subretinal fluid may be removed by perforating the choroid through the sclera, but it will usually absorb promptly if the retinal pigment epithelium is brought in contact with the retinal hole.

A variety of procedures are used to indent (buckle) the sclera and choroid so that the retinal pigment epithelium will be in apposition to the retinal hole. Selection of a particular procedure depends on the type of hole and the number of quadrants of the retina that contain holes. If a single horseshoe-shaped hole is present, a plastic implant is often placed radially upon the sclera. Multiple holes may require an encircling rod (cerclage) around the circumference of the eye (Fig. 16-25). Silicone oil or air may be injected into the vitreous cavity.

Proliferative vitreoretinopathy complicates rhegmatogenous retinal detachment. It is characterized by the growth of membranes on both surfaces of the detached retina and on the posterior surface of the detached vitreous gel. Contraction of these membranes distorts and elevates the retina, and is the most important cause of failure in retinal reattachment surgery. The abnormality originates from proliferation of retinal pigment epithelial cells that have migrated into the vitreous cavity through the retinal hole. Retinal glial cells may further contribute to membrane formation. The membrane causes shrinkage of the sensory retina so that it cannot be apposed to the pigment epithelium. Treatment is difficult and often not successful. Intravitreal silicone oil, scleral buckling, vitrectomy, and removal of membranes from the inner retinal surface are used.

Uveal effusion syndrome

Effusion of fluid between the retinal pigment epithelium and the sensory retina causes a retinal detachment without retinal breaks. The disorder affects males almost exclusively and is often bilateral. Choroidal detachment may be associated, but signs of uveitis are absent or minimal. The main symptoms are loss of vision and decrease in the superior visual field corresponding to the inferior retina. Ophthalmoscopically, when the patient is sitting up, there is a ballooning retinal detachment below; in the Trendelenburg position, the detachment shifts to the upper portion of the fundus. When a choroidal detachment is present, it forms a flat annulus around the globe between the equator and the ciliary processes. The cerebrospinal fluid has an increased pressure and protein content without pleocytosis. The subretinal fluid protein (mainly albumin) content is three times that in the plasma. The disease slowly progresses similarly but not simultaneously in each eye. The retina reattaches after months or years with or without treatment.

INJURIES

Contusions and retinal holes. Contusion may cause a variety of injuries, including retinal holes that lead to retinal detachment. A traumatic retinal hole occurs in an otherwise healthy retina—it is usually single, often horseshoe shaped, and located in the superior temporal quadrant. Eyes that have been subject to severe contusions should be studied carefully 3 and 6 months after the injury to be certain a retinal hole has not developed. It is necessary to study the fundus with wide pupillary dilation and to direct particular attention to the periphery.

Commotio retinae. Commotio retinae is a contrecoup phenomenon in which the posterior pole develops edema and hemorrhages because of a blunt contusion of the anterior segment. Vision is markedly reduced and often does not improve. Ophthalmoscopically, edema of the sensory retina obscures the retinal pigment ep-

ithelium and choroid. It may disappear spontaneously or may be followed by atrophy of the retina and choroid.

Macular holes. Macular holes are round, red holes of the fovea centralis that measure about ¼ disk diameter in size and are associated with visual acuity reduced to 20/200 or less. Although they are holes in the retina, retinal separation rarely follows. Examination with a biomicroscope indicates that the majority of the holes are cysts with a translucent anterior wall. There is no treatment.

Perforations of the retina. Perforations of the retina are usually associated with loss of vitreous and disorganization of the globe. Retinal detachment may result because the trauma stimulates proliferation of glial or mesodermal tissue, or both, causing retinal traction.

Purtscher injury. Purtscher injury is a rare abnormality in which the sudden increase in intravascular pressure associated with crushing injury of the chest causes retinal hemorrhages and edema.

Fat emboli. Fat emboli of the retinal blood vessels may be seen in fractures of long bones and pancreatitis. They have the same prognosis as emboli from other causes.

Radiant energy. The cornea and the lens transmit long visible light rays (red) and infrared with nearly 100% efficiency (see Chapters 2 and 7). These rays are usually absorbed by the retinal pigment epithelium, and the energy is dissipated by the choriocapillaris. They may cause injury to the retina if (1) the exposure is of long duration and continuous, (2) the energy is at particular wavelengths, (3) the pupil does not constrict to limit the amount of energy entering the eye, (4) the eye is nearly emmetropic so that the rays come to focus on the fovea centralis, (5) the retina is sensitized by vitamin A depletion, or (6) the retina is sensitized by drugs. The classic type of such damage follows observation of a solar eclipse, in which the pupil is dilated because of low light intensity and infrared rays are focused on the fovea centralis. Lasers provide electromagnetic energy at levels not available from natural sources. Laser energy may damage the retina, choroid, and their blood vessels through heating the tissues, protein coagulation, or through photodisruption in which high energy strips the atoms of their electrons.

Light damage (photic retinopathy) to the retina may occur in those who gaze at the sun as part of sun worship or in a psychosis. Marked pupillary constriction may prevent injury. Infants with hemolytic anemia, in whom light oxidizes the bilirubin in the skin, must have their eyes protected during phototherapy. Ocular surgeons routinely protect the retina from injury from operating lights during surgery, particularly after the insertion of an intraocular lens in cataract extraction (see Chapter 7).

Retinal poisons and toxins. Chloroquine and the phenothiazines in large doses cause a pigmentary degeneration of the central retina. Topical administration of epinephrine eyedrops in aphakic eyes also causes a maculopathy with loss of vision. In susceptible persons, a small amount of quinine may cause severe vasoconstriction of retinal arteries with the central visual field reduced to 5° to 10° in diameter.

TUMORS
Retinoblastoma

A retinoblastoma is a malignant tumor that originates in the outer nuclear layer of the retina and strongly resembles fetal retina. It is the most common intraocular tumor of childhood. It is second only to malignant melanoma of the choroid as the most common intraocular tumor of any age group.

Retinoblastoma occurs in three forms: hereditary, sporadic (nonhereditary), and chromosomal (13 q 14) deletion forms. Hereditary retinoblastoma affects both eyes, or there are multiple tumors in one eye. Patients are prone to develop other primary nonocular malignant tumors, often osteosarcoma, before the age of 35 years. Sporadic retinoblastoma affects only one eye, has a single focus, the karyotype is normal, and patients are older at the time of diagnosis than those with bilateral or multifocal tumors. As many as 15% of patients with sporadic uniocular tumors may actually have the hereditary form of retinoblastoma. In the chromosomal deletion form of retinoblastoma, there is loss of band 14 of the long arm of chromosome 13 (13 q 14).

The "two-hit" hypothesis proposes that the induction of a retinoblastoma requires two genetic changes. The locus for these changes is on the short arm of chromosome 13 (13 q 14) close to the locus for esterase D. Normally the two alleles of this locus have a regulatory or suppressor role during embryogenesis and possibly after birth. The first genetic change is inheritance of a retinoblastoma gene from an affected parent. This gene is recessive and is not expressed unless a second event occurs. The second event is the loss, inactivation, or mutation of the allele for this gene on the homologous chromosome so that there is no suppression or regulation.

Wilms' tumor, familial renal cell carcinoma, neuroblastoma, and small cell carcinoma of the lung are thought possibly to be inherited on a similar basis.

The tumor is a pale pink or white mass (Fig. 16-26) with newly formed blood vessels on its surface. There may be many independent tumors or implantation growth on the iris, cornea, or vitreous. The vitreous may contain numerous globules of dull white tumor seeds. Calcium may occur within the tumor as pearly white, sharply defined areas on the surface of the tumor or as chalky white areas with poorly demonstrated deeper edges. It is best demonstrated with computed tomography or ultrasonography. DNA is deposited in the vessel wall of retinoblastoma and is comparable to calcified material in oat cell carcinoma of the lung.

If the aqueous humor has not been frozen,

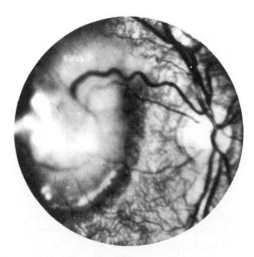

Fig. 16-26. Retinoblastoma of the right eye in a lightly pigmented 1-year-old infant. The tumor projects into the vitreous and casts a shadow on the adjacent retina. There is calcification visible at the apex of the tumor.

the aqueous humor lactic dehydrogenase level is increased in retinoblastoma and the serum-aqueous humor ratio is high in about 93% of the cases. The false-negative rate is approximately 7% and the false-positive rate about 1% when the unfrozen sample is not contaminated with hemolized blood. The alpha fetal protein and carcinoembryonic antigen is increased in some patients.

Often the tumor is first diagnosed when it has protruded far forward into the vitreous cavity, filling the entire globe, and is visible in the eye as a grayish yellow reflex behind the lens. By this time, the pupil is often fixed and the eye is blind. Less frequently, an esotropia or exotropia occurs because of poor vision. Tumor necrosis may cause a red, painful eye that may have glaucoma.

The most important diagnostic step to be taken when retinoblastoma is suspected in one eye is careful ophthalmoscopic examination of the opposite eye with the pupil widely dilated and, if necessary, the child anesthetized. All portions of the retina must be inspected, and particular attention should be directed to the periphery. In sporadic instances both parents should be examined to be certain that neither

has a spontaneously arrested retinoblastoma. Careful study of the fellow eye, when there is no involvement, must be carried out at frequent intervals until late childhood.

Treatment. Treatment is highly individualized and based mainly on the size, location, and number of tumors present (Table 16-4). Often one eye is in a well-advanced stage (groups IV or V) when the tumor is unilateral or bilateral. Usually the eye is enucleated, and the histologic diagnosis confirmed. Tumors in the fellow eye are generally treated with external beam radiation combined with photocoagulation, cryocoagulation, or a radioactive cobalt plaque sutured to the sclera adjacent to the tumor. Cytoxan and vincristine are used for 1 year after treatment in unilateral cases and cyclophosphamide and vincristine in bilateral cases.

Currently any eye in groups I, II, or III is treated even though the fellow eye is normal and both eyes are treated if small tumors are present bilaterally.

Other tumors

Vascular malformations of the retinal blood vessels, Coats disease, and phakomatoses may occur. Hypertrophy of the retinal pigment epithelium may cause a localized black area in the fundus or may occur congenitally as grouped pigmentation. Neoplastic transformation of the retinal pigment epithelium is rare.

Table 16-4. Prognostic indicators in retinoblastoma

Group I: Very favorable
  A. Solitary tumor, less than 4 disk diameters in size, at or behind the equator
  B. Multiple tumors, none over 4 disk diameters in size, all at or behind the equator
Group II: Favorable
  A. Solitary lesions, 4 to 10 disk diameters in size, at or behind the equator
  B. Multiple tumors, 4 to 10 disk diameters in size, at or behind the equator
Group III: Doubtful
  A. Any lesion anterior to the equator
  B. Solitary tumors, larger than 10 disk diameters in size, behind the equator
Group IV: Unfavorable
  A. Multiple tumors, some larger than 10 disk diameters in size
  B. Any lesion extending anteriorly to the ora serrata
Group V: Very unfavorable
  A. Massive tumors involving over half the retina
  B. Vitreous bleeding

From Ellsworth, R.M.: Current management of retinoblastoma. In Jakobiec, F.A., editor: Ocular and adnexal tumors, Birmingham, Ala., 1978, Aesculapius Publishing Co.

BIBLIOGRAPHY
General

Bec, P.: The fundus periphery, New York, 1984, Masson Publishing USA.
Birngruber, R., and Gabel, V.P., editors: Laser treatment and photocoagulation of the eye, The Hague, Netherlands, 1984, Dr. W. Junk.
Byer, N.E.: The peripheral retina in profile: a stereoscopic atlas, Torrance, Calif., 1982, Criterion Press.
Disorders of the fundus. Entire issue, Ophthalmology **91:**1431-1730, 1984.
Dixon, J.A.: Surgical application of lasers, Chicago, 1983, Year Book Medical Publishers.
Krill, A.E., and Archer, D.B.: Krill's hereditary retinal and choroidal diseases, vol. 2, New York, 1977, Harper & Row, Publishers.
L'Esperance, F.A., Jr.: Ophthalmic lasers: photocoagulation, photoradiation and surgery, St. Louis, 1982, The C.V. Mosby Co.

New Orleans Academy of Ophthalmology: Symposium on medical and surgical diseases of the retina and vitreous, St. Louis, 1983, The C.V. Mosby Co.

Robin, A.L.: Lasers in ophthalmology, Chicago, 1984, Year Book Medical Publishers.

Ophthalmoscopic findings

Bird, A.C.: Retinal edema, Surv. Ophthalmol. **28**:433, 1984.

Eagle, R.C., Jr.: Mechanisms of maculopathy, Ophthalmology **91**:613, 1984.

Miller, H., Miller, B., and Ryan, S.J.: Correlation of choroidal subretinal neovascularization with fluorescein angiography, Am. J. Ophthalmol. **99**:263, 1985.

Congenital and developmental abnormalities

Cassidy, S.B., Pasgon, R.A., Pepin, M., et al.: Family studies in tuberous sclerosis: evaluation of apparently unaffected parents, J.A.M.A. **24**:1302, 1983.

Cibis, G.W., Tripathi, R.C., and Tripathi, B.J.: Glaucoma in Sturge-Weber syndrome, Ophthalmology **91**:1061, 1984.

The Committee for the Classification of Retinopathy of Prematurity: An international classification of retinopathy of prematurity, Arch. Ophthalmol. **102**:1130, 1984.

Hardwig, P., and Robertson, D.M.: Von Hippel-Lindau disease: a familial, often lethal, multi-system phakomatosis, Ophthalmology **91**:262, 1984.

Ibayashi, H., Nishimura, M., and Yamana, T.: Avascular zone in the macula in cicatricial retinopathy of prematurity, Am. J. Ophthalmol. **99**:235, 1985.

Lewis, R.A., Gerson, O.P., Axelson, K.A., Riccardi, V.M., and Whitford, R.P.: Von Recklinghausen neurofibromatosis. II. Incidence of optic gliomata, Ophthalmology **91**:929, 1984.

Patz, A.: Observations on the retinopathy of prematurity, Am. J. Ophthalmol. **100**:164, 1985.

Perry, H.D., and Font, R.L.: Iris nodules in von Recklinghausen's neurofibromatosis: electron microscopic confirmation of their melanocyte formation, Arch. Ophthalmol. **100**:1635, 1982.

Salazar, F.G., and Lamiell, J.M.: Early identification of retinal angiomas in a large kindred with von Hippel-Lindau disease, Am. J. Ophthalmol. **89**:540, 1980.

Schaffer, D.B., Quinn, G.E., and Johnson, L.: Sequelae of arrested mild retinopathy of prematurity, Arch. Ophthalmol. **102**:373, 1984.

Vascular disorders

Berkow, J.W.: Subretinal neovascularization in senile macular degeneration, Am. J. Ophthalmol. **97**:143, 1984.

The Branch Vein Occlusion Study Group: Argon laser photocoagulation for macular edema in branch vein occlusion, Am. J. Ophthalmol. **98**:271-282, 1984.

First International Cystoid Macular Edema Symposium, April 1983, Surv. Ophthalmol. **28**(Suppl.): 431-619, 1984.

Folk, J.C., Thompson, H.S., Han, D.P., and Brown, C.K.: Visual function abnormalities in central serous retinopathy, Arch. Ophthalmol. **102**:1299, 1984.

Gutman, F.A.: Evaluation of a patient with central retinal vein occlusion, Ophthalmology **90**:481, 1983.

Kohner, E.M., Laatikainen, L., and Oughton, J.: The management of central retinal vein occlusion, Ophthalmology **90**:484, 1983.

Inflammations

Culbertson, W.W., Blumenkranz, M.S., Haines, H., Gass, J.D.M., Mitchell, K.B., and Norton, E.W.D.: The acute retinal necrosis syndrome. Pt. 2. Histopathology and etiology, Ophthalmology **89**:1317, 1982.

Dreyer, R.F., and Gass, J.D.M.: Multifocal choroiditis and paneuveitis, Arch. Ophthalmol. **102**:1776, 1984.

Fisher, J.P., Lewis, M.L., Blumenkranz, M., Culbertson, W.W., Flynn, H.W. Jr., Clarkson, J.G., Gass, J.D.M., and Norton, E.W.D.: The acute retinal necrosis syndrome. Pt. 1. Clinical manifestations, Ophthalmology **89**:1309, 1982.

Freeman, W.R., and O'Connor, G.R.: Acquired immune deficiency syndrome retinopathy, pneumocytitis, and cotton-wool spots, Am. J. Ophthalmol. **98**:235, 1984.

Fuerst, D.J., Tessler, H.H., Fishman, G.A., Yokoyama, M.M., Wyhinny, G.J., and Vygantas, C.M.: Birdshot retinopathy, Arch. Ophthalmol. **102**:214, 1984.

Gaynon, M.W., Boldrey, E.E., Strahlman, E.R., and Fine, S.L.: Retinal neovascularization and ocular toxoplasmosis, Am. J. Ophthalmol. **98**:585, 1984.

Jampol, L.M., Kraff, M.C., Sanders, D.R., Alexander, K., and Lieberman, H.: Cystoid macular edema, Arch. Ophthalmol. **103**:28, 1985.

Lyness, A.L., and Bird, A.C.: Recurrences of acute posterior multifocal placoid pigment epitheliopathy, Am. J. Ophthalmol. **98**:203, 1984.

Nussenblatt, R.B., Mittal, K.K., and Ryan, S.: Birdshot retinochoroidopathy associated with HLA-A29 antigen and immune responsiveness to retinal S-antigen, Am. J. Ophthalmol. **94**:147, 1982.

The Silicone Study Group: Proliferative vitreoretinopathy, Am. J. Ophthalmol. **99**:593, 1985.

Fluid-separating layers

The Retina Society Terminology Committee: The classification of retinal detachment with proliferative vitreoretinopathy, Ophthalmology **90**:121, 1983.

Schepens, C.L.: Retinal detachment and allied diseases, vol. 2, Philadelphia, 1983, W.B. Saunders Co.

Degenerations

Berson, E.L., Sandberg, M.A., Rosner, B., Birch, D.G., and Hanson, A.H.: Natural course of retinitis pigmentosa over a three-year interval, Am. J. Ophthalmol. **99**:240, 1985.

Bhattacharya, S.S., Wright, A.F., Clayton, J.F., Price, W.H., Phillips, C.I., McKeown, C.M.E., Jay, M., Bird, A.C., Pearson, P.L., Southern, E.M., and Evans, H.J.: Close genetic linkage between X-linked retinitis pigmentosa and a restriction fragment length polymorphism identified by recombinant DNA probe L1.28, Nature **309**:253, 1984.

Feeney-Burns, L., and Ellersieck, M.R.: Age-related changes in the ultrastructure of Bruch's membrane, Am. J. Ophthalmol. **100**:686, 1985.

Gass, J.D.M., Jallow, S., and Davis, B.: Adult vitelliform macular detachment occurring in patients with basal laminar drusen, Am. J. Ophthalmol. **99**:445, 1985.

Green, W.R., McDonnell, P.J., and Yeo, J.H.: Pathologic features of senile macular degeneration, Ophthalmology **92**:615, 1985.

Ishibashi, T., Patterson, R., Ohnishi, Y., Inomata, H., and Ryan, S.J.: Formation of drusen in the human eye, Am. J. Ophthalmol. **101**:342, 1986.

Kenyon, K.R., Maumenee, A.E., Ryan, S.J., Whitmore, P.V., and Green, W.R.: Diffuse drusen and associated complications, Am. J. Ophthalmol. **100**:119, 1985.

Moloney, J.B.M., Mooney, D.J., and O'Connor, M.A.: Retinal function in Stargardt's disease and fundus flavimaculatus, Am. J. Ophthalmol. **96**:57, 1983.

Morgan, C.M., and Schatz, H.: Idiopathic macular holes, Am. J. Ophthalmol. **99**:437, 1985.

Newsome, D.A.: Retinal fluorescein leakage in retinitis pigmentosa, Am. J. Ophthalmol. **101**:354, 1986.

Tso, M.O.M.: Pathogenetic factors of aging macular degeneration, Ophthalmology **92**:628, 1985.

Injuries

Mainster, M.A., Sliney, D.H., Belcher, C.D. III, and Buzney, S.M.: Laser photodisruptors: damage mechanisms, instrument design and safety, Ophthalmology **90**:973, 1983.

Tumors

Cavenee, W.K., Hansen, M.F., Nordenskjold, M., Kock, E., Maumenee, I., Squire, J.A., Phillips, R.A., and Gallie, B.L.: Genetic origin of mutations predisposing to retinoblastoma, Science **228**:501, 1985.

Dryja, T.P., Cavenee, W., White, R., Rapaport, J.M., Petersen, R., Albert, D.M., and Bruns, G.A.: Homozygosity of chromosome 13 in retinoblastoma, N. Engl. J. Med. **310**:550, 1984.

Gallie, B.L., and Phillips, R.A.: Retinoblastoma: a model of oncogenesis, Ophthalmology **91**:666, 1984.

Gordon, H.: Oncogenes, Mayo Clin. Proc. **60**:697, 1985.

Knudson, A.G., Jr.: The genetics of childhood cancer, Cancer 35(3 suppl.):1022, 1975.

Mukai, S., Rapaport, J.M., Shields, J.A., Augsburger, J.J., and Dryja, T.P.: Linkage of genes for human esterase D and hereditary retinoblastoma, Am. J. Ophthalmol. **97**:681, 1984.

Murphree, A.L., and Benedict, W.F.: Retinoblastoma: clues to human oncogenesis, Science **223**:1028, 1984.

17

THE VITREOUS HUMOR

The vitreous humor, a transparent tissue that has the physical properties of a gel, fills the vitreous cavity. It comprises two thirds (4.5 ml) of the volume of the eye and about three fourths of the weight. Normally it fills the entire vitreous cavity, and vitreous fibers blend with the fibrillary material of the internal limiting lamina of the retina (Fig. 17-1). Its anterior surface, the anterior hyaloid, is hollowed to conform to the posterior convexity of the lens, and a few fibers may extend between the posterior lens capsule and the anterior hyaloid (the hyaloid capsular ligament). The posterior hyaloid lines the entire retina. The base of the vitreous is a band 2 mm wide that straddles the ora serrata to provide a firm attachment of the vitreous to the retina and ciliary body. Retinal holes frequently occur along the posterior border of the vitreous base. The vitreous humor is also firmly attached to the margin but not the surface of the optic disk.

The vitreous humor consists of a peripheral cortex that contains a central region. A collagen meshwork fans out from the cortex into a more delicate meshwork in the central vitreous. Within the collagen meshwork are long, coiled hyaluronic acid molecules that retain water and give the vitreous body its viscosity. Some 99% of the vitreous humor is water. The cortical vitreous contains a few large, flat cells, hyalocytes, that function as connective tissue macrophages.

The vitreous humor is a physiologic and biologic gel. Disease, aging, and injury disturb the factors that maintain water in suspension, and the vitreous liquefies. With the loss of the gel structure, fine fibers, membranes, and cellular aggregates become visible, although they are almost transparent. In disease, blood vessels may grow from the surface of the retina or optic disk onto the posterior hyaloid and blood may fill the vitreous cavity.

Symptoms and signs of diseases

Abnormalities of the vitreous humor may cause three main symptoms: (1) material in the vitreous may be visualized when looking at a bright blue sky or pastel-shaded wall ("floaters"); (2) membranes, blood cells, or foreign material may impair image formation and reduce vision; or (3) traction by the vitreous on the sensory retina may cause light flashes when the eyes move, often with the eyes closed (photopsia), or in the dark. Floaters in the normal eye consist of protein remnants of the embryologic hyaloid vascular system. In disease, floaters consist of blood cells or abnormal collagen aggregates. Photopsia results from traction of the vitreous upon the retina and may be a sign of actual or impending retinal hole formation. Shrinkage of the vitreous causes a variety of entoptic phenomena that can be seen with the eyes closed or in the dark. As the eyes move, the shrunken vitreous gently bumps the retina, initiating a nervous impulse and perception of light.

The vitreous humor is studied with the indirect ophthalmoscope and a convex lens so that opacities are visible against the red background of the fundus. It may be studied with a biomi-

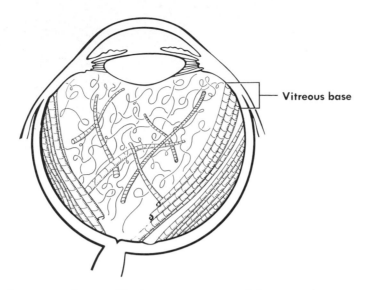

Fig. 17-1. The vitreous humor fills the vitreous cavity of the eye. The vitreous humor is firmly adherent at the ora serrata and peripheral retina (vitreous base) and the periphery of the optic disk. The surface of the vitreous humor anterior to the ora serrata is the anterior hyaloid; that adjacent to the sensory retina is the posterior hyaloid.

croscope and either a −40 diopter or a −50 diopter contact lens equipped with inclined mirrors to study the ocular periphery. Gross vitreous opacities can be seen with a direct ophthalmoscope.

DEGENERATIONS

Syneresis. This degenerative condition occurs in aging, in myopia, and after injuries and inflammation of the eye. The vitreous humor becomes partially or completely fluid, creating the appearance of membranes or strands floating freely in the fluid (Fig. 17-2). The condition is caused by release of water by the vitreous fibrillar structures, which then float in the water. These particles float across the visual line, impair vision, and may be extremely vexing. They are visible with the ophthalmoscope or slit lamp. The symptoms may be relieved by wearing an appropriate lens for any ametropia present, but no treatment will restore the normal viscosity and structure of the vitreous.

Vitreous detachment. The vitreous humor is firmly attached in the area surrounding the optic nerve. With aging, the central portion of the vitreous humor may be replaced with fluid. The peripheral cortical hyaloid may then separate from the retina and collapse the central cavity. This creates a fluid-filled, optically

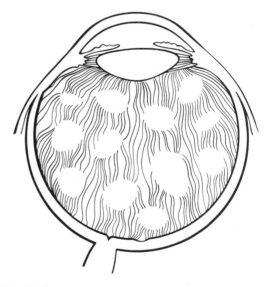

Fig. 17-2. Syneresis with fluid-filled spaces in the vitreous humor.

empty space between the retina and vitreous (Fig. 17-3). The original site of attachment to the margin of the optic disk is often marked with a ring-shaped opacity on the posterior hyaloid. Vitreous detachment occurs most commonly in women between 55 and 65 years of age. They suddenly notice a relatively large, fixed floater near the point of fixation. As the

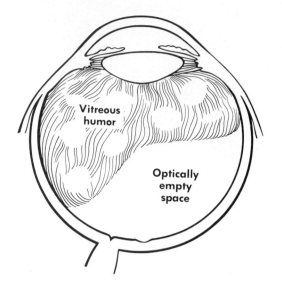

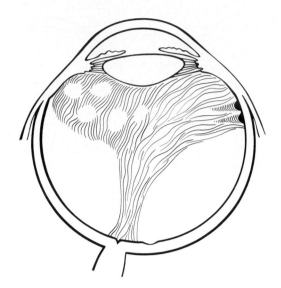

Fig. 17-3. Vitreous detachment with fluid-filled optically empty space between the retina and posterior hyaloid.

Fig. 17-4. Detachment of the vitreious humor with persistent adhesion on the right side that may cause traction on the retina and a retinal tear.

individual attempts to fix upon the floater, it darts out of the field of vision. There may be associated subjective lightning flashes, so that with the eyes closed or in a dark room a sudden movement of the eye causes a flash of light, which results either from traction or the vitreous striking the retina. On examination, one may see the floater in front of an optically empty space adjacent to the posterior retina. The fellow eye usually becomes involved within a few months. There is no effective treatment, although the floater tends to become less conspicuous with time. Detachment of the vitreous humor may cause retinal traction and retinal hole formation. Traction upon a small retinal blood vessel may cause a minute vitreous hemorrhage. At the onset of a vitreous detachment, the peripheral retina must be studied with indirect ophthalmoscopy.

Detachment of the vitreous disturbs the vitreoretinal interface and may lead to a variety of conditions that affect retinal function. Proliferative diabetic retinopathy with vitreous membranes of mesenchymal and fibroblastic origin occurs only if there is detachment of the vitreous. In simple epiretinal membranes, accessory retinal astroglia migrate from the inner layers of the retina and form a fine, cellular membrane between the retina and the vitreous. These membranes are often seen histologically in eyes removed for disease but are

clinically subtle. They rarely cause visual problems. Surface wrinkling retinopathy is probably a similar condition, but the wrinkling of the retina causes visual symptoms.

A more severe group of related conditions includes macular pucker after retinal detachment surgery, cellophane maculopathy, preretinal macular fibrosis, and retinal star folds. There has been little clinical and pathologic correlation, and it is not known whether these are the same or different conditions.

The most severe condition initiated by detachment of the vitreous is massive vitreous retraction or massive periretinal proliferation that complicates retinal detachment surgery. After surgery the detached retina develops fixed folds, and the vitreous is sprinkled with pigmented cells. There is proliferation of retinal pigment epithelium both anterior to and posterior to the sensory retina, and irreversible blindness is the usual outcome.

Vitreous adhesion is a destructive phenomenon in which contraction of the vitreous causes traction upon the retinal areas to which it is abnormally attached (Fig. 17-4). Shrinkage in the peripheral region may cause a horseshoe-shaped tear, with the flap held open by the persistent attachment of vitreous. Traction in the region of the ora serrata may be a factor in the production of peripheral retinal holes or retinal dialysis.

Hereditary degenerations. The three main forms of inherited vitreoretinal degeneration are: (1) X chromosome–linked juvenile retinoschisis, inherited as an X chromosome–linked recessive trait (see Chapter 10); (2) hyaloideotapetoretinal degeneration of Goldmann-Favre; and (3) dominantly inherited hyaloideoretinopathy of Wagner. Additionally, vitreous degeneration is seen in hereditary degenerative myopia, the facial-clefting syndromes, and some retinal and peripheral degenerative diseases.

Hyaloideotapetoretinal dystrophy of Goldmann-Favre is an autosomal recessive progressive disorder that includes a liquid vitreous humor, vitreous veils with central and peripheral retinoschisis, tapetoretinal degeneration, and complicated cataracts. Blindness results ultimately.

Dominantly inherited hyaloideoretinopathy of Wagner is associated with liquefaction and destruction of the vitreous humor with grayish-white preretinal membranes, myopia, cataracts, retinal separation, and retinal pigmentation and depigmentation.

A variety of skeletal abnormalities may occur together with a dominantly inherited hyaloideoretinopathy. The most characteristic are hereditary arthro-ophthalmopathy (Stickler) associated with progressive multiple dysplasia of the epiphyses, overtubulation of long bones, cleft lip and palate, hypermobility of joints, flattened vertebral bodies, pelvic bone deformities, and sensorineural deafness.

VITREOUS OPACITIES

Many foreign substances may be suspended in the vitreous body: (1) exogenous material, such as parasites or foreign bodies, or (2) endogenous substances, such as leukocytes or erythrocytes from the blood, pigment, tumor cells, cholesterol, or calcium salts. All cause the symptoms of floaters and may cause a severe reduction in vision. The sudden appearance of a shower of opacities suggests retinal traction on a retinal blood vessel resulting in a hemorrhage and possible retinal hole. A large opacity of relatively fixed position is less suggestive of serious disease. Whatever their appearance, examination of the peripheral fundus with pupillary dilation and indirect ophthalmoscopy is necessary to exclude a retinal hole as the cause.

Muscae volitantes. These physiologic opacities consist of residues of the primitive hyaloidal vascular system. A patient sees them in bright illumination, against a cloudless sky, or a pastel-shaded wall. They drift in and out of the visual field and dart from the field of vision when one attempts to fixate directly on them. Some patients, after first observing them, require reassurance about their universality. Correction of ametropia makes the opacities more difficult to observe.

Hemorrhage. The moment of a retinal hole may be signalled by a minute hemorrhage into the vitreous body as the vitreous traction causes a tear in the sensory retina that ruptures a retinal blood vessel. The sudden appearance of diffusely scattered dots or lines is a signal for immediate examination to locate a possible retinal hole and close it before a retinal detachment occurs.

Bleeding into the vitreous humor results from rupture of fragile, newly formed blood vessels originating from the optic disk or retina. Neovascularization may be caused by trauma, inflammation, vascular and metabolic disease, tumors, or rupture of a subhyaloid retinal hemorrhage secondary to a subarachnoid hemorrhage (Terson). The blood may be evenly dispersed throughout the vitreous humor, localized, or distributed in sheets. In a young person resorption may be rapid, but persistent or recurrent hemorrhages are followed by yellow or white debris and fibrous membranes in the vitreous humor. The symptoms depend upon the location of the vitreous hemorrhage. Peripheral hemorrhage causes floaters, whereas blood in the visual axis reduces vision and may cause a red haze. Vitreous hemorrhage may cause visual loss because of persistent opacification, inflammation, glaucoma, siderosis, or fibrous tissue proliferation and contraction that causes retinal detachment. Vitrectomy through the pars plana removes diseased or opacified vitreous and membranes.

Asteroid hyalosis. This is an involutional, mainly uniocular phenomenon that predominantly affects men, in which hundreds to thousands of stellate or discoid ("snowball") opacities are suspended throughout or in a portion of a solid vitreous. They appear creamy white when viewed with the ophthalmoscope and sparkle like Christmas ornaments in the illumination of a biomicroscope. The opacities consist of various calcium-containing lipids, and they apparently result from degeneration of vitreous fibrils. They are suspended in vitreous of normal viscosity. Although they obscure the view of the fundus, they do not indicate disease, cause symptoms, or require treatment.

Cholesterolosis bulbi. This abnormality was known during much of the twentieth century as synchysis scintillans. However, the vitreous need not be liquefied, and the crystals may occur in the iris and retina. Cholesterol crystals occur in blind eyes along with retinal detachment or may be secondary to severe ocular disease or injury. They are mainly observed in enucleated eyes. If the lens has been removed, the crystals may be observed both in the anterior chamber and in the vitreous cavity.

Persistent hyperplastic primary vitreous. The primary vitreous is a fibrillar meshwork that bridges the region between the lens vesicle and inner wall of the optic cup. At the 11 mm stage of gestation, the primary vitreous is invaded by mesoderm and intermingles with the elaborate vasa hyaloidea propria. The hyaloid vascular system begins to atrophy at the 60 mm stage, and by the eighth month of gestation, the process is completed, leaving only minute remnants visible as muscae volitantes.

Failure of the hyaloid artery to regress, combined with the hyperplasia of the posterior portion of the vascular meshwork of the embryonic lens (tunica vasculosa lentis), produces persistent hyperplastic primary vitreous. This monocular condition occurs in full-term infants. The eye fails to develop, is smaller than the fellow eye, and the initially clear lens becomes opaque. Immediately behind the lens is a pinkish-white fibrous mass that may vary in size from a small plaque to one entirely covering the posterior surface of the shrunken lens. Traction elongates the ciliary processes that extend to the mass. The equator of the lens is smaller than normal. The anterior chamber is shallow. The tissue posterior to the lens is vascular, and the vessels radiate from the center. The posterior capsule may rupture and cause cataract. Buphthalmos may develop.

The elongation of the ciliary processes, the microphthalmos, and the rupture of the posterior lens capsule occurring in one eye of a full-term, normal-weight infant distinguish the condition from microphthalmos, retinoblastoma, retinopathy of prematurity, retinal dysplasia, and congenital cataract. Computed tomography may indicate persistence of intraocular fetal vasculature.

Early removal of the lens is necessary to preserve the eye. Some vision, but usually not full vision, is retained, but without lens extraction, the eye is destined for enucleation because of glaucoma. Preferably, the lens is removed with the retrolenticular membrane intact by means of a suction-aspiration-cutting instrument introduced through the pars plana. Patients should be operated on as early as possible (1 day to 4 weeks of age). Fitting with a contact lens immediately thereafter may prevent amblyopia.

PROLAPSE OF THE VITREOUS

After intracapsular cataract extraction or incision of the posterior lens capsule after extracapsular cataract extraction, the anterior hyaloid may herniate into the anterior chamber. The severity of the herniation varies from a small opening in the anterior hyaloid to complete filling of the anterior chamber with vitreous. If an intact anterior hyaloid adheres to the corneal endothelium, a bullous keratopathy occasionally develops because of impairment of corneal deturgescence by the corneal endothelium. Treatment must be directed to surgical separation of the hyaloid from the cornea by vitrectomy. Secondary glaucoma may occur if vitreous prolapses through the pupil and prevents the passage of aqueous humor from the posterior to anterior chamber. This is treated by pupillary dilation but may require removal of the anterior hyaloid.

Loss of vitreous at the time of intraocular surgery is a serious complication because the interposition of vitreous between wound edges may lead to faulty healing and cystoid macular edema. Additionally, the firm adhesions of the vitreous base to the ora serrata combined with forward displacement of the vitreous humor may cause retinal traction and result in a retinal tear. Ophthalmic surgeons seek to prevent vitreous loss by maintaining a soft eye and avoiding increased intraocular pressure. Vitreous loss at the time of surgery is treated by means of an anterior vitrectomy to ensure that no vitreous is between the wound edges and no traction is upon the vitreous base.

VITRECTOMY

Removal and replacement of the vitreous with balanced saline solution or physiologic saline (which is soon replaced by the body fluids) is indicated in patients with vitreous opacities that cause legal blindness or in patients with complications of intraocular surgery, inflammation, trauma, or complicated retinal separations (Table 17-1). Additionally, vitrectomy is often performed when vitreous membranes reduce vision. Some legally blind patients who could benefit from the procedure are not aware of this procedure and the possible improvement in vision. Unfortunately, in many patients, the primary disorder that caused the abnormal vitreous humor may also have seriously damaged the retina or caused glaucoma so that substitution of a clear vitreous does not always improve vision.

The procedure is of no value if the retina is not functional, but cataract or severe opacification of the vitreous may make evaluation of retinal function difficult. An ideal patient is able to visualize his retinal blood vessels as a penlight moves against the lower eyelid (entoptic visualization). Bright-flash electroretinography should be normal. The visual-evoked potential to bright flash should be normal. The pupillary response and light projection should be normal. The anterior chamber angle and iris should be free of new blood vessels; glaucoma should not be present.

Unfortunately, most patients are not ideal surgical candidates. Light projection is often poor, but light perception must be present. Prognosis is poor if the electroretinogram is nonrecordable. Rubeosis of the iris or anterior chamber angle is often a contraindication. Patients with dense membranes attached to the retina or generalized retinal detachment have a poor prognosis. Eyes that have become soft and disorganized (phthisis bulbi) respond poorly. Most of the patients with a good prognosis have improved vision after vitrectomy.

Vitrectomy is done through a 3 mm incision in the pars plana (closed system) or through the conventional incision at the corneoscleral limbus (open eye). Vitrectomy through the corneoscleral limbus requires simultaneous or prior removal of the crystalline lens.

The eye retains its shape in pars plana vitrectomy. As vitreous is removed from the eye by

Table 17-1. Indications for vitrectomy

I. Persistent vitreous opacity with legal blindness
   A. Hemorrhage
   B. Vitreous amyloidosis
   C. Preretinal membranes
   D. Vitreous membranes and strands
II. Complications of cataract extraction
   A. Vitreous touch with bullous keratopathy
   B. Pupillary block glaucoma
   C. Loss of vitreous
   D. Incarceration of vitreous in wound with traction.
III. Endophthalmitis with vitreous abscess
IV. Trauma
   A. Anterior chamber reconstruction
   B. Intraocular nonmagnetic foreign bodies
V. Complicated retinal detachments
   A. Vitreous adhesion syndromes
     1. Massive vitreous retraction
     2. Localized traction
     3. Transvitreal membranes
   B. Giant retinal tears
VI. Persistent hyperplastic primary vitreous
VII. Malignant glaucoma

cutting and suction, physiologic saline is infused into the eye to balance the suction. The intraocular pressure must be maintained at a near-normal level because the eye collapses if the pressure is too low and the central retinal artery occludes if the pressure is too high. A pressure of between 25 and 35 mm Hg is considered optimal. The infusion-aspiration is combined with one of several types of scissors or rotating or chopping cutters (Fig. 17-5). (Ultrasound fragmenters, although useful in lens extraction, are usually not helpful in vitrectomy.) If the lens is present, the operation is usually carried out through a scleral incision in the pars plana about 4 mm posterior to the corneoscleral limbus in the temporal quadrant slightly above or below the horizontal meridian and its long ciliary artery. A cataractous lens is removed with the same or a slightly modified instrument.

The procedure is carried out under microscopic control, with the use of a contact lens to neutralize the corneal refraction and to view the vitreous and retina. Many types of cutters have been designed to cut membranes with minimal traction upon the retina.

The operations may be divided into those in which the anterior vitreous is removed and those in which both the anterior and posterior

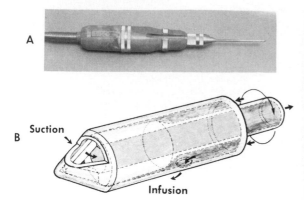

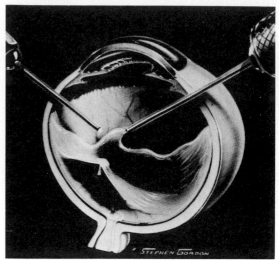

Fig. 17-5. A, The suction infusion vitreous cutter. **B,** Schema of the cutting tip. Vitreous is aspirated into the cutting port of an outer stationary tube and cut by the sharp edges of the inner rotating tube. It is then aspirated through the inner tube out of the eye. Simultaneously, the intraocular volume removed is replaced by an infusion of Ringer solution, which enters the eye through a small opening at the side of the outer tube. (Courtesy Robert Machemer.)

Fig. 17-6. Removal of a vitreous-retinal membrane using an illuminating system (*right*) and a suction-infusion vitreous cutter. The surgeon views the interior of the eye through a microscope and a contact lens. (From Boyd, B.: Highlights of ophthalmology, Panama, 1981, Clinica Boyd.)

vitreous are removed. Vitreous membranes may be removed at the same time (Fig 17-6).

Rubeosis iridis and glaucoma are the most common complications. After removal of the lens, an angiogenic factor, which is thought to be responsible for retinal neovascularization, may have easier access to the iris and may aggravate a preexisting rubeosis iridis or stimulate additional blood vessels.

Glaucoma occurs because of rubeosis iridis or obstruction of the trabecular meshwork by the cell membranes of erythrocytes (ghost cells) that persist after a vitreous hemorrhage. The cells cannot enter the anterior chamber when the lens is present; but after lens extraction and vitrectomy with rupture of the anterior hyaloid face, these cells are free to circulate through the eye. Glaucoma occurs in as many as one third of the eyes that have had vitrectomy-lens extraction. To provide clear media, every effort must be made to irrigate the vitreous cavity adequately at the time of surgery.

BIBLIOGRAPHY
General

Oyakawa, R.T., Michels, R.G., and Blase, W.P.: Vitrectomy for nondiabetic vitreous hemorrhage, Am. J. Ophthalmol. **96:**517, 1983.

Stern, W.H., Diddie, K.R., Smith, R.E., and Koelling, J.: Vitrectomy techniques for the anterior segment surgeon: a practical approach, New York, 1983, Grune & Stratton.

Opacities

Boldrey, E.E.: Risk of retinal tears in patients with vitreous floaters, Am. J. Ophthalmol. **96:**783, 1983.

Goldberg, M.F., and Mafee, M.: Computed tomography for diagnosis of persistent hyperplastic primary vitreous (PHPV), Ophthalmology **90:**442, 1983.

Murakami, K., Jalkh, A.E., Avila, M.P., Trempe, C.L., and Schepens, C.L.: Vitreous floaters, Ophthalmology **90:**1271, 1983.

Novak, M.A., and Welch, R.B.: Complications of acute symptomatic posterior vitreous detachment, Am. J. Ophthalmol. **97:**308, 1984.

Stark, W.J., Lindsey, P.S., Fagadau, W.R., and Michels, R.G.: Persistent hyperplastic primary vitreous: surgical treatment, Ophthalmology **90:**452, 1983.

Vitrectomy

Diabetic Retinopathy Vitrectomy Study Research Group: Early vitrectomy for severe vitreous hemorrhage in diabetic retinopathy, Arch. Ophthalmol. **103:**1644, 1985.

Peyman, G.A., and Schulman, J.A.: Intravitreal surgery: principles and practice, East Norwalk, Conn., 1986, Appleton-Century-Crofts.

18

THE OPTIC NERVE

The optic nerve is morphologically and embryologically a nerve fiber tract of the central nervous system. Posterior to the lamina cribrosa, its axons are sheathed in a thin layer of doubled plasmalemma derived from oligodendrocytes that form the myelin covering. The nerve is composed mainly of the axons of the ganglion cells of the retina that synapse in either the lateral geniculate body (vision) or the pretectal region (pupil). In the retina the fibers are bare axons that constitute the nerve fiber layer of the retina, but behind the lamina cribrosa they are myelinated.

The optic nerve may be divided into the following parts: (1) intraocular, (2) intraorbital, (3) intracanalicular, and (4) intracranial. The nonmyelinated intraocular portion contained within the scleral canal may be divided into three parts: (1) inner retinal, (2) middle choroidal, and (3) outer scleral.

The nerve fiber bundles are separated into columns by small fibrous astrocytes. The lamina cribrosa begins at the level of the choroidal layer and is composed mainly of astrocytes, collagenous connective tissue, and small blood vessels. Considerable attention is directed to the blood supply of the intraocular portion of the optic nerve because of its involvement in glaucoma and papilledema.

The intraocular portion of the optic nerve that is visible with the ophthalmoscope is the optic papilla, or optic disk (papilla is a misnomer because the disk is at the same level or lower than the retinal nerve fiber layer).

A central depression, the physiologic cup with its edges concentric to those of the disk, is lined with glial tissue. When glial tissue is sparse, the ophthalmoscopist can see the perforations of the lamina cribrosa. When glial tissue is abundant, the physiologic cup is absent. Sometimes a small amount of tissue projects into the vitreous as the Bergmeister papilla.

A vertical line through the center of the foveola divides the retina into nasal and temporal portions; all nerve fibers nasal to this line decussate in the optic chiasm. Temporal fibers do not decussate.

Within the orbit the optic nerve is surrounded by a continuation of the cranial meninges: an outer dura mater, an intermediate arachnoid, and an inner pia mater, which is a thin, vascularized connective tissue sheet. The collagenous pial sheath enters the nerve and divides and subdivides myelinated nerve fiber bundles into columns.

Within the orbit to the level of the lamina cribrosa, the pia mater provides the optic nerve blood supply. At the scleral level, short posterior ciliary arteries provide the blood supply, whereas the retinal surface is supplied by the branches from the central retinal artery.

SYMPTOMS AND SIGNS OF OPTIC NERVE DISEASE

The main symptom of optic nerve disease is loss of vision. If fibers composing the papillomacular bundle, which originates from the fovea centralis, are involved, visual acuity, is decreased, often with disturbances of color vision. (The central retina provides 90% of the fibers of the optic nerve.) Involvement of fibers anterior to their decussation in the chiasm causes defects in the vision of one eye only. Interference with nerve conduction in the chiasm or in the optic tract causes visual defects in both eyes.

Conduction defects in the optic nerve cause an afferent pupillary defect of the involved eye.

Pain is a prominent symptom only in retrobulbar neuritis, in which there is pain deep in the orbit when the eye is moved or when pressure is applied to the globe. The pain is combined with loss of vision and a normal-appearing disk. The causes of papillitis are often the same as the causes of retrobulbar neuritis. There is no pain, but the optic disk is swollen. In anterior ischemic optic neuropathy, vision is reduced, the optic disk is edematous and pale, often with splinter hemorrhage. The uninvolved fellow eye often has an exceptionally small physiologic cup. Loss of vision, often in both eyes, is the main symptom in posterior optic neuropathy. In papilledema there is often no disturbance of vision and diagnosis is based on the ophthalmoscopic appearance of the swollen disk and surrounding retina. The diagnosis in optic atrophy is based on correlation of an abnormal visual field with a pale abnormal optic disk.

Ophthalmoscopy plays a major role in the diagnosis of optic nerve abnormalities since the optic disk may be viewed directly. The central artery and vein are located at the center or slightly to the nasal side of the disk. A small whitish depression is located at the center of the disk (optic cup, physiologic cup), and through this one may sometimes view the lamina cribrosa. Surrounding the cup is a pink area of tissue composed of nerve fiber bundles, columns of glial cells, and capillaries, which gives a pink appearance. The margins of the optic disk are usually regular. In some normal eyes the pigment epithelium and choroid do not extend to the disk, and a crescent of sclera is visible. The transparent nerve fiber layer of the sensory retina passes over the sclera to the optic disk. In other eyes the retinal pigment epithelium terminates short of the disk so that the choroid is visible.

Attention is directed particularly to the size and shape of the physiologic cup, the surface of the disk and its color, pulsation of the central retinal vein, and the margins of the disk. Measurement of the visual acuity and determination of the visual fields are essential to accurate diagnosis. The variety of diseases affecting the optic nerve is large, and accurate diagnosis requires a complete history, neurologic examination, search for systemic disease, and aware-

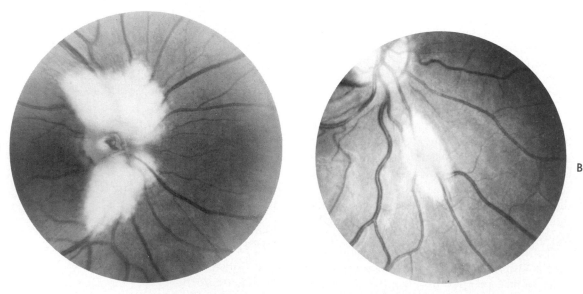

Fig. 18-1. **A,** Myelination of the optic nerve encroaching over margins of the optic disk. **B,** Small patch of myelination of peripheral retinal nerve fibers.

ness of the variety of diseases that may cause similar findings.

The cup-disk ratio is the ratio of the horizontal width of the optic cup to the horizontal diameter of the entire disk. Its main significance is in the diagnosis and management of glaucoma. A high ratio in one or both eyes is suggestive of glaucoma.

The optic nerve head has a dual blood supply from the retinal circulation and the short posterior ciliary arteries. The surface of the optic disk is nurtured mainly by retinal arteries, whereas the deeper portion derives its blood supply from the short posterior ciliary arteries. Neovascularization of the surface of the optic disk occurs in diabetes mellitus, branch and central vein occlusion, obstruction or insufficiency of the internal carotid artery, pulseless disease (Takayashu disease), and other conditions usually associated with ischemia. These vessels seem to be derived from the posterior ciliary arteries rather than from the retinal blood vessels.

As in intracranial lesions, perimetry and computed tomography are essential to accurate diagnosis.

Myelinated (medullated) nerve fibers. Myelination of the anterior visual system begins in the lateral geniculate body at 5 months gestation. It reaches the chiasm at 6 to 7 months, the intraorbital optic nerve at 8 months, and the lamina cribrosa at birth. Sometimes (0.1%) the process does not stop there but continues over the retinal surface (Fig. 18-1). Ophthalmoscopy discloses an area of white, opaque, glistening appearance with soft, feathered edges usually continuous with the optic disk.

The area of myelination involves only a small sector of the retina that is usually near the disk. The absence of pigment proliferation, the feathery edges, and the normal visual field differentiate myelinated nerve fibers from chorioretinitis. Rarely, a patch of myelinated nerve fibers is visible on the surface of the retina, and the retina surrounding the optic nerve is not myelinated. There are no symptoms or treatment.

DEVELOPMENTAL ANOMALIES

Hyaloid artery. The hyaloid artery nurtures the lens during the first 10 weeks of embryonic development. After the retinal fissure closes, the hyaloid artery enters the eye at the optic

disk and then atrophies. Occasionally a short stub of this vessel projects into the vitreous cavity from the center of the optic disk. It is usually of no clinical significance, although it may rarely cause a recurrent vitreous hemorrhage. At the 100 mm stage of fetal development, the hyaloid artery forms a fusiform enlargement, the bulb, from which retinal vessels originate. The bulb is surrounded by a small mass of glia, the Bergmeister papilla, which may proliferate and slightly elevate the central portion of the disk. Failure of the hyaloid artery to regress causes persistent primary vitreous. As one gazes at a bright background, the minute residual fragments of the hyaloid system (muscae volitantes) may be seen as faint threads.

Drusen. Two kinds of drusen (Ger. pl. *druse:* stony nodule, geode), both unlike retinal drusen, occur in the intraocular portion of the optic nerve. Common drusen are laminated, calcareous, acellular accretions. They are the result of axonal degeneration with calcification. When deep in the disk, they may give the disk margins a blurred appearance that is differentiated from papilledema by the absence of dilated retinal veins. They autofluoresce and may be seen more clearly in red-free light. In adults they enlarge and approach the surface of the disk and give it an irregular, nodular appearance (Fig. 18-2). Drusen often cause visual field defects but seldom decrease visual acuity. Hemorrhage on the disk, adjacent retina, or vitreous rarely occurs. Computed tomography demonstrates them well; the optic nerve sheaths are not distended in papilledema.

Often the retinal blood vessels trifurcate rather than bifurcate on the disk surface. Angioid streaks, pigmentary degeneration of the retina, and optic atrophy have been associated with common drusen. They are rarely familial.

The second type of drusen are giant drusen, which are astrocytic hamartomas that occur with tuberous sclerosis.

Hypoplasia of the optic nerve. This is a developmental abnormality in which the number of axons in the optic nerve is reduced. There is no reduction in the supporting tissues. It may be segmental or complete, unilateral or bilateral. Complete hypoplasia causes decreased vision in the affected eye. Visual decrease in seg-

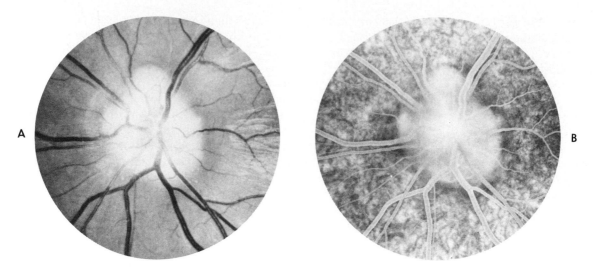

Fig. 18-2. Common drusen of the optic nerve. **A,** Blurred optic disk margins without venous congestion. **B,** Late phase of fluorescein angiography with drusen clearly evident without vascular leakage.

mental hypoplasia is variable but not as severe as in complete hypoplasia. When both eyes are affected, there is often a congenital pendular nystagmus and severely reduced vision. Bilateral optic nerve hypoplasia may be associated with agenesis of anterior midline structures of the brain, developmental delay, hypothyroidism, and decreased growth hormone. Most cases are sporadic, but some have been associated with maternal drug ingestion during pregnancy, maternal diabetes, and illness during pregnancy. Ophthalmoscopically, the optic disk appears small or tilted, a double ring of pigment may be present, and the retinal blood vessels are tortuous.

Conus. In conus, or congenital crescent, the choroid and retinal pigment epithelium do not extend to the disk. A large white semilunar area of sclera is thus seen adjacent to the disk, most commonly below in the region of the primitive retinal fissure. Defective vision, hyperopic astigmatism, and visual field defects are often present. The retinal blood vessels may be displaced to the periphery of the disk or to its lower portion.

A myopic crescent, which has a similar appearance, is located at the temporal side of the disk. It is not present at birth and is associated with degenerative myopia.

Colobomas of the optic disk. Incomplete closure of the retinal fissure causes optic nerve defects ranging from a deep physiologic cup to a pit in the optic disk to a deeply excavated optic nerve (Fig. 18-3) to a defect involving the optic nerve and a coloboma of the choroid and iris. There may be associated ocular defects and failure of the eye to develop normally. The condition is mainly unilateral, but bilateral colobomas of the optic disk occur as an autosomal dominant hereditary defect.

Pits in the optic disk are probably incomplete colobomas of the optic nerve. They are usually single and are located in the inferior temporal region of the optic disk. The pit is darker than the surrounding tissue and is usually round or oval. The pit may be shallow or as deep as 8 mm. It is from one eighth to one third the size of the disk. A small central scotoma is often present. In 30% of the patients a central serous choroidopathy develops.

Pseudopapilledema. The terms pseudopapilledema, pseudoptic neuritis, or pseudophthalmitis describe a congenital abnormality of the optic disk in which the disk margins are blurred by the heaped nerve fibers, accentuated by an excess of glial tissue. The disk has a dirty, grayish appearance with ill-defined margins, frequently most marked on the nasal side. It occurs commonly in severely hyperopic eyes. Vision is not impaired, and the retinal blood vessels are normal. The condition is not progressive and requires no treatment. Optic nerve drusen also blur the disk margin.

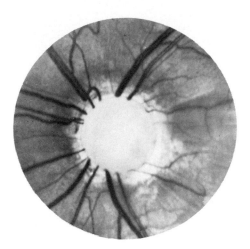

Fig. 18-3. Coloboma of the optic disk in a 19-year-old man with 20/40 vision. This condition is transmitted as an autosomal dominant defect. Patients are particularly prone to develop a central serous choroidopathy that suggests a communication between the subretinal space and the subarachnoid space.

Optociliary shunt vessels. These are markedly dilated vessels on the surface of the optic disk that occur as sequelae to chronic obstruction of veins passing through the lamina cribrosa. They may occur in meningioma, glioma, coloboma, drusen, arachnoid cysts, sarcoid of the optic nerve, and in chronic atrophic papilledema. They may follow resolution of branch vein obstruction.

Papilledema

Papilledema is a passive edema of the optic disk that results from increased intracranial pressure. The optic nerve is surrounded by the meningeal sheaths of the brain, and increased intracranial pressure may be transmitted to the subarachnoid space surrounding the optic nerve. Thus papilledema occurs only if the meningeal spaces surrounding the nerve are patent. Papilledema does not occur in eyes in which optic atrophy has destroyed most or all nerve fibers. The increased pressure in the sheaths of the optic nerve impairs but does not stop slow axonal transport that results in axonal swelling, particularly in the region of the lamina cribrosa. The swelling produces secondary. minimal changes in fast axonal transport.

Papilledema may be divided into four types: (1) early; (2) fully developed; (3) chronic; and (4) atrophic.

Papilledema begins with hyperemia of the optic disk and (usually) loss of spontaneous pulsation of the central retinal vein. The retina adjacent to the optic disk loses its light reflexes and appears deep red without luster. Small radial hemorrhages may occur on the margin of the disk. There may be indistinct blurred disk margins.

In the fully developed condition (Fig. 18-4), the nasal and temporal margins of the optic disk are blurred and its margins become grossly elevated above the surface of the retina. The retinal veins are engorged and dusky, and splinter hemorrhages occur at or adjacent to the disk margin. There may be cotton-wool spots (ischemic infarcts), hard exudates (chronic retinal edema residues), and macular hemorrhages. Capillaries on the surface of the optic disk leak fluorescein (Fig. 18-5). The swollen disk displaces the sensory retina and causes enlargement of the blind spot on visual field testing. Computed tomography shows distention of the optic nerve sheaths.

If the papilledema is not relieved, the hyperemia disappears and neuronal degeneration and gliosis give the disk a gray, milky appearance. Finally, there is an atrophic optic atrophy (secondary optic atrophy) with decreased size and prominence of the optic disk, a grayish gliosis of the disk, and sheathed, narrow retinal vessels.

Visual symptoms may be limited to transient dimness of vision, sometimes aggravated by change in head position. Other visual signs and symptoms are produced by the underlying disease that causes a papilledema.

The severity of papilledema is often proportionate to the increase in the intracranial pressure. Papilledema, however, is not an invariable accompaniment of increased intracranial pressure. When papilledema fails to develop although intracranial pressure is increased, the subarachnoid space surrounding the optic nerve is probably not patent. Similarly, if there is blockage of flow of cerebrospinal fluid from the brain to the spine in a patient with increased intracranial pressure, there may be papilledema with low pressure as demonstrated on lumbar puncture.

Papilledema is caused by a variety of disorders (Table 18-1). Brain tumors located below the tentorium are more likely to cause papilledema than those located above. Papilledema

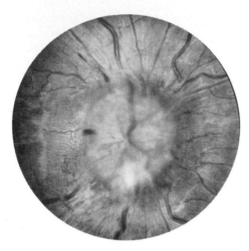

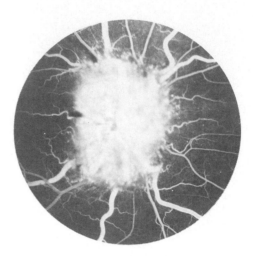

Fig. 18-4. Chronic papilledema in a 33-year-old woman with benign cerebral hypertension. Visual acuity was 20/20 in each eye, and the condition disappeared spontaneously.

Fig. 18-5. Fluorescein angiography of papilledema. Dye shows the dilated veins and outlines the hemorrhages. There is fluorescein leakage, which never occurs from normal optic disk vessels.

Table 18-1. Some causes of papilledema

  I. Space-occupying intracranial lesions
 II. Developmental disorders: craniostenosis, aqueduct stenosis (adult type), syringomyelia
III. Vascular hypertension
 IV. Microbial infections: meningitis, encephalitis, brain abscess
  V. Cranial trauma: epidural, subdural, intracranial hematoma
 VI. Intracranial vascular malformations: lateral sinus thrombosis, carotid-cavernous fistula, subarachnoid hemorrhage, dural-sinus thrombosis
VII. Toxicity: tetracycline, oral progestational agents, nalidixic acid, lead, arsenic, corticosteroid administration and withdrawal, vitamin A
VIII. Metabolic disorders: obesity, diabetic ketoacidosis, Addison disease, hypoparathyroidism, scurvy, dialysis disequilibrium
 IX. Miscellaneous: sarcoidosis, lupus erythematosus, syphilis, Paget disease, gastrointestinal hemorrhage, status epilepticus, carcinomatous meningitis, serum sickness, pulmonary emphysema
  X. Hematologc: leukemia, thrombocytopenia, pernicious anemia, polycythemia, hemophilia, leukemia, iron deficiency anemia, infectious mononucleosis
 XI. Occlusive disease posterior ciliary arteries, anterior ischemic optic neuropathy, giant cell arteritis, vascular hypertension
XII. Pseudotumor cerebri

Table 18-3. Retrobulbar optic neuropathy (without disk swelling)

Retrobulbar ischemic
   Arteritic
   Nonarteritic
Compressive
Toxic
Infiltrative
Hereditary

Table 18-2. Anterior optic neuropathy (with disk swelling)

Anterior ischemic
   Arteritic
   Nonarteritic
Compressive
   Gliomas, meningiomas
   Hamartomas
   Choristomas
   Malignant tumors
Anterior toxic
Ocular hypotony
Optic disk tumors

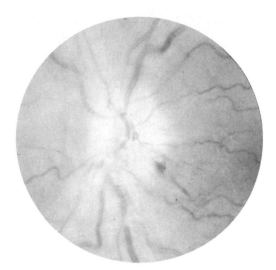

Fig. 18-6. Ischemic optic neuropathy with new small flame-shaped hemorrhage at margin of the disk.

may occur in blood dyscrasias and in hypertensive cardiovascular disease. In hypertensive cardiovascular disease, the occurrence of cotton-wool spots in the retina and the arteriolar constriction serve to distinguish hypertensive papilledema from that caused by intracranial neoplasms. Papilledema is seen in pseudotumor cerebri, congenital hydrocephalus, craniosynostosis, and after head injury. Pulmonary insufficiency, particularly that associated with cystic fibrosis of the pancreas, may cause papilledema.

Treatment must be directed to the cause. Persistent papilledema is associated with eventual loss of vision and secondary optic atrophy. Surgical decompression of the optic nerve or scleral canal is indicated to preserve vision.

Pseudotumor cerebri syndrome. Idiopathic intracranial hypertension occurs predominantly in women (2:1) and is characterized by papilledema, increased intracranial pressure, normal cerebrospinal fluid composition, and normal or small-sized ventricles. The symptoms are those of increased intracranial pressure with headache aggravated by coughing and sneezing, transient obscuration of vision, and sometimes abducent nerve palsy. Obesity and menstrual irregularity are common, but often no abnormality is evident. Hypervitaminosis A must be excluded. Treatment includes lumbar punc-

ture, acetazolamide therapy, dehydration, surgical decompression of the optic nerve, and lumbar-peritoneal shunting. Often the condition disappears spontaneously.

Optic neuropathy and optic neuritis

Optic neuropathy describes abnormalities of the optic nerve as the result of ischemia, toxins, and compression. Ischemic disorders are arteritic when they are caused by blood vessel inflammation, predominantly giant cell arteritis. They are nonarteritic or idiopathic when they occur secondary to vascular and occlusive disease. Optic neuropathy may be divided into anterior (Table 18-2) and retrobulbar ischemic neuropathy (Table 18-3), anterior and posterior toxic neuropathy, and compressive optic neuropathy.

Optic neuritis is a general term to describe involvement of the optic nerve as a result of demyelination, inflammation, or infection. When the optic disk is swollen, the neuritis may be described as papillitis; when the optic disk is normal, the condition is termed retrobulbar neuritis.

Ischemic anterior optic neuropathy. Interruption of the blood supply to the optic nerve head causes severe visual loss, visual field defects, and a pale, swollen optic disk with peripapillary hemorrhages (Fig. 18-6). The condition is noninflammatory, clearly ischemic, and involves both the optic disk and the optic nerve immediately adjacent.

Anterior ischemic optic neuropathy is divided into arteritic and nonarteritic (or ideopathic) types (Table 18-4). The arteritic type is less common (25%) and associated with inflammation of the blood vessels. The nonarteritic type involves mainly vascular occlusive disorders with impairment of circulation in the posterior ciliary arteries that supply the optic disk. Sexes are equally affected. The age distribution reflects the cause.

Visual acuity is reduced usually more severely in the arteritic type. Altitudinal visual field defects are common, often with loss of the inferior visual field. An afferent pupillary defect is present. Ophthalmoscopic examination shows a swollen optic disk that may simulate the papilledema or may be mild. Hyperemia, however, is exceptional, and the disk is usually pale. Single or multiple flame-shaped hemor-

Table 18-4. Ischemic optic neuropathy

Arteritic
    Giant cell arteritis
    Systemic lupus erythematosus
    Polyarteritis nodosum
    Allergic, postviral, immunization vasculitis
    Syphilis
    Buerger disease
    Radiation necrosis
Nonarteritic ("idiopathic")
    Accelerated hypertension
    Diabetes mellitus
    Migraine
    Carotid occlusive disease
    Polycythemia vera
    Acute hypotension
    Sickle cell abnormalities
    Atherosclerosis

rhages occur near the disk margin. Cotton-wool spots may be present.

Diagnosis and treatment must be directed to the cause.

Retrobulbar ischemic optic nerve neuropathy. This is an uncommon type of optic nerve neuropathy in which there are visual field defects, often altitudinal, combined, on occasion, with visual loss. The diagnosis is often based on exclusion of stroke or intracranial tumor. Atherosclerosis of the blood supply to the optic nerves, connective tissue disorders, diabetes mellitus, trauma, and orbital radiotherapy have been described as causes.

Anterior toxic optic neuropathy. Optic disk swelling with impaired visual acuity and visual field defects that involve both the fixation area and the blind spot (cecocentral scotoma) may follow systemic absorption of many substances. Both eyes are usually affected. Commonly implicated compounds include chloramphenicol, ethambutol, isoniazid, and lead.

Retrobulbar toxic optic neuropathy. These abnormalities are characterized by progressive, bilateral visual loss, cecocentral scotomas, and usually pallor of the temporal portion (papillomacular bundles) of the optic disk. Deficiencies of a single portion of the vitamin B complex may be responsible: B_{12} (cobalmin), B_6 (pyriodoxine), B_1 (thiamine), niacin, or riboflavin. Tropical amblyopia may occur in poorly nourished individuals in whom the food staple cassava results in cyanide intoxication. Tobacco-alcohol amblyopia is seen in heavy smokers and drinkers who are also poorly nourished. A vari-

ety of drugs have been implicated: antipyrine, digitalis, anabuse, quinine, and streptomycin.

Optic neuritis. Inflammation, demyelination, or infection may affect the optic nerve anywhere in its course from the optic disk to the optic chiasm. When the intraocular portion of the optic nerve is involved, the optic disk is swollen and hyperemic, and the condition is called papillitis or anterior optic neuritis. If the optic disk is normal, the condition is called retrobulbar neuritis. When both the optic disk and adjacent retina are affected, the condition is called optic neuroretinitis.

The main symptom is monocular loss of vision that is usually abrupt over a period of hours; rarely, visual loss progresses over several weeks. The severity of loss varies from minimal reduction to loss of all light perception. Color vision is impaired in the affected eye far more severely than visual acuity (in optic neuropathy the visual loss and impairment of color vision usually parallel each other). A central or paracentral scotoma occurs. Altitudinal defects, arcuate scotomas, and cecocentral scotomas are exceptional and suggest a neuropathy rather than a neuritis.

An afferent pupillary defect (see Chapter 14) is always present. It is detected by alternate illumination of the pupils in a dimly illuminated room. The visual-evoked response is always abnormal. In retrobulbar neuritis, computed tomography shows a diffuse swelling and enhancement of the optic nerve. Most patients are between 20 and 50 years of age; sexes are affected equally. Irrespective of the portion of the nerve involved, the causes are the same (Table 18-5).

Painless loss of vision with a central scotoma occurs in disorders affecting the fovea centralis such as cystoid edema and central serous choroidopathy. In retrobulbar neuritis an afferent pupillary defect is present, and color vision is more severely depressed than in retinal conditions. A penlight beam directed into the eye for 10 seconds does not further impair vision in optic neuritis, whereas vision is reduced one or more Snellen lines in central serous choroidopathy.

Retrobulbar inflammation of the optic nerve in the orbit where it is in close relationship with the superior rectus and medial rectus muscles causes pain on movement of the eye. There may be tenderness on palpation of the

Table 18-5. Some causes of optic neuritis

Infections
  Intraocular
    Keratitis, endophthalmitis, chronic uveitis
  Extraocular
    Orbital cellulitis
  Systemic
    Lupus erythematosus, autoimmune encephalitis, men-
      ingitis, syphilis, tuberculosis, coccidiomycosis, bac-
      terial endocarditis, measles, mumps, chicken pox,
      infectious mononucleosis, zoster
Demyelinative disease
  Multiple sclerosis
  Acute disseminated encephalomyelitis
  Neuromyelitis optica (Devic disease)
  Diffuse periaxial encephalitis (Schilder disease)
  Diffuse cerebral sclerosis (Krabbe disease, Pelizaeus-
    Merzbacher syndrome, metachromatic leukodystro-
    phy)

globe through the closed eyelids. This pain combined with loss of central vision, a central scotoma, and the absence of any ophthalmoscopic changes often suggests the diagnosis of retrobulbar neuritis. If the causative agent is removed or if the condition occurs in the course of a demyelinating disease, the inflammation may run its course in 2 to 6 weeks and a complete recovery ensues. A residue of optic atrophy affecting the papillomacular bundle may remain.

In papillitis, the disk appears smaller than normal because of diminished contrast with the surrounding retina. The disk margins are obscured, and there is dilation of retinal veins. Flame-shaped hemorrhages may occur on the surface of the disk and the adjacent retina. In severe inflammations, hard, yellow retinal deposits occur, and these may be grouped about the fovea centralis in an oval (circinate) pattern. With persistence of the swelling there may be glial tissue proliferation from the disk along the retinal vessels, and any subsequent atrophy is classified as "secondary." Ophthalmoscopically, early papilledema and early papillitis appear the same, but there is early loss of vision in papillitis. Additionally, papillitis is unilateral, and there may be inflammatory cells in the adjacent vitreous.

Children develop papillitis more frequently than adults. Elderly individuals who develop disk swelling with acute monocular loss of vision probably have anterior ischemic optic neuropathy.

The cause of optic neuritis is often impossible to determine. Optic neuritis is the initial occurrence in 15% of patients who subsequently develop multiple sclerosis. Additional symptoms develop within 4 years. About one third of patients who have multiple sclerosis develop optic neuritis sometime in the course of their disease. Even though there is no history of visual impairment in multiple sclerosis, the visual-evoked potential may be impaired.

In severe inflammations of the retina or the choroid, there is often an extension of the inflammatory process to the optic nerve. The primary disease dominates the clinical picture.

Optic atrophy

Optic atrophy is the end result of diseases or injuries to retinal ganglion cells or their axons that produces degeneration of axons anterior to the lateral geniculate body (Table 18-6). The diagnosis is based on the ophthalmoscopic appearance of a pale optic disk with defective visual function. If the lesion causing the optic atrophy is in the retina, an ascending optic atrophy occurs, which terminates in the lateral geniculate body. Descending optic atrophy follows diseases involving optic nerve fibers anterior to their synapse in the lateral geniculate body.

The chief symptom of optic atrophy is loss of central or peripheral vision. Failure to demonstrate a defect by means of confrontation fields does not exclude a visual field defect that might require extremely small stimuli to detect.

The atrophy is called primary if there is no evidence of preceding edema or inflammation. It is called secondary if there is a preceding papillitis or papilledema. The same conditions may be responsible for either a primary or a secondary optic atrophy; the sole difference is the swelling of the optic disk that precedes a secondary optic atrophy.

Primary optic atrophy. In primary optic atrophy the number of nerve fiber bundles in the optic nerve is reduced, and there is a rearrangement of the remaining disk astrocytes into dense parallel layers across the nerve head. The disk margins are distinct, and there appears to be a loss of capillaries although they are demonstrated on fluorescein angiography. The atrophy may be complete or partial. The ophthalmoscopic appearance of pallor does not parallel the severity of the visual field loss.

Table 18-6 Etiologic classification of optic atrophy

I. Glaucoma
II. Retinal ganglion cell or nerve fiber disease
  A. Pigmentary degeneration of the retina
  B. Chorioretinal degenerations, inflammations, atrophy
III. Inflammation
  A. Demyelinating disease
  B. Meningitis, encephalitis, abscess
  C. Tabes dorsalis
  D. Optic neuritis (Table 18-5)
  E. Metastatic septicemia
IV. Optic neuropathy
V. Papilledema
VI. Toxicity
  A. Chemical: arsenic, lead, methanol, ethanol, quinine, tobacco, chloroquine, ethambutol, chloramphenicol
  B. Vitamin B deficiency: beriberi, pellagra, pernicious anemia
VII. Glioma
  A. Juvenile pilocytic astrocytoma
  B. Adult malignant astrocytoma (glioblastoma)
VIII. Heredity
  A. Leber disease
  B. Dominant juvenile early infantile optic atrophy with diabetes mellitus and sometimes deafness
  C. Behr disease
  D. Glucose-6-phosphate dehydrogenase deficiency—Worcester variant
IX. Trauma

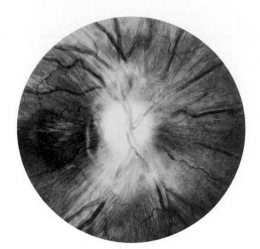

Fig. 18-7. Secondary optic atrophy.

Open-angle glaucoma is the chief cause of primary optic atrophy. After central artery occlusion or after quinine poisoning, the optic nerve may appear to be waxy white and the retinal vessels may appear as small white cords. In the late stages of retinal pigmentary degenerations, the disk appears to have a yellowish waxy color with attenuated arteries crossing it. In lesions limited to the central retina, the atrophy involves only the papillomacular bundle at the temporal margin of the optic disk.

Secondary optic atrophy. Secondary optic atrophy is preceded by swelling of the optic disk, caused by papilledema or papillitis. Ophthalmoscopically, the disk margins appear blurred, the lamina cribrosa is obscured, and there is gliosis over the surface of the disk extending to the retina (Fig. 18-7). The blood vessels may be obscured and their course distorted by scar tissue.

OPTIC NERVE TUMORS

Retinoblastomas and malignant melanomas of the choroid may extend to involve the optic nerve. Primary optic nerve tumors are uncommon.

Melanocytoma. A melanocytoma of the optic disk (Fig. 18-8) is a maximally pigmented nevus that usually occurs on the inferior temporal portion of the optic disk but may cover the entire disk. It occurs mainly in deeply pigmented individuals. It is benign and has a low malignant potential.

Glioma. Juvenile gliomas (juvenile pilocytic astrocytoma) have their onset in the first decade of life and are astrocytic hamartomas. The orbital portion of the optic nerve is involved in about half the instances, whereas the tumor is both orbital and chiasmal in the remainder. Orbital tumors cause proptosis. Loss of vision occurs irrespective of the tumor location. About 15% of patients with neurofibromatosis develop an optic nerve glioma.

Adult glioma is a rapidly progressive malignant astrocytoma (glioblastoma) that occurs in middle-aged adults and results in death within 2 years. The tumor is not related to juvenile gliomas.

Optic nerve sheath meningiomas. Meningiomas affecting the optic nerve originate either from the meningeal coverings of the nerve or extend from the cranial cavity. They cause a slowly progressive loss of vision, optic atrophy, and optociliary shunt vessels. The symptoms

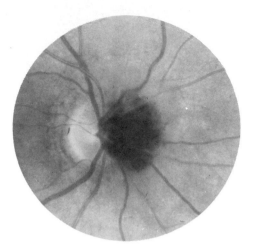

Fig. 18-8. Melanocytoma of the optic disk of the right eye.

and signs are similar to those of sphenoidal ridge meningiomas. Computed tomography demonstrates enlargement of the optic nerve. Women are mainly (5:1) affected; neurofibromatosis is present in about 15%.

BIBLIOGRAPHY
General

Brown, G.C., and Tasman, W.S.: Congenital anomalies of the optic disc, New York, 1982, Grune & Stratton.

Burde, R.M.: The neuro-ophthalmic patient, St. Louis, 1984, The C.V. Mosby Co.

Burde, R.M., Savino, P.J., and Trobe, J.D.: Clinical decisions in neuro-ophthalmology, St. Louis, 1985, The C.V. Mosby Co.

Lessel, S., and van Dalen, J.T.W., editors: Neuro-ophthalmology, vol. 3, Amsterdam, 1984, Elsevier.

Miller, N.R.: Walsh and Hoyt's clinical neuro-ophthalmology, vol. 1, ed. 4, Baltimore, 1982, Williams & Wilkins Co.

Miller, N.R.: Walsh and Hoyt's clinical neuro-ophthalmology, vol. 2, ed. 5, Baltimore, 1985, Williams & Wilkins Co.

Myelinated nerve fibers

Straatsma, B.R., et al.: Myelinated retinal nerve fibers, Am. J. Ophthalmol. **91:**25, 1981.

Developmental anomalies

Bec, P., Adam, P., Mathis, A., Alberge, Y., Roulleau, J., and Arne, J.L.: Optic nerve head drusen: high-resolution computed tomographic approach, Arch. Ophthalmol. **102:**680, 1984.

Skarf, B., and Hoyt, C.S.: Optic nerve hypoplasia in children, Arch. Ophthalmol. **102:**62, 1984.

Papilledema

Orcutt, J.C., Page, N.G.R., and Sanders, M.D.: Factors affecting visual loss in benign intracranial hypertension, Ophthalmology **91:**1303, 1984.

Repka, M.X., Miller, N.R., and Savino, P.J.: Pseudotumor cerebri, Am. J. Ophthalmol. **98:**741, 1984.

Wall, M., Hart, W.M., Jr., and Burde, R.M.: Visual field defects in idiopathic intracranial hypertension (pseudotumor cerebri), Am. J. Ophthalmol. **96:**654, 1983.

Optic neuropathy and neuritis

Beck, R.W., Savino, J., Repka, M.X., Schatz, N.J., and Sergott, R.C.: Optic disc structure in anterior ischemic optic neuropathy, Ophthalmology **91:**1334, 1984.

Feit, R.H., Tomsak, R.L., and Ellenberger, C., Jr.: Structural factors in the pathogenesis of ischemic optic neuropathy, Am. J. Ophthalmol. **98:**105, 1984.

Guyer, D.R., Miller, N.R., Auer, C.L., and Fine, S.L.: The risk of cerebrovascular and cardiovascular disease in patients with anterior ischemic optic neuropathy, Arch. Ophthalmol. **103:**136, 1985.

Repka, M.X., Svino, P.J., Schatz, N.J., and Sergott, R.C.: Clinical profile and long-term implications of anterior ischemic optic neuropathy, Am. J. Ophthalmol. **96:**478, 1983.

Shults, W.T.: Ischemic optic neuropathy, Ophthalmology **91:**1338, 1984.

Tumors

Brown, G.C., and Shields, J.A.: Tumors of the optic nerve head, Surv. Ophthalmol. **29:**239, 1985.

Grimson, B.S., and Perry D.D.: Enlargement of the optic disk in childhood optic nerve tumors, Am. J. Ophthalmol. **97:**627, 1984.

Jakobiec, F.A., Depot, M.J., Kennerdell, J.S., Shults, W.T., Anderson, R.L., Alper, M.E., Citrin, C.M., Housepian, E.M., and Trokel, S.L.: Combined clinical and computed tomographic diagnosis of orbital glioma and meningioma, Ophthalmology **91:**137, 1984.

Reidy, J.J., Apple, D.J., Steinmetz, R.L., Craythorn, J.M., Loftfield, K., Gieser, S.C., and Brady, S.E.: Melanocytoma: nomenclature, pathogenesis, natural history and treatment, Surv. Ophthalmol. **29:**319, 1985.

Rosenberg, L.F., and Miller, N.R.: Visual results after microsurgical removal of meningiomas involving the anterior visual system, Arch. Ophthalmol. **102:**1019, 1984.

Sibony, P.A., Krauss, H.R., Kennerdell, J.S., Maroon, J.C., and Slamovits, T.L.: Optic nerve sheath meningiomas, Ophthalmology **91:**1313, 1984.

19
THE LENS

The lens is a transparent, avascular, biconvex structure held in position behind the pupil by zonular fibers that originate in the crypts of the ciliary processes and insert into the periphery of the lens capsule. The lens substance is surrounded by the lens capsule, the thickest basement membrane of the body. The anterior capsule is the basement membrane for a single layer of adjacent epithelial cells. The posterior capsule is the basement membrane of lens fiber cells that have their nuclei near the equator of the lens in the nuclear bow. The majority of lens fibers have lost their nuclei, migrate inward, and form an increasingly compact tissue. A central nucleus is formed by the oldest fibers (the embryonic nucleus) and is surrounded by more recently formed lens fibers to constitute the lens nucleus. Younger fibers form the lens cortex. The lens metabolism is mainly aerobic because it has no blood vessels and minimal oxygen is dissolved in the aqueous humor and the vitreous humor that surround it. The lens is not inert, however, and remains relatively dehydrated, has actively multiplying cells at the equator, synthesizes lens proteins and membranes from amino acids derived from posterior chamber aqueous humor, and maintains a concentration gradient with high potassium, glutathione, ascorbic acid, and inositol levels.

The lens and the cornea are the main refracting surfaces of the eye. The inherent elasticity of the lens causes it to become more spherical as zonular fibers relax when the ciliary muscle contracts. This provides increased refractive power (accommodation). Because of compression of mature fibers in its central portion, the lens gradually loses its inherent elasticity, and usually by 45 years of age the change in shape in response to ciliary muscle contraction is too slight to provide adequate additional refractive power for near work (presbyopia).

The lens is transparent because most cells have no nuclei and the lens proteins have a short-range spatial order like dense liquids or glass that have no underlying lattice organization. Any loss of transparency is called a cataract, or a lens opacity, a term that is less ominous to a patient. Cataracts result from protein denaturation, increased molecular weights of proteins, water clefts and vesicles between lens fibers, increasing proliferation, and migration of lens epithelium.

SYMPTOMS AND SIGNS OF DISEASES OF THE LENS

The symptoms of diseases of the lens relate mainly to vision. In presbyopia, accommodation decreases and near vision fails. With cataract formation vision decreases for far and near. In nuclear sclerosis the index of refraction of the lens increases, thus increasing the refractive power of the anterior segment. This added power may permit the patient to read without glasses, although the myopia reduces uncorrected distance visual acuity. Central lens opacities may split the visual axis and cause an optical defect in which two or more blurred images are formed, a monocular diplopia. Opacities caused by increased water content decrease vision but the fluid may migrate or absorb, resulting in visual improvement. The coincidence of better vision in a patient receiving medication to treat cataract has led to many cataract remedies.

A partially dislocated (subluxated) lens may impair vision by providing irregular refracting surfaces. If the lens is removed from the visual axis through complete dislocation or surgery, the eye loses a major refractive element and becomes severely hyperopic. An opening in the lens capsule releases lens protein into the aqueous humor and causes uveitis and sometimes a secondary glaucoma. Marked swelling of the lens may obstruct the passage of aqueous humor from the posterior chamber to anterior chamber and cause a pupillary block glaucoma.

Ophthalmoscopic examination with a convex lens (+10D) and the pupil widely dilated shows cataracts as dark opacities against the red background of the fundus reflex. Visualizing the details and location of the opacity usually requires examination with a biomicroscope. Examination using a penlight and a condensing lens (+20D) indicates gross abnormalities.

If the lens is dislocated, the iris loses support and becomes tremulous, the condition of iridodonesis; the anterior chamber is deeper. If a lens is dislocated into the vitreous body, it may be seen with the ophthalmoscope in the region to which it has gravitated as a dark sphere that magnifies the retina beneath it or as a black globule if it is cataractous.

DEVELOPMENTAL ANOMALIES
Coloboma

In coloboma there are one or more minute notches at the equator of the lens. The disorder occurs as a congenital absence of a segment of zonule, often in association with other intraocular colobomas. Progressive colobomas occur in the course of hereditary disorders such as Marfan syndrome or Refsum disease, or after blunt trauma. The absence of a sector of zonular fibers relaxes the corresponding lens equator, which becomes a chord rather than an arc of a circle. A retinal detachment may occur. Restoration of the defective zonule is not possible.

Spherophakia (microphakia)

In spherophakia the lens is small and has increased anterior and posterior curvature. The zonular fibers are easily visible with pupillary dilation, and since the iris lacks support, it is tremulous (iridodonesis). Subluxation of the lens is common, apparently because the stretched zonule weakens and breaks. Closed-angle glaucoma occurs when the small, round lens blocks the flow of aqueous humor through the pupil. The increased refractive power of the lens causes myopia.

Spherophakia may be part of an autosomal recessive syndrome (Weill-Marchesani), which is characterized by short stature, short stubby fingers, joint stiffness, and mental retardation. The syndrome is a hyperplastic form of congenital mesodermal dystrophy, in contrast to the Marfan syndrome, which is a hypoplastic defect. Treatment by sector iridectomy is directed mainly toward the prevention of a pupillary-block glaucoma.

Lenticonus

Lenticonus is an uncommon disorder, rarely inherited as an autosomal recessive characteristic, in which a cone forms at the anterior pole of the lens. Ophthalmoscopically a dark disk ("oil globule") reflex is visible in the pupillary area. Males are predominantly affected. Anterior lenticonus with familial hemorrhagic nephritis (Alport syndrome) occurs with spherophakia and cataract.

An abnormal increase in curvature of the anterior or, more commonly, of the posterior surface of the lens (lentiglobus) is usually unilateral and causes an oil-globule ophthalmoscopic appearance.

Ectopia lentis

When the lens loses the support provided by the zonular fibers, it dislocates either into the vitreous cavity or into the anterior chamber (Fig. 19-1). If some, but not all, of the zonular fibers remain attached, they act as a hinge so that the lens is subluxated from its usual position. Examination indicates a deep anterior chamber and a tremulous iris. The symptoms are mainly optical, since absence of a major refracting element causes the eye to become markedly hyperopic and to lose the accommodation provided by the lens. Migration of a dis-

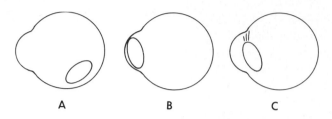

Fig. 19-1. A, Dislocation of the lens into the vitreous cavity. **B,** Dislocation of the lens into the anterior chamber, an abnormality that leads to pupillary-block glaucoma. **C,** Subluxation of the lens with the remaining zonular fibers acting as a hinge.

located lens into the anterior chamber causes an acute secondary glaucoma. A glaucoma may occur with a lens in the vitreous cavity, but the mechanism is not clear. A subluxated lens often, but not inevitably, dislocates.

The same conditions are responsible for either subluxation or dislocation. Ocular contusion may cause subluxation, particularly in an individual with latent syphilis. Deliberate dislocation, or couching, an ancient (and unwise) surgical procedure, is still practiced in some parts of the world. Subluxation/dislocation is a regular feature of Marfan syndrome (see below and chapter on diseases of the connective tissue and joints), cystathionine β-synthase deficiency, and spherophakia (Weill-Marchesani). Rarely, an autosomal recessive defect causes ectopia lentis without other somatic changes. Lens dislocation has been described in many hereditary disorders that have no enzyme deficiency but do not occur regularly. Intraocular tumors, uveitis, severe myopia, and buphthalmus may each be complicated by lens dislocation.

Sometimes a dislocated lens causes only an optical defect that is neutralized with correcting lenses. More often, secondary glaucoma, uveitis, or both necessitate removal.

Marfan syndrome. The Marfan syndrome (arachnodactyly, dystrophia mesodermalis hypoplastica) is a widespread abnormality of connective tissue transmitted as an autosomal dominant defect (see Chapter 29). Ectopia lentis occurs in most cases. The lens is often subluxated upward and temporally so that its equator can be seen in the pupil. Severe myopia is common. Hypoplasia of the iris, miosis, and anterior chamber anomalies may be present. The systemic manifestations include aortic dilation, dissecting aneurysms of the aorta, mus-

cular underdevelopment, femoral and diaphragmatic hernias, and multiple skeletal defects, particularly arachnodactyly (spider fingers).

Cystathionine β-synthase deficiency (homocystinuria). This is an autosomal, recessive disorder with major involvement of the eye, skeletal system, central nervous system, and vascular system. The severity varies markedly in different individuals, but nearly all develop subluxation of the lens between the third and tenth year of age. Excessive amounts of homocytsine are present in the blood and urine. The plasma level of cystine is reduced, cystathionine is absent, and methionine is increased.

Ectopia lentis is progressive in nearly all patients and the dislocated lens occasionally causes a pupillary block glaucoma. The lens dislocation is secondary to broken zonular fibers that appear thickened, unlike the thin, elongated fibers in Marfan syndrome. Osteoporosis causes scoliosis, vertebral collapse, genu valgum, pes cavus, and other abnormalities. Mental retardation with delayed psychomotor development occurs in about one half of patients. Thromboembolism may affect large and small arteries and veins, possibly secondary to excessive platelet adhesiveness or other abnormality of platelets. The skin and hair are fair and there is a malar flush. Many clinical features suggest Marfan syndrome, but demonstration of the cystathionine β-synthase deficiency in cultured cells distinguishes the two conditions.

There is considerable genetic heterogeneity. Cystathionine β-synthase may be entirely absent, there may be reduced enzyme activity with normal binding of the cofactor pyridoxal phosphate, and reduced enzyme activity with reduced binding of the cofactor. Patients in whom there is no trace of cystathionine β-synthase activity do not respond to administration of pyridoxine, while those with some activity benefit. Some patients have an abnormally low serum folate concentration that is aggravated by pyridoxine administration. The most common cause of homocystinuria is cystathionine β-synthase deficiency, but homocystinuria also occurs in other genetic disorders, one of which (defective synthesis of cobalamin [vitamin B_{12}] coenzymes) causes epileptiform ocular and eyelid movements.

LENS-INDUCED OCULAR DISEASE

In addition to the glaucoma resulting from deformities or displacement of the lens, secondary glaucoma may result from hypermaturity of the lens (phacolytic glaucoma) or from rapid swelling of the lens (phacogenic glaucoma). Rupture of the lens capsule may be followed by uveitis; or there may be systemic hypersensitivity to lens protein after an extracapsular lens extraction, so that liberation of lens protein in the fellow eye with cataract removed causes a severe intraocular inflammation (endophthalmitis phacoanaphylactica).

Phacolytic glaucoma. In some eyes with hypermature cataract, large mononuclear phagocytes filled with lens material obstruct the trabecular meshwork, causing a secondary open-angle glaucoma intractable to medical treatment. The possibility of this glaucoma leads surgeons to remove advanced cataracts before they become hypermature even though other ocular diseases may preclude restoration of good vision.

Phacomorphic glaucoma. A rapid swelling of the lens follows hydration of lens fibers in senile intumescent cataract and also follows either surgical or accidental rupture of the lens capsule. A secondary closed-angle glaucoma may ensue, particularly if the anterior chamber is already shallow. The glaucoma must first be controlled medically, and then the lens must be removed.

Lens-induced uveitis. Accidental traumatic rupture of the lens capsule liberates lenticular protein within the eye. Although lens proteins are relatively poor antigens, uveitis, sometimes complicated by glaucoma, may develop. Mutton-fat keratic precipitates, posterior synechiae, and, rarely, a pupillary membrane form.

Treatment consists of lens extraction and corticosteriod administration. Sometimes after extracapsular cataract extraction, the eyes appear to be sensitized to lens protein. Extracapsular lens extraction with retention of lens material in the second eye then may cause an endophthalmitis (endophthalmitis phacoanaphylactia).

Retention of the lens nucleus or of fragments of the nucleus in the vitreous cavity after extracapsular lens extraction causes a severe uveitis. The nuclear material must be removed from the eye by means of vitrectomy.

CATARACT

A cataract is any opacity in the crystalline lens. Acquired cataract is a common disorder. In the Framingham, Massachusetts study, 15% of persons 52 to 85 years of age had cataracts that reduced their visual acuity to 20/30 or less. Some one million cataract extractions are done annually in the United States, and it is estimated that 5 to 10 million individuals become visually disabled each year because of cataract. Patients who refuse surgery for operable cataracts constitute the second largest group of blind individuals in the United States.

Table 19-1. Methods of classifying cataract

I. According to age at onset
  A. Congenital
  B. Infantile
  C. Juvenile
  D. Adult
  E. Senile
II. According to location of opacity in lens
  A. Nuclear
  B. Cortical
  C. Capsular: posterior or anterior (rare)
  D. Subcapsular: posterior or anterior (rare)
III. According to degree of opacity present
  A. Immature: transparent lens fibers are present
  B. Intumescent: swelling of lens with fluid clefts
  C. Mature: entire lens has become opaque
  D. Hypermature: liquefaction of the opaque lens fiber occurs (morgagnian cataract)
  E. After-cataracts: capsular remains after lens has been removed
IV. According to rate of development
  A. Stationary
  B. Progressive
V. On basis of biomicroscopic appearance
  A. Lamellar
  B. Coralliform
  C. Punctate and many others
VI. On basis of cause

No classification of cataract is satisfactory. They may be classified on the basis of cause, age at onset, severity of opacification, or location of the opacity (Table 19-1). The most significant clinical points include (1) severity of visual impairment; (2) the likelihood of visual improvement after cataract extraction; (3) the presence of systemic disease and, if present, whether the disease is related to the cataract development (Table 19-2); and (4) local ocular

Table 19-2. Cataract with systemic disorders

I. Generalized
  A. Embryopathies (induced in utero)
    1. Maternal infection (rubella first trimester of pregnancy [associated deafness and heart disease], other viruses [cytomegalovirus, mumps, vaccinia, variola, poliomyelitis possible], toxoplasmosis, syphilis)
    2. Maternal drug ingestion, radiation
  B. Marfan syndrome (arachnodactyly, ectopia lentis, mesodermal hypoplasia)
  C. Retinal pigment epithelium degenerations (Laurence-Moon-Biedl: retinitis pigmentosa, obesity, polydactyly, hypogenitalism, deafness, ataxia, oligophrenia)
  D. Systemic infections causing uveitis with complicated cataract
II. Cutaneous
  A. Atopic dermatitis (15 to 25 years of age)
  B. Rothmund syndrome (onset 3 to 6 months of age)
  C. Incontinentia pigmenti (Werner) often with uveitis)
  D. Congenital ichthyosis or ectodermal dysplasia
  E. Siemen syndrome

III. Metabolic
  A. Diabetes mellitus (growth-onset diabetes)
  B. Galactosemia (usually shortly after birth: transferase or kinase deficiency)
  C. Lowe syndrome (oculocerbrorenal syndrome)
  D. Hypocalcemia (with tetany)
  E. Fabry disease
  F. Refsum disease
  G. Glycose-6-phosphate deficiency
  H. Increased plasma tryptophane
IV. Neurologic
  A. Hepatolenticular degeneration (sunflower cataract)
  B. Spinocerebellar ataxia, oligophrenia (Marinesco-Sjögren)
V. Muscular
  A. Myotonic dystrophy (20 to 30 years of age)
VI. Osseous
  A. Mandibulofacial dysostosis
  B. Osteitis fibrosa and skin pigmentation
  C. Stippled epiphysis
  D. Oxycephaly
VII. Chromosomal abnormalities
  A. Down syndrome
  B. 13-15 trisomy
  C. Cockayne syndrome

Table 19-3. Cataract without systemic disorders

I. Eye otherwise healthy and no systemic disease
  A. Nearly all senile cataracts
  B. Most cataracts in adults
  C. Many hereditary and congenital cataracts
II. Cataract combined with other ocular disorders but no systemic abnormalities
  A. Congenital and hereditary abnormalities (cyclopia, colobomas, microphthalmia, aniridia, persistent primary vitreous [retained hyaloid vasculature], heterochromia iridis)
  B. Acquired defects and delayed hereditary abnormalities
    1. Miscellaneous ocular diseases (glaucoma, uveitis, retinal separation, pigmentary degeneration of retina, myopia, ocular neoplasms)
    2. Retinopathy of prematurity (cataracts develop after 3 years of age)
    3. Toxicity (corticosteroids systemically or topically, ergot, naphthalene, dinitrophenol, triparanol [MER-29], topical anticholinesterase, phenothiazines)

    4. Ocular trauma
      a. Contusion (Vossius ring [pigment on anterior capsule], posterior subcapsular cataract)
      b. Laceration
      c. Retained intraocular foreign body (iron: siderosis; copper: chalcosis)
      d. Electromagnetic radiation
        (1) Infrared (iris absorption with heat coagulation of underlying lens, also true exfoliation of lens capsule)
        (2) Microwaves (focused high energy, a heating effect)
        (3) Ionizing radiation (cataractogenic dose varies with energy and type, younger lens more vulnerable)
        (4) Ultraviolet radiation
      e. Anterior ocular ischemia after retinal detachment surgery

causes in the absence of systemic disease (Table 19-3).

Cataracts present at birth may be hereditary or congenital. Cataracts that develop after birth may be associated with ocular disease, trauma, systemic disease, or aging. Aging is by far the most common cause, but aging cataracts may occur at a relatively early age.

Cataracts in which all of the protein is opaque are termed mature. If some protein is transparent, the cataract is immature. If the protein of the cortex of a mature cataract becomes liquid, the cataract is hypermature. The fluid may escape through an intact capsule and cause the lens to shrink. Swelling of the lens fibers results in an intumescent cataract.

Acquired cataract

Acquired cataracts include those that occur sporadically as a result of toxins, systemic disease, injury, damage from intraocular inflammation, and aging. Many abnormalities cause characteristic morphologic changes that may be distinguished by biomicroscopic examination (Fig. 19-2).

Symptoms. The chief symptom of acquired cataract is a gradual decrease of vision that is not associated with pain or inflammation of the eye. Double vision in one eye (monocular diplopia) may be caused by the lens opacity splitting light bundles, but this disappears with further decrease in vision. In the early stages, lights may be surrounded by a colored halo.

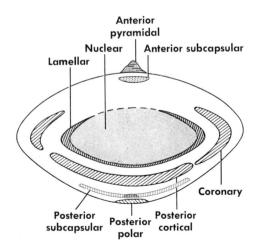

Fig. 19-2. Locations of various cataracts.

Dilation of the pupil that occurs in dim illumination improves vision. Glare and constriction of the pupil in bright illumination reduce vision, particularly in patients with posterior subcapsular cataracts that obstruct the visual axis. Patients may complain of spots in the visual field that, unlike those caused by vitreous floaters, remain fixed and do not dart about with movements of the eye. In nuclear cataracts there is often an increase in the refractive power of the lens so that patients are able to read without glasses.

Examination. Examination of the lens with the ophthalmoscope may indicate a gross opacity filling the pupillary aperture or an opacity silhouetted against the red background of the fundus (Fig. 19-3). A nuclear opacity is located centrally and usually appears larger than a posterior subcapsular opacity. A peripheral cortical opacity has the appearance of irregular spokes with the lens clear centrally. Dilation of the pupil is necessary to examine the lens adequately.

Ocular examination is particularly directed toward finding evidence of injury or inflammation to account for the lens opacity. Roentgenographic examination to demonstrate a metallic foreign body is indicated if there is a history of ocular injury followed by lens opacity. General physical examination and laboratory studies seldom suggest the cause. The main differential diagnosis involves aging, toxins, diabetes mellitus, or other systemic disorders such as hypocalcemia, myotonic dystrophy, or skin disease. Cataracts in the aged occur more commonly in patients with diabetes mellitus or high blood pressure than in others.

Special types. Many different causes of acquired types of cataract have been described: senile, toxic, traumatic, diabetic, and hypocalcemic. Some have a characteristic appearance in their early stages, but with progression it is not possible to distinguish the various types.

Senile cataract. In the Framingham, Massachusetts study, individuals with senile cataract were more likely to have increased serum phospholipid and high nonfasting blood glucose levels, as well as high blood pressure.

With aging, the lens nucleus changes include protein aggregation, increased production of insoluble protein, oxidation of sulfhydryl groups, production of nondisulfide covalent cross-links between crystalline polypeptides, increased pigmentation in the lens nucleus, and production of blue fluorescence not attributable to tryptophan. Opacities may occur in the lens nucleus, the lens cortex, or the posterior subcapsule. These changes may occur concurrently but may involve different mechanisms in different parts of the lens.

Nuclear, or hard, cataract is an accentuation of the normal condensation process in the lens nucleus. It becomes evident at about 50 years of age and progresses slowly until the entire nucleus is opaque (Fig. 19-3). Often the earliest change is an increase in the index of refraction of the lens so that there is a decrease in hyperopia or an increase in myopia. The gradual progress of this lens opacity may be associated with improved near vision. This may lead the patient to believe erroneously that vision is permanently improved—"second sight." However, as the opacity progresses, vision for both near and far gradually deteriorates. Since the opacity is located in the visual line, the vision may vary with the pupillary diameter.

A cortical, or soft, cataract involves the lens cortex. Lens fibers are either opaque or hydrated, forming clefts that run radially to create a spokelike pattern. These opacities tend to involve the equatorial region initially. They may become very marked without impairment of vision. Gradually, however, the opacities involve the central area and cause decreased visual acuity.

A posterior subcapsular opacity is the most common type of aging change. It develops gradually and causes the posterior capsule to appear as gold and white granules. Because the visual axis is obscured early, the opacity causes a disproportionate loss of vision for its density and size.

Traumatic cataract. Contusion of the eye may cause a posterior subcapsular cataract many months after the original injury, even though the lens capsule has not been grossly injured.

Rupture of the lens capsule invariably causes a cataract. If the opening is microscopic in size, there may be a minute linear opacity corre-

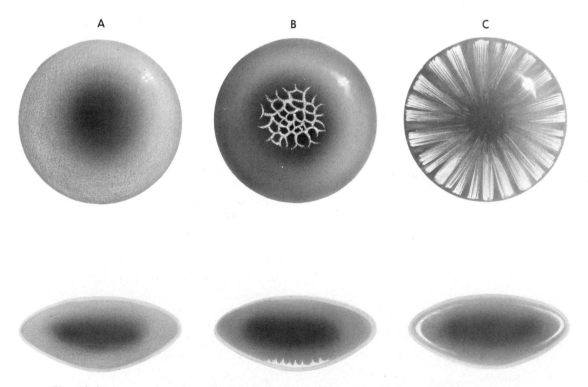

Fig. 19-3. Appearance of various types of aging cataracts. **A,** Nuclear sclerosis. **B,** Nuclear sclerosis and posterior subcapsular cataract. **C,** Nuclear sclerosis and anterior and posterior cortical cataracts.

sponding to the opening. More commonly, however, an initial posterior subcapsular opacity extends forward to involve the entire lens, and grayish lens material extrudes into the anterior chamber. An inflammation of varying severity results, and in individuals less than 25 years of age the entire lens may be autolyzed. In patients older than 25 years the nucleus remains and causes a continuing inflammation.

The effects of a foreign body within the lens depend on its size and rate of oxidation. Glass and plastics are well tolerated. Iron and copper cause characteristic opacities.

Diabetic cataract. Diabetic cataract is an uncommon type of lens opacity that occurs in poorly controlled growth-onset diabetes mellitus in the second decade of life. The opacity closely resembles "sugar" cataracts in experimental animals. The opacities are bilateral and cortical, predominantly involve the anterior and posterior subcapsular region, and consist of minute dots of varying size, usually called "snowflakes." A diabetic cataract may go to complete opacity (maturity) in less than 72 hours.

Patients with adult-onset diabetes have a slightly earlier onset of age-related cataract than do nondiabetic patients. Surgery is usually uncomplicated, but retinopathy may impair vision.

Sugar cataracts have been extensively studied in experimental animals. This type of cataract follows an increase in sugars (or pentoses given experimentally) in the lens. The excess sugar within the lens is reduced by aldose reductase to its alcohol (glucitol is glucose alcohol, also called L-sorbitol; dulcitol or galcitol is galactose alcohol). The lens capsule is relatively impermeable to sugar alcohols. Because of the excess sugar alcohol (polyol), the lens imbibes water, causing an osmotic imbalance. Eventually, increased sodium and decreased potassium levels and decreased glutathione levels lead to cataract formation. Topical administration of aldose reductase inhibitors prevents the cataract in rats.

Cataract occurs in galactosemia because of a deficiency in either hexose-1-phosphate uridyl transferase or galactokinase.

In some strains of mice a hereditary deficiency of sodium-potassium adenosinetriphosphatase (NaK ATPase) and failure of the cation pump causes cataract formation.

Hypocalcemic cataract. Cataracts thought to be the result of hypocalcemia or hyperphosphatemia develop when the blood calcium falls to a level at which neuromuscular hyperexcitability occurs. The opacities are small, discrete, and iridescent, and are located in the subcapsular region. Correction of the metabolic defect prevents their progression, and transparent lens fibers intrude between the lens capsule, causing the opacities and the cataract to appear laminated. Not every patient with hypocalcemia develops cataract, and additional metabolic factors may be contributory.

Toxic cataract. Permanent and transient lens opacities may be produced in experimental animals, particularly weanlings, by various sugars, electrolyte disturbances, and endocrine and dietary deficiencies. For the most part, the correlation with human cataract is remote, although galactose cataract occurs in infants (as well as the susceptible experimental animal) who, because of absence of the enzymes for their galactose metabolism, accumulate high levels of galactose alcohol (dulcitol) in their lenses.

Corticosteroids systemically administered in high doses for long periods, especially in arthritic patients, may cause posterior subcapsular opacities. Prolonged topical administration has the same effect with considerable individual variation. The opacity begins at the posterior pole as highly refractile, multicolored dots that impair vision. Peripheral cortical opacities then develop, but vision is seldom decreased enough to require cataract extraction.

Miotic drugs, particularly anticholinesterases, used topically to treat glaucoma or accommodative esotropia, produce anterior subcapsular opacities. These seldom progress, and they can be distinguished from aging changes only by prospective studies.

High doses of chlorpromazine produce a starshaped figure composed of granular deposits in the anterior capsular region of the lens. There are similar deposits in the cornea.

Medical treatment. Lens vacuoles may absorb spontaneously with visual improvement. Opacification does not invariably progress and does not progress at a constant rate. Thus many agents are advocated, particularly in Europe and Asia, to delay, prevent, or reverse cataract formation. Iodine salts, vitamins (particularly vitamins B, C, or E), adenosine triphosphate, various irritating drops reputed to increase ocular circulation, hormones, organ extracts, reducing agents, aspirin, and many other compounds are used. Aldose reductase inhibitors prevent the accumulation of sugar alcohols in galactosemic or diabetic animals and prevent sugar cataract formation. Photochemical changes in the lens from absorption of ultraviolet radiation, particularly in the range of 300 to 400 nm, can be prevented by protective eyeglasses.

During the period of decreasing vision, frequent and accurate refraction will maintain vision at the best possible level. When minute opacities involve the axial area, dilation of the pupil by means of a weak solution of phenylephrine (Neo-Synephrine 2.5%) or 2% homatropine may provide visual improvement. Pupillary dilation must not be used in patients with a shallow anterior chamber in whom there is danger of precipitating closed-angle glaucoma.

Surgical treatment. Extraction of the lens is indicated in the following instances: (1) when the opacity causes a visual defect that interferes with an individual's vocation or avocation, (2) if the lens threatens to cause a secondary glaucoma or uveitis, (3) to permit visualization of the fundus in order to monitor glaucoma, or (4) to permit adequate visualization of the fundus prior to photocoagulation, vitrectomy, or retinal surgery.

Many surgeons advocate surgery for monocular cataract in active individuals irrespective of the excellence of vision in the opposite eye. Binocular vision may be restored postoperatively by insertion of an intraocular lens or by means of a contact lens worn on the operated eye.

A cataract may cause glaucoma because of increased size or release of a toxic fluid in hypermaturity that causes macrophages to block the trabecular meshwork. Any opening in the lens capsule releases protein into the anterior chamber that causes a uveitis and sometimes a secondary glaucoma.

An acquired cataract may be removed in one of two ways: (1) by removal of the entire lens, including its capsule (intracapsular extraction); or (2) by removal of the anterior capsule, nu-

cleus, and cortex, with retention of the posterior capsule (extracapsular extraction). The intracapsular procedure was the method of choice from 1930 to 1980. Since then, extracapsular extraction has become increasingly more popular because of the use of posterior chamber intraocular lenses that require an intact equatorial lens capsule for support. Additionally, there is a lower incidence of cystoid macular edema with the extracapsular extraction.

Adequate anesthesia and ocular muscle immobility (akinesia) are important factors in successful surgery. Akinesia of the orbicularis oculi muscle is produced by means of a block of the facial nerve just anterior to the tragus or by infiltration of the muscle fibers with a local anesthetic. An anesthetic is also injected into the muscle cone and causes anesthesia of the eye (retrobular injection) and akinesia of the extraocular muscles. After the retrobulbar injection, massage of or pressure upon the globe reduces the intraocular pressure and decreases the danger of vitreous loss.

In the customary intracapsular lens extraction, an incision is made at the superior corneoscleral limbus. A portion of the iris may be removed, sparing the sphincter (peripheral iridectomy), or, less commonly, the peripheral and central portions of the iris may be excised (sector iridectomy).

The zonular fibers supporting the lens may be dissolved with the proteolytic enzyme alpha-chymotrypsin in individuals less than 60 years of age. In patients over 60 years of age, the zonule may be stripped by use of counterpressure. Preferences for lens removal vary widely. The lens may be frozen to a low-temperature probe (cryoprobe) or grasped by means of a suction cup and the entire lens, including its capsule, lifted from the eye. The incision is closed with fine sutures.

In the extracapsular extraction a large portion of the anterior lens capsule is excised, and the lens nucleus is removed from the eye (the anterior capsule may be opened with a YAG laser 24 hours before cataract extraction). The remaining cortex is then removed by suction-aspiration. All lens fibers are removed from the posterior capsule under microscopic observation. A posterior chamber intraocular lens is used. Some surgeons remove the lens by means of a suction-infusion instrument with the incision made through the portion of sclera adjacent to the pars plana portion of the ciliary body (lensectomy).

A soft (cortical) cataract is removed by one of the variants of mechanical disruption of the lens and aspiration (phacoemulsification). The procedure requires a small (3 mm) incision. The procedure is particularly useful in cataracts, whatever type, that occur before 50 years of age and have no nuclear sclerosis. After 50 years of age the degree of sclerosis of the nucleus determines whether or not phacoemulsification is used. The procedure is tedious in elderly patients with a hard nucleus. It is contraindicated in corneal endothelial disease and after severe uveitis. Irritation from nuclear remnants that accidentally fall into the vitreous may necessitate a vitrectomy.

Removal of the lens causes a marked reduction of the refractive power of the eye (aphakia) and impairment of the efficiency of the eye as an optical instrument. The most evident change is a severe hyperopia that cannot be neutralized by accommodation, because the lens is absent. Additionally, spherical and chromatic aberration and magnification of retinal images are increased. Irregular closure and faulty apposition of the incision may cause astigmatism.

The optical defect in aphakia may be neutralized by spectacles, a contact lens, an intraocular lens, or by surgery of the cornea to increase its refractive power (see Chapter 10). The corrective lenses worn in aphakia are maximally effective only when the patient looks through the optical center of the lens. With spectacle correction there is an annular area of blindness from 30° to 60° in the field of peripheral vision, and objects dart in and out of this field of vision. The prismatic effects of thick lenses cause image jumping and prismatic displacement of objects so that objects are not located where they appear. These prismatic effects and the magnification caused by aphakic spectacles make walking difficult. Conversely, because of the magnification, patients are frequently able to read unusually small print. Since accommodation is absent, it is necessary to wear bifocal or trifocal lenses; and because of the decreased depth of focus, the range of

clear vision for near is limited. Usually the refraction following a cataract extraction does not stabilize for several months, and a final type of lens is not prescribed until then.

Contact lenses in aphakia. Many of the optical disturbances caused by aphakia may be minimized, although not eliminated, with contact lenses. Because of the interruption of the nerve supply by the corneal incision, contact lenses are often better tolerated by cataract patients than by other patients. Conversely, many patients are unable to wear contact lenses successfully because of age, hemiplegia, parkinsonism, rheumatoid arthritis, or mental deterioration.

Extended-wear contact lenses may be used in some patients who cannot remove contact lenses daily. Dry eyes, blepharitis, and astigmatism of more than 3 diopters complicate contact lens wear. Patients are fitted after all sutures are removed, when the refraction is stable, usually about 2 or 3 months after surgery.

About one quarter of the eyes develop superficial vascularization that extends 1 or 2 mm into the cornea, usually superiorly. In patients with preexisting corneal vascularization, a soft contact lens aggravates the condition or causes vessels not carrying blood (ghost vessels) to carry blood.

Since soft contact lenses correct a maximum of 1.5 diopters of astigmatism, any greater astigmatism must be corrected by means of spectacles or rigid (hard) contact lenses.

Intraocular lens implantation. Insertion of a clear plastic lens in the pupillary space at the time of cataract extraction eliminates the optical problem of aphakia, although a reading correction is still necessary. Intraocular lenses provide binocular vision. They are indicated in patients in dusty occupations, in which contact lens hygiene is not possible, and in individuals who, because of dry eyes, shakiness, or unwillingness to try, cannot manage contact lenses. Insertion of the intraocular lens adds another step to the operation, and the intraoperative and postoperative complication rate of cataract extraction is slightly higher than if intraocular lenses were not used. They provide a better optical result than aphakic correction with spectacles.

Two types of intraocular lenses are used: (1)

anterior chamber lenses fixed in the angle of the anterior chamber, and (2) lenses that are inserted in the posterior chamber after an extracapsular lens extraction (Fig. 19-4).

A wide variety of shapes and sizes are available. The refractive power of the intraocular lens is determined preoperatively by measurement of the refractive power of the cornea with a keratometer and by measurement of the length of the eye by ultrasonography.

The major complication of intraocular lenses relates to mishaps in which the corneal endothelium is damaged, causing bullous keratopathy. Cystoid macular retinal edema (see Chapter 16) is more common after intracapsular lens extraction and lens implantation than after extracapsular lens extraction and lens implantation.

The use of intraocular lenses in children is debatable, because over the next 60 or 70 years the implant lens may become opaque. I believe that, although intraocular lenses are not indicated in children with bilateral congenital cataracts, they are indicated in some children with severe lacerations of one eye that require reconstruction of the anterior segment and lens removal.

After-cataract. The retained posterior lens capsule may become opaque after extracapsular cataract surgery. There are two main causes: (1) lens fibers adjacent to the capsule may not be fully removed at the time of cataract extraction, and (2) the anterior lens capsule that remains after capsulotomy may proliferate over the posterior capsule and obscure the visual axis.

The posterior capsule may be incised in the region of the visual axis at the time of cataract extraction. A YAG laser may be used to open the capsule at a later time.

Congenital cataract

Every individual has minute nonprogressive lens opacities that do not impair vision. Many hereditary cataracts are recognized by their characteristic structure. These opacities consist of multiple, fine, irregularly shaped opacities in the central or peripheral areas of the lens. The diagnosis is based on their morphologic characteristics as seen with a biomicroscope.

Attention in infancy is directed to cataracts severe enough to impair vision. The questions that arise include: (1) Does the opacity involve one or both eyes? (2) Does the visual decrease

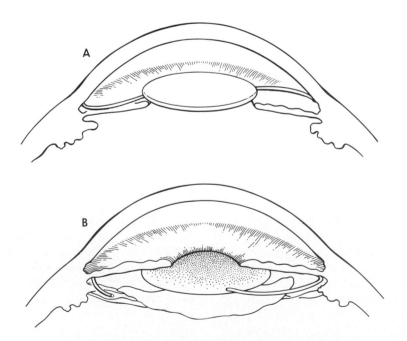

Fig. 19-4. A, Anterior chamber intraocular lens that is held in position with loop of nylon (haptics) placed in the anterior chamber angle. **B,** A posterior chamber lens placed in the lens capsule from which most of the anterior portion has been excised.

prevent normal schooling? (3) Are there associated ocular defects? (4) Are there associated systemic defects? (5) Are the lens opacities progressive? (6) What is the cause?

General physical examination shortly after birth should indicate a red fundus reflex. If a red fundus reflex is not seen with the ophthalmoscope, careful examination should be done after the pupils are dilated with 1% phenylephrine and 0.2% cyclopentolate. Ocular examination of infants may be facilitated by a hungry baby nursing or by immobilization. The fundus may be studied with a direct or indirect opthalmoscope using an infant-size goniolens (Koeppe) that also permits visualization of the lens and anterior chamber angle.

Visual acuity is difficult to assess in infants, but if opticokinetic nystagmus can be elicited, visual acuity likely will be more than 20/60 and surgery will not be required. If retinal blood vessels can be seen with an ophthalmoscope with the pupils dilated, surgery will likely not be necessary and the patient may have normal schooling.

Nystagmus, retinal or choroidal abnormalities, microphthalmia, and strabismus reduce the likelihood of good postoperative vision. Dense cataracts are often removed despite associated ocular defects inasmuch as the 20/200 corrected vision is better than preoperative vision. Conversely, corrected vision of 20/20 with aphakia is not more effective than 20/60 vision with the lens and accommodation intact.

Systemic defects should be identified and the progression of the lens opacity observed.

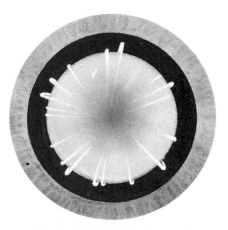

Fig. 19-5. Lamellar cataract with riders.

The medical and ocular history of other members of the family should be obtained. A family study is most rapidly initiated by examining the eyes of parents accompanying an infant. Hearing should be tested. The occurrence of supernumerary fingers and toes, gross abnormality in the development of the bones of the face or skull, or disproportion of the bones of the extremities should be noted. Flaccidity of the muscles should be investigated. Evidence of mental retardation and delayed physical development should be sought, particularly with reference to delayed psychomotor development such as failure to sit, stand, or talk at anticipated age levels.

Laboratory studies may include patient and maternal studies for antibodies against rubella, cytomegalovirus, toxoplasmosis, and syphilis. Galactosemia is excluded by appropriate enzyme testing. A reducing substance may be present in the urine. Commerical test tapes are specific for glucose and do not indicate other reducing substances in the urine. Homocystinuria may cause cataract, although it more commonly causes ectopia lentis. It is excluded by means of the cyanide nitroprusside test of urine. A positive test requires chromatography. Reducing substance and albumin may occur in the urine in the oculocerebrorenal (Lowe) syndrome, a moderately common cause of congenital cataract. Aminoaciduria occurs in a variety of congenital disorders associated with cataract. Chromosome analysis is indicated if there are widespread systemic defects in addition to cataracts.

Special types. Special types of congenital cataract include lamellar (zonular) and those associated with maternal rubella, oculocerebrorenal (Lowe) syndrome, mental retardation (Sjögren), Down syndrome (mongolism), and galactosemia.

Lamellar (zonular) cataract. The lens grows throughout life by forming successive layers. Lens fibers may become opaque because of a transient disturbance; with further growth of the lens, these fibers migrate centrally as deep concentric lamellar, or zonular, cataracts. Lamellar cataract is a common type of cataract and may develop up to 1 year after birth (Fig. 19-5). It is usually bilateral and is often transmitted as an autosomal dominant defect without any other abnormality. It consists of a series of concentric thin sheets (lamellae) of opacities surrounded by clear lens. There may be ⊃-shaped riders that extend along the edge from the anterior surface of the opacity to its posterior surface. Depending on the density of the opacity, vision may be good or markedly reduced. Vision may become worse at puberty, necessitating surgery. A unilateral lamellar cataract may follow contusion of the eye. Hypocalcemia in infancy causes a bilateral lamellar defect.

Maternal rubella. Rubella infection during pregnancy may cause widespread fetal ocular and systemic defects. The severity of the complications varies with different strains of the virus and is more severe the earlier in the pregnancy the rubella infection occurs. The lens may be entirely opaque, or there may be a central pearly white opacity. Nystagmus, strabismus, corneal opacities, microphthalmia, retinal hyperpigmentation, and glaucoma also occur. The pupil dilates poorly, and in all types of surgery, results are often unsatisfactory. The lens may harbor the virus for up to 2 years after birth, and all lens cortex should be removed at the initial operation to prevent an endophthalmitis.

Oculocerebrorenal (Lowe) syndrome. This is an X chromosome–linked recessive disorder, in which there are bilateral small lenses with dense to mature cataracts present at birth, mental retardation, growth failure, and hypotonia. Glaucoma, which is often present, may cause buphthalmos. There may be corneal scarring. A renal tubular dysfunction increases in severity with age and rickets develops secondary to hypophosphatemia.

Down syndrome. This is a frequent cause of mental retardation associated with widespread mental, systemic, and ocular defects. Cataracts develop in about 60% of the patients. Various types of cataract may occur: lamellar, posterior polar, sutural, and peripheral. For the most part, the opacities are not marked. Nystagmus may occur, and severe myopia is common.

Galactosemia. Galactosemia is a hereditary abnormality in which there is impairment of the enzymatic conversion of galactose to glucose (see Chapter 24).

Surgical treatment. Congenital cataracts should be removed as soon as it is evident that they may impair normal visual maturation. Monocular cataracts are removed the day of birth or shortly thereafter, provided the parents can manage the insertion and hygiene of an extended-wear contact lens.

The anterior lens capsule is opened with a needle knife; the lens cortex is disorganized with a knife, ultrasound, or mechanical cutter with infusion-suction; and the lens cortex is aspirated. The 3 mm incision is large enough only to admit the 20-gauge needle that contains the infusion and suction lines and auxiliary devices. If the pupil dilates poorly, it may be enlarged with a cutter. Refraction may be done as soon as the procedure is completed and an extended-wear contact lens prescribed.

Complications. Early and delayed complications are rare and related to retention of excessive cortical material that causes an iridocyclitis. The posterior capsule should remain intact, and the structural integrity of the eye is retained.

Retinal separation, previously a common cause of blindness following congenital cataract surgery, is now rare. It usually occurred 20 or more years after the operation.

Results. About 35% of patients with congenital cataracts have an associated serious eye defect that prevents good vision, even after successful lens extraction. Monocular cataract that was often not removed because of severe amblyopia may be removed the day of birth or shortly thereafter and vision corrected with an extended-wear contact lens. Some patients have 20/20 vision in each eye but no binocular vision.

BIBLIOGRAPHY
General

Alpar, J.J., and Fechner, P.U.: Fechner's intraocular lenses, New York, 1986, Thieme, Inc.

Clayman, H.M.: Intraocular lens implantation: techniques and complications, St. Louis, 1983, The C.V. Mosby Co.

Emery, J.M., and Jacobson, A.C.: Current concepts in cataract surgery: selected proceedings of the eighth biennial cataract surgical congress, New York, 1984, Appleton-Century-Crofts.

Ginsberg, S.P.: Cataract and intraocular lens surgery: a compendium of modern theories and techniques, Birmingham, 1984, Aesculapius Publishing Co.

Iliff, N., ed.: Complications in ophthalmic surgery, New York, 1983, Churchill Livingstone.

Jaffe, N.S.: Cataract surgery and its complications, ed. 4, St. Louis, 1984, The C.V. Mosby Co.

Jakobiec, F.A., and Sigelman, J.: Advanced techniques in ocular surgery, Philadelphia, 1984, W.B. Saunders Co.

Keates, R.H., Fry, S.M., and Link, W.J.: Ophthalmic neodymium YAG lasers, Thorofare, N.J., 1983, Slack, Inc.

King, J.H., Jr., and Wadsworth, J.A.C.: An atlas of ophthalmic surgery, ed. 3, Philadelphia, 1981, J.B. Lippincott Co.

Krupin, T., and Waltman, S.: Complications of ophthalmic surgery, ed. 2, Philadelphia, 1984, J.B. Lippincott Co.

Steele, A.D.M., and Drews, R.C., ed.: Cataract surgery, Boston, 1984, Butterworth Publishers.

Trokel, S.L.: YAG laser ophthalmic microsurgery, East Norwalk, N.J., 1983, Appleton-Century-Crofts.

Waltman, S.R., and Krupin, T., eds.: Complications in ophthalmic surgery, ed. 2, Philadelphia, 1984, J.B. Lippincott Co.

Cataract

Binder, P.S.: Secondary intraocular lens implantation during or after corneal transplantation, Am. J. Ophthalmol. **99:**515, 1985.

Ederer, F., Hiller, R., and Taylor, H.R.: Senile lens changes and diabetes in two population studies, Am. J. Ophthalmol. **91:**381, 1981.

Kador, P.F.: Overview of the current attempts toward the medical treatment of cataract, Ophthalmology **90:**352, 1983.

Kinoshita, J.H., Kador, P., and Catiles, M.: Aldose reductase in diabetic cataracts, J.A.M.A. **246:**257, 1981.

Liesegang, T.J.: Cataracts and cataract operations (first of two parts), Mayo Clin. Proc. **59:**556, 1984.

Liesegang, T.J.: Cataracts and cataract operations (second of two parts), Mayo Clin. Proc. **49:**623, 1984.

Ringvold, A., and Davanger, M.: Iris neovascularization in eyes with pseudoexfoliation syndrome, Br. J. Ophthalmol. **65:**138, 1981.

Straatsma, B.R., Foos, R.Y., Horwitz, J., Gardner, K.M., and Pettit, T.H.: Aging-related cataract: laboratory investigation and clinical management, Ann. Intern. Med. **102:**82, 1985.

Straatsma, B.R., Horwitz, J., Takemoto, L.J., Lightfoot, D.O., and Ding, L.L.: Clinicobiochemical correlations in aging-related human cataract, Am. J. Ophthalmol. **97:**457, 1984.

Wcate, R.A.: Senile cataract: the case against light, Ophthalmology **90:**420, 1983.

Zaidman, G.W.: The surgical management of dislocated traumatic cataracts, Am. J. Ophthalmol. **99:**583, 1985.

20

THE GLAUCOMAS

The glaucomas (Table 20-1) are a family of ocular diseases in which increased intraocular pressure may cause optic atrophy with excavation of the optic disk and characteristic loss of visual field. The degree of increased pressure that causes organic change is not the same in every eye, and some individuals may tolerate for long periods a pressure that would rapidly blind another. There are two major factors involved in the visual loss of glaucoma: (1) the intraocular pressure, which depends on the rate of production of aqueous humor and its rate of exit through the trabecular meshwork, and (2) the resistance of the intraocular portion of the optic nerve to the development of optic atrophy. This relates to its configuration, the adequacy of its blood supply, axoplasmic transport, and unknown factors.

Glaucoma is customarily divided into open-angle and closed-angle types. If the cause is evident, glaucoma is designated as secondary, but if the cause is unknown, as primary. In open-angle glaucoma the aqueous humor has free access to the trabecular meshwork, the drainage apparatus in the anterior chamber angle. In closed-angle glaucoma the root of the iris is in apposition to the trabecular meshwork, and aqueous humor cannot leave the eye. This occurs most commonly in eyes that have a shallow anterior chamber. Closed-angle glaucoma involves one of several mechanisms: (1) pupillary block in which all aqueous humor does not pass through the pupil but accumulates in the posterior chamber, causing the iris to balloon

forward to block the anterior chamber angle; (2) direct mechanical block of the anterior chamber angle by the root of the iris (plateau iris); and (3) increased size or edema of the ciliary body pressing the root of the iris forward against the trabecular meshwork.

Primary open-angle glaucoma is a disease of unknown cause previously called simple glaucoma, chronic glaucoma, glaucoma simplex, compensated glaucoma, and wide-angle glaucoma. It is characterized by three abnormalities: (1) increased intraocular pressure; (2) atrophy of the optic nerve with increased diameter, depth, or both, of the optic cup and decrease in the extent of the neuroretinal rim ("cupping"); and (3) typical visual field defects. The anterior chamber angle appears normal to direct observation, and the aqueous humor has free access to the trabecular meshwork.

Primary closed-angle glaucoma is a disorder in which an anatomic abnormality displaces the iris root anteriorly so that the peripheral anterior chamber is shallow and the entrance to the chamber angle is narrow. The entire anterior chamber may be shallow in the pupillary closure type, or the central anterior chamber may be of normal depth with the angle recess abnormally shallow in the plateau iris type. In the past it has been called acute glaucoma, congestive glaucoma, uncompensated glaucoma, angle-closure, or narrow-angle glaucoma.

Secondary glaucoma may be of the open- or closed-angle type. Secondary open-angle glaucoma occurs because of (1) fibrovascular prolif-

Table 20-1. Classification of glaucoma

Primary
  Chronic open-angle
  Glaucoma "suspect"
    Low-tension
    Ocular hypertension
  Closed-angle
    Pupillary block
    Plateau iris
      Ciliary body block
Secondary open-angle
  Pretrabecular
  Foreign cells within trabecular meshwork
  Trabecular meshwork abnormality
  Increased venous pressure
Secondary closed-angle
  Membrane contracture
  Pupillary block
  Angle shift
Developmental glaucoma
  Primary
  Secondary

eration on the anterior chamber face of the trabecular meshwork, notably in rubeosis iridis; (2) cells or tissue "clogging" the pores in the trabecular meshwork; (3) abnormalities within the trabecular meshwork from edema, trauma, or corticosteroid administration; or (4) increased pressure in the episcleral venous network into which aqueous humor drains from the canal of Schlemm.

Secondary closed-angle glaucoma occurs with one or more of the following: (1) contracture of fibromuscular membranes in the anterior chamber; (2) pupillary block with interference with flow of aqueous humor from posterior to anterior chamber; and (3) closure of the anterior chamber angle from a forward shift of the peripheral iris.

Tearing, photophobia, and blepharospasm characterize congenital glaucoma. In this disorder the increased intraocular pressure is caused by a congenital, sometimes hereditary disorder in which the anterior chamber retains its fetal configuration with the root of the iris attached to the trabecular meshwork or the trabecular meshwork covered by a membrane. The treatment is surgical.

Symptoms and signs

The symptoms of closed-angle glaucoma are mainly related to a sudden increase in intraocu-

lar pressure. There may be repeated attacks of ocular pain and blurred vision occurring after a prolonged time in darkness, after emotional upset, or after similar situations that cause pupillary dilation. The rapid increase in intraocular pressure causes an epithelial edema of the cornea that results in blurred vision and halos surrounding street lights (iridescent vision). The initial attacks are often spontaneously relieved by pupillary constriction that occurs normally during sleep or in bright illumination. (The supine position [face upward] in sleep may relieve a closed-angle attack by permitting the iris-lens diaphragm to fall away from the anterior chamber angle.) Either after repeated attacks or without previous symptoms, an acute closure of the angle occurs with reduced vision and a red, painful eye. Severe prostrating pain, usually unilateral, may be confused with migraine, impending rupture of a carotid artery aneurysm, and similar causes of hemicrania. There may be nausea, vomiting, and symptoms suggestive of an acute surgical abdominal condition.

Closed-angle glaucoma is diagnosed on the basis of (1) increased intraocular pressure combined with (2) an anterior chamber angle in which the aqueous humor does not have free access to the trabecular meshwork (closed). When the chamber angle is not closed, the pressure is normal unless previous attacks have damaged the trabecular meshwork or caused adhesions between the iris and the peripheral angle (peripheral anterior synechiae).

Open-angle glaucoma is usually asymptomatic. The intraocular pressure slowly increases over several years or more, and although it may reach a high level, corneal edema and ocular pain do not occur. In the early stages of disease the peripheral vision is not affected; any changes can be demonstrated only by careful perimetry. Measurement of the visual fields by confrontation is of little diagnostic value until late in the disease when the visual field becomes extremely constricted. Increased diameter and depth of the optic disk occurs with loss of the neuroretinal rim, pallor of the disk, and displacement of blood vessels within the cup.

Methods of examination

Several tests are of particular importance in the diagnosis of glaucoma: (1) tonometry: the measurement of ocular tension; (2) gonioscopy: the observation of the anterior chamber angle; (3) ophthalmoscopy: the evaluation of the color and configuration of the cup and neuroretinal rim of the optic disk; (4) perimetry: the measurement of visual function in the central and peripheral field of vision; and (5) photographic evaluation of the nerve fiber layer of the retina.

Tonometry. The intraocular pressure can be measured by connecting a cannula within the eye to a suitable recording instrument. It is indirectly measured by determining the ocular tension, which measures the ease with which the sclera or cornea may be indented. Ocular tension is measured by means of a tonometer. There are two basic types: (1) contact, in which the instrument is placed on the anesthetized eye, and (2) noncontact, in which an air pulse is used. The Schiøtz tonometer (Figs. 20-1 and 6-5) is an indentation tonometer that measures the amount of corneal deformation produced by a given force. The Goldmann applanation tonometer (see Fig. 6-5) measures the force necessary to flatten a given area of the cornea. Other tonometers use an electronic sensor in the tip. With contact tonometers the cornea must first be anesthetized by the instillation of a local anesthetic such as benoxinate. The indentation tonometer measures the ease with which the globe is indented by the plunger of the instrument. A soft eye is easily indented, indicating a low pressure, whereas a hard eye is indented with greater difficulty. The amount of indentation has been calibrated in enucleated eyes in millimeters of mercury pressure.

The applanation tonometer is influenced by fewer extraneous factors than the Schiøtz tonometer, but it requires greater experience and more costly equipment.

The noncontact tonometer flattens the cornea with an air pulse that increases the reflected light from the cornea. The time required to produce complete corneal flattening is related to the intraocular pressure. The time is measured electronically, and a computer in the instrument provides a digital readout of the pressure.

Normal individuals have a mean intraocular pressure of about 15 mm Hg ± 3 mm. Untreated glaucomatous eyes with field loss have a mean intraocular pressure of 22 mm Hg ± 5

mm. Intraocular pressure tends to increase with aging and to be higher in women than in men.

The ocular tension (which reflects the intraocular pressure) varies with the pulse and respiration. Additionally, the tension of the normal eye may vary by as much as 6 mm Hg during a 24-hour period. This 24-hour variation

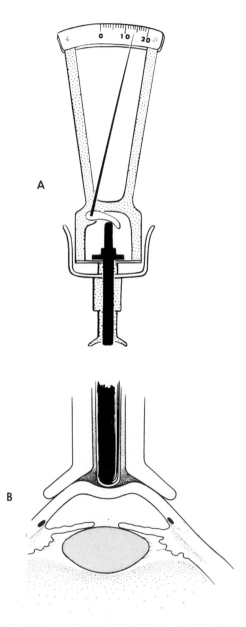

Fig. 20-1. A, Schiøtz tonometer in which the plunger, in black, measures the ease of indentation of the cornea. **B,** Indentation of the anesthetized cornea by the plunger of the tonometer to measure ocular tension.

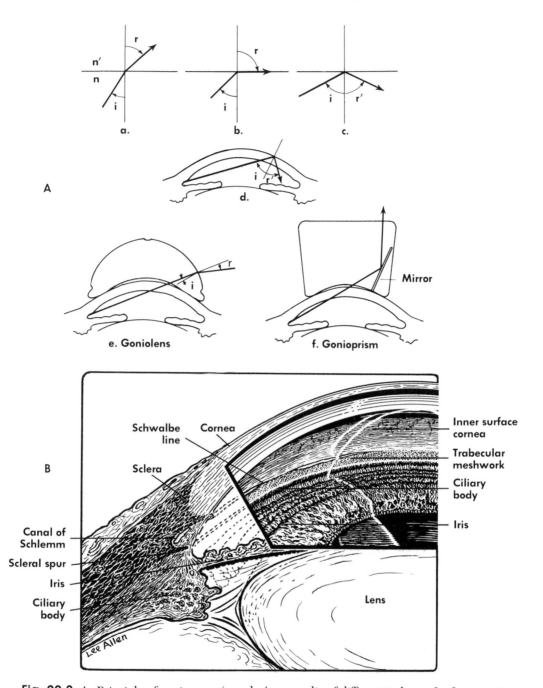

Fig. 20-2. A, Principle of gonioscopy (n and n' are media of different indices of refraction; i is the angle of incidence, r is the angle of refraction): A, Light is refracted when the angle of incidence is less than the critical angle. B, Light is refracted at 90° when the angle of incidence is equal to the critical angle. C, Light is reflected when the angle of incidence exceeds the critical angle (total internal reflection). D, Light from the anterior chamber angle is reflected back into the eye because the angle of incidence exceeds the critical angle at the junction of the cornea-air interface. E and F, Contact lenses have an index of refraction similar to that of the cornea; light that enters the lens is refracted (goniolens) or reflected (gonioprism) to the eye beyond the contact-lens-air interface. (From Shields, M.B.: A study guide for glaucoma, Baltimore, 1982, The Williams & Wilkins Co.) **B,** Correlation of chamber angle anatomy with gonioscopic appearance. The trabecular meshwork, which opens into the canal of Schlemm, is bounded anteriorly by the line of Schwalbe and posteriorly by the scleral spur. (Courtesy Lee Allen.)

(diurnal) may be much greater in individuals with glaucoma than in normal individuals. Additionally, the pressure may be increased by consumption of a large volume of fluid. The diuresis induced by ethyl alcohol may lower pressure. Adequate management of glaucoma may require measurement of tension at different hours to learn the maximum pressure. Such measurements are particularly important to individuals who seem to have glaucoma well controlled but who demonstrate progressive ocular damage.

Tonography. Tonography measures the rate at which the intraocular pressure decreases when the eye is compressed by means of an indentation tonometer resting upon it. The weight of the tonometer resting upon the eye expresses aqueous humor through the outflow channels, causing an increase in the amount of indentation by the plunger of the instrument. The tonometer is calibrated by determining the volume of the indentation. The difference between the volume at the beginning and at the end of the test is equal to the amount of aqueous humor expressed from the eye minus the amount of aqueous humor produced by the ciliary body while the tonometer rested upon it. The results are expressed as the coefficient of the facility of outflow (C), the microliters of aqueous humor expressed from the eye per minute per millimeter of mercury of intraocular pressure.

Measurement of the facility of outflow is an adjunct to other methods of diagnosis. In recent years most clinicians have not used it.

Gonioscopy. The opaque sclera and corneoscleral limbus prevent direct inspection of the angle of the anterior chamber. It is possible to see this area by means of a contact lens and mirror or a contact lens combined with a prism (Fig. 20-2). This method of inspection is of particular diagnostic importance since findings in the angle distinguish between closed-angle glaucoma and open-angle glaucoma. Closed-angle glaucoma can only be diagnosed definitely when the intraocular pressure is increased and the angle is closed. Earlier self-limited attacks of closed-angle may have produced adhesions between the iris and the angle (peripheral anterior synechiae, goniosynechiae), which suggest the diagnosis. Gonioscopy has also been used in the development of an effective surgi-

cal procedure for congenital glaucoma and in the diagnostic and therapeutic evaluation of many types of secondary glaucoma.

Gonioscopy may be direct or indirect. Direct gonioscopy uses a goniolens to neutralize the corneal refraction. The patient is in a supine position, and a light source and hand-held microscope are used. In indirect gonioscopy a gonioprism is used combined with a microscope. Direct gonioscopy causes less distortion of angle structures and permits a view of deeper structures within a narrowed chamber angle (which is also aided by the supine position). Indirect gonioscopy provides better illumination and magnification. Indentation through the sclera of the region of the ciliary body combined with gonioscopy is particularly useful.

Ophthalmoscopy. The examination of the ocular fundus in glaucoma is directed mainly to the appearance of the optic disk. The nerve fibers on the surface of the optic disk receive their blood supply from branches of the central retinal artery. These vessels anastomose with small branches of the partial arterial circle of Haller-Zinn that are derived from the short posterior ciliary arteries. Posterior to the lamina cribrosa, the blood supply is provided by the short posterior ciliary arteries and by the pial branches of the central retinal artery. Optic disk blood vessels are subjected to the intraocular pressure, and it has been hypothesized that a persistent increase of the intraocular pressure causes optic atrophy. The damage is attributed to obstruction of axoplasmic flow as a result of either mechanical displacement of the lamina cribrosa or ischemia of the disk.

Optic nerve cupping in glaucoma is the result of loss of nerve fiber axons at the level of the lamina cribrosa that first occurs at the inferior and superior margins of the optic cup. Associated with this loss is posterior and lateral displacement of the lamina cribrosa. Optic nerve cupping results in a variety of changes in the optic disk (Table 20-2).

The normal optic nerve head is slightly oval vertically. The central area may contain a depression, the cup, that is of lighter color than the surrounding nerve. In some eyes the cup is stark white and the lamina cribrosa may be seen at its base. The cup is surrounded by the orange-red neuroretinal rim, the nerve tissue between the margin of the cup and the margin of the optic disk. The central retinal artery and vein are located on the nasal side of the cup.

The size of the optic disk is determined by the size of the posterior scleral foramen, and the size of the cup is determined by the volume of glial supportive tissue. The horizontal cup-to-disk ratio (C/D) (Fig. 20-3) tends to be the same in the two eyes of an individual and to be similar in families.

As bundles of axons are lost in the optic disk in glaucoma, several patterns of increase in the size of the cup (glaucomatous cupping) may be observed (Fig. 20-4). There may be selective loss of the neuroretinal rim at the superior and inferior portions of the cup. Alternatively, the cup may enlarge, particularly at the superior and inferior temporal portions. This may appear as a symmetrical increase in the size of the

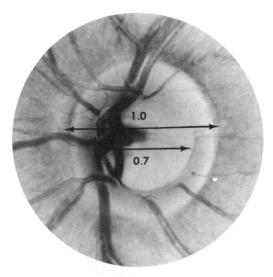

Fig. 20-3. The optic disk with the neuroretinal rim surrounding the optic cup. The horizontal cup/disk ratio is the ratio of the diameter of the cup to the diameter of the disk. In this illustration, the cup/disk ratio is 0.7.

Table 20-2. Ophthalmoscopic signs in glaucoma

Cup
    Documented increase in diameter or depth
    Cup/disk ratio more than 0.6
    Cup/disk ratio difference of more than 0.2 between
        two eyes
    Sharp margins or undermining of a large cup
    Extension of cup to disk margin
    Markedly oval cup
    Notching of cup
    Exposed lamina cribrosa
Neuroretinal margin
    Pale with cupping
Blood vessels
    Arterial pulsation
    Exposed disk vessels ("baring")
    Nasal displacement
    Splinter hemorrhages at disk margin
    Dilated veins
Miscellaneous
    Loss of retinal nerve fiber layer (red-free light)
    Peripapillary atrophy

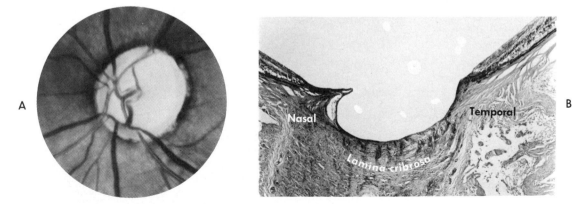

Fig. 20-4. A, Optic atrophy with glaucomatous excavation of the optic disk. The temporal neuroretinal rim has disappeared entirely because of glaucomatous atrophy. The blood vessels are displaced nasally and the blood vessels at the base of the optic cup are exposed ("bared"). **B,** Histologic section of advanced optic atrophy and glaucomatous excavation ("bean pot" excavation). The lamina cibrosa is characteristically bowed away from the eye.

cup, but often there are marked differences in the two eyes. There may be deepening of the cup with no initial increase in its diameter. All of these changes reflect loss of neural rim tissue.

Since the retinal vessels pass on the nasal side of the disk, enlargement of the cup may uncover a previously concealed vessel. It appears as a curved vessel that marks the earlier margin of the cup. Splinter hemorrhages may occur on the margin of the disk.

Evaluation of progressive disk changes caused by glaucoma is difficult. Stereoscopic visualization using a contact lens to neutralize corneal refraction and the biomicroscope is useful but may miss subtle changes. The clinician may monitor changes in the disk by careful drawings of the area of cupping in all meridians, the width of the neuroretinal rim, and the position of blood vessels. Color stereophotographs permit serial comparison. The inherent error of subjective evaluation has been mini-

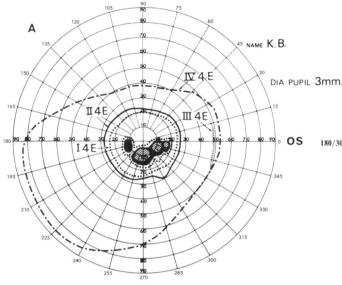

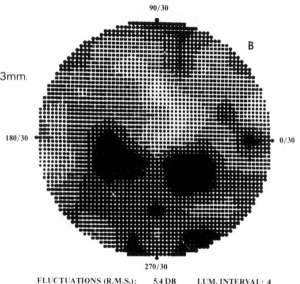

FLUCTUATIONS (R.M.S.): 5.4 DB   LUM. INTERVAL: 4

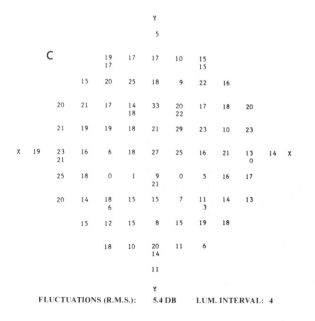

FLUCTUATIONS (R.M.S.): 5.4 DB   LUM. INTERVAL: 4

Fig. 20-5. Comparison of the Goldman, **A,** and automated (Octopus [**B** and **C**]) visual fields of the left eye *(OS)* in a patient with glaucoma. An arcuate defect is present in the inferior visual field. In **A,** the Roman numerals refer to the size of the test object (I = 0.25 mm^2; II = 0.1 mm^2; III = 4 mm^2; and IV = 16 mm^2). The Arabic numbers and letters refer to the light intensity (*4E* is the brightest intensity; *1A* is the dimmest). In **B,** a gray scale and ten gradations are used to indicate light intensity; white is dimmest and black is brightest. There are 76 points tested, each separated by 6° horizontally and 3° vertically. In **C,** a numeral scale is used to illustrate the same data as in **B.** (From Kolker, A.E., and Hetherington, J., Jr.: Becker-Shaffer's diagnosis and therapy of the glaucomas, St. Louis, 1983, The C.V. Mosby Co.)

mized but not eliminated by several quantitative measurements derived mainly from map reading devices.

If glaucomatous atrophy is not arrested, all neuroretinal rim tissue is lost. The optic disk is white, and the cup extends to the margin of the disk. The cup slopes away from the temporal margin of the disk onto a concave floor where gray stippling of the cribriform plate is seen. The nasal slope is much steeper than the temporal slope. The nerve fiber layer of the retina is reduced, particularly in regions corresponding to notched defects in the nerve tissue of the disk.

Perimetry. The appearance of the optic disk must be correlated with measurement of visual function in the peripheral and central fields of vision. Perimetry is most useful in the diagnosis of early glaucoma and in documenting the control or the progression of the disease. The visual field defect is often proportionate to the severity of the optic nerve atrophy. A skilled perimetrist correlates the optic nerve defects with the visual field abnormalities. In the early stages of glaucoma, visual field defects may be transient and manifest only when the intraocular pressure is increased. As the disease progresses, the defects become permanent.

Visual fields are measured by using kinetic (moving) and static techniques. Kinetic techniques utilize a tangent screen (see Chapter 6) or an arc or bowl perimeter. The test object moves from a nonseeing area to a seeing area, and the patient signals when it is perceived.

Static perimetry uses a nonmoving (fixed) target. In suprathreshold techniques, a target is shown for 0.5 to 1.0 second, and the points at which the patient fails to see the target are recorded. In threshold static perimetry, the intensity of the target light is increased until the patient just detects it and the intensity of the light is recorded.

A number of automated computer-assisted perimeters are now available for either screening or sensitive, complex field measurements (Fig. 20-5). Many use static techniques, utilizing either suprathreshold or threshold targets. A number of different computer programs are available. Their role in clinical management of glaucoma is currently being evaluated.

The nasal visual field is most susceptible to glaucomatous change (Fig. 20-6). It corresponds to axons that enter the temporal side of the optic nerve from the temporary periphery. These fibers are above and below the large mass of neurons that originate in the fovea centralis. The peripheral fibers do not cross a horizontal line that extends temporally from the fovea. With increased intraocular pressure, these axons, which originate from the arc-shaped area of the temporal retina, lose their function, causing a typical arcuate island of blindness called an arcuate scotoma. The fibers in the peripheral retina are also damaged, causing peripheral field defects. The central retinal fibers from the fovea centralis are more resistant to the increased pressure. Good visual acuity may be retained despite advanced glaucoma and retention of only the central 5° to 10° of visual field.

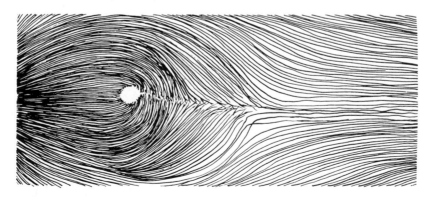

Fig. 20-6. The temporal raphe lateral to the fovea centralis. Nerve fibers do not cross the raphe, and their atrophy causes a nerve fiber bundle defect in the nasal visual field. (From Vrabec, F.: Am. J. Ophthalmol. **62**:927, 1966. Copyright Ophthalmic Publishing Co.)

A number of conditions other than glaucoma must be considered in evaluating visual opacities, and constriction of the pupil may exaggerate defects. Refractive errors should be corrected for accurate perimetry. Aging reduces the threshold sensitivity. The patient's comprehension, alertness, and cooperation, as well as the skill of the examiner, influence results.

Genetics of glaucoma

Primary open-angle glaucoma has a multifactorial, or polygenic, inheritance. The children and siblings of glaucomatous patients tend to have a higher intraocular pressure, lower facility of outflow, higher cup/disk ratio, and increased intraocular pressure when topical corticosteroids are administered. Diabetes mellitus and myopia are also risk factors that increase the likelihood of developing optic nerve disease with increased pressure. Primary open-angle glaucoma is more common in blacks than whites, produces damage at an earlier age and leads to blindness at a much greater rate.

Most patients with open-angle glaucoma develop increased intraocular pressure and a decreased outflow facility after the topical administration of 0.1% dexamethasone four times daily for 6 weeks. Continued increase in the intraocular pressure leads to optic nerve atrophy with excavation and a typical visual field defect. It is postulated that the response to topical corticosteroids is genetically determined, so that those who respond with a marked increase in pressure (4%) have a genotype with a similar allele pair for high pressure (P^H or gg). Those who do not respond (64%) have a similar allele pair for low pressure (P^L or nn), whereas those with an intermediate response (32%) are heterozygous for high and low pressure. Those who are homozygous for a high pressure response tend to have positive glucose tolerance tests and low serum protein-bound iodine and tend to be nontasters of phenylthiocarbamide.

Closed-angle glaucoma has a multifactorial inheritance related to the size of the anterior ocular segment.

Congenital, or infantile, glaucoma is transmitted as an autosomal recessive characteristic. Boys are affected twice as often as girls. Cardiac, auditory, and cerebral defects may also be present.

Primary open-angle glaucoma

Primary open-angle glaucoma (simple glaucoma, glaucoma simplex, compensated glaucoma, chronic glaucoma, or chronic simple glaucoma) is a bilateral condition in which there is an abnormal increase in the intraocular pressure in the absence of a grossly visible (with the gonioscope) obstruction between the trabecular meshwork and the anterior chamber (see Fig. 20-2). The increased intraocular pressure leads to an atrophy and excavation of the optic disk and typical defects of the visual field. In the United States open-angle glaucoma is one of the chief causes of blindness in adults. It occurs because of an abnormality in the aqueous humor outflow system between anterior chamber and the canal of Schlemm. There are varying degrees of severity, and unquestionably, many individuals have mild forms of the disease without knowing it.

Symptoms and signs. Open-angle glaucoma tends to become evident after 35 years of age. It has no particular sex predisposition. External examination of the eye does not indicate an abnormality such as that which may be recognized in closed-angle glaucoma.

Open-angle glaucoma is characterized by an almost complete absence of symptoms and a chronic, insidious course. Halos around lights and blurring of vision do not occur unless there has been a sudden increase in intraocular pressure, and many patients never have visual difficulties. Visual acuity remains good until late in the course of the disease; thus, measurement of visual acuity is of no value as a screening test.

Diagnosis. The diagnosis of open-angle glaucoma depends on demonstration of an increased intraocular pressure combined with characteristic changes in the visual field and optic disk. The increased intraocular pressure precedes the optic nerve and visual field changes by many years, and it is important that the increased pressure be diagnosed before such changes occur.

Measurement of ocular tension should be routine in all ocular examinations. The optic disk should be carefully evaluated. In the event of any change suggestive of glaucoma, perimetry is indicated. Particular attention should be directed to possible glaucoma in individuals with a family history of glaucoma or myopic individuals, in those with diabetes mellitus, and in blacks.

Medical treatment. The treatment of primary open-angle glaucoma is mainly medical. Surgery is indicated if the intraocular pressure is persistently high, if there is progression of optic disk changes, or if there is progression of visual field defects. Medical treatment is directed toward increasing outflow of aqueous humor from the anterior chamber, decreasing the secretion of aqueous humor, or both.

When increased intraocular pressure occurs with optic disk cupping and characteristic visual field defects, the need for treatment is obvious. The management of patients with increased ocular tension and normal disks and visual fields must be individualized. Patients with diabetes mellitus, a family history of glaucoma, a large optic cup, any cardiovascular abnormality, and advancing age are at increased risk to develop glaucomatous damage. Black patients are particularly vulnerable to glaucomatous damage. There is no indicator of future damage and periodic ophthalmoscopic examination with particular attention to the optic disk, visual field measurements, and tonometry may be all that is required. If the ocular tension exceeds 30 mm Hg, treatment is indicated. In individuals 65 years of age and older, treatment is indicated if ocular tension exceeds 25 mm Hg. Because pressure varies during the day, ocular pressures must be measured at different times.

Medical treatment of open-angle glaucoma presents the same difficulties as treatment of any chronic disease that has no symptoms. Miotic drugs may aggravate the visual loss caused by incipient cataract or, in younger individuals, induce a painful ciliary muscle spasm with excessive accommodation. Patients have difficulty in remembering to take their medications, a problem often aggravated when several different medications are prescribed for daily use. An alarm wristwatch may be helpful.

In well-controlled glaucoma, examination is usually indicated three times a year. The tension must be measured and the optic disks studied. At least once a year perimetry and gonioscopy must be repeated. In poorly controlled glaucoma, in which the intraocular pressure is persistently increased and there is pro-

gressive optic nerve involvement, examination is required as frequently as necessary to control the disease.

Primary open-angle glaucoma is treated with timolol (0.25% and 0.5%), an alpha$_1$ and beta$_1$ adrenergic receptor antagonist; betaxolol (0.5%), a beta$_1$ adrenergic receptor antagonist; pilocarpine (1% to 4%), a cholinergic-stimulating drug; echothiophate iodide (.03% and .06%), a cholinesterase antagonist; epinephrine (1% and 2%), an alpha and beta agonist; and acetazolamide (250 mg tablets), a carbonic anhydrase inhibitor (see Chapter 3). A number of compounds that belong to these drug classes are available. Therapy should begin with the smallest possible concentration that will maintain normal pressure and prevent optic nerve defects.

Treatment is often initiated with 0.25% or 0.5% timolol maleate, topically instilled, no more often than every 12 hours. It is contraindicated in patients with asthma, other pulmonary obstructive disease, or cardiac conduction defects. Timolol does not affect the pupil size or accommodation and is well tolerated by most patients. In some patients initial reduction of pressure is not maintained and ocular tension returns to pretreatment levels in several days. In others control of pressure is lost 3 to 12 months after treatment is begun. The drug is used widely, and depression, anxiety, and other central nervous system effects may occur. Betaxolol, a cardioselective beta adrenergic receptor antagonist, became commercially available in October 1985. It does not have the pulmonary effects of timolol and may be used in patients with pulmonary obstructive disease.

Pilocarpine (1% to 4%), the traditional medication for initial therapy, has been replaced by timolol. Therapy should begin with the smallest concentration that will maintain normal pressure and prevent optic nerve defects. Pilocarpine facilitates the aqueous outflow in open-angle glaucoma. Because of its miotic effect on the pupil, it is also used in the management of closed-angle glaucoma. Pupillary constriction often decreases vision in patients with minor cataracts. In individuals less than 40 years of age, pilocarpine often causes a transient (1 to 2 weeks) ciliary muscle spam with aching pain in the eyes and artificial or increased myopia from excessive accommodation, and because of this, timolol is preferred. Carbachol (0.75% to 3%) may be substituted for pilocarpine.

Topical instillation of epinephrine in a 0.5% to 2% solution decreases secretion of aqueous humor and improves aqueous outflow. Epinephrine is moderately irritating to the eye and may cause black adrenochrome pigmentation of the conjunctiva and maculopathy in aphakic eyes. Epinephrine solutions are used either alone or in combination with cholinergic-stimulating drugs, often pilocarpine. Propine, a conjugated epinephrine, penetrates the cornea with ease and may be used topically in a 0.1% concentration.

Echothiophate iodide (0.03%, 0.06%, 0.125%, and 0.25%) is active against the true cholinesterases of the sphincter pupillae muscle. It causes an intense miosis with a maximum effect in 4 to 6 hours that persists up to 24 hours. It is used twice daily, usually in 0.03% to 0.06% concentrations. It depletes systemic nonspecific anticholinesterases and may cause prolonged respiratory depression in general anesthesia using succinyl chloride. Toxic reactions may follow the use of procaine, which, like succinyl chloride, is hydrolized by the nonspecific anticholinesterases. It is contraindicated in closed-angle glaucoma, bronchial asthma, gastrointestinal spasm, vascular hypertension, myasthenia gravis, and Parkinson disease. Chronic topical administration may cause vesicles of the anterior portion of the lens. Children may develop pupillary cysts. Despite the contraindications, echothiophate iodide is useful in open-angle glaucoma, some secondary glaucomas, and in accommodative esotropia.

Carbonic anhydrase inhibitors reduce the secretion of aqueous humor by the ciliary processes. Acetazolamide is the drug commonly used. The drug is effective 2 hours after administration; its maximum action lasts for 6 hours. Sequels (500 mg) are effective for 12 hours. Paresthesia, with numbness and tingling of extremities, anorexia, and other side effects often require reduction of the dose or substitution of other carbonic anhydrase–inhibitor compounds.

Surgical treatment. If the intraocular pressure can be maintained at a normal level by means of drugs and if there is no progress in the severity of the glaucoma as judged by the ophthalmoscopic appearance of the optic disk and by the absence of progressive visual field defects, open-angle glaucoma is treated medically. If the intraocular pressure cannot be controlled medically and there is progress in the visual field defects and in the severity of optic atrophy, surgery is indicated.

The main surgical procedure in open-angle glaucoma, in which the trabecular meshwork is clearly visible, is laser trabeculoplasty. The argon laser is commonly used. The eye is anesthetized with a topical anesthetic, and the trabecular meshwork is viewed through an antireflective coated four-mirror gonioprism. Usually a 50 μm spot size and 0.1 second duration are used. A power setting is used that will blanch the anterior trabecular meshwork but not cause bubble formation. Usually an initial power of 400 mW is selected, and this is increased in 200 mW increments until a visible reaction is observed. The power is then reduced by 100 mW and used for treatment if it produces a reaction. individual surgical preferences vary, but often 75 to 80 applications are spaced evenly over the entire circumference of the anterior trabecular meshwork. The main immediate complication is a transient increase in intraocular pressure that may require acetazolamide or oral glycerine to control. Other complications are relatively minor: transient iritis, peripheral anterior synechiae, hyphema, and transient corneal opacities. Intraocular pressure control is achieved in about 85% of all patients, but most (75%) continue to require antiglaucoma medications. Control may be lost with passing time, and laser trabeculoplasty is not effective with additional application.

In eyes in which laser trabeculoplasty cannot be performed because of inability to see the trabecular meshwork, or if laser trabeculoplasty fails to control the intraocular pressure, a filtering operation is indicated. All filtering operations are based on creating a fistula between the anterior chamber and the subconjunctival space through which aqueous humor will flow. An incision is made into the anterior chamber, and the anterior or posterior lip may be removed so that the wound edges are not adjacent and will not be closed by cicatrix. Cauterization by heat of the scleral wound edges also prevents the wound from closing. The scleral openings into the anterior chamber are combined with a complete or peripheral iridectomy or with inclusion of a portion of the iris in the scleral wound. Alternatively, the opening may be made by means of a trephine that is 1 or 2 mm in diameter. 5-Fluorouracil, an antimetabolite, is sometimes injected into the bleb site to inhibit fibroblastic proliferation and enhance the likelihood of filtration.

Trabeculectomy is the operation of choice in many centers. An operating microscope is used, and a superficial flap of sclera is fashioned to expose the scleral side of the trabecular meshwork. A portion of the meshwork is then excised and the scleral flap replaced. A filtering bleb often develops after surgery. The chief advantage of the operation is the immediate formation of the anterior chamber after the procedure; this prevents the development of peripheral anterior synechiae. Excessively low pressure (hypotension), cystic conjunctival blebs, cataract, and bullous keratopathy occur less commonly after trabeculectomy than after other filtering operations.

Photocoagulation of the ciliary processes may reduce aqueous humor secretion but requires a widely dilated pupil.

OCULAR HYPERTENSION ("GLAUCOMA SUSPECT")

This is a condition in which the intraocular pressure is consistently high (above 20 mm Hg in both eyes) in individuals who have open angles, normal optic disks, and normal visual fields. Some physicians call this early primary open-angle glaucoma; others believe that the patient has potential glaucoma; others believe the eyes are normal but with pressures at the upper end of the distribution of normal ocular pressures. The terms apply only when both eyes are involved; if one eye has overt primary open-angle glaucoma, the fellow eye is glaucomatous, although consistently high intraocular pressure is the only sign.

Most patients do not develop abnormal disks or visual field defects. The risk of developing glaucoma, however, is greater with higher tensions, increased age, lower coefficients of outflow, or higher cup/disk ratios. When all of these factors are unfavorable, about 10% to 15% of the patients develop a visual field defect within 5 years.

Usually patients with pressures consistently less than 24 mm Hg are observed only. Patients with pressures of more than 30 mm Hg are usually treated with a beta blocker. Patients in the intermediate range are treated if they have unfavorable factors such as myopia, diabetes mellitus, vascular disease, a family history of glaucoma, and large or asymmetric optic disks.

Low-tension glaucoma

This is a condition in which the intraocular pressure is consistently normal but the optic disks show typical changes of glaucoma with characteristic visual field defects. Patients may have a history of congestive heart disease, cardiac arrhythmia, anemia, or transient ischemic attacks. The condition may reflect an imbalance between the arterial perfusion pressure of the optic disk and the intraocular pressure. It may be nonprogressive after a transient episode of vascular shock. A progressive form may result from chronic vascular insufficiency of the optic disk and be a chronic ischemic optic neuropathy.

Treatment is directed to the primary medical condition and reduction of the intraocular pressure.

Secondary open-angle glaucoma

A secondary open-angle glaucoma is any condition in which the intraocular pressure is abnormally high in one or both eyes whether or not the optic disk or visual field is abnormal. The anterior chamber angle is open, but the trabecular meshwork may be abnormal. Secondary open-angle glaucoma may be classified as (1) pretrabecular, (2) trabecular pores, (3) intratrabecular, and (4) posttrabecular (Table 20-3).

Secondary pretrabecular open-angle glaucoma occurs in rubeosis iridis (neovascular glaucoma), the iridocorneal syndromes (see chapter on uvea), in epithelial downgrowth, and with inflammatory membranes. Secondary trabecular open-angle glaucoma occurs with obstruction of the trabecular meshwork pores with erythrocytes, ghost cells, macrophages, uveal pigment, neoplastic cells, protein, zonules (after use of alpha-chymotrypsin in cataract extraction). Secondary intratrabecular open-angle glaucoma occurs with edema of the trabecular meshwork as a result of inflammation,

Table 20-3. Secondary open-angle glaucoma

Pretrabecular
  Fibrovascular membrane
    Rubeosis iridis
  Iridocorneal syndrome
  Epithelial downgrowth
  Fibrous proliferation
  Inflammatory membrane
Cells within trabecular meshwork
  Erythrocytes
    Ghost cells
  Macrophages
    Hemolytic glaucoma
    Phacolytic glaucoma
    Melanocytic glaucoma
  Neoplastic cells
  Pigment
    Pigment dispersion syndrome
    Uveitis
  Protein
    Uveitis
    Zonules after alpha-chymotrypsin
Intratrabecular
  Edema: inflammation, trauma
  Corticosteroids
Increased episcleral pressure
  Carotid-cavernous fistula
  Hemangiomas
  Orbital tumors
  Thyroid exophthalmos

---

trauma, retained foreign bodies, corticosteroid administration, and in glaucoma cyclitic crisis. Posttrabecular secondary open-angle glaucoma occurs because of increased episcleral venous pressure from vascular abnormalities, thyrotropic exophthalmos, and retrobulbar tumors.

Special types. Neovascular glaucoma results from the development of a fibrovascular membrane over the anterior chamber surface of the trabecular meshwork. The membrane originates with new blood vessel formation in the anterior chamber. Common causes include central vein closure and diabetic retinopathy. Many vascular, neoplastic, and inflammatory disorders may be responsible. The earliest sign is a faint flare in the anterior chamber because of abnormal vascular permeability. Small tufts of dilated capillaries at the pupillary margin are followed by the formation of new blood vessels on the surfaces of the iris and trabecular meshwork. Contraction of a fibrous membrane evident with larger vessels causes adhesions (peripheral anterior synechiae) between the iris and trabecular meshwork. In time the entire angle is occluded. Treatment is difficult. The eyes are often blind from the precipitating disease. Photocoagulation of the retina may cause regression of new iris blood vessels. Cryotherapy to the ciliary body may reduce intraocular pressure. Topical instillation of 1% atropine and corticosteroids and a soft contact lens may relieve pain. A retrobulbar injection of alcohol relieves pain for several months.

Heterochromic iridocyclitis (of Fuchs) is a nongranulomatous chronic anterior uveitis associated with a secondary glaucoma and frequently a posterior subcapsular cataract. Both the glaucoma and the cataract with which the uveitis is associated may be aggravated by corticosteroids used locally in the treatment of the uveitis.

Glaucomatocyclitic crisis is a unilateral acute inflammation of the uveal tract in which the signs of a rapid increase in intraocular pressure predominate. There is corneal edema with blurring of vision and marked decrease in the coefficient of outflow facility. The disease is distinguished from angle-closure glaucoma in that the angle is open. The inflammation may be confined to the trabecular meshwork with minimal inflammatory signs. Systemic indomethacin may terminate the attack.

In the pigment dispersion syndrome, there is loss of pigment from the iris pigment epithelium and a deposition of pigment on the posterior lens equator, corneal endothelium in a vertical line (Krukenberg spindle), and trabecular meshwork. There are transillumination defects of the iris. In some cases glaucoma occurs. Strenuous exercise or dilation of the pupil with medications releases pigment from the iris that obstructs the trabecular meshwork and increases intraocular pressure. Prophylactic instillation of pilocarpine prevents the pressure increase that occurs with exercise.

Contusion of the eye results in a marked immediate increase in intraocular pressure that persists for 30 to 45 minutes. If hemorrhage follows contusion, a secondary glaucoma may ensue. It results from blockage of the trabecular meshwork by erythrocytes and macrophages containing hemoglobin products. Contusion may result in tears in the ciliary body and recession of the chamber angle. The majority of such eyes do not develop glaucoma. Some develop what clinically appears to be monocular open-angle glaucoma from 1 month to 10 years after the injury.

The exfoliation syndrome (pseudoexfoliation of the lens) is characterized by deposits of a flaky, translucent material that is most noticeable on the anterior lens capsule and pupillary margin but also on both surfaces of the iris, zonules, ciliary body, vitreous, trabecular meshwork, corneal endothelium, and surrounding blood vessels in the orbit. It also is found covering the pigment epithelium of the iris, sometimes forming a layer on the anterior surface, and within the iris stroma surrounding blood vessels. It may be prominent on the basal surface of the nonpigmented ciliary epithelium and is also found on the zonules, vitreous, trabecular meshwork, corneal endothelium, and orbital blood vessels.

The exfoliative material is composed of oxytalan, a microfibrillar component of pre-elastic tissue. Its source is unknown, but oxytalan is a product of cells that normally form basement membrane. It could be part of the epithelium of either lens capsule or ciliary processes.

True exfoliation of the lens occurs in glassblowers' cataract, in which the iris absorbs infrared energy and transmits the generated heat to the lens capsule, causing a splitting of the zonular lamellae of the lens capsule.

Corticosteroid glaucoma is caused by topical and sometimes systemic administration of corticosteroid preparations. It may be self-limited and may also cause severe optic nerve atrophy and cupping with persistently increased intraocular pressure. The mechanism is unknown. It has been attributed to glycosaminoglycan deposition in the trabecular meshwork, decreased activity of phagocytes in the meshwork, and alteration of cyclic adenosine monophosphate (cAMP) in the anterior ocular segment.

Iridocyclitis causes a secondary glaucoma by blocking the trabecular meshwork with inflammatory cells, protein, and fibrin. There may be an inflammation of the trabecular meshwork (trabeculitis) causing irreversible damage to the meshwork and a permanent open-angle glaucoma. The disease course is the same as that of open-angle glaucoma.

Lens abnormalities may produce either a secondary open-angle or a secondary closed-angle glaucoma. Occasionally an intact lens dislocated in the vitreous body will be associated with an open-angle glaucoma, the mechanism of which is not evident. Lens hypermaturity and rupture of the lens capsule cause a glaucoma through the release of lens polypeptides or protein, resulting in a uveitis with secondary glaucoma.

A carotid-cavernous sinus fistula increases the episcleral venous pressure and impairs aqueous outflow resulting in increased intraocular pressure.

Rectus muscle fibrosis in thyrotropic exophthalmos increases intraocular pressure when the contralateral muscle contracts. The pressure is normal when the normal muscle is not contracting. Usually the inferior rectus muscle is restricted, and on upward gaze the intraocular pressure increases and erroneously high tensions are recorded. In downward gaze the tension is normal. Any proptosis may increase episcleral venous pressure, decrease aqueous humor outflow, and increase intraocular pressure.

Primary closed-angle glaucoma

Closed-angle glaucoma is an abnormality in which the intraocular pressure increases because the outflow of aqueous humor from the anterior chamber is mechanically impaired by contact of the iris with the trabecular drainage meshwork, the peripheral cornea, or both. The condition has been designated in the past as narrow-angle, acute congestive, and uncompensated glaucoma. No term is ideal because the intraocular pressure is normal when the angle is open and pressure is increased only when a major portion of the angle is closed. Adhesions form between the iris and trabecular meshwork and peripheral cornea (peripheral anterior synechiae or goniosynechiae), and aqueous outflow is impaired. Both eyes are involved, although one eye may develop symptoms several years before the fellow eye.

The disease occurs one quarter as frequently as open-angle glaucoma in the United States and Europe. It is more common than open-angle glaucoma among Japanese, Southeast Asians, and Eskimos. In whites it is approximately three times as common among women, but in blacks the sex incidence is equal.

The disease occurs because of an inherited anatomic defect that causes a shallow anterior chamber. The peripheral iris often inserts on the extreme anterior edge of the ciliary body, causing the anterior chamber angle to be shallow and placing the iris close to the trabecular meshwork. The cornea may be small in diameter, and the eye is hyperopic. The lens is closer to the cornea than usual, and with the normal increase in size of the lens with aging, it becomes even closer. The iris appears to bow forward so that it seems to parallel closely the posterior convexity of the cornea (Fig. 20-7). This may be observed by shining a penlight into the anterior chamber from the temporal side of the eye. A shadow, which is not present in the normal eye, is cast by the nasal portion of the relatively convex iris.

Increased intraocular pressure occurs when there is anterior displacement of the peripheral iris. This anterior displacement causes it to isolate the trabecular meshwork from the anterior chamber, preventing the exit of aqueous humor. Two conditions operating singly or together may cause this displacement: (1) impairment of aqueous humor through the pupil causes a pupillary block with accumulation of aqueous humor in the posterior chamber; causing the peripheral iris to balloon forward and crowd into the anterior chamber angle; (2) an-

terior insertion of the iris to the ciliary body (plateau iris) results in so little space between the trabecular meshwork and iris that pupillary dilation squeezes the iris against the trabecular meshwork. The central anterior chamber may be deep, although the periphery is shallow.

Patients who have an anterior chamber with a depth of 2.5 mm or less are likely candidates for the development of pupillary block glaucoma. The shallow anterior chamber may be recognized by the decreased distance between the posterior surface of the cornea and the anterior surface of the iris. Patients with such predisposition may go for many years without symptoms, and it may be impossible to provoke an increase in intraocular pressure. With aging and gradual increase in the size of the lens, the margin of safety decreases, and such patients may have attacks of increased intraocular pressure. Many patients with a shallow anterior chamber never develop symptoms of an acute increase in intraocular pressure. Such eyes, however, must be observed carefully to avoid an acute angle-closure episode. Patients should be warned, particularly concerning symptoms of blurred and hazy vision that may be combined with iridescent vision and pain. Some patients without symptoms have inter-

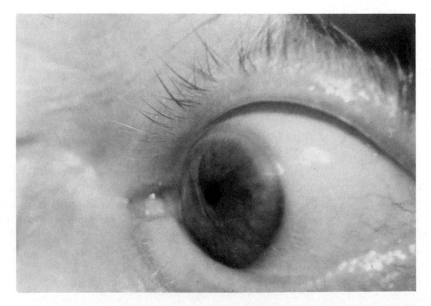

Fig. 20-7. Shallow anterior chamber angle observed from the temporal side. The diagnosis of angle-closure glaucoma requires observation of a closed-angle when the tension is increased.

mittent angle closure that causes progressive peripheral anterior synechiae, which causes a chronic closed-angle glaucoma.

Provocative testing. Provacative testing is carried out to learn under controlled conditions if an abnormal increase in ocular tension occurs combined with closure of the anterior chamber angle. The tests are often negative, even in eyes that have had pressure attacks of closed-angle glaucoma or eyes destined to have attacks. Occasionally, eyes with open-angle glaucoma respond with increased pressure to provocative tests for closed-angle glaucoma.

In the dark-room-prone test the patient is placed face down (lying with face down or sitting with head forward resting on arms or hands) in a dark room. The patient must not sleep. A positive test is an increase of pressure of 10 mm Hg or more combined with gonioscopic observation of a closed chamber angle. The headdown posture encourages an anterior shift of the iris-lens diaphragm as a result of gravity.

Topical instillation of 0.5% tropicamide produces moderate pupillary dilation. An increase of 8 mm Hg in pressure combined with a closed angle after 60 minutes is considered positive.

Acute closed-angle glaucoma. This glaucoma is often preceded by intermittent episodes of a blocked anterior chamber angle. Initially there is blurred, iridescent vision; spontaneous relief does not occur, the intraocular pressure continues to increase, and the symptoms become more severe. A ciliary type of injection (Table 20-4) is present, and there may be profuse lacrimation. Epithelial corneal edema is marked, and epithelial bullae form, giving the cornea a steamy appearance. The blood-aqueous barrier breaks down, and there is increased protein in the aqeous humor. The blood vessels of the iris stroma are dilated, and the pupil is in middilation and does not react to light. Severe systemic symptoms include nausea, vomiting, malaise, and signs suggestive of an acute abdomen. The symptoms may be aggravated by systemic absorption of drugs used in the treatment of the acute angle-closure attack.

If the attack persists, peripheral anterior synechiae form between the root of the iris and the cornea (Fig. 20-8). After several days, these synechiae almost entirely destroy the drainage meshwork. Adhesions (posterior synechiae) form between the iris and the lens, and if the attack is not relieved, necrosis of the sphincter pupillae muscle results in a permanently semidilated pupil. Fluid vesicles form in the anterior subcapsular region of the lens and may persist as white flecks (glaucoma flecks). If the condition is untreated, vision progressively de-

Table 20-4. Differential diagnosis of closed-angle glaucoma

	Angle-closure glaucoma	Acute iritis	Acute conjunctivitis
Pain	Severe, prostrating	Moderate to severe	Burning, itching
Injection	Ciliary type that is more intense near the corneoscleral limbus and fades toward fornices; not constricted with 1:1,000 epinephrine; vessels do not move with conjunctiva, are violet in color; individual vessels not distinguishable		Conjunctival type that is most intense in fornices and fades toward corneoscleral limbus; eye whitened with 1:1,000 epinephrine; vessels superficial, move with conjunctiva, are bright red; individual vessels evident
Pupil	Semidilated, does not react to light	Miotic, reaction delayed or absent	Normal
Cornea	Steamy, iris details not visible	Usually clear with deposits on posterior surface sometimes visible	Clear and normal
Secretion	Watery	Watery	Stringy pus
Onset	Sudden	Gradual	Gradual
Vision	Markedly reduced	Slightly reduced	Normal
Intraocular pressure	Increased	Normal or soft unless 2° glaucoma	Normal

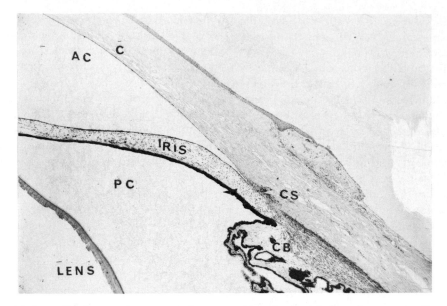

Fig. 20-8. Angle-closure glaucoma with anterior synechiae excluding the anterior chamber angle, *AC*, from the trabecular area and the canal of Schlemm, *CS*. The posterior chamber, *PC*, is larger than normal. *C*, Cornea. *CB*, Ciliary body. (Hematoxylin and eosin stain; × 38)

teriorates and a blind, painful eye develops. Optic atrophy with pallor of the nerve occurs relatively early, but excavation occurs late in the glaucoma.

Chronic primary closed-angle glaucoma. This is a type of glaucoma in which the patient never has a severe acute congestive attack but has intermittent periods of increased pressure. Symptoms may be absent, or there may be periodic subacute episodes of mild congestion and iridescent vision. Beginning superiorly, the iris gradually occludes the trabecular meshwork. Eventually the pressure is at a level of 40 mm Hg or more. The presence of peripheral anterior synechiae distinguishes the condition from open-angle glaucoma. A peripheral iridotomy may cure the condition if more than one quadrant of the angle is free of anterior peripheral synechiae. If the angle remains occluded, a filtering operation is indicated.

Diagnosis. Closed-angle glaucoma is characterized by abnormally increased intraocular pressure and a closed angle demonstrated by gonioscopy. Acute iritis and acute conjunctivitis are disorders to be distinguished (see Table 20-2).

Treatment. The patient should remain in a brightly illuminated room, and the supine (face up) position is preferable. Oral glycerine is used as a hyperosmotic agent. Intravenous acetazolamide is administered. A goniolens or cotton-tipped applicator is used to apply pressure for 30 seconds to the anesthetized cornea. This forces anterior aqueous humor toward the peripheral anterior chamber, which forces posterior aqueous humor through the pupil. Ocular tension is measured after 30 minutes, and if it is still increased, intravenous mannitol is begun. Intravenous mannitol always reduces intraocular pressure. At the conclusion of the infusion, gonioscopy is done to learn if the angle is open. Pilocarpine may then be used to constrict the pupil.

The angle-closure mechanism may be eliminated by a peripheral iridotomy in which the accumulation of aqueous humor in the posterior chamber is prevented. The laser is customarily used for this. The opening in the iris prevents the pressure in the posterior chamber from exceeding that of the anterior chamber and prevents pupillary block. Iridotomy is performed after control of the acute attack when signs of ocular congestion have disappeared.

In patients with shallow angles who have never had an attack of closed-angle glaucoma, an iridotomy probably ensures freedom from attack. Usually a laser iridotomy is done on both eyes, even if the fellow eye has never developed an acute attack.

In a patient who is having intermittent symptoms with spontaneous relief, a laser iridotomy is the operation of choice.

A laser iridotomy may be performed with one of several different types of laser. Topical anesthesia is used. A contact lens with a small condensing lens to focus the beam on the iris is used. The iridotomy is made in the mid iris on the nasal or temporal superior side. Techniques differ, depending on the type and energy of the laser.

Secondary closed-angle glaucoma

Secondary closed-angle glaucomas are those in which the iris in contact with the trabecular meshwork or peripheral cornea prevents aqueous humor from access to the trabecular meshwork (Table 20-5). It occurs in an anterior form with contraction of membranes in neovascular glaucoma, trauma, aniridia, and endothelial syndromes. Posterior forms occur with pupillary block secondary to lens abnormalities such as intumescence, subluxation, after cataract extraction because of iris-vitreous block, or a block caused by an intraocular lens. It occurs without pupillary block in ciliary block (malignant glaucoma), with cysts of the ciliary body, in contracture of tissue in retrolental fibroplasia, and persistent hyperplastic primary vitreous.

Malignant glaucoma (ciliary block glaucoma) may occur after surgery for closed-angle glaucoma or after a filtering procedure for open-angle glaucoma or cataract extraction in an individual with a shallow anterior chamber. The anterior chamber becomes shallow or obliterated, and the intraocular pressure is increased. This may occur immediately after the operative procedure or as much as 1 year later. Miotics aggravate the condition. Initial treatment consists of pupillary dilation with phenylephrine and atropine combined with acetazolamide and intravenous mannitol infusion. Medical therapy failure requires aspiration of the vitreous from the anterior chamber and its replacement with air. If the anterior chamber remains flat after surgery, a partial anterior vitrectomy with an infusion-aspiration cutter may be curative. Fluid vitreous may be aspirated from the cen-

Table 20-5. Secondary closed-angle glaucoma

Contracture of membranes in angle
  Rubeosis iridis
  Iridocorneal syndrome
  Posterior polymorphous corneal dystrophy
  Ocular contusions
Inflammatory membranes in angle
Aniridia
Pupillary block
  Lens
    Swollen (intumescent)
    Subluxated
  Iris-vitreous block (after cataract extraction)
  Complete posterior synechiae
Closure peripheral angle
  Ciliary block
  Scleral buckling
  Pan-retinal photocoagulation
  Intraocular tumors
Congenital
  Rieger syndrome
  Axenfeld anomaly
  Persistent hyperplastic primary vitreous

ter of the eye through an 18-gauge needle.

Failure of the anterior chamber to reform after cataract or glaucoma procedures and other anterior segment surgery or after a penetrating injury of the eye is a serious complication because the root of the iris comes into contact with trabecular meshwork. If the condition persists, peripheral anterior synechiae form and a secondary glaucoma occurs that is particularly recalcitrant to treatment. The condition is far easier to prevent by careful closure of ocular wounds than it is to treat once it is established.

After injury or anterior segment surgery, particularly lens extraction complicated by faulty wound healing, there may be downgrowth of conjunctival or corneal epithelium to cover the trabecular meshwork, iris, and ciliary processes and cause a severe glaucoma, often intractable to treatment.

Secondary closed-angle glaucoma caused by pupillary block occurs because of vitreous or an intraocular lens blocking the pupillary aperture after lens extraction in which the peripheral iridectomy is nonfunctional. Inflammatory adhesions of the iris to the lens or to the vitreous face in aphakia may also cause a pupillary block. Dislocation of the lens into the anterior chamber blocks the pupil and causes a similar secondary glaucoma.

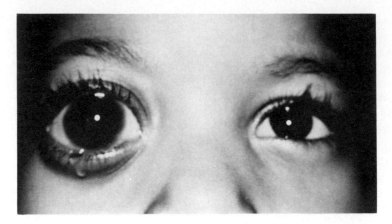

Fig. 20-9. Marked enlargement of the right eye of a 3-year-old girl with infantile glaucoma.

Table 20-6. Clinical classification of congenital glaucoma

Primary
    Developmental abnormality of aqueous outflow system.
Secondary
    Damage to aqueous outflow from maldevelopment of some other part of the eye
Primary congenital glaucoma
    Usually an isolated autosomal recessive trabecular meshwork abnormality with absence of iris recess with iris insertion
        into trabecular surface.

Table 20-7. Anatomic classification of congenital glaucoma

Trabecular meshwork abnormalities (trabeculodysgenesis)
  Flat iris insertion (most primary congenital glaucomas)
    Anterior insertion
    Posterior insertion
    Mixed insertion
  Concave iris insertion
Iris abnormalities
  Anterior stroma
    Hypoplasia (primary congenital glaucoma, Axenfeld and Rieger anomalies)
    Hyperplasia (Sturge-Weber syndrome)
  Anomalous iris blood vessels
    Superficial (usually with iris hypoplasia)
    Persistent tunica vasculosa lentis
  Full iris
    Holes, coloboma, aniridia
Corneal abnormalities
  Peripheral (mainly Axenfeld syndrome)
  Midperipheral (usually Rieger syndrome)
  Central (Peter syndrome, anterior staphyloma, anterior chamber cleavage syndrome)
  Dimensions (microcornea, macrocornea)

Modified from Hoskins, H.D., Jr., Shaffer, R.N., and Hetherington, J.: Arch. Ophthalmol. **102:**1331, 1984.

Table 20-8. Glaucoma associated with congenital anomalies

  Aniridia
  Broad-thumb syndrome
  Chromosomal abnormalities
  Homocystinuria
  Lowe syndrome
  Marfan syndrome
  Maternal rubella
  Microcornea
  Neurofibromatosis
  Pierre Robin syndrome
  Persistent hyperplastic primary vitreous
  Spherophakia
  Sturge-Weber syndrome
  Secondary glaucoma in infants
    Retrolental fibroplasia
    Tumors
      Retinoblastoma
      Juvenile xanthogranuloma
    Inflammation
    Trauma

Modified from Hoskins, H.D., Jr., Shaffer, R.N., and Hetherington, J.: Arch. Ophthalmol. **102:**1331, 1984.

Developmental glaucoma

The glaucomas present at birth or as the result of abnormal ocular development may be divided into primary and secondary types (Table 20-6). Primary developmental glaucoma results from maldevelopment of some portion of the aqueous outflow system. Secondary developmental glaucoma results from damage to the aqueous outflow system caused by maldevelopment of some other portion of the eye. Primary congenital glaucoma, the most common hereditary glaucoma of childhood, is an autosomal recessive disorder, in which the recess of the angle of the anterior chamber is abnormal and the iris inserts directly into the surface of the trabecular meshwork.

The defects interfere with drainage of the aqueous humor, causing an increase in intraocular pressure, which in turn causes stretching of the elastic coats of the eye with marked enlargement of the globe (total staphyloma [Fig. 20-9, buphthalmos]) and optic atrophy with excavation. The human globe is subject to this stretching only until about 3 years of age. Glaucoma occurring after this age does not cause enlargement of the globe and follows a course similar to adult glaucoma. Congenital glaucoma exists at and usually before birth; infantile glaucoma occurs from birth until 2 years of age; juvenile glaucoma occurs from 2 to 16 years of age. Some authors use the term *juvenile glaucoma* for the open-angle glaucoma occurring between 3 and 20 years of age.

Primary hereditary congenital glaucoma affects boys (65%) more often than girls, and the disorder is bilateral in 75% of the cases. Cardiac, auditory, and cerebral defects may also be present. Signs of infantile glaucoma may be present and even far advanced at birth or become apparent before the child has reached 3 months of age. The earliest symptoms are lacrimation, blepharospasm, and photophobia. Examination indicates a corneal edema with a ground-glass appearance that obscures the pattern of the iris. The corneal diameter increases from 10.5 to 12 mm or more, and breaks in the Descemet membrane appear as glassy lines on the back surface of the cornea. The anterior chamber is deeper than normal. Tension may be measured using topical anesthesia and the pneumotonometer. Examination under anesthesia requires agents other than ketamine, succinylcholine, or halothane. The intraocular pressure should be measured as soon as the child sleeps.

Developmental glaucoma is caused by one of three major developmental anomalies that involve (1) the trabecular meshwork, (2) the iris, (3) the cornea, or (4) a combination (Table 20-7). Anomalies of the trabecular meshwork are associated with hereditary congenital glaucoma. Hypoplasia of the iris is common in hereditary congenital glaucoma as well as Axenfeld and Rieger anomalies, while hyperplasia of the iris is seen rarely in Sturge-Weber syndrome. Corneal abnormalities are seen in Axenfeld, Rieger, and Peter anomalies, anterior staphyloma, and in anterior segment mesenchymal dysgenesis.

Glaucoma may be associated with a number of congenital abnormalities (Table 20-8). Essentially, the increased intraocular pressure involves one of the mechanisms listed above.

The preferred surgical treatment of congenital glaucoma is the goniotomy procedure, in which an incision is made into the region of the trabecular meshwork under direct visual control by using a goniolens. Trabeculotomy may be effective if goniotomies fail or cannot be performed because of a hazy cornea.

Patients must be carefully observed postoperatively to be certain the glaucoma is controlled. Intraocular pressure must be measured and the corneal diameters carefully measured with attention directed to breaks in the Descemet membrane. Successful treatment may reverse optic disk cupping. Repeated examinations are required to monitor the ocular tensions, vision, and refractive error.

BIBLIOGRAPHY
General

Belcher, C.D., Thomas, J.V., and Simmons, R.J.: Photocoagulation in glaucoma and anterior segment disease, Baltimore, 1984, The Williams & Wilkins Co.

Epstein, D.L., ed.: Chandler and Grant's Glaucoma, ed. 3, Philadelphia, 1986, Lea & Febiger.

Kolker, A.E., and Hetherington, J., Jr.: Becker-Shaffer's diagnosis and therapy of the glaucomas, ed. 5, St. Louis, 1983, The C.V. Mosby Co.

Luntz, M., Harrison, R., and Schenker, H.: Atlas of glaucoma surgery, Baltimore, 1984, The Williams & Wilkins Co.

Ritch, R.: The secondary glaucomas, St. Louis, 1982, The C.V. Mosby Co.

Shields, M.B.: A study guide for glaucoma, Baltimore, 1982, The Williams & Wilkins Co.

Open-angle glaucoma

Martin, M.J., Sommer, A., Gold, E.B., and Diamond, E.L.: Race and primary open-angle glaucoma, Am. J. Ophthalmol. **99**:383, 1985.

Secondary glaucoma

Ehrenberg, M., McCuen, B.W. II, Schindler, R.H., and Machemer, R.: Rubeosis iridis: preoperative iris fluorescein angiography and periocular steroids, Ophthalmology **91**:321, 1984.

Garner, A., and Alexander, R.A.: Pseudoexfoliative disease: histochemical evidence of an affinity with zonular fibres, Br. J. Ophthalmol. **68**:574, 1984.

Poliner, L.S., Christianson, D.J., Escoffery, R.F., Kolker, A.E., and Gordon, M.E.: Neovascular glaucoma after intracapsular and extracapsular cataract extraction in diabetic paitents, Am. J. Ophthalmol. **100**:637, 1985.

Sugar, S.: Pigmentary glaucoma and the glaucoma associated with the exfoliation-pseudoexfoliation syndrome: update, Ophthalmology **91**:307, 1984.

Methods of examination

Airaksinen, P.J., and Drance, S.M.: Neuroretinal rim area and retinal nerve fiber layer in glaucoma, Arch. Ophthalmol. **103**:203, 1985.

Balazsi, A.G., Drance, S.M., Schulzer, M., and Douglas, G.R.: Neuroretinal rim area in suspected glaucoma and early chronic open-angle glaucoma, Arch. Ophthalmol. **102**:1011, 1984.

Keltner, J.L., and Johnson, C.A.: Effectiveness of automated perimetry in following glaucomatous visual field progression, Ophthalmology **89**:247, 1982.

Lewis, R.A., Hayreh, S.S., and Phelps, C.D.: Optic disk and visual field correlations in primary open-angle and low-tension glaucoma, Am. J. Ophthalmol. **96**:148, 1983.

Wirtschafter, J.D., Becker, W.L., Howe, J.B., and Younge, B.R.: Glaucoma visual field analysis by computed profile of nerve fiber function in optic disc sectors, Ophthalmology **89**:255, 1982.

Congenital glaucoma

Hoskins, H.D., Jr., Shaffer, R.N., and Hetherington, J.: Anatomical classification of the developmental glaucomas, Arch. Ophthalmol. **102**:1331, 1984.

Photocoagulation

Belcher, C.D. III, Thomas, J.V., and Simmons, R.J.: Photocoagulation in glaucoma and anterior segment disease, Baltimore, 1984, The Williams & Wilkins Co.

Brubaker, R.F., and Liesegang, T.J.: Effect of trabecular photocoagulation on the aqueous humor dynamics of the human eye, Am. J. Ophthalmol. **96**:139, 1983.

Krupin, T., Kolker, A.E., Kass, M.A., and Becker, B.: Intraocular pressure the day of argon laser trabeculoplasty in primary open-angle glaucoma, Ophthalmology **91**:361, 1984.

Lustgarten, J., Podos, S.M., Ritch, R., Fischer, R., Stetz, D., Zborowski, L., and Boas, R.: Laser trabeculoplasty, Arch. Ophthalmol. **102**:517, 1984.

Thomas, J.V., El-Mofty, A., Hamdy, E.E., and Simmons, R.J.: Argon laser trabeculoplasty as initial therapy for glaucoma, Arch. Ophthalmol. **102**:702, 1984.

Treatment

Leier, C.V., Baker, N.D., and Weber, P.A.: Cardiovascular effects of ophthalmic timolol, Ann. Int. Med. **104**:197, 1986.

Stewart, R.H., Kimbrough, R.L., and Ward, R.L.: Betaxolol vs. timolol, Arch. Ophthalmol. **104**:46, 1986.

Wandel, T., Charap, A.D., Lewis, R.A., Partamian, L., Cobb, S., Lue, J.C., Novack, G.D., Gaster, R., Smith, J., and Duzman, E.: Glaucoma treatment with once-daily levobunolol, Am. J. Ophthalmol. **101**:298, 1986.

Weinreb, R.N., Ritch, R., and Kushner, F.H.: Effect of adding betaxolol to dipivefrin therapy, Am. J. Ophthalmol. **101**:196, 1986.

21

OCULAR MOTILITY

In humans the eyes are spaced 50 mm to 65 mm apart. Because of this horizontal separation, the image of an object is not exactly the same in each eye. The slightly different image originating in each eye is fused in the brain into three dimensions and the object is perceived as having height, width, and depth—a stereoscopic image. To provide this stereopsis the eyes must be horizontally separated, but too little or too much separation makes it impossible to fuse the image that originates from each eye. Each eye must be directed simultaneously to the same object. Each image must have about the same degree of clarity and size. Since the sensory impulse from each decussates at the optic chiasm, each side of the brain must be functional.

To fuse these two slightly different (disparate) images into one requires a sensitive sensory and motor mechanism. The sensory mechanism provides the visual sensation of form, color, and direction of the stimulus. The motor system consists of the intraocular muscles of accommodation, the pupillary response to illumination, and the extraocular muscles that align the foveola of the two eyes on the same object. The sensory and motor systems are an indivisible entity, although clinically they may be considered separately. An abnormality in either mechanism may lead to faulty alignment of the eyes, to a visual abnormality, or to both.

A complicated terminology is used to describe the motor-sensory relationships.

TERMINOLOGY

Visual axis. The visual axis is an imaginary line that connects an object in space with the fovea centralis. In a person with normal ocular, sensory, and motor systems, the visual line of each eye intersects at the object in space and there is binocular fixation. If the visual lines are not directed to the same fixation point, fixation is by one eye only. The line of direction is a line that connects an object in space with the retina. It corresponds to the visual line when it connects an object with the foveola.

Retinal correspondence. Whenever a retinal element is stimulated, the stimulus is perceived as having intensity and direction that localizes the stimulus in space. Retinal elements that project in the same direction are corresponding retinal elements. An object that stimulates corresponding retinal elements is perceived singly. If different corresponding elements of each eye receive the same stimulus, the stimulus is seen as double.

When the corresponding retinal elements are only slightly separated horizontally (disparate) and receive the same stimulus, the stimulus is perceived singly with the sensation of depth (stereopsis). Stereopsis requires the use of both eyes and is restricted to a maximum distance of about 125 to 200 meters. Monocular clues provide additional information concerning depth, including (1) motion parallax (when one looks at a scene with one eye and moves one's head or eye, far objects move more than close objects); (2) linear perspective (parallel lines seem to approach each other in the distance); (3) overlays of contours (interposition of a close object in front of a more distant object); and (4) highlights, shadows, size of close objects, and color of distant objects (bluish haze of distant mountains).

Suppression. Suppression is that condition in which the image originating on the retina of one eye does not enter consciousness. Riflemen, microscopists, and others who use one eye may, without conscious effort, intermittently ignore the image from the nonfixing eye. If the eyes do not fixate simultaneously on the same object, the stimulation of noncorresponding retinal elements causes a retinal rivalry. To avoid double vision (diplopia) there is cortical suppression of the sensory input from the deviating eye. Visual acuity may be good in each eye when used separately, but the image of the eye that is not being used is suppressed.

Amblyopia. Normal development of stereoscopic vision requires binocular, simultaneous use of each foveola during a critical time that occurs early in life. In infants with monocular cataracts this time is before 3 months of age. In the experimental animal, unilateral deprivation of vision for 2 weeks during the first 12 weeks of life causes severe structural changes in the visual system that are particularly evident anatomically in the lateral geniculate body. Visual acuity is reduced in the deprived eye. The cell layers of the lateral geniculate bodies innervated by the deprived eye are up to 30% smaller than those in the adjacent layers from the nondeprived eye. Binocularly driven cells are absent in the visual cortex that derives 90% of its input from the nondeprived eye. The decreased input from the deprived eye is caused by synaptic inhibition in the occipital cortex.

Ambylopia is a condition in which a unilateral or bilateral decrease in form vision (visual acuity) occurs that is not fully attributable to organic ocular abnormalities. It is caused (Table 21-1) by deprivation of form vision, abnormal binocular interaction, or both, during visual immaturity (birth to 6 years of age). It may be reversed in some individuals by therapeutic measures. The decreased visual acuity impairs pursuit (following) movement when the amblyopic eye is used for fixation. The visual acuity of the amblyopic eye is better when test let-

Table 21-1. Causes of amblyopia

Strabismus
  Esotropia
  Exotropia (rare)
  Hypertropia (rare)
Anisometropia
  Hypermetropia
  Myopia
  Astigmatism (rare)
  Aniseikonia (rare)
Visual deprivation
  Unilateral
    Cataract (monocular)
    Blepharoptosis
    Opaque cornea
    Hyphema
    Vitreous cloudy
    Prolonged patching (nonsupervised)
    Prolonged topical atropine
  Bilateral
    Cataract
    Nystagmus

After von Noorden, G. K.: Invest. Ophthalmol. Vis. Sci. 26:1704, 1985.

ters are viewed singly rather than in a series. In decreased illumination the visual acuity of an amblyopic eye is unchanged, whereas an eye with reduced visual acuity caused by an organic disease may show a marked decrease.

The diagnosis of amblyopia in infants and extremely young children is difficult. Measurement of the preference for fixation of the habitually fixating eye as compared with the habitually deviating eye is helpful. The habitually fixating eye is covered and then uncovered. If it immediately resumes fixation, amblyopia is probably present in the fellow eye. If the normally deviating eye maintains fixation through the next blink of the eyelids, amblyopia is unlikely. An infant may also object when the eye with better vision is covered.

The correction of amblyopia depends on the maturity of the visual system at the onset and the duration of the abnormal visual experience. Treatment is by occlusion of the better eye (Fig. 21-1) to force use of the poorer eye. Because of the sensitivity of the visual system in infants to deprivation during the first year of life, patching should follow a pattern of 3 days sound eye and 1 day amblyopic eye. Between 1 and 3 years of age, the sound eye may be patched 4 days and the amblyopic eye 1 day.

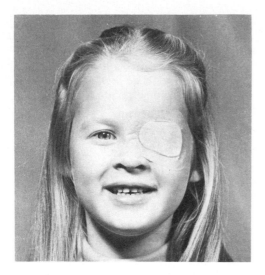

Fig. 21-1. Occlusion of the better eye to force use of the poorer eye in strabismic amblyopia.

Since the previously amblyopic eye may become the better eye and the patching may induce amblyopia in the covered eye, patients must be examined at least once every 2 weeks. After 3 years of age, the patching period may be extended if visual acuity is measured frequently. Patching is carried out until there is no further improvement in visual acuity for 3 months. If visual acuity decreases after patching is terminated, patching should be reinstituted until the visual improvement is sustained. Often this requires intermittent occlusion until the patient is 9 or 10 years of age.

Prolonged atropinization of one eye or patching of one eye for disease or injury should also be avoided in infants and children under 5 years of age. If atropinization is required, the sound eye should also be atropinized so a sensory imbalance is not produced. Occlusion amblyopia is reversible, but if occlusion is prolonged during visual immaturity, a permanent iatrogenic amblyopia may be induced.

Eccentric fixation. This is a monocular condition (usually) in which the foveola is not used for fixation because of amblyopia or an organic disease of the foveola. A special ophthalmoscope (Visuscope), which projects a fixation target on the fundus, may indicate that an area adjacent to the foveola is used for fixation rather than the foveola. The retinal area used

by each patient varies widely. The more distant from the foveola, the poorer the visual acuity. Severe eccentric fixation is evident if an eye remains deviated when the fellow eye is covered. The prognosis for visual improvement is much poorer when amblyopia is associated with eccentric fixation.

Anomalous retinal correspondence. Anomalous retinal correspondence is a binocular condition in which corresponding retinal elements do not project in the same direction. Thus the foveolas of the two eyes have different directional values so that the foveola of one eye corresponds to an extrafoveal region of the fellow eye. Abnormal retinal correspondence involves directional values of the two eyes and is sometimes associated with normal visual acuity in each eye.

When the eyes cross, the angle formed by the intersection of the visual axis of each eye is the angle of strabismus. The objective angle of strabismus is that angle measured by the prism cover test (or a similar test). The subjective angle is that angle in which the patient indicates his perception of the direction of the visual axis of each eye. When the subjective angle and objective angle are the same, normal retinal correspondence is present. If the subjective angle and the objective angle of strabismus are different, anomalous retinal correspondence is present. If the patient perceives the visual axes to be parallel (subjective angle of zero) when the visual axes are not parallel, the anomalous retinal correspondence is harmonious. If the subjective angle is not zero and does not equal the objective angle of strabismus, the anomalous retinal correspondence is nonharmonious or disharmonious.

Motor correspondence. In version movements of the eyes (see Chapter 2) the eyes move simultaneously from eyes front (primary position) to the right, left, up, or down (secondary positions). The nerve impulse for version is always sent simultaneously and equally to the muscles responsible for the movement (Hering's law of equal innervation). Thus, in rotating the eyes to the right, the right lateral rectus muscle and the left medial rectus muscle each receive an equal innervational impulse to contract. Isolated impulses to the muscles of one eye only or to a single ocular muscle do not occur.

In convergence and divergence (vergence movements) the medial recti muscles and the lateral recti muscles receive simultaneous and equal nervous stimuli for contraction and relaxation. The divergence and convergence movements align the eyes in such a way as to maintain binocular fixation and stereopsis.

Fusional vergence. This term is applied to the movements of convergence or divergence that occur when an object is imaged on slightly disparate horizontal parts of the retina.

Fusion-free position. This is the position of an eye when it is covered or when vision is otherwise obscured to eliminate binocular vision.

Duction movements. Duction movments refer to rotation of one eye: adduction (rotation nasally), abduction (rotation toward the temple), sursumduction (elevation), deorsumduction (depression), excycloduction (rotation of upper pole of cornea toward the temple), and incycloduction (rotation of upper pole of cornea nasally). Rotations in an oblique direction, such as up and in or down and out, are combinations of horizontal and vertical rotations. Duction movements are usually observed by covering one eye and directing attention to the uncovered eye.

Orthophoria. Orthophoria is the ideal condition in which the eyes are directed simultaneously to the same point of fixation at either near or far when fusion is suspended.

Heterophoria. Heterophoria is the condition in which the eyes are directed simultaneously to the same point of fixation at either near or far only when fusion is present. When fusion is interrupted, the eyes are not parallel. Exophoria refers to the tendency to medial deviation when fusion is suspended, exophoria to lateral deviation, and hyperphoria to upward deviation (the higher eye is customarily described).

Heterotropia (strabismus, squint, cross-eyes, walleyes). Heterotropia is a condition in which the eyes are not directed to the same point of fixation at either near or far, or both, despite both eyes being open and uncovered so that fusion is possible. Esotropia refers to medial deviation of the nonfixing eye. Exotropia refers to lateral deviation of the nonfixing eye. Hypertropia refers to upward deviation. The higher rather than the lower eye is designated. Cyclotropia refers to torsional deviation in which the upper end of the vetical corneal meridian deviates temporally (excyclotropia) or nasally (incyclotropia).

Esodeviation describes a medial deviation of the eye that may be an esophoria or esotropia. Exodeviation describes exophoria or exotropia.

Heterotropia (strabismus) is termed intermittent or periodic when there are periods when the eyes are parallel. It is termed constant when the eyes are never parallel. Strabismus is monocular when the same eye always deviates and the fellow eye always fixates. It is alternate when either eye deviates while the fellow eye fixates. An accommodative strabismus is one in which the degree of crossing varies with the amount of accommodation. A sensory strabismus is one in which an impairment in image formation causes the deviation.

Concomitance refers to equal deviation in all directions of gaze. A nonconcomitant deviation is one in which the deviation varies in different directions of gaze. Nonparalytic strabismus is initially a concomitant strabismus, but may become nonconcomitant because of secondary contracture, overactions, and inhibitions of muscles. At the time of onset, paralytic strabismus is always nonconcomitant but may eventually become concomitant and make it difficult to determine which muscle is weakened.

Heterotropia may be divided into (1) paralytic (nonconcomitant), in which one or more muscles are weakened so that their normal action is impaired by mechanical or restrictive factors or their nervous connections are impaired, and (2) nonparalytic (concomitant), in which there is no primary muscle impairment. Secondary overaction or underaction of individual muscles in nonparalytic strabismus may simulate a paralytic strabismus.

Diagnostic measures

The different tests to measure visual acuity, ocular movements, binocular function, and possible ocular deviation may be confusing. Worse, they may lead to the erroneous conclusion that diagnosis and management of a heterotropia is so difficult that management should be delayed until a patient is old enough to cooperate with subjective testing, thus allowing poor vision from strabismic ambylopia or other sensory abnormalities to develop. Examination and treatment are indicated in any infant whose eyes are not aligned at all times during waking hours after 6 months of age. Diagnostic measures emphasize two major areas: (1) the ocular deviation and (2) the visual (sensory) status.

Cover-uncover test. The presence or absence of a deviation is determined by the cover-uncover test (Fig. 21-2). First, the examiner observes the patient and estimates which eye is used for fixation. The patient's attention is then directed to a fixation target. In infants this may be a light or moving toy. After the age of 3 or 4 years a small picture or letters should be used to stimulate accommodation and convergence. The test should always be done for both distance and near fixation. The eye that appears to be fixing is covered for a few seconds with the palm of one's hand or some other occluder. As the eye is covered, attention is directed to the uncovered eye (Fig. 21-3). If there is no movement, binocular fixation was present before covering. If the uncovered eye moves to achieve fixation, a manifest deviation was present before covering. Attention is then directed to the covered eye as it is uncovered. If there is a movement to achieve fixation (fusional movement) and no movement of the previously uncovered eye, heterophoria

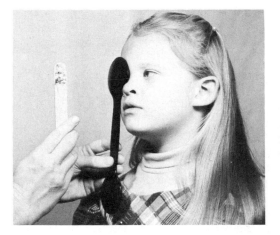

Fig. 21-2. The cover-uncover test with an accommodative target. The individual fixes on details on the target, and the eye is covered for a few seconds and then uncovered. The test should be performed for near and distance fixation and with and without corrective lenses.

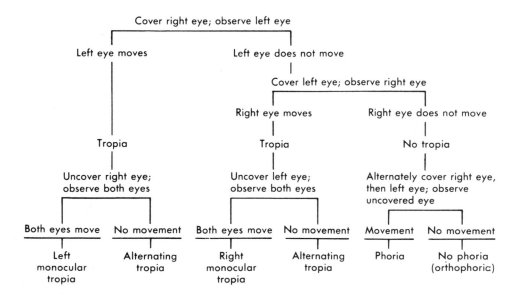

Fig. 21-3. Diagnosis of phorias and tropias by using the cover-uncover test.

is present. If there is no movement of either eye and the eye that was covered is deviated, an alternating heterotropia is present. If the eye that was covered assumes fixation and the fellow eye deviates, a nonalternating monocular heterotropia is present, and the eye that was covered is preferred for fixation.

This test is of more than theoretic importance. If either heterophoria or orthophoria is present, the patient has fusion. If heterotropia is present, the individual either is seeing double or suppressing the image from one eye.

Prism and cover test (alternate cover test). If the cover-uncover test indicates that either a heterophoria or a heterotropia is present, the prism and cover test is used to measure how much deviation is present. While the patient maintains fixation, one eye is covered and then uncovered as the fellow eye is immediately covered. Attention is directed to the movement made by the covered eye as it is uncovered. If the eye has been turned inward while under the cover and moves outward to fix when it is uncovered, either an esophoria or an esotropia is present. If the eye has been turned outward under the cover, it will move inward when the cover is removed and an exophoria or an exotropia is present.

As the eye is uncovered, it moves to place the fixation object on the fovea centralis (movement of redress). The eye moves in the direction opposite the deviation; thus, if the basic deviation is nasal, the movement of redress is toward the temple. Prisms of increasing strength are then placed in front of one eye until the movement of redress is neutralized. The movement is neutralized because the prisms move the image of the fixation object onto the foveola. To ensure maximal accommodation, small pictures or letters are used for near fixation and the 20/30 line is used for distance fixation. The test is carried out with the patient wearing corrective lenses and without correction at near and far. The cover-uncover test must be done first to distinguish between a phoria and a tropia.

Corneal reflection test. The degree of deviation may be estimated by observing the reflection of light from the cornea of the deviating eye. The cornea has a radius of approximately 5.5 mm, and each millimeter of displacement of the reflection is equal to about 7° or 15 prism

diopters of deviation of the visual axes. Thus, if the reflection from the deviating eye is at the corneoscleral limbus, the deviation is about 37.5° (5.5 × 7).

The test is more accurately performed by having the patient fixate on a small light with the examiner observing the deviating eye. Prisms are then placed in front of the fixating eye until the light reflection is centered in the deviated eye (Krimsky test).

PARALYTIC STRABISMUS

Paralytic (nonconcomitant) strabismus is a misalignment of the visual axes that results from paresis (weakness), paralysis, or restriction of one or more extraocular muscles (see Chapter 26). When the eye with normal extraocular muscles fixates, the affected eye is in the position of primary deviation. When the affected eye fixates, the normal eye is in the position of secondary deviation. The secondary deviation (affected eye fixating) is greater than the primary deviation because the affected eye requires an excess innervational impulse to maintain fixation with impaired musculature. This excess impulse is distributed to the normally acting muscles of the fellow eye (Hering's law of equal innervation) and causes an overaction.

In general, paralytic strabismus in an adult with previously single binocular vision causes double vision (diplopia), which is most marked when the eyes are rotated into the field of action of the affected muscle. Diplopia does not occur in individuals who have never developed binocular vision.

To neutralize diplopia the face may be turned, the chin elevated or depressed, and the head tilted to the right or left shoulder (ocular torticollis) (Table 21-2). In paralysis of the medial and lateral recti muscles, the face is turned toward the field of action of the paralyzed muscle, but the head is not tilted. Thus with paralysis of either the right medial rectus or the left lateral rectus muscle, the face will be turned to the left. When the face is turned to the left, the eyes move so that the right medial rectus and the left lateral rectus muscles are not contracting. With the face turned in this direction, diplopia is absent. In paralysis of the superior or inferior recti muscles, the face may be slightly turned toward the side of the paralyzed muscle. In paralysis of the oblique

Table 21-2. Head position with paralysis of an individual extraocular muscle

Muscle	Face turn		Chin		Head tilt	
	Normal side	Side of paralyzed muscle	Up	Down	Normal side	Side of paralyzed muscle
Medial rectus		√				
Lateral rectus		√				
Superior rectus		√	√			√
Inferior rectus		√		√		√
Superior oblique	√			√	√	
Inferior oblique	√		√			√

muscles, the face is turned slightly toward the noninvolved side.

The chin is elevated in paralysis of the elevators of the eye (superior recti and inferior oblique muscles) and depressed in paralysis of the depression of the eye (inferior recti and superior oblique muscles). With paralysis of the superior and inferior recti muscles and inferior oblique muscle, the head is tilted toward the side of the affected muscle. In superior oblique muscle paralysis, the head is tilted toward the normal side. When the head is tilted toward the side of the eye with the paralyzed superior oblique muscle, this eye rotates upward. (The superior oblique muscle and the superior rectus muscle are both intorters of the eye. When the head is tilted toward the normal side, an equal innervational impulse goes to both muscles and the eye turns upward because of the action of the superior rectus muscle.)

Structural anomalies of an ocular muscle, conjunctiva, or Tenon capsule may cause contracture of a muscle or prevent its antagonist from rotating the eye. The signs are those of paralysis of the normal antagonist. Thus, in thyroid myopathy, fibrosis and contracture of muscles that insert on the inferior surface of the eye prevent upward rotation. In blowout fractures of the orbit, the tissues in the inferior portion of the orbit may be trapped in the floor of the orbit and the eye cannot rotate upward. The forced duction test is necessary to diagnose a physical restriction of ocular rotation.

In the forced duction test, the conjunctiva is anesthetized with a topical anesthetic reinforced by 4% cocaine solution on a cotton pledget applied to the conjunctiva near the corneoscleral limbus. This conjunctiva is then grasped with toothless forceps, and the eye is passively rotated to determine its freedom of movement. Children may require general anesthesia.

An abnormally short superior oblique muscle tendon or contracture of the muscle after injury makes the inferior oblique muscle on the same side appear paralyzed because the eye cannot be elevated in adduction. The forced duction test indicates the contracture of the superior oblique muscle.

The retraction syndrome (of Stilling-Türk-Duane) occurs apparently because an innervational disturbance causes the lateral rectus muscle to contract instead of relax when the medial rectus muscle contracts. Electrical activity in the lateral rectus muscle may be decreased or absent in abduction. In the most common type, there is limited or absent abduction, restriction of adduction, retraction of the globe, and narrowing of the palpebral fissure when adduction is attempted. There may be elevation or depression of the globe in adduction. Women are more commonly affected (60%) than men, the left eye is more commonly affected (73%) than the right eye, and the condition is bilateral in 18% of the patients. Other ocular abnormalities include cataract, iris and pupil anomalies, peristent hyaloid artery, amblyopia, and choroidal colobomas. Labyrinthine deafness, facial defects, cleft palate, and malformations of the external ear, hands, and feet occur.

The diagnosis of the specific muscle involvement in a paralytic strabismus may be difficult. The history may indicate the cause to be injury, inflammation, tumor, aneurysm, or thyroid oculopathy. The onset of multiple sclerosis may be associated with muscle palsy. Myasthenia gravis may be limited to ocular muscles.

NONPARALYTIC (CONCOMITANT) STRABISMUS

In nonparalytic strabismus there is no extraocular muscle weakness; therefore the angle of deviation is the same in all fields of gaze. With continued deviation, however, secondary abnormalities may develop with overaction or underaction of muscles in some fields of gaze. Moreover, there may be an A or V deviation in which the angle of deviation is different in upward and downard gaze. Esotropia and exotropia are the major types of concomitant strabismus.

Concomitant esotropia

In esotropia the nonfixing eye deviates inward. It may be divided into nonaccommodative and accommodative types. Additionally, there may be combinations of these types.

Nonaccommodative esotropia. Nonaccommodative esotropia (Fig. 21-4) may be divided into those types with no abnormality of image formation and those types in which there is an abnormality in image formation (sensory interference) in one or both eyes (Table 21-3). Most patients have no obvious abnormality of ocular image formation or perception, and an anatomic factor cannot be demonstrated. The deviation appears shortly after birth. There is often a familial history of strabismus. The deviation is often more than 50 diopters and is

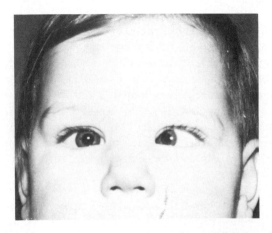

Fig. 21-4. Esotropia with the right eye fixing and the left eye deviating.

the same for both near and distance (basic esotropia). There may be a short period in which there is alternate fixation, but the deviation tends to become monocular. The angle of deviation tends to remain relatively constant and is not modified by corrective lenses or by anticholinesterase agents. Amblyopia and abnormal retinal correspondence commonly develop. The children rarely develop stereopsis or fusion even after early surgery to align the visual axes.

Often there is cross-fixation, with the infant using the left eye to look to the right and the right eye to look to the left. This fixation pattern encourages equal use of the eyes and discourages the development of amblyopia and

Table 21-3. Nonaccommodative esotropia

I. No sensory abnormality
  A. Onset at birth or shortly thereafter
  B. Familial
  C. No variation with accommodation
  D. Abnormal sensory mechanisms common
    1. Strabismic amblyopia
    2. Abnormal retinal correspondence
    3. Defective binocular vision
  E. Ocular deviation
    1. Nearly equal for near and far
    2. No effect using convex lenses
  F. Treatment
    1. Exclude neurologic and ocular disease
    2. Prevent abnormal sensory mechanism
      a. Mainly patching of eye with better vision
      b. Pleoptics (rare in United States)
    3. Surgery to correct deviation
II. Sensory interference
  A. Onset after disease or injury
  B. Possibly hereditary eye disease impairing vision
  C. No variation with accommodation
  D. Defective vision in one or both eyes
    1. Marked anisometropia
    2. Corneal opacity
    3. Monocular cataract
    4. Retinal disease
    5. Optic nerve or tract disease
  E. Ocular deviation
    1. Equal for near and far
    2. Monocular fixation using eye with better vision
    3. May develop exotropia
  F. Treatment
    1. Lenses if anisometropic (contact lenses, if necessary, as required in monocular aphakia); cataract extraction in first 24 hours of life followed by immediate contact lens wear
    2. Cosmetic surgery to straighten eyes
    3. Correction of condition causing defective vision, if possible

abnormal retinal correspondence. Cross-fixation may lead to the erroneous belief that a bilateral lateral rectus muscle palsy is present, since the child cross-fixates rather than abducts the eyes in lateral gaze. With one eye covered to prevent cross-fixation, ocular movements are full.

Some patients with congenital nystagmus and esotropia may neutralize nystagmus and improve vision by rotating the eyes to the right or left. The patient may rotate the fixing eye in a maximally adducted position to see better (nystagmus compensation or blockage syndrome). This type of esotropia usually has its onset in early infancy and is preceded by nystamus. There may be pseudoparalysis of the lateral recti muscles, and as the fixing eye moves from adduction to abduction, there is a nystagmus. Usually both eyes are adducted.

In the treatment of nonaccommodative esotropia, it is important (1) to evaluate the neurologic status of the child to exclude cerebral palsy, and (2) to exclude opacities of the cornea, lens, and vitreous, unequal refractive errors, and retinal and choroidal disease. Treatment must be started by 6 months of age. Spontaneous improvement does not occur. In cases in which amblyopia has developed, the abnormality is treated by occlusion of the habitually fixing eye to force use of the nonfixing eye. This is essential to develop central vision in each eye. Patching converts monocular strabismus to an alternating type. This conversion, a sign of visual improvement, may upset parents who believe that the crossing involved only one eye. Surgery is recommended during the first year of life to maximize fusion; although stereopsis is seldom attained, the peripheral fusion attained is often adequate to provide straight eyes for life.

Sensory interference. Children born with an abnormality that interferes with clear ocular images often develop esotropia. A severe monocular deviation is present for both near and far vision, and the child uses the better eye. It is important to diagnose the cause of the sensory disturbance and recognize individuals in whom amblyopia treatment would not be effective. A life-endangering retinoblastoma may cause sensory interference and amblyopia.

When retinal disease is present, cosmetic alignment of the eyes is the only treatment of value. This may be delayed until just before the child enters school because there is no possibility of providing binocular vision. Since there is no fusion, the eyes tend to deviate outward in later life and surgery of esotropia to make the eyes parallel in childhood may accelerate the development of exotropia (consecutive exotropia).

Accommodative-convergence/ accommodation ratio

When fixing distance objects, the visual axes are parallel and accommodation is required only to compensate for hyperopia that may be present. Fixation on an object closer than 20 feet requires convergence of the visual axes (lines) and accommodation. The amount of accommodative convergence divided by the amount of accommodation indicates the responsiveness of an individual's convergence to a particular amount of accommodation.

Accommodative convergence is measured in prism diopters. It is found by multiplying the interpupillary distance in centimeters by the distance of the object of attention expressed in prism diopters (Fig. 21-5) (the prism diopter is the reciprocal of the distance expressed in meters: ½ meter is 2 diopters; ⅓ meter is 3 diopters). Thus, if an individual without an error of refraction has an interpupillary distance of 5.5 cm and the object of attention is ⅓ meter (3 diopters) distant, he will exert 16.5 (5.5 × 3) diopters of accommodative convergence. The accommodative convergence to accommodation ratio (AC/A) is 16.5 ÷ 3 prism diopters of accommodation or 5.5. An AC/A ratio equal to the pupillary distance in centimeters is the ideal. Most individuals have a lower value but are able to maintain binocular vision by means of fusional convergence.

The AC/A ratio may be measured by the heterophoria or gradient lens method. Heterophoric testing requires measurement of the interpupillary distance. The deviation is measured for far and near while the patient has full correction of any refractive error. The following equation is then used:

$$\frac{AC}{A} = \text{Interpupillary distance (in cm)} +$$

$$\frac{\text{Deviation for near} - \text{Deviation for far}}{\text{Accommodation at near}}$$

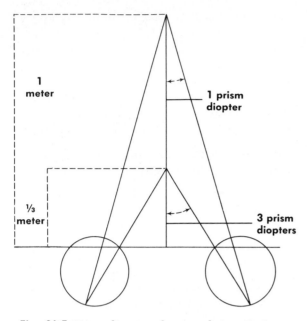

Fig. 21-5. Prism diopters of accomodation. At 1 meter the eyes must accommodate 1 prism diopter. If the eyes are 5.2 cm apart, they must exert 5.2 prism diopters of accommodative convergence.

Table 21-4. Accommodative esotropia

I. Onset after 1 year (average 2½ years)
II. Familial
III. Sensory mechanisms often normal
IV. Ocular deviation
    A. Greater for near than far
    B. Originally intermittent but tends to become constant
V. Refractive type
    A. Normal accommodative-convergence/accommodation ratio (AC/A)
    B. Decreased by convex lenses that decrease accommodation
    C. Treatment: decrease stimulus to accommodation
        1. Full hyperopic correction
        2. Biofocal lenses
        3. Miotics
        4. Orthoptic training
VI. Nonrefractive type
    A. High accommodative-convergence/accommodation ratio (AC/A)
    B. Deviation same for near and far
    C. Not decreased by convex lenses
    D. Treatment
        1. Surgery to provide alignment
VII. Combined accommodative and nonaccommodative esotropia
    A. Onset after neglected accommodative esotropia
    B. Familial
    C. Abnormal accommodative mechanisms
    D. Abnormal sensory mechanisms common
    E. Ocular deviation
        1. Monocular fixation
        2. Tends to increase initially; extropia common in adulthood
    F. Treatment
        1. Correction of accommodative component
        2. Surgery for nonaccommodative deviation

Inward deviations are positive numbers, and outward deviations are negative numbers. Thus, if the interpupillary distance is 5 cm and the deviation for near is 10 prism diopters of esotropia and for far 4 prism diopters of esotropia, the equation would read:

$$\frac{AC}{A} = 5.0 + \frac{10 - 4}{3} = 7.0$$

Alternatively, a gradient method may be used in which the amount of deviation for near is measured first with full correction and then with a concave lens over the correction. The deviation is measured by using a series of convex and concave spherical lenses, the results are plotted on a graph, and the slope of the best fitting lines is the AC/A ratio. The following formula may be used:

$$\frac{AC}{A} = \frac{\text{Deviation with concave lens} - \text{Deviation without concave lens}}{\text{Power concave lens}}$$

The AC/A ratio is not affected by eye muscle surgery or orthoptic treatment of the patient. Cycloplegics increase the ratio by impairing accommodation. Miotics lower the ratio by decreasing the need for accommodation. Bifocals decrease the need for accommodation when viewing near objects, and thus excess accommodative convergence does not occur. Spectacle-corrected refractive errors change the patient's near point of accommodation and thus affect the AC/A ratio.

Accommodative esotropia. Accommodation is the process by which the eye increases in refractive power. Accommodative esotropia is an excessive inward deviation associated with accommodation. When the individual accommodates to maintain a clear image of an object, the eyes converge excessively, and the result is esotropia.

There are two types of accommodative esotropia: (1) refractive and (2) nonrefractive (Table 21-4). Both types have their onset after 1 year of age, usually between 2 and 3 years of age. The onset is abrupt in a child who previ-

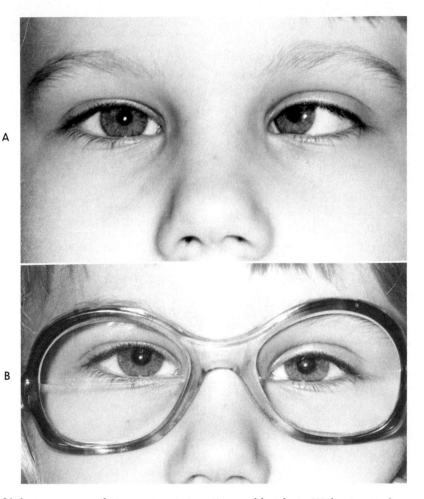

Fig. 21-6. An accommodative esotropia in a 5-year-old girl. **A,** Without optical correction, an esotropia is present. **B,** When hyperopia is corrected, the eyes are parallel.

ously had straight eyes. The deviation is brought about by an attempt to visualize objects clearly, and the amount of crossing varies with activity and fatigue. There is often a family history of ocular deviation. The esotropia is often intermittent initially and then develops into a constant type.

Examination indicates inward deviation of the eye, and this may be demonstrated with the cover-uncover test. A point of light for fixation does not stimulate accommodation adequately to demonstrate an intermittent accommodative deviation, but use of a small picture for fixation that requires accommodation makes the deviation evident. The angle of deviation, however, may be different for near and far fixation and upward or downward gaze (incomcomitance). Early in the development of the deviation there may be double vision, but this double vision usually disappears quickly as the child learns to suppress the image from the deviating eye.

Refractive accommodative esotropia. This is caused by uncorrected hyperopia combined with fusion inadequate to ensure binocular vision. The uncorrected hyperopia requires excessive accommodation to maintain a clear retinal image, which evokes excessive convergence. The inadequate fusion causes the inward deviation to become manifest (esotropia). If the fusion is adequate, the inward deviation remains latent (esophoria).

Treatment consists of full correction of the refractive error often combined with bifocal correction for near (Fig. 21-6). This may be combined with topical instillation of anticholinesterase drugs with each eye. The anticholinesterase drugs decrease the angle of deviation by facilitating ciliary muscle action, thus facilitating accommodation without excessive convergence. Since the drug facilitates accommodation, fewer nerve impulses are required for near vision, and fewer convergency impulses are generated, reducing the amount of accommodative convergence.

Often 0.06% echothióphate (Phospholine Iodide) combined with 2.5% phenylephrine is used. Phenylephrine (an adrenergic agonist) prevents the development of cysts on the pupilary border of the iris that may become so large as to interfere with vision. Echotiophate binds pseudocholinesterase and may simulate an acute abdomen in children; there may be prolonged apnea after administration of succinylcholine as a muscle relaxant in general anesthesia.

Orthoptic training is valuable for teaching the child to maintain parallel fixation without corrective lenses. This is not always an easy task, because a child may suppress the image of the deviating eye.

Nonrefractive accommodative esotropia. This is caused by a faulty synkinesis between accommodation and convergence (accommodative-convergence/accommodation ratio [AC/A]). The effort to accommodate causes an excessive convergence. With the refractive error fully corrected, there remains a marked deviation of the eyes at near.

Miotics do not modify the angle of strabismus. Nonrefractive accommodative esotropia often requires surgery.

Accommodative esotropia may be combined with a nonaccommodative esotropia, in which case surgery must be directed to the nonaccommodative portion of the esotropia.

NONPARALYTIC EXOTROPIA

The nonfixing eye deviates outward in exotropia (exodeviation) (Table 21-5). If the deviation is about the same for far and near, the exotropia is basic. If the deviation is at least 15 prism diopters more for distance than near, the deviation is a divergence excess. If the outer deviation is greater at near than distance, the deviation is a convergence insufficiency. (Deviations greater at distance than near involve divergence; deviations greater at near than distance involve convergence.) The usual type begins as an exophoria, becomes an intermittent exotropia, and sometimes (75%) progresses to a

Table 21-5. Nonparalytic exotropia

I. Exophoria → intermittent exotropia → constant exotropia
   A. Onset at birth to 5 years of age
   B. Familial
   C. No accommodative element
   D. Sensorial mechanisms proportional to binocularity established before constant exotropia (often normal)
   E. Deviation
      1. Greater for far than near
      2. Exophoria and exotropia measurements the same
      3. Aggravated by fatigue
   F. Treatment
      1. Exotropia: surgery
      2. Exophoria: observe for constant exotropia
II. Acquired exotropia
   A. Variable age of onset
   B. Often nonfamilial
   C. Deteriorated esotropia; after surgical correction of esotropia (consecutive exotropia)
   D. Sensory impairment common
   E. Ocular deviation
      1. Equal for near and far
      2. Convergence poor
      3. Often monocular fixation
   F. Treatment: surgery
III. Accommodative (uncorrected myopic exotropia)
   A. Onset after 5 years of age
   B. Familial
   C. Uncorrected myopia minimizes accommodation required for near work
   D. Sensory mechanisms normal
   E. Ocular deviation
      1. Greater for far than near
      2. Initially intermittent but tends to become constant
   F. Treatment: stimulation of accommodation by correcting myopia with lenses

manifest exotropia. Secondary exodeviations occur in the older age group as the result of reduced visual acuity in one eye and follow esotropia either spontaneously or after surgery (consecutive exotropia). Individuals with uncorrected myopia do not accommodate for clear vision at near, and the inadequate impulse to converge may cause an exotropia relieved by correcting the refractive error. In craniosynostosis the deformity of the skull places the eyes far apart, and there is often inadequate convergence that causes an exotropia.

Exophoria → intermittent exotropia → constant exotropia. This is the most common type of exotropia. It begins at birth to 5 years of age, rarely (5%) thereafter. Initially it is a large-an-

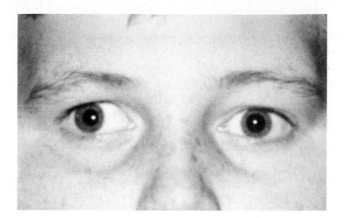

Fig. 21-7. Exotropia that began as a large-angle exophoria, passed through a stage of intermittent exotropia, and then became a constant exotropia, with suppression of the image in the deviating eye.

gle exophoria elicited by the cover-uncover test. The phoria is greater at distance than at near fixation. This period of binocularity is important in allowing normal visual development, and thus amblyopia and abnormal retinal correspondence are not as common in this disorder as in nonaccommodative types of esotropia. With growth of the face, an intermittent exotropia occurs, first at distance and then at near, brought about by fatigue and visual inattention. Suppression with inhibition of fusion leads to a constant exotropia (Fig. 21-7).

When there are long periods (75% of the time) of manifest deviation, treatment is usually surgical. Correction of myopia increases accommodation of near and provides sharp retinal images that encourage fusion. Surgical correction is indicated in infants who develop an early exotropia of more than 20 diopters with little tendency to alignment. In adults with a large-angle exotropia, surgery is indicated as soon as the diagnosis is established.

Acquired exotropia. Acquired exotropia occurs because of defective vision developing in one eye or because of a deteriorated exophoria.

Sensory impairment exotropia. Decreased vision in one eye often leads to exotropia. If the sensory loss occurs in infancy an esotropia occurs, but with passing years the eye diverges. As the eyes pass from esotropia to exotropia, there is a phase in which the visual axes are parallel, which leads to the naive belief that the esotropia has disappeared. The eyes continue to diverge more, finally developing a constant exotropia that may recur after surgery. In an older person an esotropia does not develop. Instead, soon after visual impairment, the eye diverges.

Accommodative exotropia. This is a relatively uncommon disorder that occurs because of uncorrected myopia, which decreases the need for accommodation for near work. The decrease in accommodative effort minimizes normal convergence, so the eyes tend to turn outward. Since most infants are hyperopic at birth, the condition occurs after visual maturity. Sensory anomalies are uncommon. It may occur in myopic adolescents who prefer poor vision to wearing glasses. There may be a family history of myopia. Symptoms are minimal. Examination shows an intermittent outward deviation of the eyes, which becomes constant if the condition is neglected. The wearing of concave lenses to correct the myopia is all that is required. Many individuals prefer contact lenses.

A AND V SYNDROMES

A and V syndromes are ocular deviations in which the degree of esotropia or exotropia is more marked on looking either upward or downward. An A-esotropia is greater looking upward than downward. V-esotropia is greater looking downward than upward. An A-exotropia, is greater looking downward than upward. V-exotropia is greater looking upward than downward.

The cause of the abnormality varies. In V

types of esotropia and exotropia there is often but not always overaction of both inferior oblique muscles (N III). In A types of deviation, there may be overaction of the superior oblique muscles (N IV). In overaction of the oblique muscles the adducting eye deviates upward (inferior oblique muscle) or downward (superior oblique muscle). Visual axes tend to converge in downward gaze so that in V-esotropia there may be overaction of the medial recti muscles. In V-exotropia there may be overaction of the lateral recti muscles.

A or V patterns occur in 50% of patients with esodeviations or exodeviations. The amount of deviation is measured with the prism cover test at 15° up and 25° down gaze. An A-esotropia is present if there are 15 prism diopters more esotropia in looking upward than looking downward. An A-exotropia is present if there are 15 prism diopters less exotropia on looking upward than downward. A V-esotropia is present if there are 10 prism diopters more of esotropia on looking downward than on looking upward. A V-exotropia is present if there are 10 prism diopters less of exotropia in looking downward than on looking upward.

V-esotropia is the most common, followed by A-esotropia, V-exotropia, and A-exotropia. Recession and resection of the horizontal muscles is done to correct the esodeviation or exodeviation. To enhance the effect of these procedures the new insertions of the horizontal muscles are displaced upward or downward. The medial recti muscles are always displaced toward the apex of the A or V, thus upward in A patterns and downward in V patterns. The lateral recti muscles are displaced away from the apex, irrespective of whether a recession or resection is done. Inferior oblique muscle recessions may be done if these muscles are overactive in V pattern anomalies.

PSEUDOSTRABISMUS

Pseudostrabismus is a condition in which the eyes appear crossed to the observer although they are actually aligned. The center of the pupil is usually slightly temporal to the visual axis. When the eye fixates on a penlight beam, the reflection from the cornea usually is on the nasal portion of the pupil and a positive kappa angle (Fig. 21-8, common) is present, which, if

large enough, causes the appearance of an exodeviation or decreases the apparent amount of an esodeviation. If the reflection is temporal, a negative kappa angle (rare) is present that may simulate the appearance of an esodeviation or decrease the apparent amount of an exodeviation.

In pseudoesotropia the appearance is caused by an extra fold of skin at the inner canthus of each eye (epicanthus), by a broad, flat nose, because the eyes are unusually close together, or by an oval palpebral fissure, as in Orientals. Each of these conditions conceals some of the white sclera at the medial side of the eye and simulates the appearance of an inward turned eye. The cover-uncover test, however, indicates that the visual axes are parallel, and the sole treatment is reassurance. As the child's face grows, the appearance disappears. In pseudoexotropia the appearance is caused by retinal abnormalities that displace the fovea centralis. The retinopathy of prematurity is a common cause, although preretinal membranes and other such abnormalities may be at fault.

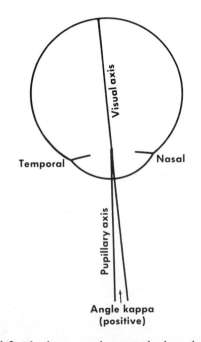

Fig. 21-8. The kappa angle created when the visual line is not in the anatomic center of the pupil. When the visual line is nasal, a positive (common) kappa angle is present. When the visual line is temporal (rare), a negative kappa angle is present.

TREATMENT OF STRABISMUS

The treatment of strabismus is directed toward (1) determining the cause, (2) development of normal visual function, and (3) alignment of the visual axes.

Determining the cause. For the first 6 months after birth, the eyes of all infants deviate at times. Most of the time the eyes are straight and remain so after 6 months of age.

If one eye deviates constantly from alignment during the first several months of life, the fundi must be examined after pupillary dilation (0.5% cyclopentolate, 1% phenylephrine). The examination is more easily done by using an indirect ophthalmoscope. The refractive error can be estimated by moving the condensing light closer and further from the eye. If there is no ocular obstacle to clear vision, such as cataract, hereditary macular degeneration, retinoblastoma, or chorioretinitis, attention is directed to preventing amblyopia (see discussion on amblyopia). If the infant uses either eye (alternates), either there is no primary ocular abnormality or it affects both eyes equally.

A strabismus that develops after the eyes have been parallel suggests either an accommodative strabismus or development of some obstacle to normal vision in the eye. The younger the infant, the more likely there is some obstacle to vision. Ophthalmoscopy and refraction are indicated. By the time an infant is 4 to 6 months old, a meaningful, complete eye examination is possible.

An esotropia that develops at about the age of 3 years is most likely the accommodative type and requires a complete examination. Particular attention must always be directed to exclusion of a paretic muscle caused by intracranial disease. Rarely a paresis of a lateral rectus muscle occurs and then disappears spontaneously. Often correcting lenses are prescribed if an accommodative esotropia cannot be distinguished from a combined accommodative-nonaccommodative type. If eyes have been parallel until the age of 3 years, there is less likelihood of amblyopia and other visual abnormalities.

Orthoptic treatment provides binocular vision through correction of suppression, amblyopia, and anomalous retinal correspondence and enhances the development of fusional amplitudes and stereopsis. Orthoptists partake in the diagnosis and nonsurgical correction of sensory and motor anomalies of the eyes under the direction of a physician. In the United States they are college-trained individuals who have specialized in orthoptics in a medical school eye department and have been certified by the American Orthoptic Council.

Eye exercises to correct an esotropia or exotropia are of no value. When convergence is insufficient, fusion exercises with base out prisms of increasing power will improve the ability to converge and relieve symptoms.

Surgery is indicated to align the visual axes and thus permit the potential for binocular vision, and to improve cosmesis. In general, one weakens overacting muscles and strengthens underacting muscles.

Correction of alignment. When vision is equal in the two eyes, it is desirable to perform symmetric surgery, normally carrying out the same surgical procedure in each eye rather than limiting the surgical correction to one eye. Usually, the better the fusion, the less surgery is required to achieve a cosmetic and functional result.

In esotropia, in which vision is approximately equal in the two eyes and in which retinal correspondence is normal, bilateral recessions of the medial recti muscles are usually preferred. In congenital esotropia with marked deviation, this is usually done at about 6 months of age.

In older patients with concomitant esotropia in which vision in one eye is poor and cannot be improved, the best results are probably achieved by resecting the lateral rectus muscle and recessing the medial rectus muscle in the amblyopic eye. If this is not adequate to align the eyes, a similar procedure may be carried out in the opposite eye.

In alternating exotropia, each lateral rectus muscle is recessed if the divergence is mainly for distance and the eyes are parallel for near, provided vision and fusion are good. If the exotropia is monocular, the deviation is the same for near and far, and fusion is poor, the initial procedure is recession of the lateral rectus muscle and resection of the medial rectus muscle in one eye.

The surgeon's aim is to perform the minimal procedure that will correct the strabismus.

However, some patients require several procedures. This commonly occurs because correction of a horizontal or vertical deviation uncovers anomalies that could not be diagnosed earlier. Usually at least 6 months should elapse between procedures to permit the correction to stablize.

MICROTROPIA (MONOFIXATION SYNDROME)

The term *microtropia* is applied to exceptionally small deviations that cause sensory abnormalities such as amblyopia, abnormal retinal correspondence, suppression of central vision, and defective stereopsis. The cover-uncover test shows no ocular movement of redress and yet, except for the sensory abnormalities, strabismus is not present. When the test is repeated with a 4 diopter prism with base either in or out, there is no recovery movement of either eye. A severe anisometropia may rarely be present, and examination with the Visuscope indicates nonfoveal fixation. In children up to 5 years of age with anisometropia, amblyopia is treated by occluding the fixing eye. Microtropia is present in nearly all nonaccommodative concomitant esotropic patients after corrective surgery and accounts for the absence of central fusion.

BIBLIOGRAPHY

Bartley, G.B., Dyer, J.A., and Illstrup, D.M.: Chracteristics of recession-resection and bimedial recession for childhood esotropia, Arch. Ophthalmol. **103:**190, 1985.

Cogan, D.G.: Neurology of ocular muscles, ed. 2, Springfield, Ill., 1978, Charles C Thomas, Publisher.

Cogan, D.G.: Neurology of the visual system, Springfield, Ill., 1980, Charles C Thomas, Publisher.

Dyer, J.A., and Lee, D.A.: Atlas of extraocular muscle surgery, ed. 2, New York, 1984, Praeger Publishers.

Helveston, E.M.: Atlas of strabismus surgery, ed. 3., St. Louis, 1985, The C.V. Mosby Co.

Helveston, E.M., and Ellis, F.D.: Pedatric ophthalmology practice, ed. 2, St. Louis, 1983, The C.V. Mosby Co.

Helveston, E.M., Ellis, F.D., Schott, J., Mitchelson, M.J., Weber, J.C., Taube, S., and Miller, K.: Surgical treatment of congenital esotropia, Am. J. Ophthalmol. **96:**218, 1983.

Leigh, R.J., and Zee, D.S.: The neurology of eye movements, Philadelphia, 1983, F.A. Davis Co.

von Noorden, G.K.: Amblyopia: a multidisciplinary approach, Invest. Ophthalmol. Vis. Sci. **26:**1704, 1985.

von Noorden, G.K.: Atlas of strabismus, ed. 4, St. Louis, 1983, The C.V. Mosby Co.

von Noorden, G.K.: Binocular vision and ocular motility: theory and management of strabismus, ed. 3, St. Louis, 1985, The C.V. Mosby Co.

22
OPTICAL DEFECTS OF THE EYE

Parallel rays of light that enter the eye are refracted by the anterior and posterior surfaces of the cornea, pass through the anterior chamber, are refracted by the various zones of the lens, and come to a focus. The position of this focus is determined by the combined refractive power of the cornea, the lens, and the surrounding media. The length of the eye determines whether the focus is in front of the retina (myopia), upon the retina (emmetropia), or whether the retina intercepts converging rays before they reach a focus (hyperopia).

The diopter, the unit of measurement of refractive power, is equal to the reciprocal of the focal length of a lens in meters. The cornea has a focal distance of 0.0233 m, and its refractive power is 1/0.0233 or 43 diopters. The refractive power of the lens at rest is about 17 diopters, with extremes of 12 and 22 diopters. Accommodation in young people increases the refractive power of the lens to a maximum of about 33 diopters. The total refractive power of the eye without accommodation is about 60 diopters, with extremes of 53 and 64 diopters. The axial length of the normal globe varies from 22 to 27 mm, with a mean of 24 mm.

Refractive errors occur because the refractive power of the anterior segment is disproportionate to the length of the eye. These two elements are usually correlated so that long eyes have less and short eyes have more refractive power, which minimizes any refractive error (Fig. 22-1). Thus it is an oversimplification to regard the myopic eye as one that is too long or a hyperopic eye as one that is too short. Instead, the refractive power of the anterior segment and the length of the globe are not correlated. Refractive errors of less than 5 diopters are generally considered to be biologic variations, and the various components of the refractive system of the anterior segment and the length of the globe follow a binomial distribution. Refractive errors of more than 5 diopters are generally considered to be pathologic and to result from developmental abnormalities of unknown origin.

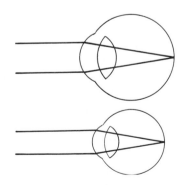

Fig. 22-1. Two emmetropic eyes. The refractive power of the anterior segment is so correlated with the length of the eye that parallel rays of light are focused on the retina. The eye below has much more refractive power than the eye above although both are emmetropic. If such a difference were present in the right and left eyes, there would be a difference of image size, called aniseikonia.

SYMPTOMS AND SIGNS OF REFRACTIVE ERROR

Decreased visual acuity, which is entirely corrected by means of lenses, is the cardinal sign of a refractive error. If vision cannot be corrected to normal by means of lenses, an organic cause must be sought to explain the decrease in vision. In myopia, vision is decreased for distance and normal for near. In hyperopia, vision may be normal or decreased for both near and far. Since accommodation may compensate for hyperopia, often no relationship exists between vision without lenses and the amount of the hyperopia.

Many different symptoms are attributed to refractive errors. Because vision and the eyes figure prominently in psychologic attitudes, symptoms may be difficult to interpret. Ocular discomfort is a vague symptom that refers to almost any unexplained sensation occurring in or about the eyes. Asthenopia, eyestrain, or visual fatigue are terms used to describe complaints related to any unpleasant symptom originating in the head or eyes, which the patient attributes to use of the eyes. These include burning, itching, increased sensitivity to light, decreased efficiency, various aches, and tiredness. Symptoms that occur even after prolonged use of the eyes are not necessarily ocular in origin. Patients may live and work in unpleasant surroundings. They tire not because of use of the eyes but because of supervisors, surroundings, tedium of routine, and the like.

Headache, irrespective of its cause, is commonly and erroneously attributed to refractive errors. If a refractive error contributes to headache, the discomfort should be related to sustained use of the eyes and relieved when the eyes are not used. It is unlikely that a headache present on awakening in the morning can be ascribed to excessive use of the eyes the evening before. Individuals living in unpleasant situations from which there is no escape may develop tension headaches that they attribute to the use of the eyes. Migraine is never caused by a refractive error.

EMMETROPIA

Emmetropia is that optical condition in which there is no refractive error so that rays of light parallel to the visual axis upon entering the eye are brought to a focus on the fovea cen-

tralis when no accommodation is exerted (Fig. 22-1). There is an exact correlation between the refractive power of the anterior segment and the axial length of the eye. Clinically, emmetropia rarely occurs, because the refractive components of the anterior segment are not exactly correlated with the axial length of the eye.

AMETROPIA

Ametropia is that optical condition in which the refractive power of the cornea and lens and the length of the globe are not correlated so that rays of light parallel to the visual axis upon entering the eye do not come to focus on the fovea centralis (Fig. 22-2). Hyperopia, myopia, or astigmatism may be present, or astigmatism may be combined with hyperopia or myopia. Ametropia is axial when it is the result of an abnormality in the length of the eye, or refractive when it is the result of an abnormality in the refractive power of the anterior segment. Ultrasonography is an easy method to determine the length of the eye. If one knows the total refractive power of the eye and its length, it is easy to determine whether ametropia is axial or refractive. Clinically, this is done in measuring the length of the eye and the curvature of the cornea to determine the appropriate power of an intraocular lens in cataract extraction.

Hyperopia. Hyperopia is that refractive condition of the eye in which, with accommodation suspended, parallel rays of light are intercepted by the retina before coming to focus (Fig. 22-3).

The condition occurs because the refractive power of the anterior segment is inadequate for

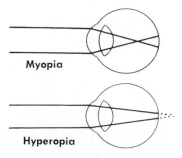

Fig. 22-2. Major types of refractive error (ametropia).

the length of the globe (refractive) or the globe is too short (axial) for the amount of refractive power present. Accommodation increases the refractive power of the anterior segment and may compensate for hyperopia and provide normal vision.

Severe degrees of hyperopia may occur with an abnormally small eye, which may range in size down to a microphthalmia. Hyperopia is induced if the fovea centralis is displaced anteriorly. Causes include orbital tumors, subretinal fluid, and intraocular tumors. Such disorders may decrease vision by a direct effect on the optic nerve or retina. Reduction of the radius of curvature of the cornea or lens or displacement of the lens backward into the vitreous body reduces the refracting power of the anterior segment and may cause an excessive degree of hyperopia. In aphakia, in which the lens is absent, hyperopia is marked and there is loss of the accommodation provided by the lens.

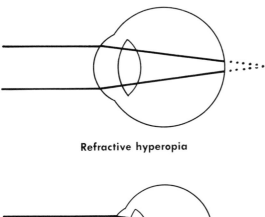

Refractive hyperopia

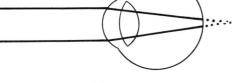

Axial hyperopia

Fig. 22-3. Hyperopia. Both eyes are hyperopic. *Top,* The eye is hyperopic because the refractive power of the anterior segment is not adequate to focus light on the retina. *Bottom,* The hyperopia occurs because the eye is too small for the amount of refractive power of the anterior segment. Accommodation may increase the refractive power of the anterior segment so that a distinct image is formed on the retina.

Hyperopia may be compensated by accommodation. If accommodation does not compensate for the hyperopia, vision is blurred. Vision is normal if the refractive error is neutralized by accommodation. Ocular symptoms may originate with excessive sustained accommodation required for clear vision. There is no direct relationship between the symptoms and the amount of accommodation required to neutralize a hyperopia. Since a portion of accommodation must be used to neutralize the refractive error for distance and additional accommodation is required for near work, the symptoms may be more marked for near work than for distance.

There are no specific signs of hyperopia. The cornea may be smaller than normal, and the globe itself may be small. This should not be confused with the appearance caused by a narrow interpalpebral fissure. Hyperopia that exceeds 5 diopters may be associated with blurring of the disk margin, called pseudopapilledema. The disk is not elevated, but the margins appear indistinct and the physiologic cup is absent. This condition is distinguished from early papilledema by the normal caliber of veins, their normal pulsation, and the absence of retinal edema and hemorrhages. Inflammation of the optic nerve at the level of the disk is usually unilateral (papillitis) and causes decreased vision, a central scotoma, and an afferent pupillary defect.

Hyperopia is classified as follows:

1. Total hyperopia is the amount of hyperopia present with all accommodation suspended, a condition produced by paralysis of the ciliary muscle by means of a cycloplegic drug.
2. Manifest hyperopia is the maximum hyperopia that can be corrected with a convex lens when accommodation is active.
3. The difference between total and manifest hyperopia is the latent hyperopia.

Since accommodation for near is related to convergence of the eyes, the increased accommodation required to neutralize hyperopia may stimulate an excessive degree of convergence. This excessive convergence is manifested as a tendency for the eyes to deviate inward (esodeviation, see Chapter 21).

Treatment of hyperopia requires an analysis of symptoms, visual acuity, and muscle balance. If visual acuity is good, muscle balance is normal, and there are no symptoms, correction of the hyperopia is not necessary, irrespective of its severity. Conversely, convex lenses are prescribed when visual acuity is decreased, when a convergence excess causes esophoria or esotropia, or when hyperopia causes symptoms.

Myopia. Myopia is that optical condition in which rays of light entering the eye parallel to the visual axis come to a focus in front of the retina (Fig. 22-4). The condition occurs (1) because the refractive power of the anterior segment is too great for the length of the eye or (2) because the eye is too long for the refractive power present. Patients with uncorrected myopia do not accommodate to improve vision because accommodation shifts the focal point even further anterior to the retina and blurs vision. Myopia may be divided into three types: (1) physiologic myopia, (2) pathologic or degenerative myopia, previously called progressive or malignant myopia, and (3) lenticular myopia. Physiologic myopia may be either refractive or axial. Degenerative myopia is axial while lenticular myopia is refractive.

Physiologic myopia, the most common type, occurs because of inadequate correlation of the refractive power of the anterior segment with the length of the globe, both of which are within their normal distribution curves. It has its onset usually between 5 and 10 years of age but may begin as late as 25 years of age. It gradually increases until the eye is fully grown, about 18 years of age. It seldom exceeds 6 diopters.

Pathologic (degenerative) myopia is an abnormality in which the axial length of the eye is excessive, primarily because of overgrowth of the posterior two thirds of the globe. Commonly, pathologic myopia begins as a physiologic myopia, but rather than stabilizing when the globe is adult size, the eye continues to enlarge.

The first ophthalmoscopic sign of degeneration is a myopic crescent of the optic disk that begins at the temporal side and progresses to surround the disk (Fig. 22-5). Staphyloma of the posterior pole causes degeneration of Bruch membrane that creates branching, reticular lines, called lacquer cracks, which may cause foveal hemorrhage. Later a subretinal neovascular membrane may develop with subsequent vascular leakage and hemorrhage. With resorption of a foveal hemorrhage, hyperpigmentation develops in the fovea centralis (Fuchs spot).

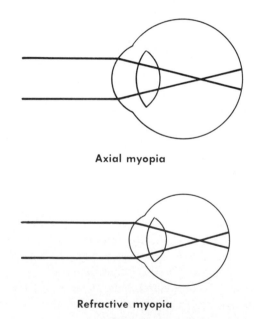

Fig. 22-4. Myopia. Both eyes are myopic. *Top,* The eye is myopic because it is too long for the amount of refractive power present. *Bottom,* The eye is myopic because the refractive power is too great for the length of the eye. Increased accommodation increases the refractive power of the anterior segment and aggravates the myopia.

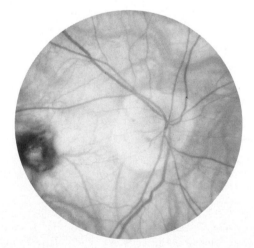

Fig. 22-5. The ocular fundus in pathologic (degenerative) myopia. The sclera is bared in the region surrounding the optic nerve, the choroid is easily visible (depigmentation in situ), and there is pigment proliferation (Fuchs spot) at the fovea centralis.

Degeneration of the retinal pigment epithelium (depigmentation in situ) and choroid exposes the sclera. The peripheral retina may show lattice degeneration and retinal breaks, increasing the risk of retinal separation. Pigment migration may simulate healed chorioretinitis.

Increase in the refractive power of the crystalline lens (lenticular myopia) increases the refractive power of the anterior segment. Such an increase occurs in uncontrolled diabetes mellitus and in nuclear sclerosis, a type of senile cataract. Drugs such as hydralazine and chlorthalidone (antihypertensives) and the phenothiazines may also increase the refractive power of the lens.

Myopia is neutralized by concave lenses. Corrective lenses should be prescribed for patients dissatisfied with poor visual acuity. Wearing corrective lenses has no apparent effect on the progression of myopia. A decrease in myopia requires a decrease in the axial length or refractive power of the eye, and this does not occur spontaneously.

If a patient with myopia is prescribed a concave lens of more refractive power than required, the patient may compensate by increased accommodation. Vision is clear, and often there are no symptoms. Such individuals may show an apparent decrease in myopia when proper lenses are prescribed. The use of a contact or bifocal lens does not affect the progression of myopia.

Tightly fitted contact lenses may temporarily reduce the corneal curvature and thus temporarily decrease the severity of myopia. The refractive error reverts to its previous state after use of the contact lens is discontinued.

Since physiologic myopia is a variation in growth, many remedies may be associated with the termination of the growth process, and credit is often given to the therapy. Studies of treatment to correct or arrest myopia have not been controlled, and double-masked methods and adequate experimental designs have been ignored. Usually there has been no matched control group or an excessive number of patients have been lost to follow-up.

Fusion of the eyelids in macaque monkeys so that form vision is impossible but light enters the eye causes axial myopia in young but not adult monkeys. The elongation of the eye is caused by an alteration of the visual input and is mediated by the nervous system. The result is similar to ocular elongation in human infants with blepharoptosis, hemangiomas of the eyelids, and opacities of the ocular media.

For decades therapy consisted of daily instillation of 1% atropine solution into the eyes. Its value has never been proved. Since this paralyzes accommodation, bifocal lenses must be used or reading must be done without glasses. Tinted lenses may be worn in sunlight, and the ocular tension must be monitored. Ocular hypertension is more common in myopia than in hyperopia, and many practitioners initiate prophylactic treatment with timolol, epinephrine, or propine at lower levels of intraocular pressure than they do in hyperopia. Patients with signs of myopic degeneration benefit from frequent optical correction of their progressive myopia to maintain clear vision. The peripheral retina must be studied carefully annually to detect retinal holes and rhegmatogenous retinal separation.

Radial keratotomy is a method of reducing the radius of curvature of the central cornea by a series of radial incisions in the peripheral cornea. Eight or sixteen incisions, each about 4 mm long, are made partially through the cornea, sparing the central cornea. Uncorrected visual acuity in myopic individuals with relatively minor degrees of ametropia is improved. Myopia is reduced by about 2.5 diopters (see Chapter 10).

Astigmatism. Astigmatism is an optical condition in which the refracting power of a lens (or an eye) is not the same in all meridians. Thus, if the refracting power of the eye is 58 diopters in the vertical and 60 diopters in the horizontal meridian, 2 diopters of astigmatism are present. Parallel rays of light do not focus at a point. To aid graphic reconstruction, one considers one focal line corresponding to the 60-diopter meridian and another corresponding to the 58-diopter meridian. The distance separating these focal lines is the interval of Sturm (Fig. 22-6). (There is actually a series of images with cylindrical lenses contributing to each.)

Astigmatism is regular when the meridians of minimal and maximal refraction are at right angles to each other and irregular when the meridians are not at right angles to each other. Ocular astigmatism is simple when one merid-

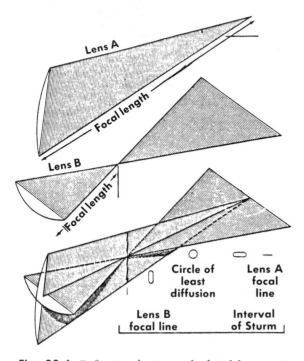

Fig. 22-6. Refraction by two cylindrical lenses, A, and B, of unequal strength. Cylindrical lens B has the greatest convexity and hence a vertical line is focused first. Parallel rays of light are focused as a line rather than as a point. The combination of two cylindrical lenses of unequal power forms two major focal lines corresponding to their refractive power. The distance between the focal lines is the interval of Sturm. A circle of least diffusion is located between the focal lines at an area where the diverging and converging tendency of the light rays is the same. It is located between the two focal lines and is closer to the stronger cylinder in proportion to the strength of the component cylinders.

ian is on the retina, simple myopic when the other meridian is anterior to the retina, and simple hyperopic when the other meridian is intercepted by the retina before coming to focus. In compound myopic astigmatism, both meridians are in front of the retina. In compound hyperopic astigmatism, both meridians are intercepted by the retina before coming to a focus. In mixed astigmatism, one focal line is focused in front of the retina and the other focal line is intercepted by the retina.

Astigmatism usually occurs because the cornea has two different radii of curvature at right angles to each other. This may occur as a biologic variant or may result from the weight of the upper eyelid resting upon the eyeball, from surgical incisions into the cornea, from trauma and scarring of the cornea, or from tumors of the eyelid such as a chalazion pressing upon the globe. Irregular astigmatism occurs in corneal scarring and in keratoconus. In keratoconus the cornea becomes cone shaped, with the apex of the cone inferonasal to the center of the cornea. Minor degrees of astigmatism may occur from variations in the radius of curvature of the lens (lenticular astigmatism). This condition is detected in patients who wear hard contact lenses that neutralize corneal astigmatism.

The symptoms of astigmatism vary considerably. A distinct retinal image cannot form (Fig. 22-7), but the circle of least diffusion may be

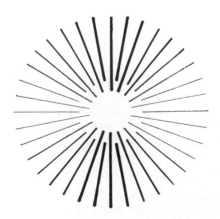

Fig. 22-7. The astigmatic dial as seen by a patient with astigmatism. The thick black lines are focused on the retina, whereas the thin lines lie in front of the retina.

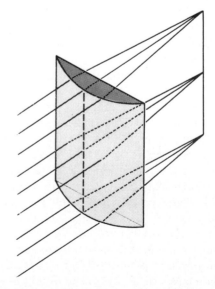

Fig. 22-8. Cylindrical lens. The line of focus parallels the axis of the lens.

imaged. Some maintain that in small degrees of compound hyperopic astigmatism, first one focal line and then the other may be focused on the retina with the constantly changing accommodation causing symptoms. Small degrees of astigmatism cause no obvious external signs. Ophthalmoscopically marked degrees of astigmatism may cause the optic disk to appear oval rather than circular.

Astigmatism is neutralized by cylindrical lenses (Fig. 22-8). The amount of astigmatism that should be corrected is debated. Some believe that even minor degrees of astigmatism require correction. If, however, visual acuity is good and there are no symptoms, correction is not indicated. Hard contact lenses may be used to correct irregular astigmatism. In keratoconus, if vision is markedly reduced and if the eyes cannot be corrected with contact lenses because of the shape of the cornea or discomfort, or both, a corneal transplant should be considered. Conversely, every patient with corneal scarring should have a trial with a contact lens before a corneal transplant is recommended.

Presbyopia. Accommodation increases the refractive power of the anterior segment through an increased curvature and thickness of the lens. The change in the shape of the lens occurs because of its inherent elasticity in response to contraction of the ciliary muscle, which relaxes the zonule. With each year of life, the lens loses some of this elasticity, decreasing the amount of accommodation. Generally, there are about 14 diopters of accommodation at 10 years of age and only 2 diopters of accommodation by 50 years of age. The decrease occurs gradually, but with only 2 diopters of accommodation, small objects viewed closer than 0.5 m from the eye are blurred.

The optical condition of decreased accommodation is known as presbyopia. The loss of accommodation occurs in all individuals, irrespective of their refractive error. However, a myopic individual may compensate for presbyopia by removing the lens that corrects the distance vision. Presbyopia is aggravated in a hyperopic individual if the lens that corrects the hyperopia is removed.

The chief symptom of presbyopia is inability to see near work distinctly. This is aggravated in dim illumination and with small print. The individual is frequently annoyed at having to place reading matter farther away from the eyes than previously. The use of nearly all accommodation for clear near vision may cause ocular discomfort. There are no external signs of presbyopia except the general appearance that indicates that the individual is more than 40 years of age.

Presbyopia is treated by means of convex lenses added to the distance correction. The power of the lens required for clear vision for near work varies with an individual's habits, age, occupation, length of arms, and accustomed distance of doing near work. Generally, the weakest possible convex lenses are prescribed to permit the individual to carry on vocational and avocational tasks. Bifocal or trifocal (multifocal) lenses are prescribed not as an additional burden to middleaged persons, but so that it will not be necessary to wear a separate pair of lenses for near and for far. If an individual requires lenses for distance, bifocal or trifocal lenses should be worn as early as they are indicated. An individual who does not become accustomed to bifocal lenses relatively early in the development of presbyopia frequently has unnecessary symptoms when multifocal lenses are prescribed in later years. If distance lenses are not required, an individual may get along nicely with lenses that correct the presbyopia solely. Nonetheless, because of the restricted focus of reading lenses, many individuals who do not need a distance correction wear bifocal lenses so that distant objects can be seen without removing the lenses.

Aphakia. When the crystalline lens is not in the visual axis, rays of light entering the eye are refracted solely by the cornea. Surgical removal of the lens is the common cause of aphakia, but dislocation of the lens out of the pupillary area may occur in systemic disease, such as Marfan syndrome, or after trauma. Since the lens is one of the two refracting portions of the eye, its removal causes severe hyperopia and a loss of accommodation.

The chief symptom is decreased vision for both far and near. Since accommodation is not possible, there are no symptoms of ocular discomfort.

The condition may be diagnosed by the loss of the reflected image from the surface of the lens and by excessive movement of the iris because of loss of support by the anterior lens capsule (iridodonesis).

Aphakia is currently corrected by means of an intraocular lens. Sometimes there is good vision for near and far without spectacles. Usually a convex lens is necessary for near work. When aphakia is corrected with ordinary spectacle lenses, the image in the aphakic eye is 25% to 33% larger than in the normal eye. If the fellow eye is normal, single binocular vision is usually not possible because of the difference in size of the retinal images (aniseikonia). The difference in image size may be reduced to somewhat less than 10% by means of a contact lens. Convex lenses, usually bifocal, are required for near vision in aphakic eyes corrected for distance with contact lenses.

Intraocular lenses are usually (80%) inserted at the time of cataract extraction. Currently an extracapsular lens extraction with a posterior chamber lens is usually selected. A secondary implant is made in aphakic eyes, usually eyes that have had an intracapsular lens extraction. An anterior chamber lens is used. Intraocular lenses provide a normal size image and obviate the optical problems of aphakia. Since there is no accommodation, a correction is required for near as in presbyopia.

ANISOMETROPIA

Anisometropia is that condition in which the refractive error of each eye is different. Minor differences are nearly universal, but when there is a difference of more than 2 diopters, the difference in image sizes of the two eyes may be the cause of symptoms. Often such patients are asymptomatic until bifocal lenses are prescribed. When the eyes are turned downward to use the bifocal segment, the difference in power of the two lenses induces a vertical prism, so that the image from each eye is on a different level. This may cause marked ocular symptoms that may be neutralized by prescribing the appropriate prism in the reading segment or by using separate lenses for near and distance.

Severe anisometropia is a common cause of amblyopia because of the developing infant's failure to use the eye with the greater refractive error. Failure of central vision to develop leads to strabismus. Even when the visual acuity can be corrected to normal with lenses, binocular vision may fail to develop; then the anisometropia produces no symptoms, because the retinal image from one eye is suppressed.

Aniseikonia. Aniseikonia is that condition in which the size or shape of the retinal images of the two eyes is different. A difference of 0.5 diopter in the refractive error gives a retinal image size difference of about 1%. Most individuals can tolerate a difference of up to 5% without ocular discomfort. Symptoms result from aniseikonia only if binocular vision is present. Thus, many individuals who have a markedly different refractive error in the two eyes do not have symptoms because they suppress the image in one eye. Patients may prefer to use only one eye when reading or watching moving objects. All symptoms are entirely eliminated by covering one eye, as is true of all disorders of binocular vision.

During the 1930s, aniseikonia was intensively studied and corrected with specially ground lenses with different curvatures on their front and back surfaces to equalize the size of the retinal images. Today equalization may be accomplished by using contact lenses of different strengths neutralized by appropriate spectacle lenses to alter the size of images.

MEASUREMENT OF THE REFRACTIVE ERROR

The presence or absence of a refractive error may be estimated by a number of methods. There may be typical ophthalmoscopic signs evident, but the measurement of the severity of ametropia by means of the ophthalmoscope is unreliable.

Visual acuity. An impression of the degree and type of ametropia can be learned by measurement of the visual acuity. If vision is 20/20 for distance, the patient is not myopic. If vision is 20/20 for distance and poorer than this for near, the patient is either presbyopic or has hyperopia not compensated for by accommodation. If vision is less than 20/20 for distance but normal for near, the patient may be myopic. Patients with a hyperopic astigmatism that would be corrected with a convex cylinder at axis 90° ("with the rule") often see the horizontal bars of letters such as E, F, and Z more clearly than they do the vertical bars of letters such as N, H, and K. The condition is reversed when the astigmatism is about 180°.

Measurement of distance visual acuity by using a pinhole in patients who do not wear corrective lenses indicates whether decreased vision is the result of an organic disease or refractive error. If vision is not improved with a pinhole, the decreased vision is probably the result of an organic disease (see Chapter 5).

Ophthalmoscopy. The estimation of ametropia by means of the ophthalmoscope may be inaccurate unless the examiner is presbyopic and unable to accommodate. In hyperopia the disk may appear smaller than normal, and a pseudopapilledema may occasionally be present. In myopia the disk may appear larger than normal. In pathologic myopia a scleral myopic crescent may be present, there may be attenuation of the retinal pigment epithelium with a prominent choroidal pattern, and there may be areas of pigment proliferation. In astigmatism the optic disk may appear oval rather than round.

Retinoscopy. Retinoscopy (skiaskopy) is an objective method of measurement of the refractive error. It is extremely accurate when carried out by a skilled examiner. The basic principle is to substitute lenses in front of the patient's eye so that emerging rays of light from the retina are brought to a focus at the examiner's eye. The light is directed into the patient's eye by means of a light source that has an aperture for observation. It is the single most useful method of measuring ametropia. It is most useful in children and in individuals who have poor discrimination or who respond slowly.

Automated refracting instruments combine electronic sensors and microcomputers to measure the refractive error either objectively or subjectively. All require a cooperative patient. Generally, they produce results equivalent to those obtained by retinoscopy.

Subjective methods. Most subjective methods for estimating refractive errors depend largely on the patient's responses to changes in lenses. In one common method, called fogging, a convex lens, much in excess of that required for distinct vision, is placed in front of the eyes until accommodation relaxes to improve vision. The power of the convex lens is then reduced until vision is at about the level of 20/40. The patient's attention may then be directed to an astigmatic dial and a concave cylinder placed with its axis at right angles to the axis found to be most dark. Subjective testing requires discrimination of moderately small changes in vision by an individual who has moderately rapid reaction times. It is most accurate in patients who are presbyopic.

Keratometry. The keratometer is an instrument used to measure the radius of curvature (K reading) of the anterior surface of the central optical portion of the cornea. In principle it measures the size of the corneal image of an object of known size that is a fixed distance from the cornea. It is used to aid in the selection of a contact lens of correct curvature.

Cycloplegia. As has been seen, accommodation may increase the refractive power of the eye by as much as 15 diopters. Paralysis of accommodation by means of drugs (cycloplegia) permits measurement of the refractive error uncomplicated by changes in accommodation. Cycloplegia is indicated in children, in patients with strabismus, in patients in whom active accommodation makes accurate measurement of the refractive error difficult, and in patients with cloudy ocular media in whom accurate retinoscopy is not possible through the undilated pupil.

Since adequate ophthalmoscopic examination is not possible through the undilated pupil, many physicians insist that a complete ocular examination include pupillary dilation and indirect ophthalmoscopy of the retinal periphery. Phenylephrine eyedrops dilate the pupil without affecting accommodation. All cycloplegic drops both dilate the pupil, through paralysis of the sphincter pupillae muscle, and paralyze the ciliary muscle responsible for accommodation. The pupils of a patient predisposed to closed-angle glaucoma should be dilated with caution, and the pupil should be constricted before the patient is dismissed.

OPTICAL DEVICES

Spectacles are a pair of lenses encircled by rims or supported by a frame connected by a bridge that rests on the nose. They have sides or temples that pass on either side of the head to the ears. Bows are the curved extremities of the temples; shoulders are short bars that attach the frame or lenses to the temples. Lenses may provide correction for hyperopia, myopia, astigmatism, presbyopia, and muscle balance. They may be impact resistant, tinted, polarized, antireflective, or various combinations.

Spectacles generally have the following functions: (1) improving vision by correction of refractive errors, (2) relieving ocular symptoms or aligning the visual axes by changing the amount of accommodation used, (3) incorporating neutralizing prisms, (4) protecting the eye from mechanical trauma or radiant energy, or (5) compensating for subnormal vision by providing magnification.

Refractive errors are neither induced nor prevented by wearing spectacles. Refractive errors are not aggravated or corrected by wearing improper lenses or by not wearing lenses at all. (Accommodative types of esotropia and exotropia may be corrected by the appropriate lens.) Some individuals prefer blurred vision to wearing spectacles. Many such individuals wear contact lenses. Some patients complain of ocular discomfort but refuse to wear corrective lenses; there is little help for them.

Lenses are prescribed to relieve the symptoms that result from an excessive accommodative effort in hyperopia. Convex lenses may not improve visual acuity. Children with either divergence or convergence anomalies caused by disorders in accommodative convergence should wear lenses to prevent intermittent crossing of one eye, which is often associated with suppression of the image in that eye and results in interference with binocular function.

Impact-resistant lenses. All optical lenses sold in the United States, unless specifically excluded by the prescriber, must be tested to resist the impact of a ⅝-inch diameter steel ball dropped from a height of 50 inches. Such impact-resistant glass lenses are either chemically treated or case hardened by heating followed by cooling. Plastic lenses do not shatter, but they scratch more easily than glass lenses. Although they are much thicker than glass lenses, some individuals prefer them because of their lighter weight. Ordinary impact-resistant lenses do not meet the safety requirements of industry, which requires a minimum thickness of 5 mm combined with an industrial-type frame that minimizes backward displacement of the lens.

Spectacle frames manufactured in the United States are constructed with fire-retardant materials, but some frames manufactured abroad are flammable. A frame constructed with a posterior lip so that the lens cannot be displaced toward the wearer's eye provides additional protection.

Absorptive lenses (sunglasses and lens tints). All spectacle lenses reflect, absorb, and transmit a portion of the electromagnetic spectrum. A crown glass spectacle lens reflects about 8%

of visible light, absorbs short ultraviolet (less than 310 nm), transmits up to 20% of longer ultraviolet (erythema producing), and nearly all the longer wavelengths (visible light and infrared). Special types of lenses may reduce or eliminate any portion of the spectrum.

Tinted lenses contain metallic oxides that selectively absorb different regions of the spectrum. Neutral gray ("smoke") lenses are often preferred because they do not distort color vision. Yellow-tinted lenses absorb all ultraviolet, are good haze filters (atmospheric haze has a high proportion of blue wavelengths), and are used as hunting glasses. Pink tints absorb 95% of ultraviolet but otherwise have transmission properties similar to clear glass. Green and brown tints absorb ultraviolet and infrared but induce some color distortion.

Glass and plastic lenses may be coated to match the color and absorptive properties of a metallic oxide-impregnated lens. The coating may be of greater density above than below or may be applied so the entire lens has a uniform appearance. Antireflective lenses are coated with a thin layer of magnesium fluoride that increases the transmission of crown glass and reduces reflections from the surfaces of lenses. Polaroid sunglasses have a thin layer of vertically oriented dicroic crystals laminated between two layers of glass. These crystals absorb plane-polarized sun rays reflected from flat horizontal surfaces (water, concrete highways) and eliminate reflective glare. Photosensitive glass darkens when exposed to ultraviolet and clears when the ultraviolet is removed. The lenses generally darken quickly in ultraviolet but clear much more slowly when ultraviolet is removed.

Infrared radiation is difficult to protect against, and in the United States the steel- and glass-making industries use manufacturing methods that prevent infrared exposure of the worker. Ultraviolet radiation is mainly absorbed by the cornea and may cause a painful superficial keratitis. Skiers, sailors, and others exposed to high levels of ultraviolet radiation should wear colored lenses to protect the cornea. Lenses designed for industrial protection should be used solely within that industry since they may markedly reduce visual acuity in other situations.

Colored lenses should not be worn at night because they reduce the amount of light entering the eye. Color-deficient individuals should wear neutral lenses, not colored lenses. Lenses with light transmission between 5% and 20% provide much comfort to patients with albinism, photophobia, aversion to light, cone degenerations, and conditions in which the pupil is dilated or the iris is absent.

Antireflective coatings, which improve the optical performance of all lenses, are recommended. Tinted and colored lenses are indicated in light sensitivity (photophobia) caused by uveitis, bacterial keratitis, and keratoconjunctivitis sicca. They are used after eye surgery, particularly cataract extraction, and when the pupils have been dilated for ocular examination.

Fishermen use polarized lenses to see beneath the water surface. Hunters use yellow glass to reduce haze. Radiologists use silenium red glasses to maintain dark adaptation outside of the dark room. Polaroid lenses reduce glare in driving. For recreation, such as golf, tennis, or hiking, a photosensitive lens or neutral density lens is useful.

Healthy eyes do not require absorption lenses, and their chief use is cosmetic—colored lenses in attractive frames used as costume jewelry, to hide cosmetic defects, or to conceal the eyes.

Contact lenses. Contact lenses are worn beneath the eyelids and in front of the cornea (Figs. 22-9 and 22-10). They may be hard or soft and vary in diameter from 7 mm (corneal) to 15 mm (corneoscleral). Several types of plastic are used to provide hard lenses, soft lenses that are oxygen- or gas-permeable, or ultrathin lenses used for extended wear.

Contact lenses are indicated for well-motivated, self-reliant individuals if they provide better vision than spectacles, in irregular corneal astigmatism, in monocular aphakia, congenital nystagmus, anisometropia, and anisokoria. They may be substituted for spectacle correction in individuals who require constant correction for clear vision in myopia, hyeropia, and aphakia. They are required by some athletes, performers, and public figures.

Bandage contact lenses are used in the treatment of epithelial erosions secondary to recurrent corneal erosion, corneal dystrophies, ocular cicatricial pemphigoid, keratitis, and alkali burns. Lenses with a colored iris painted on the surface are used cosmetically to conceal un-

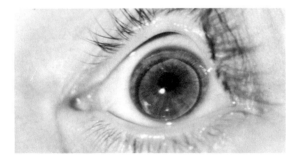

Fig. 22-9. Corneal contact lens. The lens floats on the precorneal tear film. It is outlined by shadows.

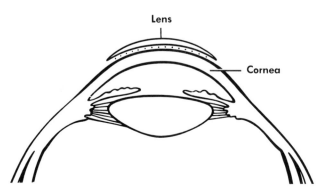
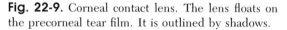

Fig. 22-10. An aspheric contact lens with a back surface that parallels the surface of the eye.

sightly corneas or change the appearance of the eyes.

Some individuals who would benefit from contact lenses are insufficiently motivated to wear them or are unable to manipulate the lenses. The lenses are contraindicated in uveitis, keratitis sicca, and neuroparalytic keratitis. Scleral lenses should not be used in glaucoma because they compress the aqueous veins. They are contraindicated in those unable to follow directions and in young children.

Contact lenses may be hard (rigid) or soft. Hard lenses have good optics, durability, are relatively easy to clean, and are readily replaceable. Moderate amounts of astigmatism may be neutralized, and they may be tinted. Most transmit oxygen poorly, require prolonged adaptation, and can seldom be used for occasional wear.

Soft contact lenses are more fragile and difficult to maintain as well as more expensive than hard lenses. A moderate amount of astigmatism is not easily neutralized, and tints are not available commercially. Most transmit oxygen well, are comfortable and easily adaptable, and may be worn intermittently.

Contact lenses may irritate patients with dry eyes, corneal dystrophies, or recurrent corneal erosion. They must not be used during active keratitis or conjunctivitis.

Hard lenses may be scleral or corneal. Hard scleral lenses are made from a cast of the patient's anterior segment and have a corneal curvature and a scleral curvature. Hard scleral lenses require a buffer solution or tears between the lens and the cornea, and wearing time is limited to prevent corneal edema (Sattler veil). Preformed hard lenses have a single radius of curvature and are worn by persons who do not tolerate a long wearing time.

Hard corneal lenses have a diameter of 7 mm to 10.5 mm. They are usually round except for bifocal lenses and those that are ground with a cylinder in the front surface when a segment is cut from the lower portion to prevent rotation. The lenses most frequently have spherical curves on both the anterior and posterior surfaces. In general, hard lenses are more uncomfortable than soft lenses and require adaptation by progressive increase in wearing time. Some individuals are unable to tolerate them. Additionally, hard lenses are more likely to cause corneal injury and change the corneal curvature, sometimes for weeks. They often provide better vision than the soft variety.

Soft contact lenses may cover only the cornea or both the cornea and a part of the adjacent sclera. They are more easily tolerated than hard lenses. Oxygen-permeable soft lenses may be worn continuously under close medical supervision and with removal for cleaning every 30 to 90 days. Soft lenses are much more useful for occasional wear (such as sports activity) and are lost less often than hard lenses. Their major deficiency is the poor correction of visual acuity, particularly in individuals with severe astigmatism. Such astigmatism may be neutralized by wearing a soft contact lens over the cornea and a hard corneal contact lens over the soft lens. Since soft contact lenses are hydrophilic, they absorb lens-cleaning solutions, medications, and chlorinated water in swimming pools and slowly release them into the tearfilm, which may cause irritation. Fluorescein, rose bengal solutions, and epinephrine stain soft lenses.

Giant cell papillary conjunctivitis is an anaphylactic hypersensitivity (type I) in which IgE immune globulins attach to conjunctival mast cells (see Chapter 9). Soft lens wearers develop excess mucus, ocular itching, and giant papillae in the tarsal conjunctiva of the upper eyelids that resemble vernal conjunctivitis. The patient must discontinue using the lenses, which should be cleaned or replaced. A different system of contact lens cleaning should be used, and the patient must follow cleaning directions meticulously. Often the condition cannot be corrected.

Superficial peripheral corneal neovascularization occurs in soft contact lens wearers if the lens is fitted so tightly that it impairs the blood supply at the corneoscleral limbus. It is necessary to replace the lens with a properly fitted lens.

Infection may be introduced into the cornea by means of a contact lens that abrades the epithelium. Ocular diseaes may be neglected by patients who believe their symptoms are caused by wearing contact lenses. Wearers must follow the manufacturer's suggestions concerning sterilization of the lenses.

Successful wear of soft or hard contact lenses requires careful, intelligent personal hygiene and cleaning of the lenses. Eye makeup must be removed daily. If creams or oils are used to remove makeup, they must be thoroughly removed from eyes, eyelids, and hands before removing lenses. The eyelashes, eyelids, and hands must be thoroughly cleaned before inserting lenses. Lenses should be stored in a clean storage case containing a sterile washing solution. Instructions for cleaning soft contact lenses must be followed meticulously.

Orthokeratology. This is the intentional alteration of the curvature of the cornea to correct myopia or corneal astigmatism by the use of a hard contact lens with a radius of curvature less than the radius of curvature of the cornea (flatter). This temporarily reduces ametropia and permits improved vision without spectacles or contact lenses for 6 to 24 hours. The contact lens then must be worn again for 6 to 12 hours to mold the cornea. The results are not predictable, and some patients are dissatisfied with the variable vision and limited period of clear vision.

Intraocular lenses. Lenses may be placed within the eye at the time of cataract extraction. An anterior chamber type lens is used after intraocular cataract extraction or as a secondary procedure. A posterior chamber lens is used after an extracapsular cataract extraction (see Chapter 19).

Reading aids for the partially sighted. Many magnifying devices that increase the size of the retinal image are available to compensate for subnormal vision. The two basic devices are (1) a Galilean telescope to bring the object closer to the observer, and (2) an optical device to bring the observer closer to the object, usually by means of a magnifier lens. This may be in the form of a spectacle lens, stand magnifier, projection magnifier, or television reader.

Diagnosis of the ocular condition that causes subnormal vision and an understanding of the occupational needs of the individual must be correlated with the selection of the mode of correction. Some patients may benefit from use of a mydriatic, others from use of a miotic. Some individuals with central retinal degeneration require high illumination, whereas others with various forms of cone degeneration see better in reduced illumination. Many patients who could be benefitted become discouraged at the long process of fitting and selection, and many practitioners lack the patience, special equipment, and optical devices required for testing.

A hand magnifier may be extremely useful. Some patients benefit from the use of a jeweler's loupe. Successful use of reading aids is correlated with the cause of loss of vision and the motivation and personality of the patient. Patients with visual reduction caused by vitreous hemorrhage and retinitis proliferans do poorly compared with those who have isolated central retinal lesions. Optimistic, self-reliant patients accept optical aids much better than those who are hostile, pessimistic, and sedentary.

BIBLIOGRAPHY
General

Adams, C.P., Jr., Cohen, E.J., Laibson, P.R., Galentine, P., and Arentsen, J.J.: Corneal ulcers in patients with cosmetic extended-wear contact lenses, Am. J. Ophthalmol. **96**:705, 1983.

Dabezies, O.H., editor: Contact lenses—the CLAO guide to basic science and clinical practice, New York, 1984, Grune & Stratton.

Elkington, A.R.: Clinical optics, Oxford, 1984, Blackwell Scientific Publications.

Faye, E.E.: Clinical low vision, ed. 2, Boston, 1984, Little, Brown & Co.

Hartstein, J.: Extended wear contact lenses for aphakia and myopia, St. Louis, 1982, The C.V. Mosby Co.

Michaels, D.D.: Visual optics and refraction, St. Louis, 1980, The C.V. Mosby Co.

Raviola, E., and Wiesel, T.N.: An animal model of myopia, N. Engl. J. Med. **312**:1609, 1985.

Refraction

Curtin, B.J.: The myopias: basic science and clinical management, Hagerstown, Md., 1985, J.B. Lippincott Co.

Reinecke, R.D., and Herm, R.J.: Refraction: a programmed text, ed. 3, East Norwalk, Conn., 1983, Appleton-Century-Crofts.

Rubin, M.L.: Optics for clinicians, ed. 2, Gainesville, Fa., 1977, Triad Scientific Publications.

Sahr, A.: Refraction and clinical optics, New York, 1980, Harper & Row, Publishers.

Spoor, T.C., Hartel, W.C., Wynn, P., and Spoor, D.K.: Complications of continuous-wear soft contact lenses in a nonreferral population, Arch. Ophthalmol. **102**:1312, 1984.

Weissman, B.A., Mondino, B.J., Pettit, T.H., and Hofbauer, J.D.: Corneal ulcers associated with extended-wear soft contact lenses, Am. J. Ophthalmol. **97**:476, 1984.

PART FOUR

SYSTEMIC DISEASES AND THE EYE

23

INFECTIOUS OCULAR DISEASES AND GRANULOMAS

The skin of the eyelids forms an effective mechanical barrier to microbial invasion; organisms (except papovavirus [warts]) must gain entrance through an arthropod vector or through a break in the skin. The glands of the eyelid may become infected if their excretory ducts are blocked. The bulbar and palpebral conjunctiva and corneal epithelium provide the same generalized defenses of mucous membranes elsewhere, combined with the mechanical defense of blinking. The reaction to infection varies from suppuration, to cellular infiltration in some viral infections, to corneal neovascularization, as for example, in congenital syphilis. Infection may rupture into the orbit through the thin walls of the nasal accessory sinuses, or organisms may be introduced through trauma. The orbital fascia effectively prevents eyelid infections from extending directly into the orbit proper. The intraocular contents may be involved in a variety of suppurative (endophthalmitis, panophthalmitis), granulomatous (sarcoid, sympathetic ophthalmia), and immune reactions (retinitis, choroiditis).

Despite constant exposure and moisture that favor microbial survival, the cornea and conjunctiva are protected by a number of systems that neutralize this innate susceptibility to infection. Evaporation of tears from the surface of the eye reduces the temperature of the ocular surface and inhibits microbial growth.

(Patching an infected eye provides an incubator for microbial growth.) Every few seconds the eyelids close and sweep across the exposed cornea and conjunctiva, keeping them moist and renewing the tear film. Blinking sweeps away microorganisms on the surface of the eye, which allows no opportunity for them to adhere to epithelial cells and colonize. The desmosomes of the epithelial cells combined with their basement membrane either prevent colonization of microorganisms or inhibit extension if colonization begins. The heterogenous collection of bacteria that populate the ocular surfaces ("normal flora") may compete for sites and substrates and minimize the opportunity for other organisms to become established.

The exposed position of the eye makes apparent its participation in various inflammatory and immune responses of the individual. Several factors, however, modify these responses, so there is no easy extrapolation of these responses to systemic events or of systemic events to the eye. The small amount of tissue involved (the entire eye weighs 7 g) may result in ocular events not being reflected in the peripheral blood or other organ systems. The cellular response that elsewhere reflects systemic defense mechanisms may reduce vision as the result of inflammatory cells and their products in the normally transparent tissues or new blood vessels in normally avascular structures. Intraocular tissue cannot usually be removed for study in the acute phases of a disorder, and many reports are based on the end stages of disease when the histologic response is no longer characteristic.

Microorganisms may be deposited on the surface of the eye from adjacent tissues and by flies, fingers, towels, eye makeup, surgical instruments, and eyedrops. After minor injury, the continuity of the epithelial surface is disrupted, and microorganisms are able to adhere to the disrupted epithelial cell layer and underlying stroma and sometimes cause infection.

The environment dictates the pattern of external eye disease in a community. Trachoma is prevalent in dry, hot deserts where flies abound and personal hygiene is poor. Onchocerciasis blinds thousands in the rain forest of Africa and Central America where the black fly is prevalent. Suppurative keratitis from bacterial, fungal, or amebic infection occurs after the commensal organisms or defense mechanisms have been disturbed by exposure, trauma, eyelid dysfunction, topical medications, or immune suppression. Herpes simplex keratitis occurs when the environment of the trigeminal ganglion that harbors the latent virus is disturbed, causing virus migration to the corneal epithelium, replication, and viral shedding.

IMMUNE AND INFLAMMATORY RESPONSES OF THE EYE

The major immune cells of ocular inflammatory disease are lymphocytes, plasma cells, mast cells, and mononuclear phagocytes.

Lymphocytes and plasma cells are located within the substantia propria of the conjunctiva, particularly within the fornices. Hyperplasia in chlamydial and viral infections causes follicles. Mucous-associated lymphoid tissue occurs between the acini of the lacrimal gland and is related to similar lymphoid tissues in other body mucosa, such as Peyer patches. The orbital tissues posterior to the orbital fascia have no lymphatic channels. Lymphocytes are not seen in the normal uvea but are prominent in nonspecific uveitis. Immune globulins occur in the uvea and corneal stroma, but are not present in the normal retina. Mast cells are located in the substantia propria of the conjunctiva, particularly at the corneoscleral limbus and peripheral conjunctiva. Degranulation of mast cells releases vasoactive substances that

cause papillary hypertrophy at the corneoscleral limbus and tarsal conjunctiva.

The mononuclear phagocyte system includes monocytes, macrophages, tissue histiocytes (including Langerhans cells), epithelioid cells, and giant cells. They originate in the bone marrow as monocytes, and enter the peripheral blood and the connective tissue. They have complement receptors, nonspecific esterase, and secrete neutral proteases and products of the arachidonic acid cascade (various prostaglandins, thromboxane). The mononuclear system modulates both B and T cells. Macrophages must process antigens to initiate an immune response.

There are two major types of lymphocytes: T cells (thymus derived) and B cells (bone marrow derived). T cells produce a wide variety of factors and mediators. One factor, the helper factor, acts on B cells to regulate their differentiation into plasma cells and immune globulin production. Another factor suppresses the differentiation of B cells into plasma cells. Cytotoxic T cells attach to and destroy target cells, such as tumor cells. T cells modify an inflammatory response through production of a variety of lymphokines: macrophage inhibition factor (MIF), inflammatory factor, macrophage aggregate factor, interferon-like factor, and transfer factor.

B cells have surface receptors for antigens. Stimulated by an antigen and aided by T-cell helper factors, they differentiate into plasma cells that produce immune globulins. There are five major classes of immune globulins (Ig): IgG, IgA, IgM, IgD, and IgE. The IgG class is divided into four subclasses.

Most antibodies belong to the IgG class. It is the most abundant immune globulin and is distributed equally between blood and interstitial tissue. It is present in tears and aqueous humor. The IgG molecule can be split by papain into three fragments. Two fragments (F_{ab}; fragment antigen binding) bind antigen. The third fragment (F_c: fragment crystalliable) fixes the IgG molecule to the surface of mast cells and phagocytes

Immune globulin A (IgA) has two classes: IgA_1 and IgA_2. Exocrine IgA is the dominant antibody of mucous membranes, including the conjunctiva. It consists of two IgA molecules joined by a secretory piece that is synthesized by the lacrimal gland and other local epithelial cells. The secretory piece (T piece for transport piece) prevents proteolysis of IgA and allows it to act as an antibody in fluids containing proteolytic enzymes. IgA does not appear to be strongly bactericidal or bacteriostatic, but may coat epithelial cells and inhibit microbial adherence.

Immune globulin M (IgM) is the largest of the immune globulins (macroglobulin) and is confined to the blood stream. It is the first type of antibody formed after encounter with an antigen. Rheumatoid factor, isohemagglutinins (anti-A and anti-B), and the antibodies against gram-negative somatic antigen (O), are the IgM type.

Immune globulin E (IgE) antigens are responsible for anaphylaxis and hypersensitivity diseases. They persist for weeks in the skin and conjunctiva bound to mast cells. Contact with the antigens leads to degranulation of the mast cells with release of the vasoactive amines, histamine, heparin, and others. IgE-forming plasma cells are concentrated in the nose and respiratory system and are involved in respiratory allergy. In the conjunctiva they are responsible for hay fever conjunctivitis and vernal conjunctivitis.

Immune globulin D (IgD) has an unknown function. Its level is raised in IgD myeloma and possibly in the Vogt-Koyanagi-Harada syndrome. In some systemic disorders, IgD antinuclear antibodies occur. It is a receptor for some antigens in B lymphocytes.

The complement system consists of a series of 18 proteins, mainly concentrated in a precursor, inactive form in the plasma. In contrast to antibody-mediated functions, the complement system acts immediately with acute inflammatory defenses once mucocutaneous barriers are interrupted. The complement system is divided into the "alternative pathway" (designated by C3, B, and D) and the "classical pathway" (designated by the capital letter C and a number 1 to 9). The alternative pathway promotes opsonization of lysis of microbes before the development of specific antibodies. Some microbes with sialic acid in their capsules (type III group B *Streptococcus*, *Neisseria meningitidis* [group band C], and *Escherichia coli*) do not activate the alternative pathway, a factor in their pathogenicity.

Only IgM and IgG can activate the classical pathway. Both pathways stimulate kinin-like activity, histamine release, chemotaxis, and neutrophil activation that result in microbial lysis.

Deficiencies in complement factors may lead to an increased susceptibility to infection. In conditions such as rheumatoid arthritis and systemic lupus erythematosus, there is excessive activation of complement pathways by physiologic mechanisms, which result in depressed levels of classical activity components in serum and synovial membranes.

MAJOR HISTOCOMPATIBILITY GENE COMPLEX

The major histocompatibility gene complex in humans consists of a cluster of genes on the short arm (6p21) of chromosome 6. (HLA is the abbreviation for this complex in humans; original studies were directed to leukocytes and HLA originally designated human or histocompatibility leukocyte antigens.) The products of these genes specify a set of antigenetically active proteins located on the surface of the cells. Every human inherits genetically unique cell surfaces and, when exposed to the cell surfaces of another individual, activates an immune response toward them. The major histocompatibility gene complex determines serologically defined antigens, generates and regulates immune responsiveness, and is associated with susceptibility or resistance to disease.

The human histocompatibility antigens are designated A, B, C, and D, and their gene loci are designated HLA-A, B, C, and D. There are 20 different allelic antigenic specifications at the HLA-A locus, about 30 at the HLA-B locus, and 6 at the HLA-C locus. These are designated HLA-A1, HLA-A3, HLA-B12, HLA-B27, HLA-C1, and the like. The HLA-D locus determines the structure of antigens that govern the mixed lymphocyte culture reactions. Eleven HLA-D locus types have been identified. There are other loci for complement and possibly other complexes.

Specific combinations of particular alleles at HLA-A, B, C, and D loci occur together on the same chromosome more frequently than expected by chance (genetic equilibrium). Thus in white individuals the HLA-A1, B8, Dw3 combination occurs much more frequently than

Table 23-1. HLA antigens and disorders with ocular abnormalities

Disorder	Antigen	Ocular disorder
Ankylosing spondylitis	B27	Uveitis
Reiter syndrome	B27	Conjunctivitis or iritis
Acute anterior uveitis	B27	Acute anterior uveitis
Pauciarticular juvenile arthritis	DR5	Uveitis, band-shaped keratopathy
Sjögren syndrome	B8, Dw3	Keratoconjunctivitis sicca
Behçet disease	B5	Ocular inflammation
Juvenile diabetes	DR4, DR3, DR2, Bf1	Ophthalmopathy
Graves' disease	B8, Dw3	Ophthalmopathy
Myasthenia gravis (without thyroma)	B8, Dw3	Ocular muscle weakness
Multiple sclerosis	DR2	Optic neuritis
Tuberculoid leprosy (Asians)	B8	Neuroparalytic keratopathy
Sympathetic ophthalmia	A11	Bilateral uveitis after injury
Birdshot retinochoroidopathy	A29	Bilateral uveitis after injury

Table 23-2. Some inflammatory mediators

Endogenous
  Plasma
    Complement cascade
    Clotting cascade
      Fibrinopeptides, fibrinolysis products
    Kinin system
      Bradykinin, kallikrein
  Tissues
    Vasoactive amines
      Histamine, heparin, serotonin
    Lysosomal products
      Proteases, cationic proteins
    Lymphokines
      Macrophage factors
      Chemotactic factors
      Mitogenic factor
      Skin reactive factor
    Arachidonic acid metabolites
      Prostaglandins, thromboxane, prostacyclin
      Slow-reacting substance of anaphylaxis
Exogenous
  Microbial products
    Endotoxin, bacterial chemotactic factor

predicted by gene frequencies of these alleles in the population. HLA-A and B influence cytotoxic T-cell specificity and might confer a selective survival advantage.

Susceptibility in many rheumatic disorders, especially sacroiliitis, spondylitis, and Reiter syndrome, is associated with HLA-B27 (Table 23-1). Only a few of those with the haplotype develop the disorder, and not all individuals with the disorder have the haplotype.

INFLAMMATION

Inflammation is the process by which the body tends to neutralize injury from microorganisms, foreign bodies, and physical and chemical irritants. It includes complex interaction between the immune, complement, vascular, hematopoietic, and kinin systems. It may be dominated by polymorphonuclear leukocytes or lymphocytic and mononuclear phagocytes. A variety of inflammatory mediators may be involved (Table 23-2).

Acute inflammation is the immediate vascular and cellular response to injury. Vasodilation, increased vascular permeability, and infiltration of leukocytes (initially neutrophils) may occur.

Chronic inflammation is a variable inflammatory response to injury. It is present as follows: (1) early in viral infection, (2) in the terminal stages of acute inflammation, and (3) as an interim in the development and resolution of granulomas. It may be related to delayed hypersensitivity (T cell-mediated hypersensitivity type IV). There may be extensive tissue necrosis mediated by macrophages stimulated by T cells or the direct action of T cells or K cells. Chronic inflammation is not always an immune response and may be stimulated by simple irritants such as small, inorganic particles.

Granulomatous inflammation consists mainly of mononuclear phagocytes. These are derived from monocytes in the circulating blood that, when in the tissues, are the source of macrophages, histiocytes, and in turn epithelial cells

Table 23-3. Immunologically mediated disorders

Type of hypersensitivity	Ocular disorder	Immune mechanism
Type I, anaphylactic	Hay fever conjunctivitis, vernal conjunctivitis, atrophy, giant papillary conjunctivitis in contact lens wearers, insect-bite reactions	IgE reacts with antigen, causing release of histamine and slow-reactive substance A from mast cells and basophils*
Type II, cytotoxic	Conjunctival cicatricial pemphigoid, Mooren ulcer, anti-tumor antibodies	IgG, IgM binds to antigen on target cell surface, promoting lysis or phagocytosis†
Type III, immune complex	Polyarteritis nodosa, scleritis, staphylococcal catarrhal ulcers, Wessely ring corneal stroma, arthus reaction, chlamydial infections, amyloidosis, serum sickness	Immune complexes (immunoglobulins + antigen) deposited in tissue to bind activated complement with release of lysosomal enzymes
Type IV, cell mediated	Corneal graft reactions, tuberculin skin hypersensitivity, sympathetic ophthalmia,‡ antiviral defense, phlyctenulosis, sarcoidosis	Sensitized T cells or macrophages react with tissue antigens

*Depleted suppressor T cells.
†Increased T-helper cells.
‡Possibly different hypersensitivity mechanisms at different stages.

and giant cells. The constituent macrophages of granulomas are replicated either rapidly or slowly. The granulomas function either to degrade or to sequester foreign substances.

Hypersensitivity is an overreaction or misdirection of the immune or inflammatory mechanism of the body to infection or antigenic stimulus (Table 23-3). Deposition of bacterial or viral antigens or the immune complexes within extraocular muscles induces orbital myositis, which has been described in Crohn disease. Autoimmunity describes the absence of tolerance of one's own cells so that an individual mounts an immune attack against himself. This is characteristic of lupus erythematosus and Sjögren symdrome, in which B- and T-cell immune responses are directed against DNA, salivary duct tissue, gastric parietal cells, and other cells.

Anaphylactic hypersensitivity (Type I or immediate type of hypersensitivity). Immune globulins of the IgE class are attached to surface receptors on mast cells. When IgE reacts with specific antigens, degranulation of mast cells with release of vasoactive amines results. Hay fever conjunctivitis is a typical reaction in

which there is massive edema in the conjunctiva. Vernal conjunctivitis and giant cell papillary conjunctivitis, in which basophils are also present, are caused by the immediate type of hypersensitivity.

Antibody-complement dependent reaction (Type II). In this hypersensitivity immune globulins are deposited in the basement membrane of mucous membrane. Helper T cells in the infiltrates are increased. A fixation and precipitation of complement or fixation without complement precipitation leads to separation of the epithelium from the substantia propria and to bullae formation. Cicatricial conjunctival pemphigoid is typical of Type II reactions.

Immune complex disease (Type III). This is a consequence of immune globulins combining with their antigen, followed by the deposition of the complex in vessel walls or connective tissues. *Staphylococcus* catarrhal keratitis and immune rings in the cornea may be caused by immune complex deposition. Fixation of complement by immune complexes results in chemotaxis or polymorphonuclear leukocytes and eosinophils. Polyarteritis nodosum, Wegener granulomatosis, and systemic vasculitis reflect complement fixation by immune complexes.

Delayed hypersensitivity T cell-mediated, cellular hypersensitivity (Type IV). In this immune reaction, effector cells with either T cells or macrophages react directly with antigens or produce lymphokines that produce the agents of the inflammatory response. T cells participate in corneal graft reaction, trachoma, and sympathetic ophthalmia.

BACTERIAL INFECTIONS

The bacterial kingdom Procaryotae is subdivided into 19 different parts based on the nature of the nucleoplasm, absences of membrane-bound cytoplasmic organelles, ribosomes of the 70S type, and a wide variety of metabolic mechanisms. Initial diagnosis of the causative organism in ocular infection is based on the Gram stain (Table 23-4).

Gram-positive organisms

Gram-positive cocci. This group includes two important families: the Micrococcaceae with the widespread genus *Staphylococcus*, and the Streptococcaceae with the genus *Streptococcus*, which has numerous species.

Staphylococci. The staphylococci are gram-positive, catalase-positive spherical cocci, often appearing in grapelike clusters in stained smears. Ocular scrapings, however, often show pairs and single cocci predominantly, together with many neutrophils. Three species are common: S *aureus*, S *epidermidis* (formerly *albus*), and S *saprophyticus*. Most strains of S *aureus* produce toxins as do occasional strains of S *epidermidis*. These two species are differentiated by the production of coagulase by S *aureus*, but noncoagulase-producing staphylococci may cause infection.

Staphylococci infection is common in chronic blepharitis, suppurative infection of the glands of Zeis (hordeolum or sty), and in infected chalazia. Staphylococcal catarrhal marginal ulcers of the cornea are a hypersensitivity reaction (Type III) to immune complexes of staphylococcal antigens or exotoxins.

Acute *Staphylococcus* conjunctivitis is less common than that caused by the *Streptococcus* and *Haemophilus* genera. Most staphylococci found in hospitals produce a penicillinase that inactivates benzyl-penicillin, phenoxy-methyl-penicillin, and ampicillin. Most nonhospital strains, however, are nonpenicillinase-producing.

Bacitracin, erythromycin, and sulfisoxazole (Gantrisin) ointments are the most useful for eyelid infections. Tetracycline (which is secreted into oil glands) is used systemically in recalcitrant infections, particularly those associated with rosacea.

Streptococci. The streptococci are gram-positive, nonmotile, spherical, ovoid, or lancet-shaped cocci, often occurring in pairs or chains. Streptococci are classified according to three schemes that overlap. Physiologically, streptococci are divided into pyogenic, viridans, lactic, and enterococcal divisions. Strains that completely hemolyze red blood cells surrounding their colonies are β-hemolytic, those that produce partial hemolysis are α-hemolytic, and those that do not hemolyze are λ-hemolytic. The Lancefield groups divide streptococci on the basis of serologically active carbohydrates. Mainly, α-hemolytic streptococci strains are not groupable serologically, but physiologically represent viridans streptococci, a cause of subacute bacterial endocarditis. β-hemolytic streptococci are pyogenic, and each belongs to a Lancefield group. Group A streptococci (β-hemolytic, St *pyogenes*) cause pharyngitis, septicemia, conjunctivitis, keratitis, rheumatic fever, and acute glomerulonephritis. Group B causes puerperal and neonatal infection, and group D causes endocarditis, urinary tract infections, and intra-abdominal inflammation (group D organisms may or may not cause hemolysis).

Streptococci may cause a pseudomembranous conjunctivitis with a tendency for corneal extension. Stromal abscess, infiltration, and ulceration may be associated with hypopyon. Diagnosis is based on culture because chain formation does not commonly occur in ocular infections. Gram stains of the organism may be confused with staphylococci.

Rheumatic fever rarely causes ocular manifestations. Glomerulonephritis caused by streptococci manifests itself in the eye only in the changes of vascular hypertension. Scarlet fever has no ocular signs except the occasional occurrence of ecchymoses and petechiae in severely ill patients after the rash appears.

Erysipelas is a recurrent, acute, hemolytic

streptococcal infection of the skin of mid-dleaged and elderly persons, usually involving the face and head. As a rule, the lesion spreads from a central focus to involve adjacent areas, which become red, glistening, swollen, and sometimes versicolored. The skin of the eyelids may be involved.

Streptococcus pneumoniae (pneumococci) are gram-positive oval- or coccal-shaped organisms that generally have tapered ends (lance-shaped) and grow in pairs. The organism is a common cause of corneal ulcers, with the lacrimal sac serving as a reservoir in chronic dacryocystitis. Pneumococcus causes a mild, acute

Table 23-4. Gram-stain of some bacteria that may cause ocular disease

Gram-positive bacteria
  Family I. Micrococcaceae
    Genus I. *Micrococcus,* sp. *luteus* (conjunctivitis)
    Genus II. *Staphylococcus,* sp. *aureus* (sty, blepharitis, conjunctivitis, keratitis, panophthalmitis); *epidermidis* (conjunctivitis and endophthalmitis)
  Family II. Streptococcaceae
    Genus I. *Streptococcus* (21 sp.), sp. *pyogenes* (conjunctivitis); *pneumoniae* (acute hypopyon keratitis, dacryocystitis); *anginosus* (beta-hemolytic streptococcus) (pseudomembranous conjunctivitis, acute hypopyon keratitis, uveitis?)
  Actinomycetes and related organisms (nonsporeforming, nonfilamentous rods)
  Coryneform group (unresolved classification problems)
    Genus I. *Corynebacterium,* sp. *diphtheriae* (membranous conjunctivitis with necrosis, postdiphtheritic paralysis [N VI and accommodation N III]); *xerosis* (in foamy secretion from inner canthus in the elderly)
  Family I. Actinomycetaceae
    Genus I. *Actinomyces,* sp. *israelii* (dacryocanaliculitis)
  Family II. Mycobacteriaceae (acid fast)
    Genus I. *Mycobacterium,* sp. *tuberculosis* (uveitis, lupus vulgaris, phlyctenules, periphlebitis); *leprae* (anterior uveitis and keratitis [lepromatous: cutaneous], ocular muscle paralysis [tuberculoid: neural])
  Family VI. Nocardiaceae
    Genus I. *Nocardia,* sp. *asteroides* (Leptothrix) (chorioretinal abscess in immune suppression, keratitis, conjunctivitis, cat-scratch fever)
Gram-negative bacteria
  Aerobic rods and cocci
    Family I. Pseudomonadaceae
    Genus I. *Pseudomonas,* sp. *aeruginosa* (necrotic keratitis)
    Uncertain genera
      Genus *Brucella,* sp. *melitensis* (goats); *abortus* (cows); *suis* (sows); *ovis* (sheep); *canis* (dogs) (uveitis? keratitis nummularis [coin-shaped]? optic neuritis?)
      Genus *Bordetella,* sp. *pertussis* (subconjunctival and retinal hemorrhages)
      Genus *Francisella,* sp. *tularensis* (necrotic conjunctival ulcer [Parinaud syndrome])
  Facultatively anaerobic rods
    Family I. Enterobacteriaceae
      Genus I. *Escherichia* (keratitis, panophthalmitis)
      Genus IV. *Salmonella* (iritis, keratitis, panophthalmitis)
      Genus VI. *Klebsiella* (keratitis, panophthalmitis)
      Genus X. *Proteus* (keratitis, panophthalmitis)
      Genus XI. *Yersinia,* sp. *pestis* (hemorrhagic chemosis)
    Uncertain genera
      Genus *Haemophilus,* sp. *influenzae* (conjunctivitis, orbital abscess in children); uncertain species: aegyptius (Koch-Weeks) (conjunctivitis)
  Cocci and coccobacilli
    Family I. Neisseriaceae
      Genus I. *Neisseria,* sp. *gonorrhoeae* (ophthalmia neonatorum and, in adults, purulent conjunctivitis); *meningitidis* (petechiae, ecchymosis, panophthalmitis); *sicca* (conjunctivitis)
      Genus III. *Moraxella,* sp. *lacunata; nonliquefaciens* (indolent ulcer, conjunctivitis)
      Genus IV. *Acinetobacter* (endophthalmitis, conjunctivitis) (Tribe Mimeae, sp. *polymorpha* obsolete)
  Endospore-forming rods and cocci
    Family I. Bacillaceae
      Genus I. *Bacillus,* sp. *subtilis* (surgical contaminant, panophthalmitis); *anthracis* (necrotic ulcer of eyelids)
      Genus III. *Clostridium* (300 sp.), sp. *botulinum* (paralysis N III, IV, VI); *tetani* (miosis, orbicularis oculi spasm)

conjunctivitis, usually in children, and is rarely associated with chronic disease.

Gram-negative organisms

Gram-negative organisms include aerobic rods and cocci of the family Pseudomonadaceae and uncertain genera, including *Brucella, Bordetella pertussis,* and *Francisella tularensis.* A large group of gram-negative facultatively anaerobic rods include those of the family Enterobacteriaceae with genera of *Escherichia, Salmonella, Klebsiella, Proteus, Yersinia,* and an uncertain genus *Haemophilus.* Neisseriaceae is the major family of gram-negative cocci and coccobacilli that includes the genera *Neisseria, Moraxella,* and *Acinetobacter (mima polymorpha).*

Pseudomonas. The pseudomonas are aerobic, gram-negative, mobile bacilli. At least 29 species are characterized, of which *P aeruginosa* causes the greatest morbidity. It produces endotoxin and proteases that inactivate complement, exotoxin A that inactivates macrophages and promotes cellular damage and tissue invasion. It occurs wherever there is moisture, is resistant to disinfectants and antimicrobial agents, and is nearly ubiquitous in the hospital environment. Its proteolytic enzymes cause a devastating liquefaction of the cornea. Less commonly, as a surgical contaminant that causes panophthalmitis. Tobramycin, gentamicin, amikacin, carbenicillin, polymyxin B, and colistin are inhibitory drugs.

Haemophilus influenzae. This is a gram-negative aerobic and facultative anaerobic coccobacillus- to rod-shaped organism that requires blood NADH for culture. It causes pneumonia, meningitis, and acute orbital inflammation in infants, usually by extension from a paranasal sinus. It may cause conjunctivitis. Some strains are resistant to parenteral penicillin and ampicillin, and patients with meningitis require simultaneous administration of chloramphenicol until sensitivity of the organism to ampicillin is established.

Haemophilus aegyptius (Koch-Weeks bacillus) causes acute or subacute conjunctivitis in tropical countries.

Neisseria and Branhamella. These genera include two important disease-producing species, *N gonorrhoeae* and *N meningitidis. Branhamella catarrhalis* and *B sicca* are generally non-

pathogenic, but may cause conjunctivitis. The genera *Moraxella* and *Acinetobacter* closely resemble *Neisseria,* but can produce rods in contrast to both *Neisseria* and *Branhamella,* which produce only cocci. Both gonococci and meningococci produce a protease for IgA, the major immune globulin of the conjunctiva.

Neisseria. This genus includes two disease-producing species, *N gonorrhoeae* and *N meningitidis.*

Neisseria gonorrhoeae. These are nonmotile, catalase- and oxidase-positive, aerobic, gram-negative cocci, which are often arranged in pairs with flattened adjacent surfaces. Pathogenic types 1 and 2 adhere to mucous membranes by means of pili and may infect the urethra, anal canal, endocervix, pharynx, and conjunctiva.

Gonorrheal conjunctivitis is a purulent inflammation of the conjunctiva (see purulent conjunctivitis) that has an incubation period of 2 to 5 days. It is a major cause of blindness, particularly in the Middle East, where it complicates trachoma. After an incubation period of 3 to 5 days, patients develop a serous discharge that quickly becomes purulent. Extreme conjunctival chemosis and periorbital edema prevent drainage of pus. The central cornea may perforate, resulting in panophthalmitis or corneal scarring.

Ophthalmia neonatorum is the term applied to any conjunctival inflammation occurring during the first 10 days of life. The most common causes in the United States are *Chlamydia trachomatis* (inclusion conjunctivitis), *Streptococcus pneumoniae, Neisseria gonorrhoeae,* and species of the *Haemophilus* genus.

Gonorrheal conjunctivitis in the adult must be treated promptly. Gram staining permits identification of the gram-negative intracellular diplococcus 48 hours before the results of cultures are available.

Gonococcemia is the most common complication of genitourinary infection. It occurs soon after infection or later during menstruation. There is fever, polyarthralgia affecting the knees, wrists, and ankles, and skin lesions varying from petechiae to necrosis. There may be a catarrhal conjunctivitis or a severe acute iridocyclitis. Reiter syndrome (urethritis, arthritis, and ocular inflammation) is a more likely cause of this triad than gonorrhea, particularly in patients with histocompatibility antigen HLA-B27. Gonococcemia is diagnosed by culture or specific immunofluorescent antibody staining of blood, cerebrospinal fluid, synovial fluid or skin lesions.

Neisseria meningitidis. This gram-negative aerobic and facultative anaerobic organism appears as a biscuit-shaped diplococcus. They are antigenically divided into the A, B, C, D, X, Y, and Z groups. Their natural habitat is the human nasopharynx, and they cause meningitis and bacteremia in susceptible individuals.

Ocular involvement during meningococcemia consists of conjunctival petechiae and ecchymosis. A purulent conjunctivitis may occur. Intraocular embolization may cause a panophthalmitis that requires prompt treatment to prevent shrinkage of the globe (phthisis bulbi). Meningitis may be associated with ocular muscle paralysis and optic nerve inflammation. The organism may cause a purulent conjunctivitis in the absence of systemic infection that is distinguished from the gonococcus by its cultural characteristics.

Acid-fast organisms

Mycobacterium. The genus *Mycobacterium* causes a number of chronic infectious granulomas in humans and animals. There are a number of nonpathogenic species. The most important human diseases caused by members of the genus are tuberculosis and leprosy.

Mycobacterium tuberculosis. This is a nonmotile, encapsulated rod that stains with difficulty, but once stained resists decolorization with strong mineral acids (acid-fast). Human and bovine varieties are pathogenic for humans, whereas murine and piscine varieties cause tuberculosis in rodents and fish but not in humans. The avian (bird) variety rarely causes human disease.

The clinical and pathologic changes of tuberculosis depend on the tissue involved and the degree of hypersensitivity of the host. Generally, the initial or primary lesion is an asymptomatic process, healing or progressing in a short time, and characterized by an inconspicuous parenchymal lesion and tissue necrosis (caseation) of the draining lymph nodes. During this period there is lymphohematogenous dissemination of the entire body. The development of cellular immunity (hypersensitivity type IV) stops the primary process and in most people the infection remains quiescent.

After a variable period of latency, hematogenous spread of the organism may cause a reaction (tuberculosis). The disease in a tuberculin-sensitive (infected) individual is more chronic than the primary type. There is severe parenchymal involvement and a minor effect on the regional lymph nodes.

As might be expected, inflammations of every portion of the eye and the adnexa have been attributed to tuberculosis. Because of the specific therapy now available, these disorders are uncommon.

The skin of the eyelids may be infected in lupus vulgaris or, more rarely, in other cutaneous manifestations of tuberculosis, each of which may spread to the conjunctiva and the cornea.

Phlyctenular disease involves the conjunctiva and the cornea. In many instances it appears to be a cell-mediated reaction to tuberculoprotein (tuberculin) or other antigens and is responsive to local instillation of corticosteroids.

Previously, chronic uveitis was often thought to be caused by tuberculosis when it occurred in an individual who was hypersensitive to tuberculin. The iridocyclitis causes mutton-fat keratic precipitates, minute nodules at the pupillary margin (Koeppe nodules), and posterior synechiae. Choroiditis destroys the adjacent retina, and inflammatory cells are released into the vitreous body. A posterior subcapsular cataract frequently develops.

Retinal periphlebitis may be complicated by neovascularization and recurrent vitreous hemorrhage. Photocoagulation of the surrounding area of periphlebitis is used to destroy new blood vessels. Vitrectomy may be used to remove unabsorbed blood.

Leprosy (Hansen disease). This disease is caused by an acid-fast rod, *Mycobacterium leprae,* similar to the agent that causes tuberculosis. There are about fifteen million cases throughout the world, and about one third of the patients have ocular complications. The infection predominantly involves the skin, superficial nerves, nose, and throat. It occurs as two principal types: (1) the lepromatous (LL, cutaneous), with depressed cellular immunity and frequent ocular involvement, and (2) the tuberculoid (TT, neural), with systemic immunity and ocular complications caused by neuroparalytic keratopathy.

The eyes are affected late in the course of the lepromatous type of disease. There may be an initial superficial infection and conjunctivitis, episcleritis, or keratitis. An insidious chronic iritis and granuloma formation cause loss of vision. Eventually, complicated cataract and ocular atrophy occur. Involvement of the skin of the brows causes alopecia of the eyebrows. Facial nerve paralysis causes ectropion of the lower eyelids and weakness in elevation of the eyebrows.

The spirochetes

Treponema pallidum. This spirochete causes acquired syphilis, usually by direct body contact. Congenital syphilis is transferred through the placenta of a pregnant syphilitic mother. Ocular involvement is seen in untreated or inadequately treated patients. Undetected syphilis is the more frequent cause of ocular inflammation. It must be considered in every instance of chronic ocular infection of unknown cause.

Acquired syphilis. Untreated acquired syphilis is divided into primary, secondary, and tertiary stages. The primary and secondary stages are infectious. The iris and the ciliary body are inflamed early in the secondary stage and late in the tertiary stage. A severe iridocyclitis is associated with a skin rash and occurs in the fourth to the sixth month after the chancre. Broad, flat posterior synechiae occur between the stromal layer of the iris and the lens.

The tertiary stage of syphilis occurs 10 or more years after the chancre, or it may never occur. It is characterized by a small number of organisms, extensive parenchymal destruction, gumma formation, and connective tissue proliferation.

Tabes dorsalis is a degenerative disease of the central nervous system characterized by signs of involvement of the posterior columns of the spinal cord and the cranial nerves. Ataxia is common, as is posterior root pain, with paroxysmal attacks at night involving the legs, abdomen, arms, and face. Slight inequality in size of the pupils and a sluggish reaction may be the only signs. Argyll Robertson pupils are diagnostic of tabes dorsalis.

Congenital syphilis. Congenital syphilis is an infection caused by *Treponema pallidum*. The infection is acquired in utero and is characterized by diffuse systemic involvement without a primary lesion. Symptoms are usually present 2 to 6 weeks after birth, but fatal lesions resembling pemphigus may be present at birth. A severe, persistent rhinitis usually develops, followed in a week by a maculopapular skin eruption. The infant's general nutrition suffers, and he is thin, snuffling, and irritable.

The clinical signs of congenital syphilis appear at puberty. The Hutchinson triad includes (1) pegged secondary dentition, particularly notching of the upper central incisors, (2) nerve-type deafness, and (3) interstitial keratitis. Other signs are collapse of the bridge of the nose as a result of necrosis of the nasal septum from syphilitic rhinitis, splenomegaly, lymphadenopathy involving the epitrochlear nodes, saber tibia, and exostosis of the tibia and the cranial bones.

Syphilitic interstitial keratitis is an inflammation of the corneal stroma that occurs with an associated anterior uveitis. The disease, which affects boys predominantly (61%), occurs between 5 and 20 years of age. It begins with anterior uveitis and corneal endothelial edema. After about 2 or 3 weeks there is acute pain, photophobia, and lacrimation. All corneal layers are affected with corneal edema and cellular infiltration of the stroma. This stage of the disease is usually short and is followed by vascular invasion of the cornea from the periphery. The invading vessels, which appear to be pushing the haze in front of them, ultimately meet to form a "salmon patch." As soon as the vessels meet, symptoms and inflammation subside. When healing is complete, faint gray lines of empty blood vessels (ghost vessels) persist in the cornea. There may be late degenerative changes, with band keratopathy, keratoconus, or secondary glaucoma. In many instances a penetrating corneal transplant will restore useful vision in healed syphilitic interstitial keratitis.

The rickettsias

This part of obligate intracellular parasites contains a large order, the Rickettsiales, and a small order, the Chlamydiales (Table 23-5).

Table 23-5. The rickettsias

Order I. Rickettsiales
 Family I. Rickettsiaceae
  Genus *Rickettsia*, sp. *prowazekii* (epidemic thyphus
   and Brill disease); *rickettsii* (spotted fever); *mooseri*
   (murine typhus)
Order II. Chlamydiales
 Family I. Chlamydiaceae
  Genus *Chlamydia*, sp. *trachomatis, psittaci*

The Rickettsiales have three families and many members. The Chlamydiales have one family and two members. All are gram-negative organisms that can multiply only within living cells. Except for epidemic typhus, in which the natural cycle is humans and lice, all other Rickettsiales have an insect vector and animal host. Chlamydiales are parasites of humans and birds that are transmitted on contact.

Rickettsiales. These organisms are transmitted by various anthropods to humans and cause an acute febrile illness and usually a skin rash. Vaccines have been prepared against some of the microorganisms, and the tetracyclines (doxocycline or minocycline) and chloramphenicol are effective therapeutically.

The ocular changes caused by infections with this family have been best described in epidemic louse-borne typhus fever (*Rickettsia prowazekii* transmitted by the human louse, *Pediculus humanus*) and Rocky Mountain spotted fever (*Rickettsia rickettsii* transmitted by animal ticks). At the onset of the disease, conjunctival hyperemia may occur, sometimes with subconjunctival hemorrhages. Marked retinal venous engorgement with edema of the optic disk and retina may occur during the second and third weeks of the fever. Venous engorgement may be severe enough to cause a retinal hemorrhage, which may rupture into the vitreous body. Cotton-wool spots and arterial occlusion may be observed.

The diagnosis of rickettsial disease depends on clinical signs in an area where the diseases are endemic.

Chlamydiales. This order has only one genus, *Chlamydia*, divided into two species, *C trachomatis* and *C psittaci*. *C trachomatis* infects the epithelial cells of the cornea, conjunctiva, pulmonary tract, urethra, and cervix of humans. *Chlamydia psittaci* infects birds and causes pneumonia in humans.

All species of *Chlamydia* have an antigen detectable by complement-fixation tests. Immunofluorescence tests for antigens and antibodies indicate that genital isolates are generally antigenic groups D to K, and ocular isolates in trachoma areas are generally antigenic groups A, B, Ba, and C. Lymphogranuloma venereum is caused by immunotypes L_1, L_2, and L_3.

The infective particle, the elementary body, enters an epithelial cell by phagocytosis. These fragile reticulate bodies are responsible for intracellular replication that develops into a crescent-shaped mass of resilient elementary bodies (inclusion bodies) that stain with specific immunofluorescence. Further multiplication ruptures the cell, and the elementary bodies are transmitted from one host cell to another.

Trachoma. Trachoma is a chronic follicular conjunctivitis caused by *C trachomatis*, which affects the upper eyelid and causes conjunctival and corneal cicatrization with blindness. The disease, which has been recognized since antiquity, affects 400 million people, 20 million are blinded. In the United States, it is prevalent mainly in Indians in the Southwest. Rural children are infected, and the combination of poverty, flies, lack of water, heat, crowding, and dust causes severe infection. Conjunctival scarring leads to distorted eyelids, which scar the cornea and cause blindness.

Communicable ophthalmia is a mixed infection in which a chronic conjunctival inflammation caused by trachoma is combined with a chronic bacterial purulent conjunctivitis. Flies transfer the infection from one child to another, and the disease becomes recurrent.

Inclusion conjunctivitis. This conjunctivitis is caused by *Chlamydia trachomatis*, which causes a urethritis in men and an asymptomatic cervicitis in women. It is a common sexually transmitted infection of the adult genital tract. Adult inclusion conjunctivitis is transmitted to the eye by fingers and fomites and occasionally by the water in swimming pools ("swimming pool conjunctivitis"). The neonate is infected during passage through the birth canal. The conjunctivitis is purulent in the newborn and muocopurulent and follicular in the adult.

Typical inclusion conjunctivitis in the neonate develops as a purulent conjunctivitis 5 to 14 days after birth. There is eyelid and conjunctival swelling, purulent discharge, and conjunctival hyperemia. The untreated disease persists 3 to 12 months and usually heals without sequelae, although there may be mild tarsal conjunctival scarring and superficial corneal neovascularization. The neonatal infection may be prevented by conjunctival instillation of erythromycin ointment at birth. It is not prevented by silver nitrate (Credé) prophylaxis. Treatment in the neonate consists of administration of tetracycline topically and erythromycin systemically for 6 weeks. The mother should be treated for cervicitis and the father for urethritis even if asymptomatic (see below.)

Adult inclusion conjunctivitis is an acute follicular inflammation with preauricular adenopathy. The follicles, unlike those of trachoma, are more marked in the lower eyelid and do not contain follicular material. Untreated, the disease may continue for months and cause corneal neovascularization and marginal infiltrates. The genitourinary tract serves as a reservoir for the infection. Treatment is by means of topically applied tetracycline ointment or drops and systemic tetracycline. Systemic erythromycin should be substituted for tetracycline in children whose permanent teeth have not erupted, in pregnant women, and in nursing mothers.

Lymphogranuloma venereum. Lymphogranuloma venereum is a contagious venereal disease manifested initially be a vesicle that bursts, leaving a grayish ulcer, followed by regional lymphadenitis that is frequently suppurative. Mild to severe constitutional signs may be present during the stage of adenitis.

Primary infection of the eyelid, occurring venereally or through accidental contamination in a laboratory worker causes an ulcerative lesion of the eyelid or conjunctiva and preauricular adenopathy (Parinaud oculoglandular syndrome). Hematogenous spread of the disease may cause uveitis, keratouveitis, or sclerokeratitis.

MYCOTIC INFECTIONS

Fungi are single-celled dimorphic (growth in two different forms in different environments) organisms characterized by the formation of mycelial filaments (hyphae) and the production of spores.

Oculomycosis is caused by many organisms that are opportunistic pathogens. The most severe fungal infections may occur in patients with no apparent immune deficiency. Fungi previously considered nonpathogenic may infect the immune-compromised individual. Trauma is a factor in more than one half of cases.

Fungi infect the eye and its adnexae in four main ways: (1) superficially to produce conjunctivitis, keratitis, and lacrimal obstruction; (2) by extension from infection in neighboring skin, paranasal sinuses, or the nasopharynx; (3) by direct intraocular introduction during surgery or by accidental penetrating trauma, particularly with plant material; or (4) by hematogenous or lymphatogenous routes in patients with pulmonary, cutaneous, or generalized mycosis.

Presumed ocular histoplasmosis is considered a common cause of uveitis. *Candida* endophthalmitis may develop in patients with indwelling catheters who receive antibiotics for a long time. Fungal, viral, bacterial, and protozoal infections may develop in immune-suppressed patients.

Superficial infection. Fungi may be introduced into the cornea by an epithelial abrasion or a foreign body, frequently consisting of vegetable matter. Instillation of corticosteroids reduces tissue resistance to infection. A fluffy white spot of inflammatory cells first appears in the anterior stroma and, with necrosis, melts into a shallow ulcer with a sterile hypopyon. There may be satellite stromal lesions. There is severe ciliary and conjunctival injection, but corneal neovascularization is absent or occurs later. The necrosis gradually involves the entire cornea, which may perforate.

The main causative organisms are *Fusarium*, *Aspergillus*, and *Candida*. Other causative fungi include *Acremonium (Cephalosporium)*, *Penicillium*, and *Coccidioides immitis*. Treatment is by local and systemic antifungal agents. Medical therapy is frequently not effective, and the cornea does not heal until covered with a conjunctival flap.

A fungus conjunctival inflammation usually occurs secondary to keratitis. In tropical areas, *Rhinosporidium* may produce polyps of the conjunctiva.

Unilateral, persistent tearing with patent lacrimal passages characterizes infections of the canaliculus. The lower canaliculus is usually involved. The punctum is dilated, and its margins elevated and inflamed. There is tearing and itching with a slight conjunctivitis medially. Diagnosis is commonly not made until a lacrimal probe grates against concretions of hardened colonies of fungi in the involved canaliculus.

The skin of the eyelids may be involved by any of the fungi that cause a dermatomycosis. Extension of fungus infection into the orbit may cause a cellulitis or, because of involvement of the optic nerve, a retrobulbar neuritis. Some inflammatory granulomas of the orbit may also be caused by fungi.

Intraocular infection. Fungal endophthalmitis after intraocular surgery occurs because of fungal contamination from the air in the operating room, from the surgical instruments and solutions, or from the conjunctival sac and eyelids of the patient. Mucormycosis extends directly from the nasal pharynx in debilitated patients who have ketoacidosis.

A variety of fungal infections of the uvea and retina are seen in patients with immune suppression after organ transplant. Fungal endophthalmitis has an incubation period of several weeks to several months and follows an indolent course. The anterior vitreous and uvea are predominantly involved. The aqueous humor is clouded with inflammatory cells, and a hypopyon may be present. Small gray-green areas or white infiltrates resembling small balls of cotton are present in the anterior vitreous. The pupils gradually fill with an inflammatory mass, and the vitreous humor is converted to a granuloma. The therapeutic effect of antifungal agents is variable and unpredictable. Removal of the vitreous humor by vitrectomy may save the eye by reducing the number of organisms and inflammatory cells present and permitting increased penetration of drugs.

Slow, indolent progression distinguishes mycotic endophthalmitis from bacterial endophthalmitis.

Rhino-orbitocerebral phycomycosis. This is a rapidly lethal infection caused by fungi such as *Mucor, Basidiobolus, Mortierella,* and *Rhizopus.* The nose or nasopharynx is the usual route of entry. The infection occurs in debilitated individuals with ketoacidosis, who develop facial swelling, proptosis, eyelid edema,

and total ophthalmoplegia and blindness. Coma develops, and death occurs within 1 week. Mucormycosis occurs in adults with diabetes mellitus, whereas the other species may be the cause in debilitated infants and children. The infection occurs in individuals with severe underlying disease, commonly diabetes with ketoacidosis, or leukemia, carcinomatosis, or bacterial infection. The inhaled spores initially cause a nasopharyngitis with infarction of vessels to the skin that causes a black, ulcerated eschar on the skin, palate, or nasal mucous membrane. Visual loss, proptosis, and ophthalmoplegia occur. Facial or orbital pain in a susceptible individual or coma in a diabetic patient that does not respond to metabolic correction are important signs. Treatment consists of systemic antifungals and antibacterials, extensive surgical debridement, and correction of acidosis.

Many fungi may cause a choroiditis or retinitis in patients receiving corticosteroids and immunosuppressive agents to suppress graft rejection. *Aspergillus* and *Candida* are the most commonly involved causal organisms. More uncommon are *Nocardia, Coccidioides,* and others. Men are more commonly affected than women. An unrelated renal donor, increasing age, and leukopenia all predispose the individual to infection. Ocular involvement is not severe, and attention may be directed to the eyes because of decreased vision. The mild chorioretinitis causes minimal cellular reaction, and there is little tendency for extension.

Hematogenous *Candida* endophthalmitis may follow antibiotic therapy, immunosuppressive therapy, cardiac and abdominal surgery, use of intravenous catheters, and drug abuse. The organisms may be in the bloodstream without causing parenchymal involvement, and treatment is not required. Sometimes systemic *Candida* may be diagnosed by a chorioretinitis, which reflects an underlying systemic candidiasis. The chorioretinitis consists of many white, fluffy, circumscribed exudates with a filamentous border located in the choroid and retina and extending into the vitreous. Additional ocular lesions include retinal hemorrhage, hypopyon, iritis, papillitis, and ciliary body abscess. Patients may be asymptomatic or have loss of vision, pain, and redness. The histologic lesion is a combination of suppurative and

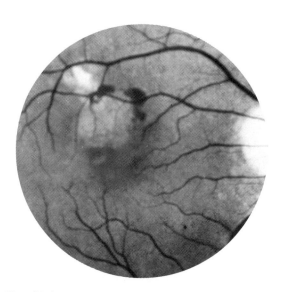

Fig. 23-1. Central retinal lesion of presumed ocular histoplasmosis in a 61-year-old woman in whom the lesion was inactive for many years. The dark material above is intraretinal blood; the inferior darkish material is greenish on ophthalmoscopy and constitutes subretinal neovascularization. The whitish area is retinal edema.

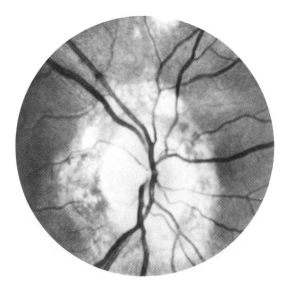

Fig. 23-2. Peripapillary chorioretinitis and the punched-out atrophic lesion (above) of presumed histoplasmosis syndrome in a 33-year-old woman.

granulomatous inflammation that begins in the choroid and extends into the retinal pigment epithelium and overlying retina. Antifungal agents are used to treat patients with ocular or systemic *Candida* infections, but patients with candidemia only are not treated.

Presumed ocular histoplasmosis. Histoplasmosis is a mild to lethal systemic disease caused by *Histoplasma capsulatum*. It manifests itself mainly as an asymptomatic acute primary respiratory tract infection or rarely as a chronic pulmonary disease with cavitation that resembles tuberculosis. Uncommonly the disease is disseminated, with widespread systemic involvement. Infection is common in rural dwellers of the Mississippi Valley and the great river valleys of South America, Africa, and Asia, but it is rare in Europe. The fungus is common in soil contaminated with bird droppings.

The presumed ocular histoplasmosis syndrome consists of a subretinal neovascular membrane in the region of the fovea centralis and atrophic areas of chorioretinal atrophy that follow chorioretinitis adjacent to the optic disk (peripapillary) and in the peripheral fundus. The lesions do not occur in patients with clinically systemic histoplasmosis, but affected individuals have a skin hypersensitivity to histoplasmosis. The organism has never been identified in the eye, but all laboratory tests suggest that the syndrome is associated with histoplasmosis, most likely on a hypersensitive rather than infectious basis.

The areas of chorioretinal atrophy ("histo spots") develop after disseminated chorioretinitis, usually in the second and third decades of life. The peripheral and peripapillary lesions remain quiescent. An atrophic spot in the region of the fovea centralis may develop a subretinal neovascular membrane 10 to 20 years later. Progression of the membrane destroys the fovea centralis. Without treatment, the neovascular membrane involutes in about 2 years.

The triad of presumed ocular histoplasmosis consists of a lesion of the central retina (Fig. 23-1) combined with a healed (usually) chorioretinitis adjacent to the optic disk and a peripheral atrophic area ("histo spots") (Fig. 23-2).

The chorioretinal lesions vary in size from a minute dot to an area as large as the optic disk.

Initially, these appear as yellowish-orange oval or circular areas having indistinct, soft borders. The inflammation may disappear or progress, and areas of different degrees of activity are seen in different parts of the eye. There are no inflammatory cells in the vitreous, and the inflammation may develop over a period of months.

The central retinal lesion is heralded by a collection of fluid between the choriocapillaris of the choroid and the Bruch membrane that causes a metamorphopsia with little or no decrease of visual acuity. The neovascular membrane appears as a dark, greenish-gray, circular or oval area. Frank bleeding occurs in the subretinal space and breaks into the sensory retina, often in a crescentic hemorrhage at the periphery of the lesions. Blood eventually spreads out into the sensory retina, causing loss of vision. The lesion eventually becomes inactive, with a hypertrophic pigmented scar. About half of the eyes have vision of less than 20/200.

Involvement of the peripheral retina may not be diagnosed. Most attention is directed to the central lesion, which impairs vision. The lesions adjacent to the optic disk and peripheral lesions may develop subretinal neovascular membranes.

Treatment is unsatisfactory. Complete destruction of the neovascular network by means of photocoagulation arrests the central lesion. Incomplete destruction does not stop the progress of the membrane toward the fovea centralis. Photocoagulation cannot be directed to new blood vessels beneath the fovea centralis because it destroys the overlying retina. Amphotericin B used effectively in progressive disseminated histoplasmosis is ineffective in presumed ocular histoplasmosis.

VIRAL INFECTIONS

Viruses (Table 23-6) are intracellular parasites that infect and cause disease in all living organisms. Human viruses, which range in size from 17 nm (picornavirus) to 300 nm (poxvirus), demonstrate marked species and organ specificity. They contain macromolecular cores of either ribonucleic acid (RNA) or deoxyribonucleic acid (DNA) that are necessary for transcription of genetic information. Virus absorption to a cell surface is through specific carboxyl and sulfhydryl chemical groups. The vi-

rus enters the cell by pinocytosis and loses its protective covering. Thereafter, it depends on its host cell for all or a portion of its enzymatic requirements. The virus may remain latent in the cell without causing any sign, or it may be stimulated into replication by a physiologic, biochemical, or environmental change or trauma.

After the virus enters a susceptible cell, the cell nucleus is stimulated to produce interferon, which is released through the cell wall. The interferon enters other cells and stimulates them to release a transitional inhibitory protein that binds to cellular ribosomes and alters them in such a way that any virus DNA or RNA entering the cell is not translated, thus preventing the virus from replicating. Virus multiplication activates B and T lymphocytes; macrophages and polymorphonuclear leukocytes migrate to the area, producing inflammation. The proteins of the virus capsid stimulate B lymphocytes and T lymphocytes. The immune globulins of plasma cells prevent infection by viruses before they enter cells. Activated T lymphocytes release lymphokines that attract T lymphocytes, macrophages, and other factors of the cell-mediated inflammatory process. In herpes virus disease, cell-mediated immunity is the most important means of defense.

Virus diseases associated with petechial hemorrhages may cause subconjunctival hemorrhage or ecchymosis of the eyelids. Iridocyclitis may occur with any viremia but may go undiagnosed because of the mildness of the iridocyclitis and the severity of the systemic disease. Viruses affecting the skin, such as the virus of warts may involve the eyelid margin and cause a secondary chronic conjunctivitis or keratitis. Respiratory tract viruses may migrate through the nasolacrimal passages to cause conjunctivitis or keratoconjunctivitis. Viruses that affect the mucous membranes, such as herpes simplex, infect the conjunctiva and corneal epithelium. Viruses that affect the central nervous system may interfere with the motor nerves to the eyes and cause extraocular muscle palsies. Virus infections may cause an optic neuritis or papillitis.

The adenoviruses and herpesviruses infecting the conjunctiva and cornea may be cultured by swabbing the conjunctiva or cornea with a

Table 23-6. Virus disease and the eye

Generic name and nucleic acid	Prototype virus	Systemic disease	Ocular disease
Herpesvirus (DNA)	*Herpesvirus hominis*		
	Type 1	Rarely encephalitis	Keratitis, blepharitis, retinitis
	Type 2	Genital warts; encephalitis	Rarely keratitis
	Varicella-zoster	Chickenpox (children)	Vesicles of eyelids, conjunctiva
		Zoster (adults)	Ophthalmic zoster: keratitis, uveitis, episcleritis, muscle palsies
	Epstein-Barr	Infectious mononucleosis	Conjunctivitis; uveitis; optic neuritis; dacryoadenitis
		Burkitt lymphoma	Orbital metastasis
	Cytomegalovirus	Brain damage	Necrotizing retinitis
Adenovirus (DNA)	Types 1, 2, 3, and 5	Respiratory tract disease	None
(31 human and 17 animal serotypes)	Types 3, 14, and 21	Respiratory tract disease	None
	Types 3 and 7 (4 and 14 rare)	Pharyngoconjunctival fever	Conjunctivitis
	Types 8 and 19 (11 rare)		Epidemic keratoconjunctivitis
Poxvirus (DNA)	Variola	Smallpox	Keratitis
	Vaccinia	Vaccination	Keratitis
	Molluscum contagiosum	Multiple warts	Chronic conjunctivitis, keratitis
Papovavirus		Warts	Keratitis (wart on eyelid)
Myxovirus (RNA)	Rubeola	Measles	Mild uveitis
Paramyxovirus (RNA)	Influenza	Influenza	Slight conjunctivitis
Arenovirus (RNA)	Togavirus: rubella	Mild evanescent rashes, fever	Congenital: microphthalmia, cataract, rubella retinopathy
		Pregnancy: fetus affected with deafness, heart defects	
Arbovirus (RNA)	Group A	Encephalitis; tick fever	Secondary to CNS syndromes
	Group B	Dengue; encephalitis	
	Group C		
	Ungrouped	Hemorrhagic fever	
Picornavirus (RNA)	Enteroviruses	Poliomyelitis	Secondary to CNS involvement
	Polioviruses	Fever	Hemorrhagic conjunctivitis (Enterovirus 70)
	Enteroviruses	Aseptic meningitis	Secondary CNS involvement
	Coxsackieviruses and echoviruses		
	Rhinoviruses	Common cold	Conjunctivitis
Retrovirus (RNA)	Human T cell lymphotropic (Type III)	Acquired immune deficiency syndrome	Cotton-wool patches, retinal hemorrhages, cytomegalic virus retinitis

cotton-tipped applicator moistened with culture medium. Optimally, specimens are inoculated promptly into tissue culture. Virus particles may be recognized by electron microscopy. The type of adenovirus may be determined by using a specific antiserum and fluorescent microscopy.

Herpesvirus. This is a group of DNA-type viruses grouped together mainly by their similarities when viewed with an electron micro-scope. The main members of the group are (1) *Herpesvirus hominis* type 1 (ocular, skin) and type 2 (genital), (2) varicella-zoster virus of children (chickenpox) and adults (zoster), (3) Epstein-Barr virus (infectious mononucleosis and Burkitt lymphoma), and (4) virus of cytomegalic inclusion disease. Monkey B disease is a subclinical herpes infection in monkeys but a fatal disease in the accidentally infected human.

Herpesvirus hominis. Herpesvirus hominis includes two subtypes that are distinctly different. Type 1 produces lesions of the mouth, cornea, central nervous system, and the skin above the waist. Type 2 is transmitted as a venereal infection and involves the genitalia and the skin below the waist. However, in about one third of patients between 15 and 24 years of age, herpesvirus type 1 invades the genital region. Similarly, herpesvirus type 2 involvement of the mouth and cornea may be seen.

Primary (type 1) infection usually occurs after 6 months of age, when maternal antibodies have disappeared. As a rule, there is gingivostomatitis along with adenopathy, fever, and malaise. In most cases, the primary infection either does not cause clinical signs or is so minor as not to be recalled. After the primary disease, the virus may remain latent in ganglia, particularly the gasserian (N V). If atopic eczema is present a severe, widespread disease may occur (eczema herpeticum, Kaposi varicelliform eruption). Systemic infection in those without antibodies may cause meningoencephalitis. Visceral herpes simplex usually occurs in newborns infected by their mothers who have recurrent herpetic vulvovaginitis.

After the primary lesion, subsequent disease is entirely local and without systemic signs. Reactivation and migration of the virus causes vesicles on an erythematous base that occur at the same site in each individual. The most frequent manifestation is a fever blister (herpes labialis, herpes facialis, "cold sore"), which often infects a mucocutaneous junction. Reactivation causes an initial sensation of burning and irritation at the involved site followed by reddish papules that vesiculate within 24 hours. The vesicles then become purulent (frequently with localized adenopathy), scale, and heal without a scar.

The eye may be the site of a primary infection in a child. More commonly it is the site of recurrent (reactivation) disease. Primary infection of the eye occurs in children and begins as a unilateral follicular conjunctivitis with a preauricular adenopathy and malaise. The disease may be confined to the conjunctiva, or the cornea may be involved with superficial punctate erosions or a single vesicle. Both types develop into a typical dendritic (branching) keratitis.

The herpesviruses are reactivated by stress, fever, ultraviolet light, and iatrogenic and disease-related immunosuppression. There is an initial foreign body sensation in the eye, and the unfortunate experienced patient usually knows the disease has recurred. Vesicles are present early but are usually ruptured by the time the patient is seen, and a dendritic pattern can be demonstrated on the cornea with the instillation of 2% sterile fluorescein. Treatment is by mechanical removal of epithelium and administration of antiviral agents.

Chickenpox (varicella). Chickenpox is an acute contagious disease characterized by a vesicular exanthem involving predominantly the hands and trunk. It develops in crops over a period of 1 to 5 days and is associated with malaise and fever. In adults a varicella pneumonia may develop. Vesicles may occur on the eyelids and rarely on the conjunctiva and the cornea. A mild iridocyclitis may occur.

Zoster. Zoster is an infectious process of the dorsal root or extramedullary cranial nerve ganglia and is characterized by a circumscribed vesicular eruption and neurologic pain in the areas supplied by the sensory nerves extending to the affected ganglia. Chickenpox is the primary infection in the nonimmune host. The virus then remains latent in the sensory ganglia for the life of the patient. If immunity is impaired, the virus replicates and migrates along sensory nerves to the skin or eye causing the lesions of zoster. Zoster is most common after 50 years of age, but also occurs in younger individuals. It may appear in the course of severe and debilitating systemic illness, and patients with lymphosarcoma and reticulum cell sarcoma are particularly susceptible.

Herpes zoster ophthalmicus is an infection and inflammation of that portion of the skin and eye innervated by the gasserian ganglion that receives fibers from the ophthalmic division of the trigeminal nerve (N V). The disease is first manifested by a severe, unilateral, disabling neuralgia in the region of distribution of the nerve. Several days later there is a vesicular eruption with much swelling and tenderness. The vesicles rupture, leaving hemorrhagic areas that heal in several weeks and leave deep-pitted scars. Pain disappears in about 2 weeks, but in a small percentage of cases a postherpetic neuralgia that is resistant to treatment persists for many years. Zoster usually increases immunity so much that the virus remains permanently latent.

The eyelids may be swollen and tender, but involvement of the globe itself is seen in only about half the patients. Ocular involvement is usually heralded by a vesicle on the tip of the nose, an area innervated, as is the cornea, by the nasociliary nerve.

Zoster lesions of the cornea occur in two forms: (1) acute epithelial keratitis and (2) corneal mucous plaque keratitis. Acute epithelial keratitis is characterized by small, fine, multiple dendritic or stellate lesions in the peripheral portion of the cornea. They are always associated with conjunctivitis and resolve within 4 to 6 days. Corneal mucous plaque keratitis appears as a whitish-gray, sharply defined plaque on the surface of the cornea that can be lifted with ease. This line usually occurs 3 to 4 months after the onset of the cutaneous lesion.

Superficial and deep corneal opacities occur. Anterior uveitis causes folds in Descemet membrane and keratic precipitates. Episcleritis may occur. The disease may persist for months and slowly regress, leaving a residue of round corneal infiltrates in the anterior corneal stroma that may be followed by corneal scarring. Secondary glaucoma occurs in about 20% of the patients and paresis of extraocular muscles in about 10%.

Treatment is often unsatisfactory. Elderly patients should not be exposed to children with chickenpox. Local corticosteroids and atropine appear helpful. In previously healthy individuals, systemic corticosteroids may relieve an attack and prevent postherpetic neuralgia. In debilitated patients, the corticosteroids may cause a fatal dissemination of the virus. The remote possibility that this might occur in an otherwise healthy patient leads many to believe that corticosteroids are contraindicated. Antiviral medications are of no value. Many nonspecific remedies have been proposed.

Infectious mononucleosis. Infectious mononucleosis is a contagious disease with a benign, though frequently protracted, course: it is usually caused by the Epstein-Barr virus. Fever and pharyngitis occur initially, and there is associated lymphadenopathy and hepatitis with or without icterus. Atypical lymphocytosis is associated with some forms. There is a high serum concentration of heterophilic antibodies against sheep erythrocytes as well as development of antibodies against the Epstein-Barr virus.

Follicular or membranous conjunctivitis, subconjunctival hemorrhages, nodular episcleritis, uveitis, nummular keratitis, periorbital edema, optic neuritis, retinal edema, and hemorrhages have been described. In some epidemics, lacrimal gland inflammation (dacryoadenitis) is prominent. It causes a painful swelling, with redness of the outer one third of the upper eyelid and typically S-shaped curve of the upper eyelid margin. Involvement of the central nervous system may cause extraocular muscle paralysis, nystagmus, hemianopsia, and disturbances of conjugate movement.

Treatment is symptomatic, and the disease is usually self-limited.

Cytomegalic inclusion disease. This is a widespread, frequently asymptomatic disease caused by a virus of the herpes group. Symptomatic cytomegalic inclusion disease is relatively. common in immune-compromised patients after organ transplant or cancer chemotherapy. It occurs in 25% of fatal cases of the acquired immune deficiency syndrome (this chapter). Congenital infection causes mental retardation and sensorineural deafness in 10% of infected newborns.

Infantile cytomegalovirus disease manifests itself by jaundice, hepatosplenomegaly, purpura, and erythroblastic or hemolytic anemia. The neural lesions vary from a few cytomegalic cells to an extensive, multifocal, necrotizing, hemorrhagic and granulomatous encephalitis. These lesions may be followed by calcification. Some patients recover, but may have severe brain damage, mental deficiency, microcephaly, epilepsy, cerebral palsy, hydrocephalus, or deafness.

The ocular lesion varies from an isolated area of chorioretinitis to one that disorganizes the globe. The diagnosis is based on the demonstration of larger than normal cells, with typical inclusions found in the urine, saliva, tears, or any tissue specimen. In the mother of an affected child, a complement-fixing antibody titer equal to or greater than 1:64 is diagnostic. The affected infant demonstrates a rising titer after 4 months of age.

An acute cytomegalic necrotizing retinitis

may cause irreversible retinal damage and loss of vision in adults. Men are affected more frequently than women. It occurs frequently in clinically advanced acquired immune deficiency syndrome (AIDS). Other causes include transfusion, direct spread from other patients, and reactivation of a latent infection. Treatment with an acyclovir-like guanine nucleotide resolves the retinitis, but the inflammation recurs when treatment is stopped.

In renal transplant patients the infection is often superimposed upon a retina already damaged by vascular hypertension. There are hard yellow deposits, retinal edema, hemorrhages, and vascular occlusion. An optic atrophy may follow. The infection is self-limited. Effective therapy is not available. A cytomegalic viremia is fairly common in renal transplant patients judging by increasing titers of antibodies and excretion of the virus in the urine, but ocular infection is rare.

Cytomegalic virus mononucleosis is an acute febrile illness with splenomegaly, hepatic involvement, and atypical lymphocytes. The heterophil test is negative, and Epstein-Barr antibodies do not develop.

Adenovirus. The group of adenoviruses is composed of at least 31 serologically distinct human types of large DNA viruses and 17 animal serotypes. The virus causes respiratory tract disease primarily in infants and children and in military recruits.

Adenovirus types 8 and 19 cause epidemic keratoconjunctivitis in adults. In children, type 8 causes systemic disease with fever, respiratory or gastrointestinal signs, and a conjunctivitis without corneal opacities. Adenovirus types 3, 4, and 7 usually cause an acute respiratory disease, pharyngoconjunctival fever, and simple follicular conjunctivitis. Adenovirus types 1, 2, 5, and others cause a febrile pharyngitis.

Pharyngoconjunctival fever. Pharyngoconjunctival fever is an acute sporadic or epidemic disease that affects all age groups, but predominantly children. It occurs in all seasons of the year but is more common in summer and is often associated with infection transmitted in swimming pools. The incubation period is 5 to 7 days, and the disease persists 1 to 2 weeks. Clinical manifestations vary markedly in different individuals and in epidemics. A usually

mild nasopharyngitis is associated with a cervical or maxillary lymphadenopathy. A fever that may reach 39° C persists 3 to 14 days. Headache referable to the sinuses, catarrhal otitis, lassitude, malaise, and sometimes gastrointestinal disturbances occur.

The conjunctivitis is acute, sometimes nonpurulent, and monocular. Follicle hyperplasia is marked in the lower cul-de-sac. Chemosis and injection are most marked over the palpebral conjunctiva. Preauricular lymphadenopathy may be present.

Adenovirus type 3 is most commonly implicated but other types have been found on culture. The serum of affected patients contains group-specific complement-fixation bodies.

Epidemic keratoconjunctivitis. Adenovirus types 8 and 19 cause epidemic keratoconjunctivitis in the United States. This is an acute infectious corneal disease spread by the ocular secretion or by eyedrops contaminated with organisms. In Japan, adenovirus type 8 causes an acute systemic disease in children with a conjunctivitis of varying severity without producing corneal opacities. The disease is usually associated with fever, malaise, gastrointestinal and upper respiratory tract symptoms, and a follicular conjunctivitis. Other children exposed to the disease develop the same disease, but exposed adults develop epidemic keratoconjunctivitis. An immunofluorescent test detects the adenoviral group antigen in conjunctival secretions and in culture. Treatment is symptomatic.

Molluscum contagiosum. Molluscum contagiosum is a tumor caused by a large poxvirus and is characterized by the development of multiple discrete nodules in the epidermal layer of the skin. The nodules are often pearly white and painless, with an umbilicated center in which a small white cone can be seen. Humans are the only host of the virus; children are infected most frequently, and the lesion is prevalent in some regions. The nodules may occur on the skin of the eyelids and on the eyelid margins. If located on the eyelid margins, virus material may be released into the conjunctival sac and cause conjunctivitis or keratitis. Excision of the nodule is the treatment of choice. Histologically, large intracytoplasmic inclusion bodies occur within acanthotic epidermis.

Verrucae (warts). Verrucae are contagious viral tumors characterized by the development of one or more cutaneous masses that have a rough surface made up of many fine projections. When located on the eyelid margin, the lesions scrape the cornea or debris contaminates the tear film and causes a chronic epithelial keratitis and conjunctivitis. Children may develop conjunctival papillomas. Removal of the nodules from the eyelid margin is necessary to heal the keratitis.

Measles (rubeola). Measles is a contagious, infectious viral (RNA) disease characterized by prodromal symptoms of fever, cough, conjunctivitis, upper respiratory tract infection, and Koplik spots on the buccal mucosa, followed in 3 to 5 days by a maculopapular cutaneous rash. The conjunctivitis is nonpurulent and may be associated with Koplik spots, particularly on the semilunar fold. The cornea has multiple punctate epithelial erosions, which cause a severe photophobia. The photophobic patient is made more comfortable by either darkness or colored glasses. Permanent corneal scarring does not occur unless there is secondary bacterial infection.

Sometimes measles or another acute contagious disease of childhood is the precipitating event in the appearance of strabismus. The primary cause of the squint is already present, and the disease seems only to accelerate its appearance or to transform an intermittent or latent type into a continuous type of strabismus.

Immunization has almost eliminated measles in the United States. During the incubation period, the administration of gamma globulin may prevent or modify the disease in the nonimmune individual. Subacute sclerosing panencephalitis is a slow viral infection caused by either the rubeola virus or a closely related virus.

Mumps. Mumps is an acute contagious viral (RNA) systemic disease characterized mainly by a painful enlargement of the salivary glands, most commonly the parotid gland, and, after puberty, by orchitis. Lymphocytic meningitis, pancreatitis, and involvement of other viscera rarely occur.

Transient corneal edema decreases visual acuity. There are no associated ocular inflammatory signs. A uveitis or dacryoadenitis may occur. The only sign of meningeal involvement may be optic neuritis, or there may be widespread extraocular muscle palsy.

Rubella (German measles). Rubella is a mild contagious disease characterized mainly by an evanescent, maculopapular skin eruption beginning on the face and neck, spreading to the trunk and extremities, and fading in 3 days. There may be mild pharyngitis and postauricular adenopathy, sometimes accompanied by slight fever, malaise, lassitude, and myalgia.

Conjunctivitis is common and consists of bilateral bulbar chemosis and injection. Keratitis is exceptional.

Rubella causes severe congenital defects in infants of mothers who contract the disease early in pregnancy. The virus is unique because it interferes with the translation of DNA and RNA and subsequent polypeptide synthesis and organogenesis. Infection between the second and sixth weeks of pregnancy causes cardiac malformation, microphthalmic cataract, and pigment epithelium degeneration. Infection any time during the first trimester of pregnancy up to the fifth month may cause deafness and mental retardation with extensive brain necrosis. A chronic virus infection may persist as long as 3 years after birth, causing further systemic deterioration as well as serving as a nidus of infection for pregnant mothers.

Retinitis and congenital cataract are the most common ocular disorders. Microphthalmia results from infection early in pregnancy. Fetal uveitis causes iris atrophy, which may prevent pupillary dilation.

The cataract is usually nuclear, cortical (complete), and bilateral. Aspiration of the cataract may be followed by chronic endophthalmitis centered around lens remnants, with the severity proportional to the amount of lens cortex remaining in the eye. Inability to dilate the pupil complicates lens extraction. A sector iridectomy, which is almost always indicated, often results in significant visual improvement. The pupil may be enlarged with vitrectomy cutting instruments.

The retina has a mottled appearance (salt-and-pepper), which is caused by hyperpigmentation and hypopigmentation of the retinal pigment epithelium. The optic disks and blood vessels are normal. Fluorescein angiography shows a diffuse hyperfluorescence throughout the posterior eyegrounds, reflecting a widespread loss of pigment of the retinal pigment epithelium. Vision and electroretinography are normal.

Prevention of rubella infection in pregnant women has eliminated rubella embryopathy. Children should be immunized with rubella vaccine to minimize transmission and so that girls will be immune when they reach childbearing age. The vaccine can infect the fetus and may be used in sexually active women only when pregnancy can be excluded (as during menstruation or immediately after childbirth) and continued nonpregnancy can be ensured for 3 months. After immunization, the hemagglutination-inhibition test indicates the presence or absence of immunity to rubella.

Picornaviruses. This family consists of two genera, the genus *Enterovirus* and the genus *Rhinovirus*, an important agent of the common cold. The genus *Enterovirus* is subdivided into polioviruses, coxsackieviruses, and echoviruses. Newly discovered members are no longer classified as coxsackieviruses or echoviruses but are numbered serially beginning with enterovirus number 68. The polioviruses cause acute anterior poliomyelitis. Bulbar poliomyelitis may cause external ophthalmoplegia with opsoclonus. The coxsackieviruses and echoviruses may cause an aseptic meningitis (viral meningitis) in which there may be paralysis of muscles innervated by the oculomotor and abducent nerves together with papilledema.

Hemorrhagic conjunctivitis. This is a specific violent inflammatory conjunctivitis first reported in Africa in 1969. The infection has spread eastward and was endemic in Florida. It is caused by a member of the picornavirus group, enterovirus 70.

Acquired immune deficiency syndrome

The acquired immune deficiency syndrome (AIDS) is a disease of the immune system that is caused by a retrovirus, human T-cell lymphotropic virus type III (HTLV-III). The virus infects helper T cells, and the depression in cellular immunity is associated with recurrent opportunistic infections and neoplastic diseases. The depression of cellular immunity is marked by lymphopenia; high IgG, IgM, and IgA levels; reduction in the T-helper to T-suppressor cell ratio; decreased mononuclear cell responses to antigens, mitogens, and alloanti-

gens; and an absolute reduction in T-helper lymphocytes.

Opportunistic infections are caused by members of protozoal, helminthic, fungal, bacterial, and viral groups. Pneumonia, caused by the parasite *Pneumocystic carnii*, is the most frequently encountered life-threatening infection. Kaposi sarcoma, a rare dermatologic vascular tumor, is the most common malignancy; B-cell lymphomas and primary lymphomas of the central nervous system have been reported. AIDS is the most severe manifestation of HTLV-III infection, but there appears to be a wide range of milder conditions, including a transient mononucleosis-like syndrome, persistent generalized lymphadenopathy, and various hematologic syndromes.

In the United States the disease is most common among three population groups: (1) homosexual or bisexual men with multiple sexual partners; (2) intravenous drug abusers who share needles; and (3) hemophiliacs who have received clotting factor concentrates. AIDS is transmitted primarily through sexual contact. Transmission by blood products is rare as blood is now screened for antibody to HTLV-III. Tears and saliva of infected persons may contain the virus, and the virus has been isolated in the conjunctiva and corneal epithelium of overtly clinically healthy individuals. HTLV-III antibody testing of the blood is indicated in each person from whom donor tissue is obtained (the test may be negative for 6 to 8 weeks after infection).

AIDS has a latent period of 6 to 8 years. Clinically, it is associated with fever, malaise, diarrhea, weight loss, cough, and dyspnea. Physically, there may be lymphadenopathy, hepatosplenomegaly, herpetic or other skin disease, oral-pharyngeal thrush, and retinal cotton-wool patches. Patients must be examined for evidence of secondary syphilis; cytomegalovirus or Epstein-Barr virus mononucleosis; disseminated mycobacterial, fungal, *Toxoplasma gondii* infections; and lymphoma.

Ocular signs include neoplasms and infectious and noninfectious lesions. Noninfectious retinopathy consists of cotton-wool patches and retinal hemorrhages, either alone or in combination. These lesions may suggest the diagnosis in the proper clinical setting but do not correlate with the patient's clinical course. Kaposi sarcoma rarely (5%) affects the conjunctiva. Intracranial involvement may cause abnormalities of ocular motility. Retrobulbar optic neuritis may occur independently or in association with retinitis.

The most common infectious lesion of the eye is cytomegalic virus retinitis (in 25% of fatal cases). It appears as a hemorrhagic retinitis with granular white areas of retinal necrosis. Treatment with an acyclovir-related nucleotide results in resolution of the retinitis and disappearance of the viremia, but the conditions recur when the medication is stopped. Ocular toxoplasmosis is not seen, and *Candida, Cryptococcus*, herpes simplex, and *Mycobacterium avium-intracellulare* rarely involve the eye.

PROTOZOAN AND METAZOAN INFECTIONS

The animal kingdom may be divided into two subkingdoms, the protozoan and the metazoan. The protozoa are classically divided into amebas, flagellates, ciliates, and sporozoans. Diseases caused by protozoa include amebic dysentery, leishmaniasis, malaria, toxoplasmosis, and trypanosomiasis. The metazoa consist of all multicelled animals whose various types of cells are not generally capable of independent existence. The metazoa range in complexity from simply arranged sponges to the highly specialized structure of humans. Human infection by metazoa is chiefly by parasitic worms and some members of the phylum Arthropoda that are transmitters of disease. The larvae of flies are parasitic and may multiply in living tissue, causing myiasis. The adult fly is not a parasite.

The eye and adnexa may be affected by direct invasion of either the adult or larval form, by toxins elaborated by worms or released with death, or by impairment of the health of the host. Diagnosis is based on immunologic studies, on the recovery of the parasite and its larvae or eggs, and on skin tests. A systemic eosinophilia occurs with massive invasion.

Protozoan infections

Toxoplasmosis. Toxoplasmosis is an infectious disease caused by an obligate intracellular protozoan, *Toxoplasma gondii*. The organism is capable of infecting a wide range of mammals,

birds, and reptiles. The cat is the definitive host. Transmission occurs readily after ingestion of toxoplasmosis cysts in meat or oocysts from cat feces.

Two types of disease occur: congenital and acquired. The congenital disease is characterized by a bilateral necrotizing neuroretinopathy and brain necrosis. Acquired infections may be asymptomatic or cause a lymphadenopathy, fever, and malaise. In patients who have neoplasms of the lymphatic system or who are being treated with immunosuppressive drugs, acquired toxoplasmosis causes severe damage to the brain, muscles, heart, liver, or lungs. Regardless of the time of onset, most ocular toxoplasmosis is congenital.

Congenital toxoplasmosis occurs in utero during the first 7 months of pregnancy. The mother transmits the infection to the fetus, which may result in an abortion or stillbirth or an infant with clinical signs of toxoplasmosis. About half of infected infants do not have clinical signs of toxoplasmosis but may develop recurrent retinochoroiditis between 10 and 20 years of age. The eyes and central nervous system are usually affected, and the severity varies widely. Visceral and muscular involvement predominates in some infants.

Ocular toxoplasmosis occurs as focal, self-limited, recurrent retinochoroiditis and as a diffuse, chronic inflammation resulting in progressive visual loss. Severe congenital toxoplasmosis causes microphthalmia, necrotizing retinitis and choroiditis, optic atrophy, iritis, visual loss, and vitreous disorganization. Central nervous system necrosis causes nystagmus and extraocular muscle palsy.

Infants with less severe toxoplasmosis infections have areas of chorioretinal atrophy with retinal pigment proliferation in both eyes. If the fovea centralis is involved, esotropia may occur or the eyes may be straight although vision is poor. The inactive lesions are sharply demarcated, and contiguous areas of chorioretinal atrophy have pigmented borders (Fig. 23-3), which are located mainly at the posterior pole. The vitreous is clear, and there is no active inflammation. The retinal lesions in some children remain quiet throughout life. In others, inflammation recurs 10 to 20 years later in an area adjacent to a healed lesion and there is severe exudation into the vitreous. Immediate treatment is essential if the fovea centralis is threatened because the necrotizing retinopathy may destroy the remaining fovea centralis.

The active ocular lesions vary considerably in an adult who was infected in utero but without clinical evidence. The inflammation occurs because of rupture of a pseudocyst and infection of adjacent cells. There is a generalized nonspecific retinochoroiditis with many vitreous exudates and veils. The retinal and choroid atrophy with surrounding pigment proliferation of infantile inflammation is rarely seen. The disease tends to be bilateral, recurrent, and chronic. Treatment is often difficult because organisms are encysted, and tissue edema, inflammation, granuloma formation, and relative avascularity prevent access of the drugs to the organisms. *Toxoplasma* antibody titers are low.

The treatment of choice for systemic or ocular toxoplasmosis is pyrimethamine (Daraprim) and triple sulfonamides. Pyrimethamine is effective in therapy because it inhibits folic acid metabolism of the protozoa. To prevent bone marrow depression, patients should be given folinic acid, which *Toxoplasma* cannot convert to folic acid. Oral and sub-Tenon injection of clindamycin may be substituted for pyrimethamine. Minocycline may be used. In the absence of an acute systemic disease, the ocular inflammation is usually treated with corticosteroids. Retrobulbar corticosteroids may cause a severe inflammation.

Metazoan infections

The main metazoan infections of humans are caused by worms and flukes. The major conditions with ocular changes are caused by roundworms (nematodes) and tapeworms (cestodes). Generally, two types of infection occur: (1) the intestinal form, in which the mature worm is attached to the bowel wall, and (2) the visceral, or somite, form, in which the larva of the parasite is present in several tissues and organs.

Nematodes (roundworms). There are an estimated 500,000 species of nematodes that may become parasitic in virtually all arthropods, mollusks, plants, and vertebrates. Typically, nematodes are elongated, cylindric worms that taper more or less at the head and tail and have a complete digestive tract. They vary from minute filiform worms to 1.5 m in length. Most human infections are acquired by ingestion of the eggs, but hookworm and *Strongyloides* larvae actively invade the skin.

Ocular infection occurs because of invasion of the eye by the larvae of nematodes that are parasitic in lower animals, most commonly the roundworms of the dog and cat.

Visceral larva migrans. This term is applied to the invasion of nematode larvae into tissues other than the skin. The common roundworm of the dog and, less frequently, of the cat *(Toxocara canis* and *Toxocara cati)* are common causes of ocular disease. Visceral larva migrans also describes the disease produced by the wandering worms of *Ascaris lumbricoides* and other nematodes.

Toxocariasis is acquired by the ingestion of *Toxocara* eggs that contain the infective second-stage larvae. The eggs are excreted by puppies and lactating bitches and require 2 or 3 weeks' development in the soil before becoming infective. The eggs hatch in the patient's small intestine, and the larvae migrate to the liver through the portal circulation. Some may enter the lungs and then the sys-

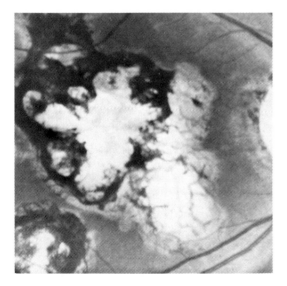

Fig. 23-3. Recurrent toxoplasmosis in a 39-year-old woman. Vision in this eye is counting fingers at 2 feet. There are a series of contiguous lesions, some with marked pigment proliferation and others so severe that the pigment epithelium has been destroyed and the sclera may be seen.

temic circulation. When larvae exceed the diameter of a blood vessel, they actively bore through the vessel wall. Many larvae become encapsulated and may produce infection years later when the capsule ruptures.

The clinical picture of toxocariasis varies with the number of eggs ingested, the frequency of reinfection, and the distribution of larvae. Typically, visceral larvae migrans is seen in boys, aged 6 months to 4 years, who have contact with puppies and eat dirt (geophagia). There is a fever, pallor, coughing or wheezing, lassitude, anorexia, and weight loss. There may be hepatomegaly, pruritic eruption over the trunk and legs, and transient subcutaneous nodules. Most patients have a leukocytosis with 50% to 90% eosinophils and high immunoglobulins IgG and IgM.

Ocular involvement occurs at an average age of 7.5 years, rather than 6 months to 4 years as with visceral larva migrans. Ocular lesions rarely occur in patients with concurrent or previous history of visceral larva migrans. Ocular involvement is usually unilateral and may cause visual loss, strabismus, and eye pain. The lesion varies from a granuloma of the posterior pole to severe endophthalmitis. A granuloma appears as a white, round lesion, about the size of the optic disk, in the retina or pars plana (Fig. 23-4). Traction lines in the retina radiate from the lesion. Fibrous bands may extend from the central retina to the pars plana. Rarely, the larvae can be seen. The lesion may be flat, or it may protrude into the vitreous cavity. Multiple retinal granulomas, posterior uveitis, vitreous hemorrhage, and optic atrophy may occur. A granulomatous retinitis may be confused with a retinoblastoma. Peripheral retinitis may cause an inflammatory falciform of the retina. Rarely the optic disk is invaded by the larva.

Increased titer of the enzyme-linked immunosorbent assay (ELISA) test, prepared with larval antigens and using serum that has been absorbed on *Ascaris* antigen, is high diagnostic. The indirect hemagglutination and bentonite flocculation tests are less diagnostic. With only ocular involvement, the tests may be negative because relatively few larvae migrated and the host's immune defense was inadequately stimulated.

Corticosteroids minimize hypersensitive reactions, but antibodies may be useful in decreasing secondary infections. Diethylcarbamazine relieves symptoms and shortens convalescent time in patients with visceral larva migrans. Children with pica should not be exposed to contaminated environments and infected dogs and cats.

Ascaris lumbricoides. *Ascaris lumbricoides* is the giant intestinal roundworm that affects children predominantly. There is no intermediate host, and infection occurs because of ingestion of eggs. The eggs hatch in the bowel, and the migrating larvae may cause pneumonia, encephalitis, or meningitis. Infection of the eye causes an intraocular inflammation that varies in severity from iridocyclitis to endophthalmitis. *Ascaris* larvae in the lungs break through the pulmonary capillaries to enter the air alveoli and then the pharynx, where they are swallowed. They develop into mature worms in the intestinal tract.

In the bowel the worm may be asymptomatic or cause intestinal disorders varying in severity from mild colic to obstruction and perforation. Sensitization to the worms or their products may cause allergic manifestations, mainly asthma or urticaria.

The ocular inflammation of the larval migration is nonspecific but may be suspected because of the violent ocular tissue reaction often combined with an eosinophilia, depending on

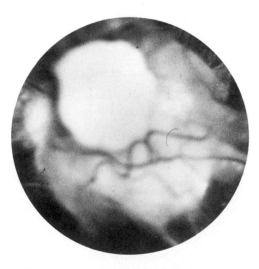

Fig. 23-4. Granuloma of the retina in toxocariasis. The white mass extends into the vitreous cavity and obscures the optic disk.

the number of worms in the circulation. Enucleated eyes have the pathologic appearance of either Coats disease or endophthalmitis. The larvae may be found in histologic sections.

Necator americanus. *Necator americanus* (common hookworm) is a nematode common in the southeastern United States. There is no intermediate host. In moist soil, eggs develop into larvae that readily penetrate the skin. The cutaneous invasion produces a severely pruritic cutaneous eruption, "ground itch." The larvae ultimately reach the lungs, enter the pharynx, and are swallowed. They develop into mature worms in the intestinal tract. An anemia develops, along with malaise, fever, and anorexia. The disease is diagnosed by discovery of ova in the stools. Treatment is with tetrachloroethylene.

The ocular signs are those described in visceral larva migrans. In the past, *Toxocara canis* infections were considered to be caused by the hookworm. The anemia may be associated with retinal hemorrhage.

Trichinosis. Trichinosis is an infestation of striated muscles by the larvae of the nematode *Trichinella spiralis*, which infects a wide group of animals of which swine are the chief human reservoir.

The encysted larvae are ingested in undercooked pork and develop in the intestine into sexually mature adults. Eggs develop and hatch in the female nematode, which release about 1,500 larvae over a 6-week period. The larvae enter the general circulation about 7 days after an individual has eaten infected meat and are widely distributed to all tissues. In severe infestations, there is muscle weakness and pain, remittent fever, and edema that is frequently localized to the orbit, particularly the upper eyelid. Ocular muscle involvement causes pain on ocular rotation. There may be subconjunctival hemorrhage.

Muscle tenderness, eosinophilia, and orbital edema suggest the diagnosis. The larvae may be found in biopsy specimens 10 days after infection. The intradermal skin test becomes positive about the third week after infection.

There is no specific therapy. Corticosteroids suppress the acute inflammation.

Filariasis. The filariae are slender, threadlike nematodes that have a tendency to inhabit a particular part of the human body. The female worms produce embryos, microfilariae, which live in the blood or skin. Bloodsucking arthropods, their intermediate hosts, spread the infection.

Onchocerca volvulus. Ocular onchocerciasis (river blindness) is a chronic filarial infection that occurs endemically in Mexico, Guatemala, Venezuela, and central Africa. It has been estimated to affect more than 40 million people and in some communities blinds as many as 40% of the adult population. The infection is transmitted from person to person by bites of infected black flies of the genus *Simulium* (buffalo gnats). Infected larvae are injected into the skin or subcutaneous tissue, which causes nodules (cercoma) of pathognomonic appearance.

The microfilariae of *Onchocerca* may be seen beneath the bulbar conjunctiva or as squirming yellowish threads in the aqueous humor. Microfilariae in the cornea cause a superficial punctate keratitis. Foreign body granuloma formation opacifies the cornea. Inflammation of the iris is common, and generalized atrophy of its pigmented layers gives it a spongy appearance. The posterior segment lesion is variable. It occurs rarely in areas where there is adequate dietary vitamin A. There is circumscribed atrophy of the choroid, clumping of retinal pigment, perivascular sheathing, and an associated optic atrophy. Death of the microfilariae causes a severe inflammatory lesion.

Treatment with a new single-dose parasiticide, ivermectin, is clearly superior to diethylcarbamazine. One oral dose is administered once or twice a year. Diethylcarbamazine (Hetrazan) is effective against the microfilaria but not the adult worm. The death of many microfilariae within the eye may cause severe side effects, and complications limit its use. Control of the disease is being attempted by the use of insecticides to eliminate the vector in small streams.

Loiasis. *Loa loa* (African eye worm) is a threadlike nematode measuring 30 to 70 × 0.3 mm. It lives in the subcutaneous tissue of humans, travels from place to place beneath the skin, and causes a creeping itch sensation. The disease is seen in the west and central parts of Africa. The vectors are day-biting flies. The worm is responsive to warmth, and in persons sitting before a fire, the worms move to the warm face and eyes.

The adult worm looks like a piece of surgical catgut beneath the conjunctiva or swimming in the anterior chamber. There is local irritation, chemosis, and lacrimation, all of which disappear quickly when the worm moves to deeper tissues. The subconjunctival worm may be removed by capturing it with a ligature.

Calabar swellings are painless, edematous, subcutaneous nodules that occur as an allergic reaction to metabolic products of the worm or from injured or dead worms. Systemic antihistamines give relief. Diethylcarbamazine (Hetrazan) eliminates microfilariae from the blood. Ivermectin is likely effective.

Cestodes (tapeworms). Tapeworms cause illness in humans in either of two stages of their life cycle: (1) the adult stage in which the mature worm is attached to the intestinal wall, and (2) the larval stage in which there are enlarging larval cysts in various tissues. The intestinal type may cause no symptoms or only symptoms of gastrointestinal disturbances. The visceral type follows ingestion of tapeworm eggs, which hatch in the intestine and release larvae that penetrate the bowel wall and spread the infection through the bloodstream. The two main types of visceral involvement with tapeworms are (1) echinococcus, or hydatid, cysts and (2) cysticerocosis.

Echinococcosis (hydatid disease). Echinococcus cysts form part of the inflammatory response to the larvae of *Echinococcus granulosus*, a minute tapeworm that infects dogs and cats. Ingestion of the contaminated feces by swine, cattle, or humans leads to hydatid cysts of the liver, lungs, kidney, brain orbit, eye, and other organs. The cyst develops into hundreds of adult worms. The cyst development is slow and resembles the symptoms of a slowly developing tumor. The contained fluid is highly irritating and infectious, and the cysts should not be evacuated. Orbital cysts, which are more common than intraocular cysts, cause a proptosis with related signs. The intraocular cyst appears as a white pea-sized mass within the vitreous body, or there may be progressive, solid retinal detachment. Surgical excision is the only effective therapy, and care must be taken not to rupture the cyst and release toxic and infectious fluid.

Cysticercosis. Cysticercosis in humans is caused by infection with eggs of *Taenia solium* (pork tapeworm) or *Taenia saginata* (beef tapeworm). Humans become the intermediate host by ingestion of the eggs in human feces, contaminated food, or water. The cyst is usually 0.5 to 1 cm in diameter and can develop in almost any tissue within the body. Most commonly, lesions within the cerebrum, the subarachnoid space at the base of the brain, or in the ventricles cause the signs and symptoms of an expanding tumor. There may be headache, papilledema, decreased vision, hemiparesis, and seizures. The cyst in the eye appears as a translucent oval body 6 to 18 mm in length, without a capsule, in which the head of the larva may be seen as a white spot. It may occur in the choroid, causing a retinal detachment, float free in the vitreous humor or anterior chamber, or be found beneath the conjunctiva or in the orbit. Removal is the only therapy, but rupture of the cyst is followed by a violent inflammation.

Ophthalmomyiasis. Invasion of the eye by the larval form (maggot) of flies of the order Diptera is caused by deposition of the eggs or larvae on the ocular surface by the adult fly, a secondary vector such as a tick or mosquito, or by the patient's fingers. The maggots bore their way into the eye, come to lie in the anterior chamber or vitreous cavity, and cause an endophthalmitis or iridocyclitis. Reduced vision occurs because of the maggot in the visual axis or from inflammation, invasion of the optic nerve, foveal hemorrhage, or serous retinal detachment. A subretinal maggot may cause an ophthalmoscopically spectacular tracing of hypopigmented tracks of chorioretinal atrophy.

SARCOIDOSIS

Sarcoidosis is a chronic idiopathic disease characterized by the widespread occurrence of epithelioid cell granulomas. The granuloma resembles a tubercle but is without caseation and either resolves or is converted into an avascular, acellular hyaline tissue. Often it contains refractile or apparently calcified bodies in its giant cells. Mediastinal and peripheral lymph nodes, lungs, liver, spleen, skin, eyes, phalangeal bones, and parotid glands are most commonly affected. There is impaired cell-mediated immunity (T lymphocytes) and increased serum immunoglobulins (B lymphocytes). Most patients in the United States are black, and sarcoid is more prevalent in the southeastern states in both whites and blacks. It is more frequent in women than in men, and most patients are between 20 and 40 years of age.

Sarcoidosis occurs in an acute, active form and in a persistent fibrotic form. Abrupt, transient polyarthralgia and erythema nodosum are the first signs in the acute form in individuals 30 years of age or younger. There is an acute, severe anterior uveitis with many mutton-fat keratic precipitates and early formation of broad, flat, posterior synechiae. Sarcoid nodules may appear in the iris stroma or at the pupillary margin.

"Snowball" opacities of inflammatory exudates of the vitreous humor occur in posterior uveitis. There may be a retinal periphlebitis, with the focal accumulations of exudates described as resembling candle-wax drippings. Sarcoid nodules may appear in the choroid, in the retina, or on the optic nerve head. Inflammation of the pars plana portion of the ciliary body occurs frequently, resulting in cells in both the vitreous cavity and anterior chamber.

Acute uveitis, combined with erythema nodosum and bilateral hilar lymphadenopathy, constitutes Lofgren syndrome. Uveoparotid fever, which consists of uveitis, parotid gland enlargement, and sometimes facial nerve palsy, constitutes Heerfordt disease.

In the active, acute form of sarcoidosis, a granulomatous reaction occurs 4 weeks after the injection of an antigen prepared from the spleen of a patient with acute sarcoidosis (Kveim-Siltzbach skin test). There is a hydroxyprolinuria, increased serum angiotensin-converting enzyme, hypercalcemia, and hypercalciuria.

Chronic sarcoidosis has an insidious, poorly recognized onset with symptoms of cough, dyspnea, and hemoptysis. Fever, weight loss, and arthralgia may be the initial signs. Uveitis, cutaneous plaques, papules, subcutaneous nodules, peripheral lymphadenopathy, lassitude, fever, and malaise may occur. Lupus pernio may be present with skin plaques, scars, and keloids.

A chronic nonspecific granulomatous uveitis occurs that is resistant to treatment. Cataract and secondary glaucoma often complicate the uveitis. Keratoconjunctivitis sicca occurs frequently. The lacrimal and parotid glands may be enlarged. The Kveim-Siltzbach test if often negative. Hydroxypolinuria, increased serum angiotensin-converting enzyme, hypercalcemia, and hypercalciuria occur rarely. Bone cysts occur most frequently in the hands and feet and rarely in the temporal or frontal bones or hard palate.

Intracranial sarcoidosis is clinically evident in 5% of the cases; there are lesions in the central nervous system in 15% of autopsy cases. The basal leptomeninges, the region of the hypothalamus and pituitary, and the cranial nerves, especially the facial nerve, are affected. Granulomatous optic neuropathy, retrobulbar neuritis, or both may cause papillitis and optic atrophy. Papilledema may reflect increased intracranial pressure or occur spontaneously. Optociliary shunt vessels may be prominent on the nerve head. Optic atrophy may result from optic nerve inflammation, compression, or glaucoma secondary to intraocular inflammation.

In all types of sarcoidosis the inferior conjunctival fornices may contain minute, translucent, slightly yellow, elevated lesions resembling follicles (Fig. 23-5). Serial section of such a lesion and skilled pathologic interpretation provide diagnostic material.

Keratoconjunctivitis sicca occurs frequently.

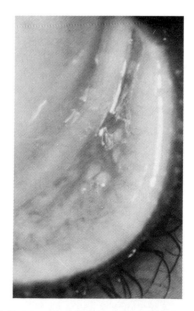

Fig. 23-5. Sarcoid nodules in the inferior cul-de-sac of a 23-year-old woman with advanced sarcoidosis.

Pseudotumor of the orbit may occur. The lacrimal and salivary glands may be enlarged.

Corticosteroids are the main treatment. The prognosis is good without relapse after treatment in the acute form. The prognosis is poor in the chronic form, and relapse is common. Uveitis is treated with both topical and systemic prednisone and topical atropine.

WHIPPLE DISEASE

Whipple disease is a multisystem disorder that occurs predominantly in middle-aged men in whom there is intestinal malabsorption. There is diarrhea, abdominal pain, fever, arthritis, weight loss, and anemia. The small bowel mucosa contains foamy macrophages that stain brilliant magenta with PAS stain. Within and adjacent to the macrophages are small rod-shaped structures that appear to be the microorganisms responsible for the disorder. They decrease or disappear after treatment with antibiotics. In 10% of the cases there is central nervous system involvement that may cause gaze palsy, nystagmus, and ophthalmoplegia. Uveitis, typical macrophages, inflammatory cells in the vitreous, retinal hemorrhages, and papilledema may occur.

BIBLIOGRAPHY
General

Allansmith, M.R.: The eye and immunology, St. Louis, 1982, The C.V. Mosby Co.

Arruga, J., Valentines, J., Mauri, F., Roca, G., Salom, R., and Rufi, G.: Neuroretinitis in acquired syphilis, Ophthalmology **92:**262, 1985.

Belshe, R.T., editor: Textbook of human virology, Littleton, Mass., 1984, PSG Publishing Co.

Darrell, R.W.: Virus diseases of the eye, Philadelphia, 1985, Lea & Febiger.

Friedlander, M.H.: Allergy and immunology of the eye, New York, 1979, Harper & Row, Publishers.

Garner, A.: Specific ocular manifestations of immunological processes. In Garner, A., and Klintworth, G.K., editors: Pathobiology of ocular disease: a dynamic approach, New York, 1982, Marcel Dekker.

Garner, A., and Klintworth, G.K.: Pathobiology of ocular disease: a dynamic approach, New York, 1982, Marcel Dekker.

Mandell, G.L., Douglas, R.G., Jr., and Bennett, J.E., editors: Principles and practice of infectious diseases, ed. 2, New York, 1985, John Wiley & Sons.

Nelson, L.B.: Pediatric ophthalmology, Philadelphia, 1984, W.B. Saunders Co.

O'Connor, G.R., and Chandler, J.: Advances in immunology and immunopathology of the eye, New York, 1984, Masson Publishing U.S.A.

Rahi, A.H.S.: Immunological processes in disease: general principles. In Garner, A., and Klintworth, G.K., editors: Pathobiology of ocular disease: a dynamic approach, New York, 1982, Marcel Dekker.

Smolin, G., and O'Connor, G.R.: Ocular immunology, Philadelphia, 1981, Lea & Febiger.

Smolin, G., Tabbara, K., and Whitcher, J.: Infectious diseases and the eye, Baltimore, 1984, Williams & Wilkins Co.

Spaide, R., Nattis, R., Lipka, A., and D'Amico, R.: Ocular findings in leprosy in the United States, Am. J. Ophthalmol. **100:**411, 1985.

Theodore, F.H., Bloomfield, S.E., and Mondino, B.J.: Clinical allergy and immunology of the eye, Baltimore, 1983, Williams & Wilkins, Co.

Viruses

Fauci, A.L., Masur, H., Gellman, E.P., Markham, P.D., Hahn, B.H., and Lane, H.C.: The acquired immunodeficiency syndrome: an update, Ann. Intern. Med. **102:**800, 1985.

Felsenstein, D., D'Amico, D., D.J., Hirsch, M.S., Neumeyer, D.A., Cederberg, D.M., Miranda, P., and Schooley, R.T.: Treatment of cytomegalovirus retinitis with 9-(2-hydroxy-1-[hydroxymethyl] ethoxymethyl) guanine, Ann. Intern. Med. **103:**377, 1985.

Fields, B.N., Knipe, D.M. Chanock, R.M., Melnick, J.L., Roizman, B., and Shope, R.E., editors: Virology, New York, 1985, Raven Press.

Francis, D.P., and Petricciani, J.C.: The prospects for and pathways toward a vaccine for AIDS, N. Engl. J. Med. **313:**1586, 1985.

Fujikawa, L.S., Salahuddin, S.Z., Ablashi, D., Palestine, A.G., Masur, H., Nussenblatt, R.B., and Gallo, R.C.: Human T-cell leukemia/lymphotropic virus type III in the conjunctival epithelium of a patient with AIDS, Am. J. Ophthalmol. **100:**507, 1985.

Kaufman, H.E., Centifanto-Fitzgerald, Y.M., and Varnell, E.D.: Herpes simplex keratitis, Ophthalmology **90:**700, 1983.

Kestelyn, P., Van de Perre, P., Rouvroy, D., Lepage, P., Bogaerts, J., Nzaramba, D., and Clumeck, N.: A prospective study of the ophthalmologic findings in the acquired immune deficiency syndrome in Africa, Am. J. Ophthalmol. **100:**230, 1985.

Inflammation

Jakobiec, F.A.: Ocular inflammatory disease: the lymphocyte redivivus, Am. J. Ophthalmol. **96:**384, 1983.

Kaplan, H.J., and Waldrep, J.C.: Immunologic insights into uveitis and retinitis: the immunoregulatory circuit, Ophthalmology **91:**655, 1984.

Lobue, T.D., Deutsch, T.A., and Stein, R.B.: *Moraxella nonliquefaciens* endophthalmitis after trabeculectomy, Am. J. Ophthalmol. **99:**343, 1985.

Sandor, E.V., Millman, A., Croxson, T.S., and Mildvan, D.: Herpes zoster ophthalmicus in patients at risk for the acquired immune deficiency syndrome (AIDS), Am. J. Ophthalmol. **101:**153, 1986.

Sarcoid

Beardsley, T.L., Brown, S.V.L., Sydnor, C.F., Grimson, B.S., and Klintworth, G.K.: Eleven cases of sarcoidosis of the optic nerve, Am. J. Ophthalmol. **97:**62, 1984.

Campo, R.V., and Aaberg, T.M.: Choroidal granuloma in sarcoidosis, Am. J. Ophthalmol. **97:**419, 1984.

Karcioglu, Z.A., and Brear, R.: Conjunctival biopsy in sarcoidosis, Am. J. Ophthalmol. **99:**68, 1985.

Whipple disease

Avila, M.P., Jalkh, A.E., Feldman, E., Trempe, C.L., and Schepens, C.L.: Manifestations of Whipple's disease in the posterior segment of the eye, Arch. Ophthalmol. **102:**384, 1984.

Protozoa and Metazoa

Edwards, K.M., Meredith, T.A., Hagler, W., and Healy, G.R.: Ophthalmomyiasis interna causing visual loss, Am. J. Ophthalmol. **97:**605, 1984.

Greene, B.M., Taylor, H.R., Cupp, E.W., Murphy, R.P., White, A.T., Aziz, M.A., Schulz-Key, H., D'Anna, S.A., Newland, H.S., Goldschmidt, L.P., Auer, C., Hanson, A.P., Freeman, S.V., Reber, E.W., and Williams, P.N.: Comparison of ivermectin and diethylcarbamazine in the treatment of onchocerciasis, N. Engl. J. Med. **313:**133, 1985.

Kazacos, K.R., Raymond, L.A., Kazacos, E.A., and Vestre, W.A.: The raccoon ascarid: a probable cause of human ocular larva migrans, Ophthalmology **92:**1735, 1985.

Semba, R.D., Day, S.H., and Spencer, W.H.: Conjunctival nodule associated with onchocerciasis, Arch. Ophthalmol. **103:**823, 1985.

Shields, J.A.: Ocular toxocariasis: a review, Surv. Ophthalmol. **28:**361, 1984.

Mycotic disease

Feman, S.S., and Tilford, R.H.: Ocular findings in patients with histoplasmosis, J.A.M.A. **253:**2534, 1985.

Ferry, A.P., and Abedi, S.: Diagnosis and management of rhinoorbitocerebral mucormycosis (phycomycosis): a report of 16 personally observed cases, Ophthalmology **90:**1096, 1983.

Ishibashi, Y., and Kaufman, H.E.: Corneal biopsy in the diagnosis of keratomycosis, Am. J. Ophthalmol. **101:**288, 1986.

Schlaegel, T.F., Jr., and Weber, J.C.: The macular in ocular toxoplasmosis, Arch. Ophthalmol. **102:**697, 1984.

24

HEREDITARY DISORDERS

Human inheritance is determined by genes, the units of genetic information, that are encoded in the deoxyribonucleic acid (DNA) of chromosomes, Each normal human has 23 pairs of chromosomes, which contain about 50,000 pairs of genes. Genes that occupy the same position (locus) on an identical pair of chromosomes (autosome) are alleles. When both members of a pair of alleles are identical, the individual is homozygous for that gene pair; when they are different, the individual is heterozygous. The genotype describes the genetic constitution of an individual. The phenotype describes those actual physical, physiological, and biochemical characteristics of an individual, which are determined by his genotype.

Each human cell (except gametes formed in meiosis) has 22 pairs of homologous (autosomal) chromosomes and one pair of sex chromosomes, which are homologous in the female (XX) and dissimilar in the male (XY). Each parent contributes 22 autosomal chromosomes and one sex chromosome to each normal offspring. A male offspring receives a Y chromosome from his father and an X chromosome from his mother. A female offspring receives an X chromosome from each parent.

MENDELIAN INHERITANCE

Genetic disorders are of three main types: (1) gene defects, (2) chromosomal disorders, and (3) multifactorial disorders. Gene defects are caused by a mutant gene—a gene in which a permanent heritable change in genetic material has occurred. If the gene defect can be fully expressed in the phenotype by a gene present on only one chromosome of a homologous pair of chromosomes, the defect is dominant. If the gene defect requires a mutant gene at the same locus of each of a pair of homologous chromosomes, the defect is recessive. If the defect is carried on sex chromosomes, it is sex-linked or X chromosome-linked. Autosomal defects are transmitted on the 22 pairs of nonsex chromosomes. Both males and females are affected, and both can transmit the abnormality to both sons and daughters.

Autosomal dominant disorders are those conditions that can be expressed in the heterozygous states. In families with 100% penetrance (regular dominance), the trait appears in every generation, the trait is transmitted to 50% of the offspring, there is an equal sex incidence, and unaffected persons do not transmit the trait to their children. Some autosomal dominant genes do not affect an individual although the gene is inherited from a parent, a lack of penetrance. Other autosomal dominant genes are not fully expressed in the phenotype, a variable expressivity that may cause a formes frustes of the disease.

Autosomal dominant disorders are manifested from one generation to the next. Except in the instance of fresh mutations, each affected individual has a parent that is affected and may have affected siblings. An affected individual and a normal mate will transmit the gene to half of their offspring; both sexes will be equally affected. Autosomal dominant conditions involve mainly structural or nonenzymatic proteins. Generally, the disorders are less severe than those occurring with autosomal recessive traits. Autosomal dominant ocular disorders (Table 24-1) include most corneal dystrophies, aniridia, some congenital cataracts, some retinitis pigmentosa pedigrees, and vitelliform macular degeneration (Best disease). Bilateral retinoblastomas, previously considered an autosomal condition, constitute a special class of an autosomal recessive gene activated by another genetic change.

Autosomal recessive traits are transmitted by clinically normal phenotypes, each of whom contributes an abnormal gene. The carrier of a single defective gene (heterozygous), while clinically normal, may show minimal evidence of the defect such as an enzyme deficiency that occurs in carriers of Tay-Sachs disease or galactosemia. When both parents are heterozygous for a recessive trait, one fourth of the offspring will be homozygous for the abnormal allele, one fourth will be normal, and one half will be heterozygous for the recessive trait. The offspring of those affected do not demonstrate the trait, although all are carriers of the abnormal gene. Most inborn errors of metabolism are autosomal recessive disorders, as are some instances of retinoblastoma, oculocutaneous albinism, and retinitis pigmentosa (Table 24-2). In general, those affected with autosomal recessive conditions have clinically more severe abnormalities than those involving dominant inheritance. Since related individuals are more likely to be heterozygous for the same abnormal gene, consanguinity is more likely to produce offspring affected by a recessive disorder.

Defects that are carried on the sex chromosomes may be heterozygous or homozygous in the female and hemizygous in the male. The female, with two X chromosomes, and being either heterozygous or homozygous, can demonstrate either recessive or dominant behavior of a trait. An abnormal X chromosome is always expressed in the male, whether dominant or recessive, because there is no corresponding X chromosome to suppress expressivity of the abnormal X chromosome. The homozygous female transmits an abnormal X chromosome to all her children. Her sons will express the trait, and her daughters will be carriers and transmit the trait. The heterozygous female transmits an

Table 24-1. Some autosomal dominant disorders with ocular signs

Albinism, ocular (rarely)
Aniridia
Cataract (some)
Corneal dystrophies (most)
Marfan syndrome
Neurofibromatosis, (some)
Oculocutaneous albinism (rarely)
Osteogenesis imperfecta
Retinitis pigmentosa (some)
Telangiectasia ataxia
Tuberous sclerosis
Vitelliform retinal degeneration (Best)
von Hippel-Lindau disease

Table 24-2. Some autosomal recessive conditions with ocular signs

A-beta-lipoproteinemia
Albinism, oculocutaneous
Alkaptonuria
Alpha-lipoprotein deficiency (Tangier)
Cerebrohepatorenal syndrome (Zellweger)
Cystinosis, benign
Galactosemia
Gaucher disease
Glycogenesis, generalized (Pompe)
Gyrate atrophy retina and choroid
Hepaticoglycogenesis (Gierke)
Homocystinuria
Lysosomal storage diseases
Nephropathic cystine storage disease (Lignac-Fanconi syndrome)
Phytanic acid storage disease (Refsum)
Retinitis pigmentosa (most)
Retinoblastoma (appears clinically to have autosomal dominant heredity)
Sulfite oxidase deficiency
Tyrosinemia type II

abnormal X chromosome to one half of her sons and daughters. The hemizygous male transmits an abnormal X chromosome only to his daughters.

The male has one X chromosome and thus carries only half the complement of X chromosome-linked genes found in the female. There can be no father-to-son transmission, because the male transmits an X chromosome to his daughters and a Y chromosome to his sons. All daughters of an affected male will inherit the defective gene (Table 24-3). Half the children of the daughter will inherit the defective gene. The abnormality will be expressed in the sons,

Table 24-3. Some ocular conditions assigned to chromosome X

Albinism, ocular	Macular dystrophy
Albinism, deafness	Microphthalmia
Alport syndrome	Mucopolysaccharidosis
Anophthalmos	(Hunter type II)
Cataract	Night blindness
Cerebral-oculo-acoustic syndrome	Norrie disease
Choroideremia	Nystagmus
Color vision deficiency	Oculocerebral
Deutanomaly	syndrome (Lowe)
Protanomaly	Ophthalmoplegia
Fabry disease	Optic atrophy
Glucose-6-phosphate deficiency	Retinitis pigmentosa
dehydrogenase	Retinoschisis
Incontinenti pigmenti	Telecanthus
Iris hypoplasia	

while the carrier daughters (first generation carriers) will transmit the gene to one fourth of their sons. An X chromosome-linked disease is evident in the female when the condition is recessive and there are allelic genes on the X chromosome. A recessive gene may be expressed if only one X chromosome is present, for example, Turner syndrome.

The Y chromosome in the male seems devoid of genetic information beyond male sex characteristics. The X chromosome contains genetic information and, since the female derives one X chromosome from each parent, there is an excess of genetic material. This excess is compensated in each cell by a random inactivation of one of the X chromosomes. Thus every female cell has one active and one inactive X chromosome (Barr body) that is derived from one or the other parent. The active paternal cells may manifest themselves in some X chromosome-linked disorders. For example, in X chromosome-linked ocular albinism, the carrier mother's iris may transilluminate. In choroideremia the mother's peripheral fundus is pigmented.

Multifactorial inheritance governs many characteristics such as height, color, refraction, and intelligence that vary over a wide range. Many genes on many chromosomes are responsible. There is no sharp distinction between normal and abnormal phenotypes. Proof of this type of inheritance is difficult to establish, but strabismus, some refractive errors, glaucoma, and many other conditions are examples.

CHROMOSOMAL ABNORMALITIES

Chromosomal abnormalities result from an abnormal number of chromosomes or from alterations in one or more chromosomes. In numerical anomalies individuals have 45 or 47 chromosomes rather than the normal complement of 46. In some fatal chromosome abnormalities, the number of chromosomes may be $46 + (23)^n$. Abnormalities of the sex chromosomes X or Y may produce individuals with 45, 47, 48, 49, or 50 chromosomes. There must be at least 22 pairs of autosomal chromosomes for normal gestation.

In addition to numeric changes, there may be structural changes in chromosome composition, which occur when there is chromosomal breakage followed by reconstitution in an altered order. There are several types: deletions, duplications, inversions, translocations, and isochromosomes. Deletions involve loss of chromosomal material. Duplications indicate addition of chromosomal material. Inversions involve a reversal of the order of sequence in a chromosome. Translocations involve the transfer of one chromosome to another that may be reciprocal when the exchange between chromosomes is without addition or loss of chromosomal material, or insertional, in which a segment of chromosome is annealed to a nonhomologous chromosome. (Chromosome parts are classified as follows: p is the short arm; q is the long arm; R is the ring; and number is the band number and position from the centromere.)

With all abnormalities of autosomal chromosomes, there may be low birth weight for gestational age, mental retardation, and failure to thrive. Hypertelorism, small palpebral fissures that slant downward and inward, blepharoptosis, strabismus, epicanthus, corneal opacities, colobomas of the iris and choroid, microphthalmia, or anophthalmia may occur.

Demonstration of a chromosomal abnormality or assignment of a gene to a specific location on a specific chromosome involves several methods: pedigree analysis, gene dosage techniques, somatic cell hybridization, and recombinant DNA techniques. These studies have led to a variety of ocular abnormalities being assigned to a specific chromosome (Table 24-4).

Table 24-4. Eye disorders that have been mapped to specific chromosomes

Chromosome		Disorder
X	x q	Ocular albinism
	x q	Retinoschisis
	x q 28	Color vision deficiency
		Deutan, protan
	x q 26 − x q 28	Mucopolysaccharidosis type II
	x q 22 − x q 24	Fabry disease
	x p	Ichthyosis
	x p 11.3 − 11	Retinitis pigmentosa
1	1 p 32 − 1 p 34	Fucosidosis
	1 p	Coppock cataract
	tentative	Retinitis pigmentosa
2	2 p 23 (tentative)	Aniridia
	2 p (tentative)	Optic atrophy (Kjer type)
3	3 p 12 − 3 q 13	Generalized gangliosidosis
4		Anterior segment dysgenesis
	4 q 23 − 4 q 27 (tentative)	Reiger syndrome
5	5 q 13	Sandhoff disease
	5 q	Mucopolysaccharidosis type VI
6		Diabetes mellitus, type I
	tentative	Paget disease, bone
7	7 p	Mucopolysaccharidosis type VII
9	9 p 12 − 9 p 13	Galactosemia
	tentative	Waardenburg syndrome
11	11 p 13	Aniridia, Wilms tumor
	tentative	Congenital glaucoma
	tentative	Albinism, tyrosinase-negative
13	13 q 14	Retinoblastoma
15	15 q 22 − 15 q 25.1	Tay-Sachs
16	16 q (tentative)	Posterior polar cataract
17	17 q	Galactokinase deficiency
19		Mannosidosis
	19 p terminal − 19 q 13	Myotonic dystrophy
22	22 q 13.31 − 22 q terminal	Metachromatic dystrophy
	22 p terminal − 22 q 11	Cat-eye syndrome

p = short arm of chromosome.
q = long arm of chromosome.
After Mets, M.B., and Maumenee, I.H.: The eye and the chromosome, Surv. Ophthalmol. **28:**20, 1983.

Deletion syndromes

Partial deletion of the short arm of chromosome 4 (46,XX[female] or 46,XY[male] 4 p-[Wolf-Hirschorn]) is associated with profound mental and growth retardation, hypertelorism (simulating exophthalmos), blepharoptosis, exotropia, epicanthal folds, and coloboma of the iris. Hemangioma of the brow is common, as are cryptorchidism and hypospadias.

Deletion of the short arm of chromosome 5 (46,XX or 46,XY,5p − 14 or − 15) is characterized by a high-pitched, weak, shrill catlike cry (cri du chat) of the infant during the first few weeks of life, the result of laryngomalacia.

There is severe mental and growth retardation with microcephaly. The infant's face is round, the inner canthus is higher than the outer, and epicanthus, hypertelorism, and alternating esotropia are present.

Deletion of the short arm of chromosome 13 (46,XX or 46,XY, 13p −) is associated with aniridia and Wilms tumor.

Deletion of the long arm of chromosome 13 (46,XX or 46,XY,13 − q) is associated with retinoblastoma, agenesis of the thumbs, and imperforate anus. In some patients there are uveal colobomas, cataract, microphthalmia, and blepharoptosis.

Deletion of the short arm of chromosome 18 (46,XX or 46,XY,18p −) is associated with mental retardation, hypertelorism, epicanthal folds, strabismus, blepharoptosis, and rarely with cataract. Deletion of the long arm (46,XX or 46,XY,18q −) is associated with midface hypoplasia and frequent eye defects, such as glaucoma, strabismus, nystagmus, tapetoretinal degeneration, and optic atrophy.

Numerical variation syndromes

Trisomy 21 syndrome. Trisomy 21 syndrome (47,XX or 27,XY, −21 [Down syndrome]) is the most common chromosomal disorder and is the most common cause of mental retardation that can be recognized at birth. Over 90% of affected individuals have trisomy 21 so that their chromosome count is 47; others have a normal chromosome number, but extra chromosome material is present. The parents have a normal karyotype. There is a gradual linear increase in incidence with increasing maternal age and a rapid logarithmic type of increase after about 33 years of age. In mothers 20 to 30 years of age, the risk increases from about 1 in 2,000 live births to 1 in 900. At 35 years of age, the incidence rises to 1 in 350 and by 40 years to 1 in 110. After 46 years of age, the risk increases to 1 in 25.

About 3.5% of patients with Down syndrome have a normal chromosome complement of 46, but extra chromosomal material is attached to another chromosome, often chromosome 14. Study of the parents of such a patient indicates that one of them, usually the mother, has 45 chromosomes with a new chromosome formed by fusion of chromosome 21 and chromosome 14 (Robertsonian translocation [45,XX, −14, −21, +(tHq21q)]). In mosaic Down syndrome, patients have a mixture of cells with 45 and 47 chromosomes. Symptoms are milder, depending on the proportion of abnormal cells. Maternal age is of no importance in cases of translocation or mosaicism.

There are numerous typical physical findings: hypotonia; mental retardation; open mouth with thick protruding tongue; dental hypoplasia, hypoplasia of the nasal bones; angular overlapping helix, prominent antihelix, and small or absent earlobe, and excessive skin on the nape of the neck. Lips are broad, irregular, fissured, and dry. Hands are short and broad, and the fifth finger is usually abbreviated. Intelligence quotients range from 15 to 70. Acute leukemia and congenital heart defects are common.

The palpebral fissure is almond-shaped, the outer canthus is higher than the medial canthus (mongoloid slant), and epicanthal folds are present. The iris is hypoplastic, and in early life, white areas are present (Brushfield spots). Cataract occurs in about 60% of the patients. Esotropia, nystagmus, myopia, and blepharitis are common. Teenagers may develop keratoconus, often complicated by an acute corneal hydrops (edema) that heals with severe scarring.

Irrespective of the refractive error or the degree of skin or iris pigmentation, the fundus appears ophthalmoscopically as it does in myopic or blond individuals. The pigmentation of the retinal pigment epithelium and choroid is scanty, and the choroidal vasculature is easily visible. The large number of retinal vessels crossing the disk margin give it a pinker color than usual.

Trisomy 18 syndrome. Trisomy 18 syndrome (47,XX or 47,XY + 18 [Edward syndrome]) is second only to Down syndrome in frequency. Ocular hypertelorism, prominent epicanthal folds, and blepharophimosis are common. There may be microphthalmia, uveal colobomas, corneal opacities, congenital glaucoma, and abnormal optic disks.

Trisomy 13 syndrome. Trisomy 13 syndrome (47,XX or 47,XY +13 [Patau syndrome]) includes severe psychomotor retardation, arhinecephaly, sloping forehead, cleft lip and palate, ocular hypertelorism, absent eyebrows, renal defects, and capillary hemangiomas. There are numerous ocular abnormalities: microphthalmia; coloboma of the iris, choroid, and optic nerve; retinal dysplasia; optic nerve hypoplasia; persistent hyperplastic primary vitreous; cataract; cyclopia; corneal opacity; and intraocular cartilage. Embryonic or fetal hemoglobin is common. Few affected infants live more than a year.

Turner syndrome. Patients with Turner syndrome (45,XO,45X monosomy, gonadal dysgenesis) receive an X chromosome from the mother but lack the X chromosome from the father. They are unambiguously female but have infantile genitalia, primary amenorrhea, infertility, and a short stature. They have the same incidence of color vision deficiency as is seen in normal males. Additionally, strabismus, blepharoptosis, blue sclera, cataract, and corneal arcus occur in more than one third.

Cat-eye syndrome. This is an abnormality with a supernumerary fragment with the long arm of chromosome 22 (46,XX or 46,XY + 22 pter or 22 q 11). There is a coloboma of the iris combined with anal atresia. There is severe motor retardation, hypertelorism, antimongoloid slant of the palpebral fissures, microphthalmia, and sometimes optic atrophy. Preauricular skin tags and fistulas, abnormal ears, congential heart disease, and renal abnormalities occur.

LYSOSOMAL STORAGE DISEASE

A lysosomal storage disease is an abnormality in which one of the acid hydrolase enzymes enclosed within the lysosome body is absent or defective and causes an accumulation of partially degraded metabolite. Approximately 35 inherited disorders are classified as lysosomal storage disease; in 20 of these the severe deficiency of a specific lysosomal hydrolase enzyme is known. In many, electron microscopic study of the conjunctiva will indicate abnormal lysosomes.

The lysosomes are intracellular organelles containing many hydrolases that degrade biologic compounds in a mild acid medium. In living cells, these enzymes are confined within the lysosome and can act only on material taken up by the cell. Four types of lysosomes are recognized: a primary lysosome and three types of secondary lysosome.

A primary lysosome is a small intracellular body that contains acid hydrolases that are synthesized by ribosomes. These enzymes accumulate in the granular endoplasmic reticulum and penetrate the Golgi apparatus, which forms an envelope containing the enzymes. A secondary lysosome is formed with either material already present in the cell or material engulfed by the primary lysosome by either phagocytosis or pinocytosis. The engulfed material is progressively digested by hydrolytic enzymes within the lysosome. If digestion is

not complete, the secondary lysosome forms a residual body. In some cells these residual bodies are eliminated from the cell. In other cells they may be retained and accumulated. The autophagic vacuole is a lysosome responsible for degradation of material produced within the cell.

The acid hydrolases of the lysosome are responsible for breaking ester bonds; glycosidases act at glycocytic linkages; phosphatases, sulfatases, and proteases act similarly. Additionally, different nonlysosomal particles called *peroxisomes* are rich in perioxidases and catylases. These enzymes are important in abnormalities such as neuronal ceroid lipofuscinosis, in which lipid material accumulates.

The lysosomal disorders may affect skeletal growth, mental development, and central nervous system development. The severity varies greatly. They may be associated with characterisitic facial changes. In some individuals there may be cloudy corneas; degeneration of the retinal ganglion cells with optic atrophy and a cherry-red spot at the fovea centralis. Other individuals develop pigmentary retinal degeneration.

The enzyme deficiency can be detected in cultured fibroblasts of the affected individual or by prenatal testing. The tissue-culture growth medium will indicate the enzyme deficiency, and electron microscopy will demonstrate the abnormal lysosomes (Fig. 24-1). Tears, urine, hair follicles, leukocytes, and fibroblasts have been used for enzyme assay. In the mucopolysaccharidoses, the abnormal storage substance may be detected intermittently in urine. Heterozygote screening for hexosaminidases A and B deficiency has been developed in many cities in the United States.

Sphingolipidoses

The sphingolipids are complex lipids that are important components of brain, nerve, and many membranes. Each contains one molecule of sphingosine, one molecule of an 18- to 26-carbon fatty acid, and a polar head group (Fig. 24-2). The combination of sphingosine and the fatty acid is called a ceramide. There are three major groups of sphingolipids: (1) sphingomyelines, the most abundant, which contain phosphorylcholine or phosphoroethylanolamine as the polar head group; (2) neutral sphingolipids, which contain one or more sugars in the polar head group; and (3) acidic glycosphingolipids (gangliosides), which contain one or more molecules of sialic acid in the polar head group.

The sphingolipidoses are genetically determined metabolic defects characterized by the

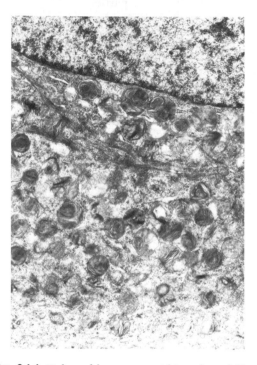

Fig. 24-1. Enlarged lysosomes within cultured fibroblasts in a lysosomal storage disease. All affected tissues show similar accumulation, and enzyme deficiency may be demonstrated in the culture media. (×19,000).

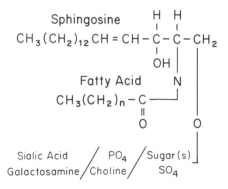

Fig. 24-2. General chemical structure of the sphingolipids.

accumulation of excessive quanitities of fatty substances in various tissues, giving rise to visceral, neural, and ocular manifestations. There are at least nine sphingolipid disorders, and a different complex lipid accumulates in each. The abnormality occurs because of a deficiency of the enzyme necessary for the degradation of the excess lipid (Table 24-5). With the exception of Fabry disease, which is an X chromosome-linked recessive abnormality, each of the conditions is transmitted as an autosomal recessive. Most result because each parent is a heterozygote. The enzyme deficiency may be demonstrated in cultured fibroblasts of parents or by assay of cultured fetal fibroblasts.

Niemann-Pick disease. Niemann-Pick disease (sphingomyelin lipidosis) is a collective term for a group of disorders in which there is widespread accumulation of sphingomyelin and cholesterol in the reticuloendothelial and nervous systems and in the parenchymal cells of many organs. There are at least six phenotypes: A, B, C, D, E, and F. Each has a deficiency of a sphingomyelinase isoenzyme.

The conditions are transmitted as autosomal recessive traits and tend to involve persons of Jewish parentage (46%). Type A (classical infantile form) and type C (late infantile or juvenile form) are the most common.

In type A (acute infantile), which may occur prenatally, poor feeding may be the earliest sign, followed by retarded mental and physical development. Nearly every organ may be infiltrated with sphingomyelin, and there is enlargment of the liver and spleen, abdominal distention, infiltration of lymph nodes and bone marrow, fever, and yellow-brown skin discoloration. There is a cherry-red spot in one or both retinas, cloudy corneas, and brown discoloration of the lens. The conjunctival stroma contains inclusions.

Type C (mixed type) has a later onset than type A and a more prolonged course, but eventually there is widespread neurologic involvement and death. Retinal cherry-red spots occur occasionally, but the lens and cornea are spared. Conjunctival inclusions are found in both the epithelium and stroma.

Accumulation of neutral sphingolipids. The main sphingolipidoses involving the accumulation of neutral sphingolipids are galactosyl ceramide lipidosis (Krabbe), diffuse angiokeratoma

(Fabry), and glucosyl ceramide lipidosis (Gaucher).

Galactosyl ceramide lipidosis. Galactosyl ceramide lipidosis (globoid cell leukodystrophy, Krabbe disease) is an inherited abnormality of a sphingolipid that is normally concentrated in the myelin sheath. It has its onset in the first 6 months of life and results in death from emaciation at 1 or 2 years of age. The disease begins with irritability and progresses to motor and mental deterioration. There is spasticity early, but patients become flaccid later. Blindness caused by optic atrophy occurs commonly. Deafness is common. There is no storage of

Table 24-5. Summary of lysosomal disorders

Disorder		Enzyme deficiency	Metabolite primarily affected
Sphingolipidoses			
G_{M1} gangliosidosis		β-Galactosidase	G_{M1} ganglioside, fragments from glycoproteins
Krabbe disease		β-Galactosidase	Galactosyl ceramide
Tay-Sachs disease		Hexosaminidase A	G_{M2} ganglioside
Sandhoff disease		Hexosaminidases A and B	G_{M2} ganglioside, globoside
Gaucher disease		β-Glucosidase	Glucosyl ceramide
Fabry disease		α-Galactosidase	Trihexosyl ceramide
Metachromatic leukodystrophy		Arylsulfatase A	Sulfatide
Niemann-Pick disease		Sphingomyelinase	Sphingomyelin
Farber disease		Ceramidase	Ceramide
Mucopolysaccharidoses			
Type	Eponym		
MPS I H	Hurler	α-L-iduronidase	Dermatan sulfate, heparan sulfate
MPS I S (formerly MPS V S)	Scheie	α-L-iduronidase	Dermatan sulfate, heparan sulfate
MPS I H-S	Hurler-Scheie	α-L-iduronidase	Dermatan sulfate, heparan sulfate
MPS II	Hunter	Idurontate sulfatase	Dermatan sulfate, heparan sulfate
MPS III A	San Fillipo	Heparin-N-sulfatase	Heparan sulfate
MPS III B	San Fillipo	N-acetyl-α-D-glucosaminidase	Heparan sulfate
MPS IV	Morquio	Hexosamine 6-sulfatase	Keratan sulfate
MPS VI	Maroteux-Lamy	Arylsulfatase B	Dermatan sulfate
MPS VII	Sly	β-Glucuronidase	Dermatan sulfate, heparan sulfate
Disorders of glycoprotein metabolism			
Fucosidosis		α-L-Fucosidase	Fragments from glycoproteins, glycolipids
Mannosidosis		α-Mannosidase	Mannose containing glycoproteins, glycopeptides, and oligosaccharides
Aspartylglycosaminuria		Amidase	Aspartyl-2-deoxy-2-acetamido glucosylamine
Other disorders with single enzyme defect			
Pompe disease		α-Glucosidase	Glycogen
Wolman disease		Acid lipase	Cholesterol esters, triglyceride
Acid phosphatase deficiency		Acid phosphastase	Phosphate esters
Multiple enzyme deficiencies (inherited as a single gene defect)			
Multiple sulfatase deficiency		Sulfatases (arylsulfatase A,B,C: steroid sulfatases; iduronate sulfatase; heparan N-sulfatase)	Sulfatide, steroid sulfate, glycosaminoglycans
Mycolipidosis		Almost all lysosomal enzymes deficient in cultured fibroblasts; present extracellulary	Glycosaminoglycans and glycolipids
Disorders of unknown cause			
Cystinosis		Accumulation of cystine in lysosomes	Cystine
Mucolipidoses I, IV		Ultrastructural evidence of lysosomal storage	Unknown

sphingolipids in tissues, but there is an absence or deficiency of β-galactosidase, which normally degrades galactosyl ceramide that result from myelin turnover. The globoid cell is characteristic. It resembles a large epithelial cell and occurs in demyelinated regions.

Diffuse angiokeratoma. Diffuse angiokeratoma (Fabry disease) is a recessive X chromosome-linked lysosomal storage disease that results from a deficiency of the enzyme α-galactosidase A. This defect leads to the progressive accumulation of the glycosphingolipid trihexosyl ceramide, particulary in the endothelial cells of blood vessels. Symptoms occur in early childhood. There are episodes of excruciating pain in the extremities, fever, and angiokeratomatous skin lesions, particularly affecting the thighs and genitalia. Venous aneurysmal dilations and tortuosity on the inferior bulbar conjunctiva occur in both hemizygous males (78%) and heterozygous females (46%). The retinal veins are more tortuous than normal and sometimes segmentally dilated. Central retinal artery or vein occlusion may occur. There are cream-colored whorl-like opacities in the cornea at the level of the Bowman zone in all hemizygotes and most heterozygotes (88%). A granular anterior subcapsular cataract occurs in some hemizygotes, and a white posterior subcapsular branching opacity resembling a herpetic dendrite occurs in both hemizygotes (37%) and heterozygotes (14%). Myopia occurs frequently, especially among heterozygotes.

Renal transplantation can prevent death in the third and fourth decades. Galactose-free diets reduce the chemical substrate, and kidney transplants increase enzyme activity.

Glucosyl ceramide lipidosis. Glucosyl ceramide lipidosis (Gaucher disease) includes at least three disorders characterized by the accumulation of glucosyl ceramide in the reticuloendothelial system because of a deficiency of the enzyme, β-glucosidase. Diagnosis requires demonstration of the deficiency in white blood cells, histiocytes, or cultured fibroblasts.

Type 1, the most common, may manifest itself at any age. Bleeding, thrombocytopenia, and intermittent infection occur, but there are no neurologic signs. Bone lesions are common. Minor pingueculas occur.

The acute neuropathic (infantile) type develops before 6 months of age, and there is widespread neurologic involvement with mental retardation, spasticity, hepatosplenomegaly, and eventually death from intercurrent infection. Ocular signs are secondary to cranial nerve involvement.

Type 3, or subacute Gaucher disease (juvenile), has its onset after 6 months of age, and survival is from 2 to 20 years. The disease is dominated by the effects of an increasing mass of Gaucher cells in the liver, spleen, lymph nodes, and bone marrow. There is hepatosplenomegaly and lymphadenopathy, bone lesions causing spontaneous fractures, and involvement of the spleen and bone marrow, with resultant pancytopenia often necessitating splenectomy. The skin is pigmented. Ultimately there is interference with blood cell formation and death from intercurrent infection.

There may be loss of voluntary eye movements, which is compensated for by head movements in response to visual stimuli (oculomotor apraxia) and other motor anomalies. Discrete white dots, which vary in size from just visible to 0.1 mm, may be scattered throughout the posterior fundus. They appear to be situated on the surface of the retina or in the inner retina. Large brown pingueculae, with their base on the corneoscleral limbus, have been described.

Gangliosidoses. The glycosphingolipids of the brain are localized primarily in synaptic membranes. Disorders occur because of a metabolic defect resulting from deficiencies of ganglioside glycohydrolases. The disorders include G_{M1} gangliosidosis types I and II, G_{M2} gangliosidosis, hexosaminidase A and B deficiency (Sandhoff disease), G_{M2} gangliosidosis with hexosominidase A deficiency (Tay-Sachs disease), and juvenile G_{M2} gangliosidosis. Progressive motor and mental deterioration begins early in life, and death occurs in childhood. All are autosomal recessive conditions. In each there is storage of a specific ganglioside and absence or deficiency of a specific enzyme. The heterozygote may be detected by decreased enzyme activity in the serum, and prenatal diagnosis is possible by amniocentesis.

Tay-Sachs disease, Sandhoff disease, and juvenile G_{M2} gangliosidosis involve storage of the same material, ganglioside G_{M2}. This compound is normally degraded by two enzymes, hexosaminidase A and B. In Tay-Sachs disease, hexosaminidase A is absent and hexosaminidase B is deficient; in Sandhoff disease both hexosaminidase A and B are markedly deficient; and in juvenile G_{M2} gangliosidosis there is moderate deficiency of hexosaminidase A and normal hexosaminidase B.

G_{M1} *gangliosidosis types I and II.* These types of gangliosidosis involve storage of the G_{M1} ganglioside because of deficiency of lysomal β-galactosidase in the brain.

G_{M2} *gangliosidosis with hexosaminidase A deficiency (Tay-Sachs disease).* This is the most common type of gangliosidosis. It is an autosomal recessive disorder and has an onset with motor weakness 3 to 6 months after birth. the most common initial symptom is a startled reaction to sound (hyperacusis). The infants often have long eyelashes, fine hair, and a delicate pink coloring. Vision is affected early. There is inattentiveness, failure to move the eyes, or strabismus. Ophthalmoscopic examination may be normal initially, but soon the fovea centralis shows a whitish area ophthalmoscopically that is approximately 2 disk diameters in size, with a small reddish foveola area (cherry-red spot). Retinal and optic atrophy is followed by blindness. As neurologic involvement progresses, convulsions or a state of decerebrate rigidity may occur. Death from bulbar involvement usually occurs at about 30 months of age.

Storage of gangliosides in the retinal ganglion cells causes the normally transparent retina to appear white at the posterior pole where the ganglion cells are several layers thick. The cherry-red spot results from the normal appearance of the choroidal circulation at the fovea centralis, where the inner retinal layers are absent. Changes in the brain include enormously swollen and distorted ganglion cells.

With a light microscope, the neurons of the central, autonomic, and somatic nervous systems appear enormously swollen and distended. Electron microscopically, the neuronal deposits consist of concentric membranes called membranous cytoplasmic bodies. Nerve fibers are demyelinated, which contributes to the optic atrophy.

The disorder has a carrier frequency of one in 30 for Ashkenazic (European) Jews and one in 300 for non-Jewish individuals.

Sandhoff disease. This condition is similar to Tay-Sachs disease, but tubular epithelial cells contain lipids. It is distinguished from Tay-Sachs disease by the severe deficiency of hexosaminidase A and B.

Juvenile G_{M2} *gangliosidosis.* Onset is between 2 and 6 years of age, with ataxia, dysarthria, seizures, and eventual decerebrate rigidity. Cherry-red spots and blindness occur late, and patients die between 5 and 15 years of age.

Ceramidase deficiency (Farber lipogranulomatosis). This disorder involves accumulation of ceramide, and in severely affected persons, a deficiency of acid ceramidase has been demonstrated. Soon after birth, infants develop swollen, tender joints and a hoarse weak cry because of deposition of ceramide in the joints and larynx. Ceramide concentration in the tissue is markedly increased, and G_1 ganglioside is increased in nerve tissue. Birefringent glycolipid may be found in the retinal ganglion cell layer, and retinal cherry-red spots have been described.

Metachromatic leukodystrophy. This is a group of autosomal recessive disorders in which an arylsulfatase A deficiency causes sulfatides to accumulate in myelin sheaths and cerebral white matter. There is massive urinary excretion of sulfatides. Late infantile, juvenile, adult, and variant forms with multiple sulfatase deficiencies have been described.

Weakness, ataxia, dysarthria, ocular muscle palsies, nystagumus, and severe mental retardation occur. Optic atrophy and grayish infiltration of the central retina with foveolar cherry-red spots lead to blindness. Membranous lysosomal residual bodies are confined to the ganglion cells of the retina and central nervous system. Material that stains red with toluidine blue (metachromasia) is found in urinary sediment and in ganglion cells, including those of the retina.

Cherry-red spot–myoclonus syndrome. In this autosomal recessive condition, cherry-red spots develop at the foveola before 10 years of age. Myoclonus then develops. Violent jerks may be precipitated by voluntary movements, the thought of movement, light touch, passive joint movements, and sound, but not by light. There is no dementia or neurologic deterioration, although decreased vision has been described. The lysosomes of retinal ganglion cells, cortical neurons, neurons of the nyenteric plexus, hepatocytes, and Kupffer cells

Table 24-6. Mucopolysaccharide storage diseases

Type	Eponym	Skeletal dysplasia	Mental retardation	Somatic changes	Corneal clouding
MPS I H	Hurler	Severe	Severe	Severe	Severe
MPS I S (formerly MPS VS)	Scheie	Slight	Slight to normal	Aortic regurgitation	Severe
MPS I H-S*	Hurler-Scheie	Moderate	Moderate	Moderate	Moderate
MPS II	Hunter†				
	A. Severe	Severe	Severe	Severe	None
	B. Mild	Moderate	Slight to normal	Moderate	With aging
MPS III A	San Fillipo	Slight	Severe		None
MPS III B	San Fillipo	Slight	Severe		None
MPS IV	Morquio	Severe	Slight to normal	Aortic regurgitation	Moderate
MPS VI	Maroteux-Lamy	Severe	Normal	Aortic regurgitation; hydrocephalus	Severe
MPS VII	β-Glucuronidase deficiency	Moderate	Moderate	Aortic regurgitation	Severe

*Heterozygous with mutant Hurler gene on one allele and mutant Scheie gene on other.
†Hunter syndrome is inherited as an X chromosome–linked recessive trait; all others are autosomal recessive. Optic atrophy has been reported in all. Pigmentary degeneration of the retina has been described in all but IV and VI.

store a material that resembles a lipofuscin material. Hepatocytes, Kupffer cells, and possibly cortical neurons store material containing polysaccharide. There is decreased neuraminidase activity for α-1-*N*-neuraminosyl galactose linkages.

Mucopolysaccharide storage diseases

The acid mucopolysaccharides are a group of related long unbranched compounds that contain two types of alternating monosaccharide units. Seven acid mucopolysaccharides have been described: hyaluronic acid, chondroitin, chondroitin-4-sulfate, chondroitin-6-sulfate, dermatan sulfate, keratan sulfate, and heparin sulfate. They are major components of cell coats, cartilage, bone other connective tissues, and intracellular cement substances. These compounds are degraded by a series of enzymatic steps. A deficiency of an enzyme leads to the storage of mucopolysaccharide in the tissues, causing characteristic clinical syndromes (Table 24-6).

Hurler syndrome (MPS-1-H) is a widespread systemic disorder usually evident within 6 months after birth. It is characterized clinically by skeletal deformities, limitations of joint movements, hernia, hepatosplenomegaly, cardiac abnormalities, deafness, mental retardation, and diffuse corneal clouding. Dermatan sulfate and heparin sulfate are found in urine and tissues, and dermatan sulfate is found in fibroblasts. There is increased ganglioside in the brain and absence of α-L-iduronidase in the tissues.

Typically the patient has a large and bulging head, the bridge of the nose is flattened, the nostrils are broad, and the nose is flattened, the nostrils are broad, and the posterior pharynx is occluded. The children are mouth breathers and have markedly carious teeth and a fetid breath. The facies are apathetic, the tongue is enlarged, and the facial features are coarse (Fig. 24-3). The neck is short, and the head appears to rest directly upon the thorax. Kyphosis is common, as are deformities of the vertebrae. The broad hands have stubby fingers, and on roentgenologic study, the terminal phalangeal bones are hypoplastic. Limitation of extension of the joints is striking. The abdomen is protuberant. Roentgenographic examination reveals a long and shallow sella turcica.

Clouding of the cornea is characteristic. The subepithelial area has the appearance of

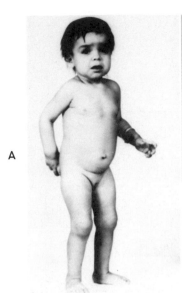

A

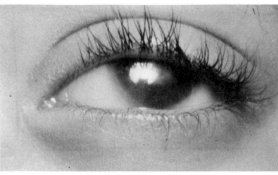

B

Fig. 24-3. A, Typical appearance of a patient with mucopolysaccharidosis (Hurler syndrome). **B,** The cloudy corneas of the mucopolysaccharidosis.

slightly glazed glass. The central cornea is more cloudy than the periphery, although histologically (Fig. 24-4) the deep epithelial layers of the periphery are more involved. The normal tension, absence of tearing, failure of the globe to enlarge, and associated physical changes exclude glaucoma as a cause of the corneal clouding. Rarely, increased intracranial pressure occurs, but the papilledema cannot be seen through the cloudy cornea. There is retinal infiltration with mucopolysaccharides and an extinguished electroretinogram.

Dermatan sulfate and keratan sulfate are found in the urine and tissues. Fibroblasts synthesize dermatan sulfate, an abnormality that permits diagnosis by means of culture of amniotic fluid. There is increased ganglioside in the brain and decreased β-galactosidase in tissues. Treatment currently is directed toward replacement of "Hurler corrective factor" found in normal plasma and containing α-L-iduronidase.

Mucopolysaccharidosis I-S (Scheie) is a less severe condition, but patients have marked clouding of the corneas.

Mucopolysaccharidosis II-H (Hunter syndrome) is inherited as an X chromosome-linked recessive trait. The patients clinically resemble those with Hurler disease, but clinical manifestations are less severe and the corneas are grossly clear, although there may be

slight corneal haze in adulthood. Patients may survive into adulthood, and mental retardation may not occur. Laboratory findings resemble findings of type I-H.

Macular corneal dystrophy (Groenouw type II hereditary corneal dystrophy) is an autosomal recessive disorder involving only the cornea. It is characterized by slowly progressive visual loss caused by the accumulation of a mucopolysaccharide within keratocytes. There is no abnormal urinary excretion of mucopolysaccharides, and skin fibroblasts do not demonstrate an abnormal mucopolysaccharide metabolism. It is regarded as a local tissue abnormality.

Other lysosomal storage diseases

Fucosidosis. This is an autosomal recessive lysosomal disease characterized by the absence or profound deficiency of α-L-fucosidase, resulting in a widespread accumulation of fucose-containing glycosphingolipids, glycoproteins, and glycosaminoglycans, together with an increased excretion of fucosides in the urine. Clinically, severe and mild phenotypes have been distinguished. The severe form causes a progressive psychomotor retardation and a moderate chrondrodystrophy that somewhat resembles the mucopolysaccharidoses. Death occurs between 3 and 5 years of age. Survival to adolescence and beyond has been reported in the mild phenotype.

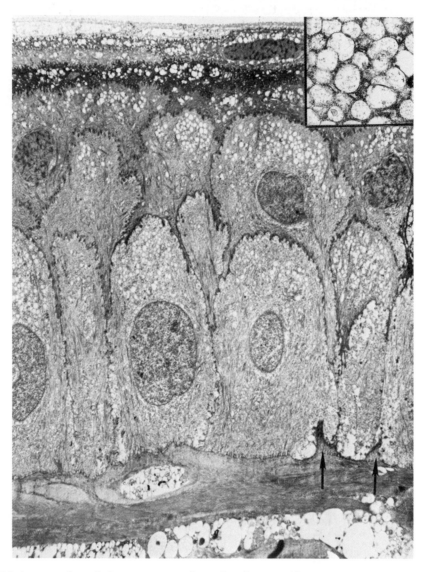

Fig. 24-4. Corneal epithelium in mucopolysaccharidosis I with numerous intracellular lysosomes (inset, × 17,000) filled with dermatan sulfate and keratan sulfate I. The Bowman membrane is destroyed, and the scarred anterior stroma sends projections *(arrows)* into the epithelium. Keratocytes have numerous lysosomes. (Electron micrograph ×1800.) (From Tripathi, R.C., and Ashton, N.: Application of electron microscopy to the study of ocular inborn errors of metabolism. In Bergsma, D., Bron, A.J., and Cotlier, E., editors: The eye and inborn errors of metabolism, New York, Alan R. Liss for The National Foundation— March of Dimes, BD:OAS **12**(3):69-104, 1976.)

The skin changes of angiokeratoma corporis diffusum occur, and there are thin and tortuous veins in the conjunctiva and ocular fundus. Conjunctival biopsy shows cytoplasmic inclusions resulting from overloading of the lysosomes. The endothelial cells of blood capillaries are filled with abnormal inclusions. Stored material is pathognomonic, and there may be clear vacuoles containing finely reticular material similar to that in mucopolysaccharidosis and less numerous dark inclusions. Sodium and chloride levels in the sweat are high and in the range encounted in cystic fibrosis.

Mannosidosis. This is a lysosomal storage disease that resembles mucopolysaccharidosis clinically and is caused by tissue deficiency of α-mannosidase A and B, resulting in accumulation of mannose-rich glycoproteins, glycopeptides, and oligosaccharides in tissues and urine. There is a prominent metopic suture and coarse facies. Patients may demonstrate cardiac dysfunction, hepatosplenomegaly, and gibbus deformity. Connective tissue defects may include hernias, diastasis recti, and testicular hydrocele. Initial rapid growth is followed by slow growth, susceptibility to infection, and decreased serum immunoglobulins. Lens opacities develop in infancy in many patients. The usual opacity is located in the posterior cortex and appears ophthalmoscopically as radiating spokes of a wheel. A milder phenotype causes punctate lens opacities.

Mucolipidosis. This is a group of lysosomal storage diseases in which neither the storage substance nor the deficient enzyme has been recognized. All have inclusions in cultured fibroblasts. In mucolipidosis II (inclusion cell or I-cell disease), cloudy corneas were present in only one of ten patients. Except for this group, most patients have corneal clouding, skeletal dysplasia, mental retardation, and coarse facial features. Some have retinal degeneration. Death in adolescence is common.

Amaurotic familial idiocy. This obsolete term was used to describe both gangliosidosis and the neuronal ceroid lipofuscinosis (infra). In gangliosidosis the ganglion cell layer of the retina accumulates gangliosides, causing a cherry-red spot. The remaining layers of the sensory retina are normal, and the electroretinogram is normal. Neuronal ceroid lipofuscinosis is a peroxidase deficiency in which the ocular changes involve mainly the photoreceptors and retinal pigment epithelium. Optic atrophy is secondary to intracranial abnormalities. The electroretinogram is nonrecordable.

Neuronal ceroid lipofuscinosis. Neural ceroid lipofuscinosis (Batten disease) is an autosomal recessive accumulation of ceroid lipofuscin in neurons. The disease may be divided into acute and chronic types plus an intermediate transitional and an atypical form. In the chronic form there is widespread deterioration of the rods and cones and the retinal pigment epithelium, attenuation of blood vessels, and optic nerve atrophy. The condition closely resembles that seen in retinitis pigmentosa. The central retina has a granular appearance, and there may be peripheral pigment deposition. Motor and mental deterioration happens slowly, and visual loss may be the initial symptom.

The acute disease is ushered in by rapidly progressive, drug-resistant, mixed, often predominantly myoclonic seizures. Rapid mental and motor deterioration follows, together with ocular changes similar to those in the chronic form. The transitional form combines the clinical and pathologic features of the acute and chronic disease forms with similar ocular changes. No visual impairment occurs in the atypical forms.

The disease occurs because of a peroxidase deficiency that may permit oxidation of unsaturated long chain fatty acids so that photoreceptor synthesis is impaired.

The following types occur: congenital (Norman Wood), infantile (Haltia-Santavouri), late infantile (Bielschowsky-Jansky), juvenile (Vogt-Spielmeyer, Sjögren), and adult (Kufs). There is a deposit of autofluorescent pigments in neurons and other cells that has a characteristic ultrastructural "fingerprint" pattern. There are low levels of docoshexaenoic acid in peripheral leukocytes.

HEPATOLENTICULAR DEGENERATION

Hepatolenticular degeneration (Wilson disease) is an autosomal recessive disorder of impaired copper excretion that results in a chronic copper toxicosis. It is never clinically manifest before the age of 5 years and may remain latent until the fifth decade. Tissue deposition of copper causes degenerative changes in the liver (cirrhosis), brain (particularly the basal ganglia), cornea (Kayser-Fleischer ring), kidneys, and joints. Hepatic or cerebral signs usually dominate the clinical picture. The rust-colored ring at the periphery of the cornea occurs in most patients. Rarely it may be the sole sign of the disease.

Initially Wilson disease is most likely to produce the symptoms and signs of liver disease. As copper is released from overloaded necrotizing hepatocytes, it accumulates in the brain, eye, kidney, bones, and joints. Acute or chronic hepatitis, cirrhosis, or portal hypertension may occur. Hepatitis with hemolytic anemia is more likely to be caused by Wilson disease than any other condition.

Cerebral signs involve the following: (1) degeneration of the nucleus lentiformis (the part of the corpus striatum comprising the putamen and globus pallidus that lies just lateral to the internal capsule), with spasticity, rigidity, dystonic deformities, disturbances of gait, dysarthria, dysphagia, or drooling; or (2) Westphal disease with tremor a major symptom. The sole manifestation may be a psychotic illness, usually of abrupt onset. The patient may have a bizarre personality, with grossly inappropriate social behavior, deterioration of schoolwork, a severe neurosis, or a disorder indistinguishable from schizophrenia or manic-depressive psychosis. Personality disorders may occur in the absence of motor involvement, and jacksonian epilepsy or hemiplegia may occur, as may a coma that persists for several weeks.

Cirrhosis of the liver, which may occur before neurologic involvement, varies from mild signs of hepatic dysfunction to portal hypertension, esophageal varices, and hepatic coma.

Kidney involvement may cause aminoaciduria (predominantly of cystine but without calculi), albuminuria, impaired concentrating capacity, glycosuria, alkaline urine, increased uric acid excretion, low serum uric acid level, hyperphosphaturia, low serum phosphate level, and osteomalacia.

The Kayser-Fleischer ring consists of a green to yellow or brown ring at the corneoscleral limbus at the level of Descemet membrane. The peripheral margin of the ring always sharply ends at the termination of Descemet membrane (Schwalbe line). The ring begins in the upper portion of the cornea and extends circumferentially. It consists of dense accumu-

lations of unequal-sized copper granules in Descemet membrane. Copper is only visible in Descemet membrane, although the corneal stroma contains a markedly increased amount of copper. Gonioscopic examination may be necessary to see the ring in early corneal involvement. Its early recognition is important because specific therapy can prevent hepatic and neurologic involvement.

Less common is a sunflow cataract involving the anterior and posterior capsules. With biomicroscopy it appears as a powdery deposit of brilliantly colored material in browns, reds, blues, greens, and yellows that is located in the visual axis with deposits radiating peripherally, resembling the petals of a sunflower.

Nystagmus, cranial nerve palsies, and other ocular movement disorders do not occur despite extensive cerebral degeneration. Night blindness and degenerative changes in the peripheral retina seem to be unrelated to the primary disorder; however, retinal function has not been systemically studied.

The diagnosis may be confirmed by the determination of the concentration of ceruloplasmin in the serum. The Kayser-Fleischer corneal ring is pathognomic. A determination of the 24-hour urinary secretion of copper or histologic and copper analysis of a needle biopsy sample of the liver may be diagnostic.

Treatment consists of a low-copper diet, general management of hepatic cirrhosis, and administration of D-penicillamine, which chelates copper and increases its excretion. Successful treatment results in disappearance of the lens deposition followed by disappearance of the corneal ring and amelioration of hepatic and neurologic symptoms.

The diagnosis of asymptomatic Wilson disease in siblings of affected patients is important because specific treatment dramatically improves what would otherwise be an inevitably fatal course.

MENKES KINKY-HAIR DISEASE

Menkes kinky-hair disease is an X chromosome-linked recessive hereditary disorder characterized by early psychomotor deterioration, seizures, spasticity, hypothermia, pili torti, late bone changes resembling scurvy, and fragmentation of internal elastic lamina causing vascular tortuosity. Levels of serum copper,

copper oxidase, and ceruloplasmin are abnormally low. A defect occurs in the intracellular transport of copper in the gut epithelium. Initially the eye develops normally, but later degeneration of ganglion cells takes place with loss of nerve fibers and optic atrophy. Eyelashes and eyebrows may be broken. Mitochondria of surviving ganglion cells and photoreceptor inner segments are markedly swollen, with an electron-dense substance in the matrix of the mitochondria and pigment epithelium. The elastic tissue in Bruch membrane is reduced.

CEREBROHEPATORENAL SYNDROME (ZELLWEGER)

Cerebrohepatorenal syndrome (Zellweger) is an autosomal recessive multisystem disorder that includes primary dysgenesis of the central nervous system, hepatic interstitial fibrosis, and multiple cysts of the renal cortex. There are abnormalities of neuronal migration and demyelination that cause macular hypotonia, seizures, and psychomotor retardation. Liver involvement causes jaundice, hepatomegaly, hypoprothrombinemia, and gastrointestinal hemorrhage. The forehead is high and bulging, the orbits are widely separated, the palpebral fissures are oblique, and epicanthal folds are present. There may be corneal opacification, glaucoma, cataract, Brushfield spots, nystagmus, rudimentary or irregular optic disks, narrow retinal blood vessels, and irregular retinal pigmentation. Bilateral corneal edema is associated with paracentral iridocorneal adhesions and focal attenuation of Descemet membrane. Selective degeneration of the outer nuclear layers and photoreceptors occurs mainly in the central retinal region.

Liver enzymes and serum iron levels are high; there is a deficiency of catalase-containing organelles (peroxisomes) that catalyze the biosynthesis of glycerol-ether lipids. Death occurs before 1 year of age, often within 3 months of birth.

INCONTINENTIA PIGMENTI

Incontinentia pigmenti is an X chromosome-linked dominant systemic disorder that affects only the carrier female. It is lethal for male embryos. Beginning at birth, there is recurrent skin inflammation with blisters that resolve spontaneously leaving irregularly pigmented atrophic scars on the trunk, legs, and scalp. There may be partial alopecia, delayed dentition, and malformed teeth. Mental retardation, seizures, and spastic paralysis may occur.

About one sixth of the affected individuals have a retinal dysplasia with rosettes and fibrous tissue that cause a total nonrhegmatogenous retinal detachment. Esotropia, optic atrophy, cataract, blue sclera, nystagmus, and hyperpigmentation of the conjunctiva and retina may occur. The retinal blood supply may terminate at the equator with a zone of arteriovenous anastomoses and fibrovascular proliferation. Neovascularization may require photocoagulation to prevent tractional retinal separation.

CONGENITAL PROGRESSIVE OCULOACOUSTIC CEREBRAL DYSPLASIA (NORRIE)

This is an X chromosome-linked recessive abnormality in which boys are born blind with a gray-yellow or opaque vascularized retrolental vascular mass in each eye. The pupils are dilated, the iris is hypoplastic, and posterior synechiae and ectropion of the pupillary fringe are present. Falciform folds of the retina, retinal detachment, and vitreous hemorrhage may occur. Corneal degeneration begins at about 1 year of age, followed by cataracts at 2 years of age. In early childhood the eyes begin to shrink (phthisis bulbi). Deafness occurs in about 33% and mental retardation in 66% of those affected. The ocular changes resemble those of trisomy 13 syndrome.

DISORDERS OF AMINO ACID METABOLISM

The major disorders of amino acid metabolism that affect the eye (Table 24-7) involve mainly the intermediate metabolism of either tyrosine or methionine. In albinism the biosynthesis of melanin from tyrosine is impaired because of a deficiency of tyrosinase or because of failure of tyrosine to enter cells containing tyrosinase. In alkaptonuria homogentisic acid produced in the metabolism of phenylalanine and tyrosine accumulates because the enzyme homogentisic acid oxidase is missing. In phenylketonuria (an abnormality associated with minimal ocular signs) plasma phenylalanine in-

Table 24-7. Disorders of amino acid metabolism (other than albinism) that have ocular signs

Disease	Defect	Systemic involvement	Eye involvement	Laboratory findings
Alkaptonuria (homogentisic acid accumulates)	Absence of homogentisic acid oxidase	Arthritis (late), pigmentation (ochronosis of cartilage and connective tissue), heart disease	Ochronosis of sclera and cornea	Homogentisic acid in urine (dark-colored urine if alkaline)
Homocystinuria (homocysteine not converted to cystathionine; homocystine accumulates)	Deficiency of cystathionine synthetase (in metabolism of methionine to cysteine)	Mental retardation, seizures, malar flush, fair skin, thromboembolism	Dislocated lenses, cataract, severe myopia	Homocystine in urine
Phenylketonuria (phenylalanine excess)	Absence of phenylalanine hydroxylase (oxidation of L-phenylalanine to tyrosine)	Mental retardation, epilepsy, restlessness, hyperactive tendon reflexes, tremors	Light-colored iris, photophobia	Increased plasma phenylalanine, phenylpyruvic acid in urine
Tyrosinemia type II	Deficiency of p-hydroxyphenyl pyruvic acid oxidase	Painful hyperkeratosis of palms and soles, brain damage	Painful keratopathy	Excess tyrosine in plasma and urine
Sulfite oxidase deficiency	SO_3 to SO_4	Brain damage	Dislocated lenses	Excess sulfocysteine
Gyrate atrophy	Ornithine amino transferase deficiency	None	Gyrate atrophy choroid, cataract, myopia	Excess plasma ornithine

creases because L-phenylalanine is not oxidized to tyrosine. In homocystinuria there is a defect in the metabolism of methionine to tyrosine. In tyrosinosis a metabolic abnormality results from excess tyrosine in the blood.

Many of these disorders, as well as galactosemia and Wilson disease, either induce or are associated with a renal transport defect (Table 24-8) that leads to a generalized aminoaciduria, glycosuria, and phosphaturia of the Lingac-Fanconi syndrome.

Gyrate atrophy of the retina and choroid is associated with an excess excretion of ornithine in the urine.

Albinism. Albinism is a hereditary disorder characterized by a reduction or absence of melanin pigmentation in the eyes, skin, and hair, or in the eyes only. The complexion is fair, the hair white, and there is reduced vision, nystagmus, and photophobia. Conditions of hypopigmentation in which vision is normal and nystagmus is absent are not albinism but are called "albinoidism," of which there are many kinds. Several are associated with deafness. Melanocytes are normally located at the epidermal-

dermal junction of the skin, in the hair bulb, in the pia-arachnoid meninges, inner ear, choroid, ciliary body, and retinal pigment epithelium. The melanocytes of the retinal pigment epithelium (and its anterior extension, the iris pigment epithelium) originate in the outer layer of the optic cup. All others originate from melanoblasts of the neural crest that migrate to peripheral sites during embryonic life. Melanocytes are absent in prealbinism but present in normal numbers in albinism. In albinism there is a failure of melanin synthesis, resulting in widespread disorders of the skin, eyes, lateral geniculate body, and other structures.

Albinism may be divided into two main types: oculocutaneous and ocular. *Oculocutaneous albinism* has at least six varieties, which are divided into tyrosinase-negative and tyrosinase-positive on the basis of pigment formation by hair follicles incubated with L-tyrosine. Patients with tyrosine-negative oculocutaneous albinism lack tyrosinase in all tissues. Patients who are tyrosinase-positive may have a defect in the biochemical activation of the enzyme, an intracellular inhibitor, or a defective feedback control mechanism. Clinical severity, genetic data, and biochemical criteria further distinguish the basic types of albinism.

Tyrosinase-positive involvement is more common among blacks than whites, whereas tyrosinase-negative oculocuatneous albinism has about the same incidence in both races.

Oculocutaneous albinism. In tyrosinase-negative albinism there is no clinically detectable pigment in the eyes, skin, or hair. There is no tyrosinase activity in any tissue. The iris is gray-blue and translucent to light directed through the sclera (transillumination). There is a prominent red reflex from the fundus, and the eye appears pink. The fovea is hypoplastic, and there is no central light reflex from the foveola. Visual acuity is at the level of 20/200 or less with no tendency to improvement with aging. There is a severe nystagmus and severe photophobia. Strabismus is present in about 90% of tyrosinase-negative albinos. Esotropia is most common (80%); the eyes diverge in the remaining individuals. The strabismus and nystagmus are aggravated by prolonged exposure to bright sun. The hair is snow-white and the skin is pink-white. The irides may be translucent in white individuals heterozygous for tyrosinase-negative albinism (60%); in black individuals the irides are generally normal (75%).

In tyrosinase-positive albinism some melanin pigment is evident in the eyes, hair, and skin. Pigmentation may increase with age. Infants resemble tyrosinase-negative albinos, but with aging the phenotype extends from the appearance of tyrosinase-negative albino to lightly pigmented individuals. The hair is usually white in infancy and darkens to yellow or light tan with age. The eyes tend to darken with age. The iris in whites transilluminates in infancy, often with spokes. In blacks the iris appears normal. Nystagmus is present in all, but is less severe than in tyrosinase-negative albinism. Visual acuity is reduced but tends to improve with age.

Ocular albinism is an X chromosome–linked deficiency of pigmentation limited to the uvea and retinal pigment epithelium. The hemizygous male is severely affected, whereas the homozygous female has minor pigmentary changes of the iris and retina. It occurs in three forms: (1) X chromosome-linked with normal color vision, (2) X chromosome-linked with less

severe hypopigmentation than form 1, and (3) X chromosome-linked with an associated protanomalous color defect but in which the female carriers do not have the mosaic fundus changes of form 1. The first type is closely associated with the Xg blood group. Rarely, ocular albinism occurs with either an autosomal dominant or autosomal recessive inheritance.

The severity of depigmentation varies, and the fundus may resemble a blond fundus with the choroidal vasculature visible. The foveal reflex is absent. The iris transmits light to a variable degree. Some but not all female carriers have a partial iris transillumination and may have coarse pigment in the midperiphery of the fundus. The pigmentation of the fundus of the female carrier may be caused by lyonization of the X chromosome. The associated pendular nystagmus may be diagnosed as a congenital nystagmus rather than being recognized as the result of the ocular albinism. The outstanding symptom is photophobia with extreme intolerance to light. Ophthalmoscopic examination indicates a bright orange-red reflex with prominent choroidal vessels that are normally obscured by the retinal pigment epithelium. The retinal blood vessels are normal.

Autosomal recessive ocular albinism is characterized by decreased vision, photophobia, nystagmus, diaphanous irides, and light yellow fundi. The parents sometimes have diaphanous irides.

Individuals with tyrosinase-negative albinism and ocular albinism have misrouted retinal ganglion cell axons so that some temporal fibers decussate at the chiasm rather than remain on the same side. The visual-evoked potential to monocular stimulation is abnormally small. The lateral geniculate body is abnormal, with fusion of adjacent layers that receive the abnormal crossed fibers. In normal humans, the lateral geniculate body has six layers. In human albinism, instead of six layers there are three, the result of fusion between adjacent layers.

Treatment of albinism is directed toward accurate correction of the refractive error and the strabismus if present. The use of a strong reading addition for near work may be helpful. Colored lenses are used to reduce the amount of light entering the eye. Contact lenses with a central clear area surrounded by a pigmented area simulate the appearance of the normal pupil and iris but do not improve vision. They are helpful in reducing photophobia.

The Hermansky Pudluk syndrome consists of tyrosinase-positive oculocutaneous albinism, hemorrhagic diathesis caused by defective platelets, and accumulation of ceroidlike material in the reticuloendothelial system, oral mucosa, and urine. The hair is white to dark red-brown, the iris is blue-gray and not translucent, and the albino red reflex is present. Nystagmus, photophobia, and decreased vision may occur. The amplitude of the electroretinogram is decreased.

The Cross syndrome of oculocerebrohypopigmentation shows blond hair, white skin, small eyes, cloudy corneas, and a coarse, jerky nystagmus. Infants have severe mental retardation and are unable to sit unaided. Gingival fibromatosis develops with eruption of primary teeth.

The Chédiak-Higashi syndrome is a fatal disease of childhood with partial oculocutaneous albinism and giant melanosomes in tissues; giant lysosomal peroxidase-positive granules in leukocytes, Schwann cells, and other tissues; and a marked susceptibility to infection.

Alkaptonuria and ochronosis. Alkaptonuria is an autosomal recessive disorder in which homogentisic acid, produced in the metabolism of phenylalanine and tyrosine, accumulates because of the absence of the enzyme homogentisic acid oxidase. Homogentisic acid is a normal intermediate in the metabolism of tyrosine, and the enzyme responsible for its oxidation is normally present in the liver, kidney, and possibly other tissues.

In affected individuals, homogentisic acid is actively excreted by the kidney and appears in the urine (alkaptonuria) in large amounts. It causes the urine to have a dark color or to become dark after standing, provided the urine is alkaline and large amounts of ascorbic acid are not simultaneously excreted. Homogentisic acid reduces Benedict reagent and may give false-positive tests for reducing substance in the urine.

Clinically alkaptonuria is characterized by homogentisic acid in the urine and generalized pigmentation of cartilage and other connective tissue (ochronosis), which in turn causes arthritis. The pigmentation is most prominent in the

eyes, ears, and nose, and it becomes evident between 20 and 30 years of age. The ocular pigmentation is the result of deposits of homogentisic acid metabolites in the collagen bundles of the cornea, sclera, and elastic tissue of the conjunctiva, which degenerate. The deposits appear on both globes in the palpebral fissure just in front of the insertions of the horizontal recti muscles; they are oval and have a slate-gray pigmentation. Biomicroscopy of the cornea discloses tiny round, golden brown deposits at the level of the Bowman zone within the palpebral fissure. The concha and the antihelix of the ears are a drab blue-gray. There is a tendency toward valvular heart disease, calcification of the heart valves, and atherosclerosis; myocardial infarction is a common cause of death.

Tyrosinemia II (Richner-Hanhart syndrome). This is an autosomal recessive oculocutaneous disorder in which plasma tyrosine levels are high and there is increased urinary tyrosine. There is a deficiency of hepatic tyrosine amino transferase. Ocular changes occur during the first months of life with lacrimation, photophobia, and ciliary injection. Corneal erosions and ulcers (Fig. 24-5), sometimes with corneal and conjunctival plaques, lead to neo-

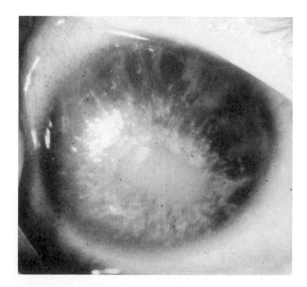

Fig. 24-5. A 4-week-old male infant with bilateral corneal ulcerations secondary to tyrosinemia II. (Courtesy Robert P. Burns, M.D., University of Missouri, Columbia.)

vascularization. The associated poor vision may lead to exodeviation and nystagmus. The skin of the palms and soles develops painful blisters or erosions that crust and become hyperkeratotic. Mental retardation occurs occasionally. A low tyrosine and phenylalanine diet is used successfully and may prevent ocular deterioration and mental retardation.

Cystathionine β-synthetase deficiency (homocystinuria). This is an autosomal recessive disorder of the metabolism of methionine to cysteine, which is caused by deficiency of the enzyme cystathionine β-synthetase. There are severe skeletal abnormalities and a marked tendency to thrombosis. Death from pulmonary embolism may occur during general anesthesia. Ectopia lentis is present in nearly all patients after 10 years of age (Chapter 19). There may be a secondary glaucoma and cataract. Lattice degeneration of the retinas may cause rhegmatogenous retinal detachment. Patients with some cystathionine β-synthetase activity respond favorably to pyridoxine (B_6) therapy. Those who do not respond should be treated with a low-methionine diet supplemented with L-cysteine.

Sulfite oxidase deficiency. This is an autosomal recessive disorder caused by a deficiency of sulfite oxidase that oxidizes sulfite (SO_3) to sulfate (SO_4). The deficiency involves dislocated lenses, mental retardation, and progressive cerebral palsy.

Renal tubule transport defects. Cystine storage disease (Lignac-Fanconi syndrome) and the oculocerebrorenal syndrome (Lowe) are caused by impaired tubular reabsorption (Table 24-8). This results in an excessive amino acid excretion and secondary complex metabolic disturbances often associated with rickets and ocular changes.

Cystine storage disease (Lignac-Fanconi syndrome). Childhood, or nephropathic, cystine storage disease occurring early in life is characterized by widespread deposition of L-cystine crystals in the kidneys, liver, spleen, bone marrow, lymph nodes, conjunctiva, cornea, and uveal tissues. Cystine accumulates within lysosomes until crystals form and the cell dies.

The disease becomes evident between the fourth and sixth months of life. Polyuria and polydipsia caused by faulty resorption of water from the renal tubule result in dehydration. Failure to grow, emesis, recurrent fever, a severe form of rickets resistant to vitamin D in the usual doses, and chronic acidosis result. An aminoaciduria involves many amino acids. There is progressive kidney damage, and chronic glomerulonephritis develops. There may be a terminal vascular hypertension and ophthalmoscopic signs of severe vascular hypertension, including papilledema. Death usually results from uremia or intercurrent infections.

Crystalline deposits occur in the conjunctiva and the cornea. Good illumination and magnification are required for their demonstration because of their small size. They appear as tinsellike, fine refractile crystals or fine white dots uniformly scattered over the entire cornea, predominantly in the anterior stroma (although the corneal dots have the same clinical appearance as the conjunctival crystals, they do not have the same x-ray diffraction pattern and may not be cystine). In the conjunctiva the crystals are superficial and tend to aggregate in the walls of blood vessels. Photophobia is marked, but visual acuity seems normal. Ophthalmoscopically there is peripheral retinal patchy depigmentation and pigment clumps that often form small rings. The retinal pigmentary changes precede corneal and conjunctival involvement.

Treatment is directed toward correction of the acidosis and dietary supplementation of phosphate and potassium. Only the amount of vitamin D that is required to correct the rickets should be given. Supplementary calcium may be necessary until the skeleton is normal, but hypercalcemia must be prevented. A cystine-free diet may be helpful. In advanced stages, renal transplant is indicated.

The renal changes of the disorder also occur in galactosemia, Wilson disease, fructose intolerance, tyrosinemia, and the oculocerebrorenal syndrome.

Benign cystinosis. Benign cystinosis is an autosomal recessive disorder in which cystine crystals are found in the eye and bone marrow. There are no kidney signs or retinal pigmentation. The cystine level is much lower than in the nephropathic type. Attention is usually directed to the disorder only when the crystals are seen in the cornea and conjunctiva.

Table 24-8. Renal tubule transport defects

Disease	Defect	Inheritance
Nephropathic cystine storage disease (Lignac-Fanconi syndrome)	Abnormal compartmentalization of cystine	Autosomal recessive
Benign cystinosis	Same as nephropathic	Autosomal recessive
Oculocerebrorenal syndrome (Lowe)	Not known	X chromosome–linked recessive

Table 24-9. Disorders of carbohydrate metabolism

Disease	Defect	Inheritance
Galactosemia	1. Deficiency of hexose-1-phosphate uridyl transferase	Autosomal recessive
	2. Galactokinase deficiency	Autosomal recessive
Hepatorenal glycogenosis (Gierke)	Deficiency of glucose-6-phosphatase	Autosomal recessive
Generalized glycogenosis (Pompe)	Deficiency of alpha-glucosidase (?), deficiency of acid maltase (?)	Autosomal recessive (?)
Glucose-6-phosphate dehydrogenase deficiency		X chromosome-linked

Oculocerebrorenal syndrome (Lowe). This is an X chromosome-linked recessive abnormality in which the affected male demonstrates hypotonia, mental retardation, osteoporosis, and failure to thrive. There is a renal tubular acidosis and aminoaciduria. Cataracts are present at birth and may involve the entire lens or be confined to the fetal nucleus. The female carrier has punctate lens opacities. Congenital glaucoma occurs in slightly more than 50% of the males. The poor vision causes nystagmus and strabismus. The pupil may be miotic and may not dilate with mydriatics.

Miscellaneous disorders. An abnormal aminoaciduria is often seen in patients with congenital cataract or in those with congenital glaucoma. In one large family, central retinal degeneration was seen in 25 of 70 members with aminoaciduria. In another group composed of individuals with mental retardation and congenital cataract, there was an excessive urinary excretion of glycine and alanine. The metabolic basis of these disorders has not been determined.

Spherophakia and dislocated lenses have been seen in hyperlysinemia associated with growth and mental retardation, seizures, and muscular asthenia. Imidazole aminoaciduria was associated with pigmentary retinopathy and mental retardation in one family. Increased urinary oxalic acid with pigmentary retinopathy has been described.

DISORDERS OF CARBOHYDRATE METABOLISM

Diabetes mellitus is clinically the most important abnormality of carbohydrate metabolism. Galactosemia (Table 24-9) is an abnormality in which there is failure to convert galactose to glucose and lactose. The glycogen storage diseases do not have prominent ocular changes; but in Gierke disease, peripheral corneal

Systemic involvement	Eye involvement	Laboratory findings
Vitamin D–resistant rickets, acidosis, polyuria, dehydration, infection	Cystine crystals in conjunctiva and cornea, retinal pigmentation	Aminoaciduria, glycosuria, hypophosphatemia, elevated alkaline phosphate
None	Corneal and conjunctival crystals	Normal Aminoaciduria, proteinuria
Rickets, mental retardation, hypotonia	Congenital cataract, glaucoma, corneal opacities	

Systemic involvement	Eye involvement	Laboratory findings
Mental retardation, hepatosplenomegaly, vomiting, dehydration	Cataracts	Reducing substance in urine (galactose), albuminuria, aminoaciduria, erythrocyte deficiency of hexose-1-phosphate uridyl transferase
None	Cataracts	Reducing substance in urine, erythrocyte deficiency of galactokinase
Retarded growth, adiposity, hepatomegaly, eruptive zanthomas	Peripheral corneal glycogen deposition	Hypoglycemia, hyperglyceridemia, hypercholesterolemia, acidosis, hyperuricemia
Lethal, anorexia, muscle weakness, tongue enlargement, cardiac and CNS involvement	Clinically negative, but glycogen deposition in eye	Requires muscle biopsy
Hemolytic anemia	Color vision deficiency, optic nerve atrophy, cataract	Decreased enzyme activity, anemia

clouding has been noted, and in Pompe disease, glycogen is found in retinal ganglion cells, corneal endothelium, pericytes of the retinal capillaries, extraocular muscles, and ciliary muscle.

Galactosemia. Galactosemia is an autosomal recessive abnormality in which there is impairment of the enzymatic conversion of galactose to glucose. Galactose is a hexose that differs from glucose in the configuration of the hydroxyl group of the fourth carbon. It is a component of many complex polysaccharides, but normally nearly all dietary galactose is converted to glucose by two series of reactions. It is first phosphorylated by the enzyme galactokinase to yield galactose-1-phosphate.

$$ATP + D\text{-galactose} \rightarrow ADP + D\text{-galactose 1-phosphate}$$

Galactose-1-phosphate is converted to uridyl diphosphogalactose by one of two reactions. In

adults, but not infants, the reaction is catalyzed by galactose-1-phosphate uridylyltransferase.

$$D\text{-Galactose 1-phosphate} + UTP \leftrightarrows$$
$$UDP\text{--}D\text{-galactose} + PP_i$$

In infants it is catalyzed by hexose-1-phosphate uridylyltransferase.

$$UDP\text{--}D\text{-glucose} + D\text{-galactose 1-phosphate} \leftrightarrows$$
$$UDP\text{--}D\text{-galactose} + D\text{-glucose 1-phosphate}$$

There are two types of galactosemia: (1) galactokinase deficiency, which is uncommon, and (2) hexose-1-phosphate uridyl transferase deficiency, the more common type.

Galactokinase deficiency galactosemia is an autosomal recessive disorder in which galactose is not metabolized and is excreted either unchanged or as galactose alcohol (galactitol) through the action of aldose reductase. Bilateral cataract appears to be the sole physical abnormality. The diagnosis is based on an absence of galactokinase in erythrocytes, high blood galactose level, and galactosuria.

The uridyl transferase deficiency is transmitted as an autosomal recessive disorder. The afflicted children are usually normal at birth, but cataracts have been found in the fetus at the fifth month of gestation. Usually, shortly after birth as the infant begins to ingest milk, he develops feeding problems along with vomiting, diarrhea, and failure to thrive. Progressive cataracts occur, initially with an increase in nuclear refractive power (as in senile nuclear sclerosis) and with the appearance of a drop of oil in the center of the lens. In other cases a zonular type of opacity develops. If galactose is removed from the diet, cataracts either will not develop or, if present, will not progress. The cataracts appear to develop from the conversion by aldose reductase of excess galactose in the lens to its alcohol, which diffuses poorly through the lens capsule and causes imbibition of water.

Systemically, there is hepatomegaly along with abdominal distension and sometimes jaundice and ascites. Cirrhosis may develop. Mental retardation is evident early. Albuminuria, aminoaciduria, and impaired liver function may be present.

Treatment involves exclusion of milk and other galactose-containing foods from the diet. Soybean milk or casein hydrolysate is usually substituted. If treatment is instituted early, mental retardation, cataract formation, and impairment of hepatic function may be avoided.

Glucose 6-phosphate dehydrogenase deficiency. This is an X chromosome-linked recessive disorder involving primarily erythrocytes and manifesting itself after ingestion of primaquine and other antimalarials, after exposure to naphthalene, or during bacterial or viral infections. The deficiency leads to a deficiency of NADPH, an essential reducing agent of erythrocytes. More than 150 variants of human glucose-6-phosphate dehydrogenase have been described. Its most common variants are the Western type, occurring predominantly in blacks, and the type found in the Mediterranean area. It is of ophthalmic interest because of the similarity of the anaerobic metabolism of the lens and the erythrocyte.

Protanomaly and deuteranomaly occur commonly in the disorder. The genes for protos and deuteros perception appear to lie relatively far apart on the X chromosome, with the gene for glucose-6-phosphate dehydrogenase between them. Optic atrophy of an X chromosome-linked type has been described. The level of glucose-6-phosphate dehydrogenase in the lens parallels that of the erythrocyte, but although cataract has been described, its incidence is only slightly higher than in the normal black population.

DISORDERS OF LIPID METABOLISM

The plasma lipoproteins function as vehicles to transport lipids in plasma, an aqueous solution in which lipids are poorly soluble. The five main classes of lipoprotein are as follows: (1) chylomicrons; (2) very low-density lipoproteins (VLDL) or pre-beta lipoproteins; (3) intermediate-density lipoproteins (IDL); (4) low-density lipoprotein (LDL); and (5) high-density lipoprotein (HDL). The protein portion of lipoproteins are apoproteins of which there are at least ten types, designated by letters A to E and Roman numerals.

Ingested dietary fats are emulsified in the duodenum by bile salts, hydrolyzed by pancreatic lipase, and then diffuse into the intestinal cell mucous membrane. The lipids, largely glycerides, are transported by chylomicrons through the intestinal lymphatics and thoracic duct to the bloodstream. They are hydrolyzed by the enzyme lipoprotein lipase in the liver, heart, adipose tissue, and other tissues, and the constituent fatty acids are resynthesized into triglycerides (triacylglycerols).

Defects of lipoprotein metabolism manifest themselves mainly in cardiovascular disorders. Several, however, show ocular abnormalities that vary from corneal arcus, stromal opacities, pigmentary degeneration of the retina, to premature central retinal artery atherosclerosis. Plasma allowed to stand overnight at 4° C often provides useful data.

A-beta-lipoproteinemia. A-beta-lipoproteinemia (Bassen-Kornzweig syndrome) is an autosomal recessive disorder in which there is defective formation of apoprotein B. This causes decreased or absent chylomicrons, low-density lipoprotein, and high-density lipoprotein. A generalized defect of cell membranes occurs that predominantly involves the central nervous system and the erythrocyte. There is anemia, abnormally shaped erythrocytes (acanthocytosis), intestinal malabsorption, posterior spinocerebellar tract degeneration, and retinal degeneration. Serum cholesterol and triglycerides are markedly reduced.

Intestinal malabsorption in infancy causes retarded growth, abdominal distention, diarrhea, and steatorrhea. Malabsorption becomes less severe in childhood, but degeneration of the posterior lateral columns and cerebellar tracts causes muscle weakness, ataxia, tremor, weakness, and nystagmus. Pigmentary degeneration of the retina is evident at 8 to 10 years of age. There is pigment clumping in the central retinal region and bright dots in the periphery. Night blindness parallels the retinal degeneration. Cataract may occur. Progressive palsy of the medial recti muscles along with exotropia, dissociated nystagmus on lateral gaze, mild blepharoptosis, and ophthalmoplegia have been described in about one third of patients.

Treatment is directed toward dietary fat restriction and administration of vitamins A and E.

Familial alpha-lipoprotein deficiency (Tangier disease). This is an autosomal recessive disorder that impairs the synthesis of apoprotein A II, a structural component of high-density lipoprotein. This supplies apoprotein C II that activates lipoprotein lipase. As a result, less chylomicrons and very low-density lipoprotein triglycerides are hydrolyzed. Plasma cholesterol is low and plasma triglycerides are high. Cholesterol esters are stored in the reticuloendothelial system, causing a hepatosplenomegaly and lymphadenopathy. The tonsils are enlarged and have an orange color and a peculiar odor. In adults the corneas may be diffusely infiltrated with fine dots visible only with the biomicroscope. Blepharoptosis and ocular muscle palsies with diplopia occur after childhood. Homozygous patients develop psychomotor retardation, polyneuropathy, and pigmentation degeneration of the retina.

Hyperlipoproteinemia. Ocular signs of hyperlipoproteinemia include lipemia retinalis, corneal arcus, xanthelasma, and ophthalmoscopic signs of atherosclerosis of the central retinal artery.

Lipemia retinalis is a transient abnormality of the appearance of the blood vessels that occurs because of an excessive amount of chylomicrons in the plasma. The blood vessels of the ocular fundus appear orange-red in color and the arterial light reflex disappears. There is no diminution in vision. It occurs in familial hyperchylomicronemia (type I hyperlipoproteinemia) in which there is a deficiency of lipoprotein lipase. Lipemia retinalis occurs in carbohydrate-induced very low-density lipoproteinemia, as seen in uncontrolled diabetes, pancreatitis, and alcoholism, more commonly than in type I hyperlipoproteinemia.

Corneal arcus (gerontoxon, arcus senilis, embryotoxon) is a deposition of phospholipid and cholesterol in the corneal stroma and anterior sclera. Generally, it appears as a deep, sharply defined, yellowish-white ring, frequently incomplete, in the cornea concentric to the corneoscleral limbus (Fig. 24-6). It involves the entire thickness of the cornea but is usually most marked in Descemet membrane and least marked in the midstroma. The area nearest blood vessels is clear, but when corneal neovascularization is present, the opacity affects that area preferentially.

Xanthelasma is a cutaneous deposition of lipid occurring most commonly in the skin of the eyelids near the medial canthus.

Phytanic acid storage disease (Refsum disease, heredopathia atactica polyneuritiformis). This is an autosomal recessive disorder in

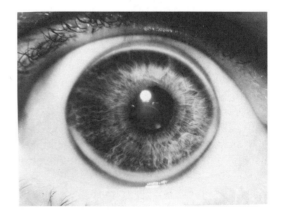

Fig. 24-6. Corneal arcus begins at the corneal periphery above and below and progresses to involve the entire corneal circumference.

which patients accumulate phytanic acid, a 20-carbon branched chain fatty acid, because of a deficiency of phytanic acid α-hydroxylase. Phytanic acid is derived entirely from dietary sources, mainly dairy products and ruminant fats. Chlorophyll in green vegetables contains phytal, the precursor of phytanic acid, but it is not significantly converted to phytanic acid in humans.

The major clinical findings are pigmentary degeneration of the retina, cerebellar ataxia, peripheral polyneuropathy, and high cerebrospinal fluid protein. Retinal pigmentary degeneration, night blindness, and constricted visual fields always occur. In 90% of the patients, there is a peripheral neuropathy, motor weakness, muscular atrophy, loss of deep tendon reflexes, and loss of superficial sensation to pain, touch, or temperature. Onset is in childhood, but diagnosis may be delayed until midlife. The retinal changes are followed by lower eyelid weakness, foot drop, and loss of deep tendon reflexes. Ataxia, intention tremor, and nystagmus indicate cerebellar involvement. There may be mild ichthyosis, miotic pupils, anosmia, and nonspecific changes in the electrocardiogram.

Long remissions occur and exacerbations are triggered by fever, surgery, and pregnancy. Improvement may follow long-term exclusion of dietary dairy fat and cattle fat, but the slow course and tendency to spontaneous remission make evaluation difficult.

A thin layer of lipid occurs in standing urine and serum when the phytanic acid level is markedly increased. Cultured fibroblasts of homozygotes indicate the absence of phytanic acid α-hydrolase.

Cerebrotendinous xanthomatosis. Cerebrotendinous xanthomatosis is an abnormality of cholesterol metabolism in which there are juvenile cataracts, xanthomas of the Achilles tendons, moderate mental retardation, and cerebellar ataxia. Ataxia occurs after puberty and is followed by pseudobulbar paralysis, which results in death. The blood cholesterol level is normal or minimally increased, but dihydrocholesterol (cholestanol), which is cholesterol without its 5,6 double bond, is deposited in the tendons. The condition appears to be an autosomal recessive disorder.

BIBLIOGRAPHY
General

Cohn, R.M., and Roth, K.S.: Metabolic disease: a guide to early recognition, Philadelphia, 1983, W.B. Saunders Co.

Franceschetti, A., François, J., and Babel, J.: Chorioretinal heredodegenerations, Springfield, Ill., 1974, Charles C Thomas, Publisher.

Grouchy, J.D., and Turleau, C.: Clinical atlas of human chromosomes, ed. 2, New York, 1984, John Wiley & Sons.

Harley, R.D., editor: Pediatric ophthalmology, ed. 2, Philadelphia, 1983, W.B. Saunders Co.

Smith, D.W., and Jones, K.L.: Recognizable patterns on human malformation: genetic, embryologic, and clinical aspects, ed. 3, Philadelphia, 1982, W.B. Saunders Co.

Stanbury, J.B., Wyngaarden, J.B., Fredrickson, D.S., Goldstein, J.L., and Brown, M.S., editors: The metabolic basis of inherited disease, New York, 1983, McGraw-Hill Book Co.

Heredity

Mets, M.B., and Maumenee, I.H.: The eye and the chromosome, Surv. Ophthalmol. **28**:20, 1983.

Shapiro, M.B., and France, T.D.: The ocular features of Down's syndrome, Am. J. Ophthalmol. **99**:659, 1985.

Lysosomal storage disease

Armstrong, D., Koppang, N., and Rider, J.A., editors: Ceroid-lipofuscinosis (Batten's Disease), Amsterdam, 1982, Elsevier Biomedical Press.

Cogan, D.G., Kuwabara, T., Kolodny, E., and Driscoll, S.: Gangliosidoses and the fetal retina, Opthalmology **91**:508, 1984.

De Venecia, G., and Shapiro, M.: Neuronal ceroid lipofuscinosis, Ophthalmology **91**:1406, 1984.

Hayasaka, S., Nakazawa, M., Okabe, H., Masuda, K., and Mizuno, K.: Progressive cone dystrophy associated with low α-L-fucosidase activity in serum and leukocytes, Am. J. Ophthalmol. **99**:681, 1985.

Naumann, G.: Clearing of cornea after perforating keratoplasty in mucopolysaccharidosis Type VI (Maroteaux-Lamy syndrome), N. Engl. J. Med. **312**:995, 1985.

Palmer, M., Green, W.R., Maumenee, I.H., Valle, D.L., Singer, H.S., Morton, S.J., and Moser, H.W.: Niemann-Pick disease—type C, Arch. Ophthalmol. **103**:817, 1985.

Riedel, K.G., Zwaan, J., Kenyon, K.R., Kolodny, E.H., Hanninen, L., and Albert, D.M.: Ocular abnormalities in mucolipidosis IV, Am. J. Ophthalmol. **99**:125, 1985.

Hepatolenticular degeneration

Deiss, A.: Treatment of Wilson's disease, Ann. Intern. Med. **99:**398, 1983.

Scheinberg, I.H., and Sterlieb, I.: Wilson's disease. In Smith, L.H., editor: Major problems in internal medicine, vol. 23, Philadelphia, 1985, W.B. Saunders Co.

Cerebrohepatorenal syndrome (Zellweger)

Cohen, S.M., Brown, F.R. III, Martyn, L., Moser, H.W., Chen, W., Kistenmacher, M., Punnett, H., de la Cruz, Z.C., Chan, N.R., and Green, W.R.: Ocular histopathologic and biochemical studies of the cerebrohepatorenal syndrome (Zellweger's syndrome) and its relationship to neonatal adrenoleukodystrophy, Am. J. Ophthalmol. **96:**488, 1983.

Dattu, N.S., Wilson, G.N., and Hajrn, A.K.: Deficiency of enzymes catalyzing the biosynthesis of glycerol-ether lipids in Zellweger syndrome: a new category of metabolic disease involving the absence of peroxisomes, N. Engl. J. Med. **311:**1080, 1984.

Amino acid metabolism

Gobernado, J.M., Lousa, M., Gimeno, A., and Gonsalvez, M.: Mitochondrial defects in Loew's oculocerebrorenal syndrome, Arch. Neurol. **41:**208, 1984.

Goldsmith, L.A.: Tyrosinemia II: lessons in molecular patho-physiology, Pediatr. Dermatol. **1:**25, 1983.

Kaiser-Kupfer, M.I., Ludwig, I.H., de Monasterio, F.M., Valle, D., and Krieger, I.: Gyrate atrophy of the choroid and retina: early findings, Ophthalmology **62:**394, 1985.

Kinnear, P.E., Jay, B., and Witkop, C.J., Jr.: Albinism, Surv. Ophthalmol. **30:**75, 1985.

Simon, J.W., Kandel, G.L., Krohel, G.B., and Nelsen, P.T.: Albinotic characteristics in congenital nystagumus, Am. J. Ophthalmol. **97:**320, 1984.

Lipid metabolism

Weleber, R.G., Tongue, A.C., Kenneway, N.G., et al.: Ophthalmic manifestations of infantile phytanic acid storage disease, Arch. Ophthalmol. **102:**1317, 1984.

25

ENDOCRINE DISEASE AND THE EYE

The endocrine and nervous systems provide the major pathways for transfer of information between cells in different parts of the body. Hormones of the endocrine system regulate the rate at which enzymes and other proteins are manufactured, affect the enzymes of metabolic pathways, or alter the permeability of cell membranes. Hormones bind to specific receptors either within the cell (steroid and thyroid hormones) or on the cell surface (hypothalamus and pituitary hormones, adrenalin, and insulin). Those that enter the cell directly combine with receptors that regulate the transcription of genes by the cell nucleus to synthesize specific enzymes and proteins. Hormones that bind to the receptors on the cell surface activate adenylate cyclase, which converts adenosine triphosphate into cyclic adenosine monophosphate (cyclic AMP). The cyclic AMP is then released into the cell cytoplasm, where it signals the cell to produce the characteristic action of the cell. The hormone is considered the first messenger, and the cyclic AMP the second messenger. The cyclic AMP is degraded by the enzyme phosphodiesterase into a physiologically inactive form of AMP.

THYROID GLAND

The hypothalamus secretes a thyrotropin-releasing hormone (TRH), which stimulates the release of the thyroid-stimulating hormone (TSH) by the pituitary gland. Pituitary TSH binds to receptors located on the surface of follicular cells of the thyroid gland. Binding of the TSH to its receptor activates adenylate cyclase, which increases the amount of intracellular cyclic adenosine monophosphate (cAMP), which mediates most of the biologic actions of TSH. These include (1) iodide trapping by the thyroid follicular cells; (2) oxidation of iodide to iodine (I_2); (3) iodination of the amino acid tyrosine; (4) coupling of iodinated tyrosine within thyroglobulin to form the thyroid hormones T_3 (triiodothyronine) and mainly T_4 (tetraiodothyronine); (5) storage of T_3 and T_4 within the colloid and release into the circulation of the thyroid hormones. In the healthy individual thyronine (T_4) is the main thyroid hormone released into the circulation. It is bound mainly to serum thyroxine-binding globulin (TBG) and in minor amounts to prealbumin and albumin. It is monodeiodinated to the active T_3, mainly in the liver, kidneys, and brain. Triiodothyronine, the molecule with metabolic activity, is active only in its free form (normal, 1.0 to 3.1 nmol/L). Free T_3 crosses cell membranes and binds to receptors mainly in the cell nucleus and induces the transcription of specific genes and the synthesis of specific proteins and enzymes. (Receptors for the thyroid hormone are located both in the cell plasma membrane and the mitochondrial membrane within the cell. Unlike the steroid hormones, T_3 enters the cell nucleus unbound to a receptor.)

Thyroid-stimulating immunoglobulins are antibodies to the normal receptor sites of the thyroid-stimulating hormone (TSH) on the surface of thyroid follicle cells. These antibodies may mimic the biologic action of TSH on the thyroid function. Depending on the assay method, the activity is called variously "human thyroid stimulator," "human thyroid adenyl cyclase stimulator," thyroid-stimulating antibody, or thyroid-stimulating immunoglobulin. Long-acting thyroid stimulator (LATS) refers to a particular bioassay in the mouse.

The occurrence of thyroid-stimulating antibody in patients who have hyperthyroidism suggests that the disease is initiated by an autoimmune abnormality. Current theories relating to the pathogenesis of autoimmune hyperthyroidism relate to (1) an abnormality of the HLA-DW3 genotype (in whites) that impairs T-suppressor lymphocyte function and permits B lymphocytes to synthesize immune globulins against TSH receptor sites, and (2) depression of T-suppressor lymphocyte function through stress or aging that permits B lymphocyte synthesis of TSH receptor antibodies.

THYROTOXICOSIS

Thyrotoxicosis is a systemic abnormality that results from the effects of an excessive concentration of thyroid hormones in the blood, usually endogenous in origin. It causes sympathomimetic and calorigenic effects. The sympathomimetic effects include nervousness, tremor, diarrhea, retraction of the eyelids, and failure of the upper eyelid to follow the globe in downward gaze (eyelid lag). The calorigenic effects cause an increased basal metabolic rate with increased appetite, weight loss, increased heat production that simulates mechanisms to promote heat loss such as tachycardia, and increased skin circulation.

Graves' disease was originally described as a triad of hyperthyroidism, ophthalmopathy, and pretibial myxedema. To these may be added a thyroid gland not regulated by the thyroid-stimulating hormone of the pituitary but is stimulated by an immune globulin to TSH receptor sites of the thyroid follicle.

The onset of the systemic disease is usually marked by fatigue, tachycardia, and, despite increased appetite, weight loss. There may be a fine tremor of the fingers and tongue, heat intolerance, and excessive sweating. The systolic blood pressure increases, atrial arrhythmias occur, and the pulse pressure widens; in individuals over 40 years of age there may be

cardiac failure. Muscle weakness may be severe, but true myasthenia gravis rarely occurs.

Total serum thyroxine (T_4), measured by radioimmunoassay, is the usual initial screening test and is not altered by iodine in the serum. In conditions in which there is increased or decreased T_4 binding, a serum free thyroxine (T_3) is usually reliable. In about 5% of thyrotoxic patients, in whom total T_4 is normal, a total serum triiodothyronine (T_3) will indicate an abnormality (colloquially, T_3 thyrotoxicosis). The thyrotropin-releasing infusion test is of value when T_3 and T_4 are within normal range and if a subtle abnormality is suspected (euthyroid Graves' disease). A basic serum sample is obtained and 200 to 400 μg of thyrotropin-releasing hormone is infused intravenously over a 1-minute period. A second serum sample is obtained 30 minutes after the infusion. In normal thyroid function the serum thyrotropin increases 100%. In patients with primary hyperthyroidism there is no increase. Assay of thyroid-stimulating immunoglobulins is indicated rarely in the differential diagnosis of exophthalmos. It indicates an autoimmune thyroid disease.

Ocular signs. In somewhat more than half the patients with hyperthyroidism, eye signs (ophthalmopathy) (Table 25-1) appear sometime in the course of the disease. These may be unilateral or bilateral and mild or severe. They may precede frank hyperthyroidism or may occur long after the thyroid abnormality has been ameliorated. The severity of ocular signs does not parallel any currently recognized clinical or laboratory manifestation of the disease or any abnormality of the thyroid, pituitary, or other endocrine glands. The ocular changes involve (1) retraction of the eyelids and (2) an increase in the volume of the orbital contents, causing the eyes to protrude (Fig. 25-1). In some patients, contracture of extraocular muscles occurs, often associated with signs of congestion of the orbital contents. Rarely, optic neuropathy occurs. The ocular changes may follow a 2- to 3-year course and rarely may not regress with control of the thyrotoxicosis.

The initial eyelid change of hyperthyroidism is usually retraction of the upper eyelid. The sclera in the 12 o'clock meridian is exposed, and there is widening of the palpebral fissure and infrequent blinking, which causes a wide-

Table 25-1. Ocular signs of thyroid dysfunction

I. Eyelids
  A. Eyelid retraction (Dalrymple)
    1. Increased by attentive gaze (Kocher) or by conjunctival instillation of epinephrine; decreased by adrenergic blockage (guanethidine locally or block of superior cervical ganglion); forehead does not wrinkle on upward gaze (Joffroy)
  B. Eyelid lag (von Graefe)
    1. Delay of upper eyelid in following globe in downward gaze (common in thyrotoxicosis of any cause)
    2. Jerky downward movement of eyelid (Boston)
  C. Infrequent blinking (Stellwag); staring appearance (Dalrymple)
  D. Miscellaneous signs
    1. Globe lags behind upper eyelid on upward gaze (Means)
    2. Lower eyelid lags behind globe on upward gaze (Griffith)
    3. Increased pigmentation of skin (Jellinek)
II. Orbital congestion*
  A. May be associated with fullness of eyelids (Enroth)
  B. May prevent eversion of upper eyelid (Gifford)
III. Exophthalmos
  A. Bilateral* or unilateral*
    1. Eyelid retraction exaggerates or simulates appearance
  B. Compressible
    1. Common type in thyrotoxicosis
  C. Solid (noncompressible)
IV. Extraocular muscles
  A. Contracture of ocular muscle usual
    1. Inferior rectus muscle prevents upward gaze
    2. Ophthalmoplegia (Ballet)
  B. Weakness of convergence (Möbius)
V. Corneal involvement
  A. Irritation from rapid drying of precorneal tear film
  B. Keratitis from failure of eyelids to cover cornea adequately (keratitis e lagophthalmos)
  C. Keratitis from rapidly developing exophthalmos
VI. Optic nerve disease
  A. Papillitis or retrobulbar neuritis
  B. Papilledema
    1. Neuroretinal edema

*May occur at any stage of thyroid dysfunction.

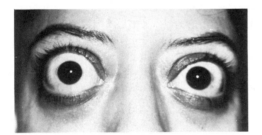

Fig. 25-1. Extreme exophthalmos and eyelid retraction in a 29-year-old woman who developed the condition gradually without signs of orbital congestion or ocular muscle weakness.

Fig. 25-2. Computed tomography of the orbits demonstrating increased size of medial recti muscles in hyperthyroidism.

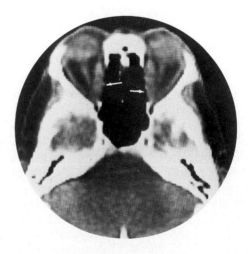

eyed, staring appearance. There is often failure of the upper eyelid to follow the globe in downward gaze (eyelid lag).

The eyelid signs of thyroid disease may result from (1) sympathetic overactivity, which causes many of the eyelid signs; (2) increased volume of the orbital contents; or (3) fibrosis of extraocular muscles, levator palpebrae superioris, and the Müller sympathetic muscles. Sympathetic overactivity and contraction of the smooth muscles of the eyelids cause retraction. The smooth muscle in the orbit of humans is too scanty to produce exophthalmos when stimulated. Eyelid retraction in hyperthyroidism does not always parallel the increase in T_3 that potentiates the action of epinephrine. The adrenergic nervous system may contribute to upper eyelid retraction and the eyelid lag in downward gaze, but it does not have a role in the pathogenesis of exophthalmos. Eyelid signs may be unilateral or bilateral and differ in severity. They may occur in the absence of exophthalmos and often precede it. They are more sensitive to amelioration of the thyroid overactivity than is the exophthalmos. Persistance of eyelid retraction after amelioration of thyrotoxicosis in sleep and general anesthesia suggests that excessive sympathetic stimulation of Müller's muscle is not the sole cause.

When severe exophthalmos develops rapidly, the globe is not protected by the eyelids and an exposure keratitis occurs (keratitis e lagophthalmos), which can lead to corneal necrosis.

Many histopathologic changes increase the volume of orbital contents. Few orbits have been studied histologically, and there is inadequate evidence to conclude that the process is the same in all patients. The ocular muscles are inflamed, may increase three to six times in mass, and have a pale, swollen, pink appearance. Lymphocytes and plasma cells infiltrate the tissues, and there is deposition of glucosaminoglycans. These increase the water content of the orbital tissues and may be responsible for the exophthalmos. Eventually, fibrous tissue replacement occurs. The cause is not known, but there are specific autoantibodies directed against plasma membranes of extraocular muscles. These immune globulins are distinct from thyroid-stimulating antibodies and other antibodies directed against thyroid gland components.

Computed tomography demonstrates one or more enlarged extraocular muscles in nearly every case of thyroid exophthalmos (Fig. 25-2). Cushing syndrome and acromegaly that cause endocrine exophthalmos do not show muscle enlargement. Often the inferior recti muscles are markedly enlarged, but all muscles may be affected. Demonstration of such muscle enlargement constitutes an important diagnostic method in Graves' disease. Ultrasonography may demonstrate ocular muscle thickening and diffuse swelling of orbital fat.

The intraocular pressure varies by more than 3 mm Hg in different directions of gaze. Usually it is higher on upward gaze. Nearly all patients (93%) with exophthalmos show the increase after 10 years compared to 60% during the first year. Any contracture of an ocular muscle will cause the increase, such as myositis and ocular muscle entrapment in orbital floor fractures.

Exophthalmos. Both orbits are usually involved in thyroid disease, although one orbit may be more markedly involved than the other. The exophthalmos develops gradually or suddenly after eyelid retraction, with increased prominence of the eyes, sensitivity to light, and conjunctival hyperemia. If the exophthalmos increases slowly, extreme degrees may develop, whereas signs of orbital congestion develop if the increase is rapid. Exophthalmos has not been produced in experimental animals by the administration of thyroid or pituitary hormones (corticotropin [ACTH], gonadotropin, growth hormone, and prolactin). Patients with exophthalmos have antibodies to the plasma membrane of ocular muscles. They do not have antibodies to the plasma membranes of skeletal muscle elsewhere in the body.

Orbital congestion. Signs of marked orbital congestion may develop quickly (Fig. 25-3). The eyelids become puffy and full. The conjunctiva becomes chemotic and injected. The conjunctival vessels may be so congested as to suggest conjunctivitis. Chemosis of the palpebral conjunctiva may be marked, and the closed eyelids may not entirely cover the globe. Edema of the conjunctiva may cause ectropion, and tearing becomes a prominent

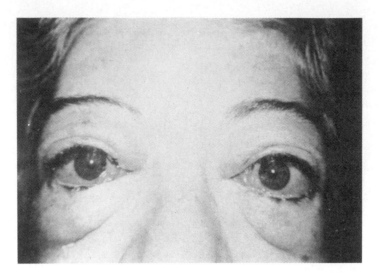

Fig. 25-3. Orbital congestion with eyelid edema, chemosis, and rapidly developing exophthalmos in a 57-year-old woman.

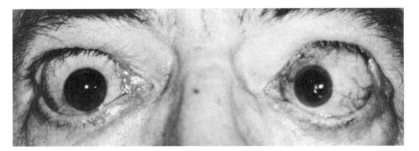

Fig. 25-4. Fibrosis of multiple extraocular muscles in a 68-year-old man. There is contraction of both medial recti muscles and both inferior recti muscles, along with severe exophthalmos and eyelid retraction.

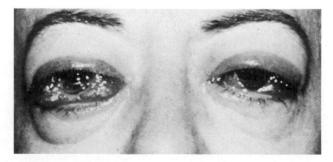

Fig. 25-5. Keratitis e lagophthalmos that developed after amelioration of hyperthyroidism in a 25-year-old woman. Loss of the eye was prevented by lateral (Berke) decompression of the orbit combined with a temporary tarsorrhaphy.

symptom. Orbital congestion may occur without exophthalmos, but more often there is a rapid increase in exophthalmos during this period. If the cornea is not protected by the eyelids, keratitis e lagophthalmos develops, causing rapid loss of vision and loss of the eye from corneal necrosis if it is not effectively treated.

Extraocular muscle fibrosis. An extraocular muscle fibrosis may develop at any time in the course of Graves' disease. Severe congestion of the orbit may mechanically limit ocular movement. If there is interference with the Bell phenomenon, in which the globe is rotated upward and outward with eyelid closure, the cornea may be exposed. A weakness of convergence follows mechanical inefficiency of the medial recti muscles in rotating the exophthalmic globes inward.

Extraocular muscle fibrosis may develop any time in the course of Graves' disease and most commonly follows adequate and appropriate treatment of moderately severe exophthalmos. Any extraocular muscle may be fibrosed. Most commonly, the inferior rectus muscle contracts, which prevents upward rotation of one or both eyes and causes a vertical diplopia. Fibrosis of multiple extraocular muscles (Fig. 25-4) may limit ocular rotation so that the head must be turned or tilted to move one eye to the primary position.

Muscular fibrosis and contraction is differentiated from a muscle weakness by the forced duction test. In a contracture of the inferior rectus muscle, the superior rectus muscle appears weakened since the eye cannot be elevated. The forced duction test indicates that contracture of the inferior rectus muscle prevents elevation of the globe.

Optic nerve involvement. In some individuals, papilledema, papillitis, or retrobulbar neuritis may develop. There are associated visual field changes characteristic of the involvement: enlargement of the blind spot, central scotomas, and sometimes peripheral field constriction. Vision is markedly reduced in patients with papillitis and in those with retrobulbar neuritis.

Patients who develop optic nerve complications may have restriction of ocular movements and varying degrees of exophthalmos. Optic neuropathy, like other ocular involvements of

Graves' disease, may develop after the hyperthyroidism has been corrected. Large amounts of systemic corticosteroids are used in therapy. Treatment must be continued for long periods; the corticosteroid dosage may be titrated against the maintenance of the visual acuity. Orbital decompression or radiation therapy of the orbits is used if corticosteroids fail or are contraindicated.

Euthyroid Graves' disease. Some patients develop the ophthalmopathy of Graves' disease with no sign of thyroid overactivity. Often thyroid-stimulating immunoglobulins are present, and some patients subsequently develop thyrotoxicosis. Other patients apparently lack the thyroid reserve to respond to excessive stimulation by these antibodies and never develop thyrotoxicosis.

Medical treatment. Treatment of the ocular changes of thyroid disease is difficult. Relief of thyrotoxicosis usually minimizes eyelid retraction, and the exophthalmos appears to regress, although it may well increase 1 or 2 mm. Despite the increase, the eyes seem less prominent without the eyelid retraction. If ocular signs are marked, antithyroid drugs or radioactive iodine should be used in small, fractionated doses to avoid rapid changes in the thyroid status. If the ocular signs of Graves' disease are present without clinical signs of hyperthyroidism, antithyroid treatment is not indicated.

Decreased orbital edema may follow sleeping with the head of the bed elevated on 5-inch blocks. Instillation of artificial tears during the day may minimize discomfort. Prevention of corneal desiccation by covering the eye with a shield or by use of ophthalmic ointments may help if the eyelids do not cover the eyes in sleep. Spectacles prevent foreign bodies from lodging on the exposed eye. Hypothyroidism should be corrected. Corticosteroids given systemically in large doses must be carefully monitored.

Surgical treatment. Loss of vision in Graves' disease occurs because of either keratitis e lagophthalmos (Fig. 25-5) or optic neuritis. Keratitis usually requires orbital decompression or tarsorrhaphy, whereas the optic neuritis often responds to systemic corticosteroids. In severe orbital congestion with exposure of the cornea, orbital decompression is the treatment of choice.

Cosmetic improvement of exophthalmos that persists after correction of the hyperthyroidism is not fully satisfactory. If the exophthalmos developed gradually and congestion is not present, a lateral blepharoplasty narrows the palpebral fissure and improves the cosmetic appearance. Retraction of the upper eyelid persisting after correction of the hyperthyroidism has been adequately treated by recessing the Müller smooth muscle of the eyelid. In severe cases, implantation of preserved sclera into the eyelid provides additional correction.

Correction of the fibrous replacement of an extraocular muscle is often disappointing. The procedure must be delayed until spontaneous improvement is unlikely, usually a year or more after the onset of the muscle weakness. The fibrosed muscle can then be recessed.

MULTIPLE ENDOCRINE NEOPLASIA

Multiple endocrine neoplasia includes three distinct disorders of neural crest differentiation. Multiple endocrine neoplasia (MEN) type IIb (III) consists of medullary thyroid carcinoma and pheochromocytoma (as does MEN, type II or IIa) with marked dysmorphic changes. Prominent, enlarged, non-myelinated corneal nerves occur in all patients with type IIb. Additionally, conjunctival neuromas, thickened eyelids, thickened conjunctival nerves, prominent eyebrows, and impaired pupillary reaction may occur. The body habitus resembles Marfan syndrome. Medullary thyroid carcinoma secretes calcitonin, and pheochromocytomas develop. The corneal nerve thickening permits diagnosis before the development of neoplasms and unusual physical features.

PARATHYROID GLANDS

The level of ionic calcium and inorganic phosphate in the body is regulated by parathyroid hormone and 25-OH vitamin D. Calcitonin, the hormone of parafollicular cells (C-cells) of the thyroid gland, may not be physiologically important in humans.

Primary hyperparathyroidism. This condition causes kidney stones and bone disorders, which result from hypercalcemia and hypophosphatemia. Calcium crystals may be deposited in the cornea and conjunctiva and, rarely, in the choroid.

Hypercalcemia and hypophosphatemia. In hypercalcemia and hypophosphatemia, calcium crystals are deposited in the cornea and conjunctiva. In the cornea, the deposits are in the Bowman zone and within epithelial cell nuclei. They are usually most marked near the corneoscleral limbus in the palpebral fissure (band keratopathy). The conjunctiva is injected, particularly in the palpebral fissure, and glistening crystals may be seen with the biomicroscope. The crystals disappear when the blood calcium level becomes normal.

Calcification in otherwise normal eyes is seen in juvenile rheumatoid arthritis (Still disease), hyperparathyroidism, milk-alkali syndrome, sarcoidosis, hypervitaminosis D, Graves' disease, posturemic phosphate depletion, widespread malignant disease, and myeloma. Calcium deposition occurs locally in pathologic conditions of the eye such as uveitis, corneal scarring, and phthisical eyes.

Hypoparathyroidism. Decreased secretion of the parathyroid hormone results in a lowered serum calcium level, an increased serum phosphorus level, and decreased urinary excretion of both calcium and phosphorus. A decreased serum calcium level causes tetany and neuromuscular hyperexcitability. In milder cases there is numbness and tingling of the extremities or in the area around the lips. Hoarseness may occur. In more severe cases carpopedal spasm and laryngeal stridor are seen. Generalized convulsions are common. Latent tetany is elicited by the Chvostek sign, in which tapping the finger over the facial nerve causes twitching of the muscles of the mouth and, in severe cases, of the nose and eyelids. Carpal spasm follows nerve ischemia when the blood supply to the arm is reduced for 3 minutes by a sphygomomanometer cuff (Trousseau sign).

Cataracts develop when the blood calcium falls to a level at which neuromuscular hyperexcitability is observed. Lens changes are bilateral and involve lens fibers predominantly in the subcapsular region. As lens damage progresses, small, discrete, punctate opacities and crystals of different shapes and colors develop in the cortical lens near the equator. Similar opacities may be found in myotonic dystrophy, cretinism, and Down syndrome. Cataracts do not always develop with hypocalcemia and the mechanism is unknown.

Calcification of basal ganglia, increased intracranial pressure, and papilledema may occur in hypoparathyroidism. Hypoparathyroidism with convulsive seizures and papilledema must be distinguished from an intracranial space-occupying lesion.

Children with idiopathic hypoparathyroidism (girls 2:1) develop chronic recurrent keratoconjunctivitis with corneal neovascularization. Superficial moniliasis involving the face and nails occurs simultaneously; later an adrenal insufficiency develops that may be fatal (78%).

DIABETES MELLITUS

Diabetes mellitus (Gr. *diabetes*, a siphon; *mellitus*, honey) is a heterogeneous, genetically determined group of disorders characterized by a disorder of glucose homeostasis. There are long-term complications that involve the eyes, kidneys, nerves, and blood vessels, combined with thickening of basement membranes. Diabetes mellitus and glucose intolerance may be classified into a number of genetically and clinically distinct types.

Insulin-dependent diabetes mellitus (IDDM, type I) has an abrupt onset, with thirst, increased appetite, excessive urination, and weight loss occurring over a period of several days. The age of onset peaks at 12 years, but the disorder may occur at any age. Previously this disorder was called juvenile or growth-onset diabetes mellitus, or ketosis prone, or brittle diabetes mellitus. Ia antigen, which is coded for by the HLA-D region of chromosome 6, may be present while functional beta cells are still present. The antigen disappears when beta cells no longer secrete insulin. A viral-induced autoimmune destruction of beta cells is considered likely. Immunosuppression trials in the early stages are currently underway. All patients require insulin eventually.

Noninsulin-dependent diabetes mellius (NIDDM, type II) usually begins in middle life or beyond. There is a resistance to glucose utilization by all insulin-responsive tissues, but all patients secrete some insulin. Nonetheless, this group is subject to the same complications as insulin-dependent patients. The typical patient is overweight. Patients do not develop ketosis and oftentimes weight reduction reduces blood glucose to normal levels. Many patients, however, require treatment with insulin. Noninsulin-dependent diabetes mellitus was formerly called adult-onset, or maturity-onset diabetes mellitus. Maturity-onset diabetes of the young occurs with an autosomal dominant heredity pattern.

Other types of diabetes mellitus include those found with increased frequency in other conditions such as pancreatic and hormonal abnormalities, disorders induced by drugs or chemicals, abnormalities of insulin receptors, certain genetic syndromes, and malnourished populations. Formerly this group was called secondary diabetes mellitus.

Diabetes is the major systemic disease that causes blindness in the United States and is the leading cause of blindness in individuals 40 to 60 years of age. The rate of blindness among diabetic persons is 20 times that of the general population. There is a much higher risk of blindness from diabetes in nonwhite women than in either white women or white men. Nonwhite men have the lowest risk of blindness from diabetes.

Disease of the capillaries and small vessels (microangiopathy) causes retinopathy, nephropathy, and neuropathy. Accelerated atherosclerosis, possibly resulting from microangiopathy of the vasa vasorum, causes coronary insufficiency and myocardial infarction as well as ischemia of the extremities with gangrene of the feet.

Close control of hyperglycemia is an essential part of preventing or forestalling diabetic oculopathy, nephropathy, and neuropathy. Possibly close control has no effect after the lesions begin and is only effective in preventing the initial lesions. Additionally, there may be different metabolic pathways in different tissues in various individuals so that the effects of hyperglycemia vary.

Many of the ocular complications of diabetes can be effectively treated if seen at an early stage. Thus every diabetic patient should have an annual thorough eye examination, including study of the peripheral fundus using an indirect ophthalmoscope or a three-way ophthalmoscopic prism and biomicroscope.

Retinopathy

Retinopathy is the most important ocular manifestation of diabetes (see Table 25-2). The introduction of insulin in 1921 followed by the sulfonamides in 1937 and the antibiotics thereafter prevented premature death of diabetic persons from coma or infection. Since then the ocular, renal, and cardiovascular complications have emerged as the chief complications of the disease. Diabetic retinopathy is not a result of concurrent atherosclerosis or vascular hypertension but is severely aggravated by uncontrolled hypertension.

The prevalence of diabetic retinopathy is related to the duration of the disease, the onset of which can be accurately known in the insulin-dependent type and only estimated in the noninsulin-dependent type. The prevalence of retinopathy is 7% in patients with diabetes for less than 10 years, 26% in patients with diabetes for 10 to 14 years, and 63% in patients with diabetes for more than 15 years.

The severity of the retinopathy generally parallels the duration of the disease, poor glycemic control (particularly within 5 years after onset), proteinuria, impotence, and heavy alcohol consumption. Smoking, obesity, and severity of the diabetes appear to be unrelated. Diabetic control has little effect once the retinopathy begins. The severity and rapidity of involvement of the two eyes may be unequal, and even in the same eye one area may progress while another recedes. Severe proliferative diabetic retinopathy develops more frequently in younger men, and blindness is more common in men than women before the age of 45 years.

The retinopathy affects the retinal capillaries, particularly between the superior and inferior temporal blood vessels. The choriocapillaris never participates in the retinopathy, although there is thickening of the choriocapillaris basement membrane.

Visual acuity is a poor index of the severity of the retinopathy. A single lesion impairing the foveola will reduce form vision, possibly to the level of legal blindness. Conversely, extensive peripheral proliferative retinopathy may severely restrict the peripheral field of vision,

but good central vision may be retained. Vitreous hemorrhage from relatively minor neovascularization may severely reduce vision, but vitreous hemorrhage that spares the visual axis may allow good central vision.

Grading the severity of changes in diabetic retinopathy is difficult. In clinical studies photographs of the patient's fundus are compared with standard photographs. In controlled studies, the retina is often "mapped" with a collage of fundus photographs and changes are specifically described. In advanced diabetic retinopathy, even though the fundus can be seen adequately by indirect ophthalmoscopy, the quality of fundus photographs is poor because of opacities in the ocular media.

The earliest lesion of the diabetic retina is degeneration of the intramural pericytes of retinal capillaries. These pericytes are strikingly responsive to insulin in comparison to smooth muscle and endothelial cells of the aorta and retinal microvessels. They probably regulate regional blood flow. Their loss may lead to weakening of the capillary wall, loss of endothelial cells, and failure of the capillary to carry blood. An aldose reductase inhibitor (Sorbinol)

Table 25-2. Diabetic retinopathy

A. Background retinopathy (nonproliferative)
  1. Intraretinal microangiopathy
    a. Loss of pericytes
    b. Microaneurysms
    c. Capillary occlusion
    d. Increased permeability with plasma leakage and retinal edema (hard exudates)
      (1) Macular edema
      (2) Peripheral edema
B. Preproliferative retinopathy
  1. Chronic retinal edema (hard yellow exudates)
  2. Cotton-wool patches (soft exudates)
  3. Intraretinal microvascular abnormalities
  4. Dilated, tortuous, kinked intraretinal blood vessels
C. Proliferative retinopathy
  1. New blood vessels
    a. Peripheral
      (1) Focal
      (2) Generalized
    b. Optic disk
    c. Both peripheral and disk
  2. Vitreous hemorrhage secondary to new blood vessels
  3. Fibrovascular proliferation
  4. Retinal traction
    a. Retinal detachment

(see galactosemia) prevents capillary basement thickening in rats fed a diet with galactose as their major source of carbohydrates. A controlled clinical trial currently seeks to learn the effect of aldose reductase inhibitors on diabetic retinopathy.

Retinopathy may be divided into (1) background retinopathy, and (2) proliferative (neovascular) retinopathy (Table 25-2). Except for new blood vessel formation in proliferative retinopathy and their sequelae, the retinal lesions are similar. Older noninsulin-dependent diabetic persons tend to have more retinal microangiopathy of the central retina and macular edema than younger, insulin-dependent diabetic persons who tend to have more neovascular proliferation of the peripheral fundus. Increased vascular permeability and occlusive vascular disease are more common in the noninsulin-dependent type. In both background and proliferative retinopathy, there are microaneurysms, dot and blot hemorrhages (intraretinal and preretinal) (Fig. 25-6), hard exudates, soft exudates (cotton-wool patches of acute retinal ischemia), retinal microangiopathy, increased vascular permeability, retinal edema, capillary dilation, tortuosity, telangiectasis, and irregularities of caliber and configuration.

Background retinopathy. Retinal microaneurysms occur most often in ocular lesion of diabetes. They also occur in retinal vein closure, Coats disease, arterial hypertension, pernicious anemia, dysproteinemia, and other systemic disease. Only in diabetic retinopathy do so many occur. Those associated with diseases other than diabetes are located on the arterial side of the capillary circulation in the periphery rather than on the venous side at the posterior pole as in diabetes. Microaneurysms occur rarely in tissues other than the retina in diabetes mellitus.

Microscopically, microaneurysms consist of minute spherical or ovoid distentions ranging from 20 μm to 200 μm in size, located on the venous side of the capillary network at the level of the inner nuclear layer. The resolving power of the direct ophthalmoscope is approximately 70 μm to 80 μm. Thus the majority of retinal microaneurysms are not seen with the ophthalmoscope. This is evident when the retina is viewed after intravenous injection of fluorescein (Fig. 25-7) or is seen histologically after trypsin digestion of the retina. Microaneurysms may become hyalinized and appear ophthalmoscopically as white dots.

Ophthalmoscopically, microaneurysms are minute, round, sharply circumscribed, red bodies that appear similar to hemorrhages.

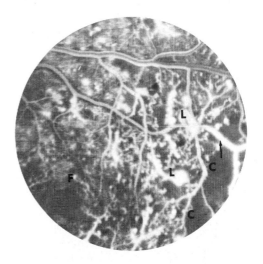

Fig. 25-7. Fluorescein angiography (early venous phase) of the left fundus of a 27-year-old woman with insulin-dependent diabetes mellitus. There are numerous microaneurysms and dilated, kinked, tortuous retinal blood vessels with areas of capillary nonperfusion *(C)* and capillary leakage *(L)* causing retinal edema. The wall of a branch of the superior temporal artery leaks fluorescein *(arrow)*, indicating endothelial damage. The foveola *(F)* is not affected, and visual acuity is 20/20.

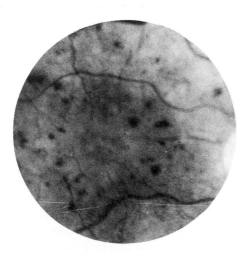

Fig. 25-6. Background retinopathy with preponderance of blot and dot hemorrhages.

They may be distinguished from deep small hemorrhages by their unchanging appearance, their usual location far from blood vessels, and their sharp borders.

Microaneurysm formation is preceded by loss of pericytes (mural cells) in the blood vessel wall. Their loss may signal failure of autoregulation of the vascular tone and may be followed by capillary dilation and microaneurysm formation. There is concurrent increase in macroglobulins leading to red blood cell aggregation and platelet clumping that impairs capillary perfusion and causes retinal ischemia.

Microaneurysms are permeable to large molecules and cause retinal edema in the area surrounding them. Near the region of retinal edema may be hard yellow exudates (Fig. 25-8) that consist of lipid-laden macrophages and cholesterol. If the microaneurysms are obliterated with laser photocoagulation, the exudate disappears and becomes white. The development of such edema deposits in the fovea is a serious complication because function cannot be entirely restored as retinal edema is reversed.

Retinal microangiopathy is an abnormality in which microaneurysms and failure of capillary perfusion cause edema and dilated abnormal intraretinal vasculature. If located near the foveola, there may be early impairment of central vision even though the retinopathy is not advanced. Argon laser photocoagulation of the areas of microangiopathy, but not the fovea, is indicated as soon as it occurs.

Possible causes of capillary closure include loss of capillary tone, microthrombi, blood sludging, platelet aggregation, edema of the surrounding retina, reduced capillary perfusion pressure, and endothelial proliferation. These result in the channeling of blood into remaining capillaries that dilate and become collateral vessels that carry blood past areas of capillary closure. With fluorescein angiography, additional capillary abnormalities such as fusiform aneurysms, capillary leakage, and dilation of capillaries are seen. Clinically, they are associated with severe progressive retinal edema. Fluorescein angiography may demonstrate small and large areas of capillary nonperfusion.

The retinal hemorrhages of diabetes do not differ from hemorrhages seen in other conditions. Small round hemorrhages are located in the inner nuclear layer of the retina, the cells

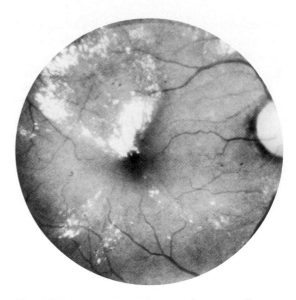

Fig. 25-8. A circinate deposit that typically surrounds an area of intraretinal, microvascular abnormalities.

of which are arranged so compactly that the hemorrhage cannot spread. Most hemorrhages are larger than microaneurysms and tend to disappear.

Flame-shaped hemorrhages are located in the nerve fiber layers of the retina; their shape reflects the distribution of the nerve fibers. Similar hemorrhages are seen in hypertension, blood dyscrasias, papilledema, and central vein obstruction.

Preretinal hemorrhages spread between the internal limiting membrane and the nerve fiber layer of the retina or between the internal limiting membrane and the vitreous (subhyaloid). Some may show a fluid level with bed rest. Acute trauma and subarachnoid and subdural hemorrhage may produce a similar hemorrhage. Preretinal hemorrhages may burst into the vitreous body, causing immediate obscuration of vision.

The deposits of diabetes are divided into hard yellow exudates (chronic edema residues), hard exudates, and soft exudates (cotton-wool patches). Hard yellow exudates surround an area of retinal edema that surrounds microaneurysms. They appear as yellowish waxy areas that coalesce, become confluent, and may form a ring (Fig. 25-9). They are composed of cholesterol crystals and lipid-laden macro-

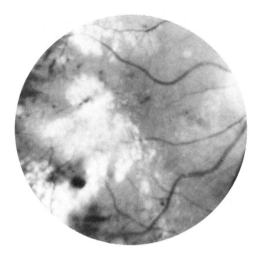

Fig. 25-9. Background retinopathy with preponderance of hard yellow exudates. Exudates affecting the foveola markedly reduce vision.

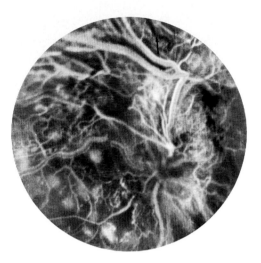

Fig. 25-10. Fluorescein angiography of severe neovascularization at the optic disk. A major retinal vein is occluded additionally *(arrow).*

phages in the outer plexiform layer. Hard deposits are residues of hard yellow deposits that remain after the retinal edema disappears.

Soft deposits, or cotton-wool patches, are microinfarcts in the nerve fiber layer of the retina secondary to acute vascular insufficiency and occlusion of terminal arterioles. The lesions are smaller than those of vascular hypertension and may be overlooked. They do not occur after retinal neovascularization.

Dilation of retinal veins occurs sometime before or during the course of nearly every instance of retinopathy. All of the veins or only a branch becomes engorged and dilated, and there may be a granular blood flow. There may be dilated segments of veins ("beading"). Although the picture resembles an impending central vein closure, the veins pulsate normally with pressure on the globe, and there are no adjacent retinal hemorrhages.

Maculopathy or foveola impairment involves a sequence of microaneurysms, capillary obliteration, development of intraretinal collateral vessels, intraretinal hemorrhages, an increased vascular permeability with breakdown of the blood-retina barrier resulting in hard yellow exudates, microcystic edema, and cysts of the foveola. Both eyes are usually similarly affected. Microaneurysms cannot occur in the capillary free zone, but they cause edema with hard yellow exudates at the periphery of the

edematous retina, impairing the foveola and reducing vision.

Proliferative retinopathy (Fig. 25-10). The development of new blood vessels in and anterior to the retina heralds a serious change in the visual prognosis of diabetic retinopathy. The vessels originate most commonly from a retinal vein near an arteriovenous crossing at the posterior pole and next most commonly from the surface of the optic disk. The superior temporal vein is the most common retinal location; the inferior temporal, superior nasal, and inferior nasal veins are involved in that order of frequency.

Initially a fine network of vessels develops. These vessels have a minimal fibrous component, are extremely permeable, and increase in length, caliber, number, and complexity. Proliferation of the associated connective tissue causes increasing intervascular opacification. The vessels involute and decrease in size and number as the fibrous tissue becomes more opaque and dense.

As long as the vitreous remains in contact with the inner limiting membrane of the retina, the new vessels spread as a flat sheet on the inner retinal surface (Fig. 25-11). If the vitreous contracts, fibrovascular tissue adherent to its retinal surface is torn loose and may rupture blood vessels, resulting in a vitreous hemorrhage. Traction on the fibrovascular tissue by

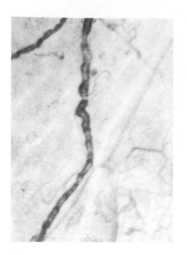

Fig. 25-11. Beading of a retinal vein with extensive neovascularization on the inner surface of the retina.

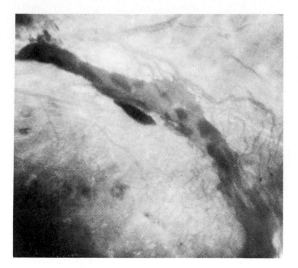

Fig. 25-12. Preretinal hemorrhage with slight hemorrhage escape into the vitreous originating from an area of retinal neovascularization.

contracting vitreous may cause a tractional, nonrhegmatogenous retinal detachment. If the vitreous is already detached when neovascularization occurs, the blood vessels extend into the vitreous cavity and may cause hemorrhage, but since there are no vitreous attachments, tractional retinal hemorrhages do not occur.

The process of fibrovascular proliferation followed by vascular involution and fibrous proliferation and contraction continues for many years. Eventually, the new vessels are not apparent, and large white fibrous traction bands extend from the surface of the disk to the vascular arcades. Much, if not all, of the retina may be detached. If, however, the foveola remains attached, some patients may maintain excellent visual acuity despite extensive fibrous and tractional retinal detachment.

Vitreous hemorrhage (Fig. 25-12) may cause sudden loss of vision or, when less dense, a mist of red may obscure vision. In young individuals, it may be quickly absorbed, but often after repeated episodes or in elderly persons the blood may persist indefinitely. The hemorrhage may produce a black ophthalmoscopic reflex or cause all fundus details to be blurred. As the blood absorbs, large vitreous floaters are visible. Vitreous hemorrhage always has a serious visual prognosis, because it often reflects vitreous contraction and the onset of the final stages of proliferative retinopathy.

Vitrectomy removes vitreous blood and sev-

ers fibrin bands that cause traction detachment of the retina. The instrumentation is complex, and the procedure is difficult. Nevertheless, many patients who were previously considered to be hopelessly blind can benefit from vitrectomy.

Treatment. Although careful control of diabetes during the first 5 years of the disease may reduce the severity or delay the onset of retinopathy, it apparently has little or no effect on the established condition. Currently, prophylactic use of aspirin, accurate control of blood glucose by use of an insulin pump, administration of aldose reductase inhibitors, and retinal photocoagulation are used.

Photocoagulation of the retina is indicated for treatment of new blood vessels of the retina, optic disk, or both. Background retinopathy is treated if it involves or threatens to involve the foveola, irrespective of severity. Local microaneurysms (focal retinopathy) have a better prognosis than diffuse retinopathy. The visual results depend upon the integrity of the foveola and the location, extent, and duration of retinal edema and exudates.

The argon laser is usually used in combination with a biomicroscope and contact lens, which neutralizes the corneal refraction and permits visualization of the fundus. A three-mirror contact lens permits visualization of the peripheral fundus. The foveola is not photocoagulated, and usually burns are not placed any closer than 0.25 disk diameters (375 μm) to the center of the capillary free zone. The area between the fovea centralis and the disk is photocoagulated cautiously to avoid damage to the nerve fibers of the papillomacular bundle.

New blood vessels more than 1 disk diameter from the optic disk are treated with focal photocoagulation. Often the new blood vessels are near the first bifurcation of the superior temporal vein. The origin of the new blood vessels is surrounded for a distance of about 0.2 disk diameter with photocoagulation of sufficient intensity to produce a slight opacification (coagulation) of the sensory retina. Major blood vessels are not photocoagulated. Treatment is continued until new blood vessels no longer carry blood and may have to be repeated. In general, focal photocoagulation produces better results than panretinal photocoagulation.

In patients with blood vessels either on the optic disk or next to it, scatter coagulation is usually followed by involution of the vessels, with the fibrous component becoming more prominent. Involution occurs with photocoagulation of a single quadrant, but panretinal photocoagulation may be required. Since extensive destruction of the peripheral retina impairs dark adaptation and peripheral vision, I limit initial photocoagulation to the region of the major blood vessels and the area temporal to the fovea centralis. If new blood vessels have not regressed in 2 weeks, the peripheral retina is ablated. The region encompassed by the superior and inferior temporal vascular arcades is not photocoagulated unless involution does not occur.

Intraretinal microvascular abnormalities in the area next to the foveola cause a rim of hard yellow exudates or retinal edema to reduce vision. Photocoagulation of the vascular component resolves the edema and exudates and, if done promptly, improves vision.

Other ocular manifestations

Diabetes mellitus causes a variety of changes in the eye and its function. Nearly every ocular structure may be affected (Table 25-3).

Rubeosis of the iris. Rubeosis of the iris (Fig. 25-13) is a vascular proliferation of the iris vessels that first becomes evident at the pupillary margin and in the anterior chamber angle. It also occurs spontaneously and following cen-

Table 25-3. Ocular complications of diabetes mellitus other than retinopathy

I. Fundus
   A. Optic nerve atrophy, edema
   B. Lipemia retinalis
II. Oculomotor nerves
   A. Neuropathy with muscle paralysis (pupil frequently spared in N III involvement)
III. Visual acuity
   A. Transient variations in refraction
   B. Photopsia and diplopia in cerebral hypoglycemia
   C. Decreased accommodation
   D. Depressed in cataract, vitreous hemorrhage, capillary nonperfusion adjacent to foveola, deposits in foveola, and foveal microangiopathy
   E. Blindness from tractional retinal detachment, massive vitreous retraction
   F. Diplopia in ophthalmoplegia caused by neuropathy
IV. Intraocular pressure
   A. Decreased in acidosis
   B. Increased in neovascular glaucoma
V. Conjunctiva
   A. Sludging of blood; tortuous, constricted blood vessels
VI. Cornea
   A. Wrinkling of Descemet membrane
   B. Decreased corneal sensation (trigeminal nerve neuropathy)
   C. Impaired healing
   D. Abnormal epithelial basement membrane, delayed wound healing
   E. Punctate keratopathy
VII. Iris
   A. Hydrops of pigment epithelium (transient glycogen storage, disappears with normal blood glucose)
   B. Rubeosis iridis
   C. Transmission defects in pigment epithelium
VIII. Lens
   A. Variation in refractive power (hyperglycemia)
   B. Snowflake ("sugar") cataract (insulin-dependent diabetes)
   C. Premature onset of senile cataract

tral vein closure. If glaucoma occurs, it is often resistant to both medical and surgical treatment.

Hydrops of the iris. Glycogen may accumulate in the pigment epithelium of the iris. Alcohol-fixed sections of eyes that have been enucleated during a period of high blood glucose concentration indicate the glycogen in dilated, vacuolated cells (Fig. 25-14). Clinically, the condition may be suspected by observing the release of pigment into the anterior chamber after dilation of the pupil or after iridectomy in diabetic persons.

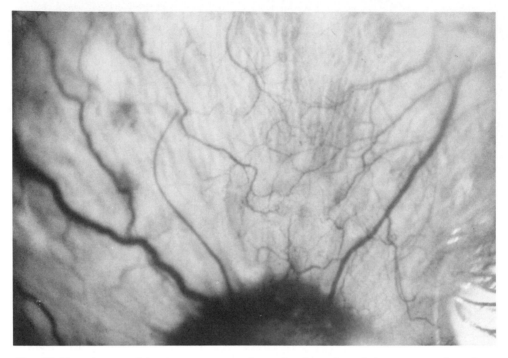

Fig. 25-13. Rubeosis of the iris in a man with insulin-dependent diabetes. Secondary glaucoma as the result of neovascularization of the anterior chamber angle did not develop.

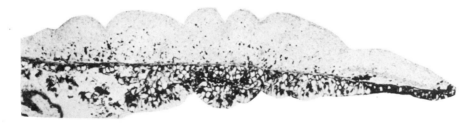

Fig. 25-14. Hydrops of the iris with the accumulation of glycogen in cystlike spaces in the pigment epithelium of the iris.

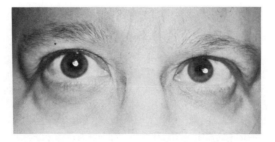

Fig. 25-15. Paralysis of the left lateral rectus muscle in a 62-year-old woman with noninsulin-dependent diabetes mellitus.

Diabetic cataract. The lens may be involved in diabetes by transient changes in refractive power, early and more frequent senile cataract, and juvenile diabetic cataract ("sugar" cataract).

Cataracts secondary to diabetes occur rarely 10 to 20 years after the onset of insulin-dependent diabetes. Diabetic cataract develops rapidly and decreases vision soon after its onset. Both eyes are involved, often simultaneously. Typically, the opacity consists of small flaky opacities (snowflakes) and water clefts located in the anterior or posterior cortex immediately beneath the lens capsule. Control of the diabetes with restoration of normal blood glucose levels stops progression of the opacity. In persistent hyperglycemia a complete (mature) lens opacity may form within 48 hours, but progress is usually more gradual. Diabetic retinopathy may prevent good vision after cataract extraction.

Neuropathy. Paralysis of ocular muscles innervated by the third or the sixth cranial nerve (Fig. 25-15) occurs relatively rarely in diabetes. Characteristically, a middle-aged to elderly individual with mild overt diabetes or chemical diabetes has a sudden onset of diplopia and muscle paralysis associated with a homolateral headache of an intensity severe enough to lead one to suspect intracranial aneurysm. There may be a history of previous Bell palsy or similar neurologic disease. Neuropathy involving other areas may or may not be present. Signs of meningeal irritation do not occur. If the third cranial nerve is involved, the pupil will most likely be spared (in 17 of 24 cases), in contrast to pupillary paralysis, which occurs commonly in cerebral tumors and aneurysms. The paralysis disappears spontaneously within several weeks if the diabetes is of short duration, or it persists up to 6 months if the diabetes has been present for a long time, particularly if it has been poorly controlled.

Unilateral frontal headache and oculomotor paralysis are characteristic of aneurysms of the intracranial portion of the carotid artery. The sparing of the pupil, the laboratory signs of diabetes, normal spinal fluid, and absence of meningeal irritation suggest that the disease is caused by diabetes.

Other causes of ophthalmoplegia besides intracranial aneurysms include tumors (roentgenographic changes), leukemia (blood count), ophthalmoplegic migraine (history), head trauma, demyelinating disease (painless onset), myasthenia gravis (painless onset), and cerebrovascular disease. The cornea may become less sensitive, reflecting a trigeminal neuropathy, particularly in diabetes of long duration.

Variations in refractive error. Hyperglycemia may be associated with or followed by increased refractive power of the lens, resulting in a change in the refractive error in the direction of myopia. Restoration of the blood glucose level to normal reverses the process. The refractive power of the lens decreases and the refractive error changes in the direction of hyperopia. The exact mechanism of the change is not known, but it is assumed that during hyperglycemia there is an increased glucose content of the lens cortex with imbibition of water, causing the lens to become thicker and thus increasing its refractive power.

The visual acuity parallels the change in refraction. Refraction during hyperglycemia varies, often markedly, from that during an interval of normal blood glucose concentration. Paralysis of accommodation by means of a cycloplegic drug does not affect the induced refractive error. Corrective lenses, often quite different from those usually worn, improve vision to normal. Diagnosis is not difficult in a known diabetic, but the variation in refraction and visual acuity may be the first indication of diabetes mellitus, particularly in the insulin-dependent individual.

A similar change in refractive power may be produced in nondiabetic individuals by drugs, particularly sulfonamide derivatives. An actual change in the total refractive power of the eye, as occurs in diabetes, should be differentiated from that occurring with sustained accommodation (spasm of accommodation), which is neutralized with drugs that paralyze accommodation.

Subjective visual symptoms. During periods of hypoglycemia, patients with diabetes mellitus without organic changes in the eyes may complain of photopsia or of double vision during periods of hypoglycemia. These symptoms are presumably of cerebral origin and are abolished by increasing the blood glucose level.

Intraocular pressure. Ciliary body secretion is sensitive to the plasma bicarbonate level. A low intraocular pressure is associated with diabetic acidosis, and the ocular hypotension may be augmented by the concurrent dehydration.

Glaucoma in diabetes is a complication of rubeosis of the iris. Open-angle glaucoma occurs more commonly in patients with diabetes mellitus, but proliferative retinopathy occurs less commonly in diabetic patients with glaucoma.

Lipemia retinalis. Lipemia retinalis is an uncommon abnormality of the ocular fundus that occurs when the triglyceride concentration of the blood exceeds 2,000 mg/dl and is combined with increased low-density lipoproteins. Ophthalmoscopically, the blood column of the retinal vessels is salmon-pink against the choroidal background. The contrast between the size of arteries and the veins of the fundus is lost, and the vessels become engorged. If the triglyceride concentration exceeds 3%, the color of the blood column changes from salmon-pink to cream. The choroidal background looks pink rather than red. Vision is not affected, and there are no ocular symptoms.

The condition occurs most commonly in diabetic acidosis, usually in insulin-dependent diabetes. It may also occur in familial and secondary hyperlipidemia.

Recognition of the ophthalmoscopic pattern may establish a presumptive diagnosis of diabetic coma. More often a milky, opalescent serum is noted in blood removed for laboratory testing, and the fundi are then studied.

Associated renal changes

Insulin-dependent diabetes commonly causes death from renal failure in the fifth decade of life. The fundi of many of these patients show a combination of diabetic retinopathy with superimposed changes of severe vascular hypertension. There may be papilledema, diabetic retinopathy, cotton-wool patches of hypertension, and angiospasm.

BIBLIOGRAPHY
Thyroid

Brennan, M.W., Leone, C.R., Jr., and Janaki, L.: Radiation therapy for Graves' disease, Am. J. Ophthalmol. **96:**195, 1983.

De Groot, L.J., Larsen, P.R., Refetoff, S., and Stanbury, J.B.: The thyroid and its diseases, ed. 5, New York, 1984, John Wiley & Sons.

Faryna, M., Nauman, J., and Gardas, A.: Measurement of autoantibodies against human eye muscle plasma membranes in Graves' ophthalmopathy, Br. Med. J. **290:**191, 1985.

Felberg, N.T., Sergott, R.C., Savino, P.J., Blizzard, J.J., Schatz, N.J., and Amsel, J.: Lymphocyte subpopulations in Graves' ophthalmopathy, Arch. Ophthalmol. **103:**656, 1985.

Feldon, S.E., Lee, C.P., Muramatsu, S.K., and Weiner, J.M.: Quantitative computed tomography of Graves' ophthalmopathy, Arch. Ophthalmol. **103:**213, 1985.

Feldon, S.E., Muramatsu, S., and Weinger, J.M.: Clinical classification of Graves' ophthalmopathy, Arch. Ophthalmol. **102:**1469, 1984.

Gamblin, G.T., Harper, D.G., Galentine, P., Buck, D.R., Chernow, B., and Eil, C.: Prevalence of increased intraocular pressure in Graves' disease—evidence of frequent subclinical ophthalmopathy, N. Engl. J. Med. **308:**420, 1983.

Gorman, C.A., Waller, R.R., and Dyer, J.A., editors: The eye and orbit in thyroid disease, New York, 1984, Raven Press.

Hurbli, T., Char, D.H., Harris, J., Weaver, K., Greenspan, F., and Sheline, G.: Radiation therapy for thyroid eye diseases, Am. J. Ophthalmol. **99:**633, 1985.

Panzo, G.J., and Tomsak, R.L.: A retrospective review of 26 cases of dysthyroid optic neuropathy, Am. J. Ophthalmol. **96:**190, 1983.

Waller, R.R.: Eyelid malpositions in Graves' ophthalmopathy, Trans. Am. Ophthalmol. Soc. **80:**855, 1982.

Diabetes

Constable, I.J., Knuiman, M.W., Welborn, T.A., Cooper, R.L., Stanton, K.M., McCann, V.J., and Grose, G.C.: Assessing the risk of diabetic retinopathy, Am. J. Ophthalmol. **97:**53, 1984.

Early Treatment Diabetic Retinopathy Study Research Group: Photocoagulation for diabetic macular edema, Arch. Ophthalmol. **103:**1796, 1985.

Fett, J.W., Strydom, D.J., Lobb, R.R., Alderman, E.M., Bethune, J.L., Riordan, J.F., and Vallee, B.L.: Isolation and characterization of angiogenin, an angiogenic protein from human carcinoma cells, Biochemistry **24:**5480, 1985.

Frank, R.N.: On the pathogenesis of diabetic retinopathy, Ophthalmology **91:**626, 1984.

Friedman, E.A., and L'Esperance, F.A., editors: Diabetic and renal-retinal syndrome, vol. 2, prevention and management, New York, 1982, Grune & Stratton.

Kollarits, C.R., Kiess, R.D., Das, A., Hall, A.M., Jordan, E.L., Jr., and Donovan, J.E.: Diabetic retinopathy and insulin therapy in a rural diabetic population, Am. J. Ophthalmol. **97:**709, 1984.

Little, H.L.: Treatment of proliferative diabetic retinopathy: long-term results of argon laser photocoagulation, Ophthalmology **92:**279, 1985.

Little, H.L., Jack R.L., Patz, A., and Forsham, P.H. editors: Diabetic retinopathy, New York, 1983, Thieme-Stratton.

McDonald, H.R., and Schatz, H.: Grid photocoagulation for diffuse macular edema, Retina **5**:65, 1985.

McDonald, H.R., and Schatz, H.: Visual loss following panretinal photocoagulation for proliferative diabetic retinopathy, Ophthalmology **92**:388, 1985.

Moss, S.E., Klein, R., Kessler, S.D., and Richie, K.A.: Comparison between ophthalmoscopy and fundus photography in determining severity of diabetic retinopathy, Ophthalmology **92**:62, 1985.

Olsen, T., Ehlers, N., Nielsen, C.B., and Beck-Nielsen, H.: Diabetic retinopathy after one year of improved metabolic control obtained by continuous subcutaneous insulin infusion (CSII), Acta Ophthalmol. **63**:315, 1985.

Rand, L.I., Krolewski, A.S., Aiello, L.M., Warren, J.H., Baker, R.S., and Maki, T.: Multiple factors in the prediction of risk of proliferative diabetic retinopathy, N. Engl. J. Med. **313**:1433, 1985.

Srikanta, S., Ganda, O.P. Eisenbarth, E.S., et al.: Islet-cell antibodies and beta-cell function in monozygotic triplets and twins initially discordant to type I diabetes mellitus, N. Engl. J. Med. **308**:322, 1983.

Turner, G.S., Inglesby, D.V., Sharriff, B., and Kohner, E.M.: Natural history of peripheral neovascularization in diabetic retinopathy, Br. J. Ophthalmol. **69**:429, 1985.

26

THE CENTRAL NERVOUS SYSTEM AND THE EYE

Many different disorders of the central nervous system involve the eye or its adnexa, cause ocular symptoms, or both. Although some are immediately evident, many require extensive study and testing to diagnose. Even the most cursory physical examination should indicate that the pupils are round and equal and react directly and consensually to light, that the eyes move normally in all directions, and that the optic disks are flat and of normal color.

PUPILS

The pupils are normally round and approximately equal in size. Both pupils constrict when the retina of one eye is stimulated with light. The pupil is not round if it is adherent to the lens or cornea or after surgical excision of the pupilary margin (iridectomy).

Lesions affecting the afferent pupillary pathway, such as in optic atrophy or optic neuritis, impair pupillary constriction to light (see Chapter 14). Horner syndrome is caused by interruption of the sympathetic nerve fibers to the dilatator pupillae muscle. The pupil is miotic and does not dilate when cocaine is instilled into the eye; there is an associated blepharoptosis and failure of sweating of the face on the involved side. Adie syndrome involves parasympathetic postganglionic nerves of the ciliary ganglion in which the pupil is larger than its fellow and pupillary constriction is absent or delayed. Argyll Robertson pupils (miotic and irregular pupils that fail to constrict to light but constrict to convergence) occur in tabes dorsalis.

Unilateral mydriasis and coma after head injury suggest a skull fracture on the side of the dilated pupil. Tumor, aneurysm, and head injury are more likely to compress pupillary fibers and to cause pupillary dilation (mydriasis) than are diabetic neuropathy or meningitis. With midbrain hypoxia, the pupils dilate, but otherwise the pupils constrict in coma. Pupils dilated by topical instillation of drugs such as atropine, ocular injury, or closed-angle glaucoma do not constrict after instillation of 1% pilocarpine. Pupils dilated because of oculomotor nerve disease or injury constrict readily after pilocarpine instillation.

OCULAR MOVEMENTS

The motor nerves to the eye may be involved in a variety of abnormalities caused by trauma, hemorrhage, cerebral edema, ischemia, inflammation, neoplasm, aneurysms, or demyelination. Impairment of a motor nerve or its nucleus results in a failure of the eye to move in the field of action of the muscle or muscles they innervate. A strabismus is present and, if binocular vision is developed, there is a diplopia. Inability to move both eyes in the same direction (right or left, up or down) is a gaze palsy. Strabismus or diplopia do not occur. Sometimes a gaze palsy and isolated ocular muscle palsy occur simultaneously.

Oculomotor nerve. Complete paralysis of the oculomotor nerve (N III) causes a blepharoptosis of the upper eyelid (levator palpebrae superioris) and paralysis of the medial rectus, superior rectus, inferior rectus, and inferior oblique muscles (external ophthalmoplegia). The pupil is dilated (mydriasis) and does not constrict to light or convergence, and there is loss of accommodation (cycloplegia). Mydriasis and cycloplegia constitute an internal ophthalmoplegia. When the unimpaired fellow eye fixes, the paralyzed eye rotates outward because of the intact action of the lateral rectus muscle (N VI). Oculomotor nerve paralysis caused by an aneurysm or neoplasm often involves the pupil as well as ocular muscles (total ophthalmoplegia); when caused by a medical condition such as diabetic neuropathy, the pupil is spared. The pupil and the ciliary muscle are usually not affected in lesions in the oculomotor nerve nucleus. Ophthalmoplegia caused by a lesion in the brain stem is often associated with lesions of other cranial nerves.

Involvement of the fibers of the oculomotor nerve passing through the red nucleus causes Benedikt syndrome, in which there is homolateral oculomotor paralysis, contralateral dyskinesia, and contralateral intention tremor of the arm only. There may be an associated contralateral hemianesthesia.

Involvement of axons near the ventral surface of the brain in the cerebral peduncle interrupts pyramidal fibers and causes Weber syndrome, which results in homolateral oculomotor nerve paralysis, contralateral hemiplegia, and paralysis of the tongue and lower part of the face.

Interruption of the oculomotor nerve in the cavernous sinus is likely to be associated with involvement of the fourth and sixth cranial nerves. Involvement in the superior orbital fissure may impair sympathetic nerve fibers, so that pupillary dilation is not conspicuous.

The peripheral oculomotor nerve is likely to be involved in aneurysms of the circle of Willis, tumors of the base of the brain, meningeal carcinomatosis, and chronic meningitis caused by zoster, syphilis, or tuberculosis. The nerve is usually spared in purulent meningitis, which is more likely to involve the sixth cranial nerve.

All motor nerves to the eye are involved in cavernous sinus thrombosis, and the motor involvement is likely to precede pupillary involvement. The syndrome of the superior orbital fissure involves all the motor and sensory nerves of the eye, including the sympathetic nerves. It may be produced by suppuration in the sphenoidal sinus, skull fracture, hemorrhage, or tumor.

Aberrant regeneration of the nerve fibers after paralysis of the third cranial nerve may cause a pseudo–von Graefe phenomenon in which the fibers originally distributed to the inferior rectus muscle innervate the levator palpebrae superioris muscle. When an attempt is made to look downward, the inferior rectus muscle is ineffective, but the upper eyelid elevates. Aberrant regeneration of the branch intended for the medial rectus muscle into the innervation of the sphincter pupillae muscle causes constriciton of the pupil when an attempt is made to adduct the eye. If nerve fibers destined for the superior rectus muscle abnormally regenerate into the levator palpebrae superioris muscle, attempts to elevate the eye are associated with excessive elevation of the eyelid. With closure of the eyelids, for example, in sleep, an abnormal Bell phenomenon occurs in which the upper eyelid elevates rather than closes.

Trochlear nerve. Disorders of the trochlear nerve (N IV) affect the superior oblique muscle, which rotates the eye downward when it is adducted. Diplopia is particularly marked in reading. The affected eye is higher than the sound eye; the head is tilted to the sound side, the face is rotated to the sound side, and the chin is depressed. The head in this position is moved to the field of action of the muscle so as to minimize double vision. When the head is tilted to the affected side, the affected eye moves higher. (The superior rectus muscle and the superior oblique muscle are intorters of the eye and rotate the 12 o'clock meridian of the cornea inward.) When the head is tilted to the affected side, each muscle is stimulated equally to intort the eye. Since the superior oblique muscle is paralyzed, the unaffected superior rectus muscle elevates the affected eye.

After superior oblique muscle paralysis, there may be early secondary contracture of the inferior oblique muscle. This results in a hypertropia in upward gaze that is larger than that in downward gaze.

Abducent nerve. Disorders of the abducent nerve (N VI) to the lateral rectus muscle cause inability to turn the eye laterally beyond the midline. The unopposed action of the medial rectus muscle causes esotropia. When attempts are made to abduct the eye, the palpebral fissure may widen. The long intracranial course of the nerve and its angulation over the sphenoidal bone make it vulnerable in skull fractures, increased intracranial pressure, and purulent meningitis.

Gradenigo syndrome is caused by an osteitis of the petrous tip of the pyramidal bone and follows mastoid and middle ear infections on the homolateral side. It is associated with sixth cranial nerve paralysis, pain on the same side of the face from fifth cranial nerve involvement, and deafness. Acoustic neuromas (neurofibromatosis) are associated with deafness, sixth cranial nerve paralysis, facial paralysis caused by seventh cranial nerve involvement, and papilledema.

Gaze palsy. Supranuclear lesions in the frontal lobe result in inability to direct the eyes to the contralateral side. The eyes rotate toward the side of the lesion. In bilateral lesions of the frontal lobe the patient is unable to turn the eyes in any direction but is able to maintain fixation and following movements. (Thus in testing for abnormalities in conjugate ocular movements [gaze] the examiner should observe the voluntary movements of the eyes and not have the patient follow the movements of a test object).

Internuclear ophthalmoplegia. When the paramedian pontine reticular system commands the eyes to turn to the right or left, the ipsilateral abducent nucleus is stimulated and the stimulus ascends via the medial longitudinal fasciculus to the contralateral medial rectus muscle subnucleus of the oculomotor nucleus (Fig. 26-1). Disruption of the medial longitudinal fasciculus disconnects the oculomotor subnucleus that innervates the medial rectus muscle from the abducent nucleus. Then on horizontal gaze to the right or left, the abducting eye (ipsilateral lateral rectus muscle) rotates

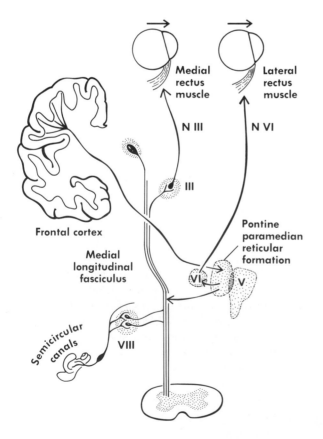

Fig. 26-1. The medial longitudinal fasciculus connects the pontine paramedian reticular formation with the subnucleus of the contralateral oculomotor nerve (III) that serves the medial rectus muscle. On conjugate horizontal gaze to the right, impulses originate in the left frontal optomotor cortex. They decussate in the region of the internal capsule to synapse in the pontine paramedian reticular formation. Impulses pass to the abducent nucleus on the same side and to the medial longitudinal fasciculus on the opposite side. This impulse passes to the portion of the oculomotor nucleus serving the left medial rectus muscle. In internuclear ophthalmoplegia a lesion in the medial longitudinal fasciculus impairs transmission from the pontine paramedian reticular formation to the contralateral medial rectus muscle.

laterally but may demonstrate a coarse jerk nystagmus. The adducting eye (contralateral medial rectus muscle) remains in the primary position since the signal through the medial longitudinal fasciculus does not reach its nucleus. Convergence, which is not mediated by impulses through the medial longitudinal fasciculus, may or may not be affected. In early internuclear ophthalmoplegia, adduction may be slowed and there is an exodeviation in lateral gaze to the side of the lesions and orthophoria in primary gaze.

Bilateral internuclear ophthalmoplegia in young adults is most commonly caused by multiple sclerosis. In older individuals occlusive vascular disease is most common. It also occurs with brain-stem tumors, syphilis, encephalitis, and trauma and may be simulated by myasthenia gravis. Unilateral internuclear ophthalmoplegia is the result of an infarct of a small branch of the basilar artery. Internuclear ophthalmoplegia involves conjugate horizontal gaze only.

Tumors in the midbrain or the pineal body produce Parinaud syndrome, in which there is supranuclear conjugate palsy of vertical gaze (inability to elevate or to depress the eyes on command). Often the pupils are dilated and do not constrict to light; papilledema is usual.

A lesion in the pontine center for lateral gaze that is located near the abducent nucleus causes inability to direct the eyes to the side of the lesion with the eyes rotating to the opposite side.

Oculomotor apraxia is a gaze abnormality in which the eyes rotate in a direction opposite to which the head turns. After the head turn stops, the eyes rotate to the object of fixation. It may occur in ataxia-telangiectasia, Gaucher disease, or as an isolated defect.

OPTIC NERVE

Atrophy of the optic nerve may be complete or partial and may be caused by diseases within the eye that affect ganglion cells or their axons in the retinal nerve fiber layer or diseases outside the eye that affect axons in their course to the lateral geniculate body. These lesions are localized as prechiasmatic, chiasmatic, and those of the optic tract. Prechiasmatic lesions affect one eye only unless two lesions affect the two optic nerves.

Optic atrophy, hemianopsia, and reduced visual acuity suggest a lesion of the optic tracts or chiasm. Optic nerve atrophy preceded by papilledema or inflammation is called secondary; if without prior papilledema, it is called primary.

Inflammation of the optic nerve (termed retrobulbar neuritis when involving the optic nerve posterior to the eye or papillitis when involving the intraocular portion of the optic nerve) is nearly always monocular and reduces visual acuity. In the retrobulbar variety there are no ophthalmoscopic signs of the disorder, but the pupil does not constrict to light.

Papilledema is usually bilateral, does not impair vision early in its course, is never present when the lamina cribrosa is clearly visible, and is associated with absence of spontaneous or induced retinal vein pulsation.

Increased intracranial pressure

The symptoms of increased intracranial pressure are severe bioccipital and bifrontal headaches that awaken the patient from sleep or are present at awakening. The headache is deep, steady, and dull and is aggravated by coughing, sneezing, or defecating, all of which increase intracranial pressure. Typically, the headache is relieved by vomiting, which occurs without nausea and may or may not be projectile. Signs include sphincter incontinence, mental torpor, and unsteady gait. Late vagus nerve effects are slowed pulse, lowered pulse pressure, and increased respiratory rate. There is a clouding of consciousness that varies from a delirium to a psychosis, or somnolence to deep coma.

The main ocular sign of increased intracranial pressure is bilateral papilledema. In the absence of ocular or orbital disease, the most likely cause is a space-occupying lesion. Many brain tumors do not cause increased intracranial pressure or are diagnosed before it develops. Other ocular signs of increased intracranial pressure occur relatively late. Extraocular muscle paresis, particularly unilateral lateral rectus muscle paralysis, occurs late and is not of localizing value. Initially pupillary constriction to light and convergence is normal, but later it is lost.

The oculomotor nerve may be compressed at the tentorial notch in herniation of the temporal lobe, which causes unilateral mydriasis and loss of the direct and consensual light pupillary reflex. Later paresis of the levator palpebrae superioris muscle causes blepharoptosis followed by paresis of other muscles innervated by the oculomotor nerve.

VISUAL PATHWAY

The visual field is the loci of objects or points in space that can be perceived when the head and eyes are kept fixed. Prechiasmal lesions affect vision in one eye only. A lesion immediately anterior to the chiasm may cause a severe visual field defect in the ipsilateral eye and a minor temporal field defect in the fellow eye because the inferior nasal fibers of the fellow retina bend into the opposite nerve. A lesion of the chiasm involves decussating nasal fibers and causes loss of vision in the temporal portion of each field, a bitemporal field defect, or, if complete, a bitemporal hemianopsia. A chiasmal lesion that is predominantly lateral may cause a hemianopic defect in the temporal field of only one eye.

Lesions posterior to the chiasm involve nerve fibers that originate from the temporal retina on the ipsilateral side and from the nasal retina on the contralateral side. The visual field defect is bilateral, a homonymous defect. If complete, it is hemianopsia (half blindness: visual fields are always described in terms of the blind portion of the field). Disturbances of the nasal retina cause temporal visual field defects; disturbances of the temporal retina cause nasal visual field defects (see Chapter 5). Partial defects that do not involve the entire half of the visual field may be congruous or incongruous. Congruous defects are the same in size, shape, and intensity in the visual field of each eye. They occur in lesions in the geniculocalcarine tract that extends from the lateral geniculate body to the visual cortex. Generally, lesions of the parietal or occipital lobes cause congruous defects. Incongruous visual field defects are bilateral but different in each eye. They occur in lesions in the optic tract, lateral geniculate body, and temporal lobe.

INTRACRANIAL MASS LESIONS

Primary and metastatic tumors of the brain, intracranial aneurysms, hematomas, granulomatous inflammations, and parasitic cysts may cause increased intracranial pressure and headache and may induce localizing neurologic defects. Primary brain tumors may be divided into gliomas, meningiomas, vascular tumors such as angiomas and hemangioblastomas, pituitary tumors, congenital tumors such as craniopharyngioma, teratomas, and adnexal tumors that originate in the pineal body and choroid plexus. Metastatic tumors constitute 10% to 25% of all brain tumors and may originate from almost any primary tumor, most commonly the lung in men and the breast or lung in women.

Gliomas composed of malignant glial cells are the most common primary brain tumor. Glioblastoma is the most rapidly growing and causes brain necrosis and edema. Astrocytomas are slower growing and are often associated with cysts. Oligodendrogliomas are clinically similar to astrocytomas. Medulloblastomas are highly malignant tumors of the cerebellum and mainly tumors of childhood. An ependymoma develops from ependymal cells in the walls of ventricles.

A meningioma is a slow-growing connective tissue tumor of the dura mater. Sphenoidal ridge meningiomas may include structures at the apex of the orbit or they may invade the orbit. Meningioma of the intraorbital portion of the optic nerve sheath causes proptosis and shunt vessels on the optic disk.

Angiomas are slow-growing congenital vascular malformations. Hemangioblastomas are slow-growing vascular neoplasms most commonly found in the cerebellum. They may be associated with angiomatosis of the retina and cysts of the kidney and pancreas (von Hippel-Landau syndrome).

Intracranial granulomatous inflammations include tuberculosis, toruloma, sarcoidosis, usually of the meninges, and syphilitic gumma.

Cystcercosis caused by the larva of *Taenia salium* or *Taenia sagnita* may cause single or multiple cerebral masses.

Focal symptoms. The brain differentiates from the hollow dorsal neural tube that forms three vesicles (Table 26-1). The structures derived from the forebrain (prosencephalon) are located above the tentorium (supratenorial), while those derived from the hindbrain (rhombencephalon) are located below the tentorium

Table 26-1. Embryonic origin of some brain parts

Supratentorial
  Prosencephalon (third ventricle and lateral ventricles)
    Cerebrum (frontal, parietal, temporal, and occipital lobes)
    Optic vesicles, optic nerves and tracts
    Olfactory bulbs
    Diencephalon
    Pineal gland
    Pituitary gland
    Thalamus
    Hypothalamus
Intermediate between supratentorial and infratentorial
  Mesencephalon (cerebral aqueduct)
    Cerebral peduncles
    Nuclei nerves III, IV, anterior V
    Corpora quadrigemina
      Superior, inferior colliculi, nerve VIII (cochlear)
Infratentorial
  Rhombencephalon (fourth ventricle)
    Cerebellum
      Vermis
    Pons (part of medulla)
      Nerve V, medial longitudinal fasciculus, nerves VI, VII
    Medulla oblongata
      Nerves VIII (vestibular), IX, X, XI, XII

Table 26-2. Pituitary adenomas*

Hematoxylin-eosin staining
  Eosinophilic (acromegaly: growth hormone)
  Basophilic (Cushing syndrome, adrenocorticotropic hormone, expansion of pituitary adenoma after adrenalectomy [Nelson syndrome])
  Chromophobic (with increased prolactin synthesis, amenorrhea, or impotence but no galactorrhea; with preceding plus galactorrhea [Forbes-Albright syndrome])
  Miscellaneous (multiple hormone production: acromegaly, growth hormone, prolactin, and adrenocorticotropic hormone; thyroid-stimulating hormone: hyperthyroidism or hypothyroidism)

*Histologic and functional characteristics are not this well correlated.

(infratenorial). Structures derived from the midbrain (mesencephalon) may be in a supratentorial or infratentorial location.

Supratentorial tumors. Structures derived from the forebrain include the cerebral hemispheres (frontal, temporal, parietal, and occipital lobes), the chiasm, the pituitary gland, the anterior and middle fossa, and the diencephalon. Visual field defects are common, as are optic atrophy and papilledema. Disturbance of ocular movements is less common than with infratentorial lesions.

Chiasmal syndrome. Computed tomography and radioimmunoassay of pituitary and other endocrine hormones make the progression of lesions that cause the chiasmal syndrome less likely than before. The syndrome consists of optic atrophy combined with bitemporal visual field defects. It is caused by impairment of nerve conduction in the axons that decussate in the chiasm from the nasal one half of each retina. Often the optic nerve atrophy and visual field defect are more advanced in one eye than in the other. The common causes of the chias-

mal syndrome are pituitary adenomas, craniopharyngiomas, and meningioma of the tuberculum sallae. Rarely sarcoidosis, metastatic carcinoma, and Hand-Schüller-Christian disease are causes.

Pituitary adenomas. Pituitary adenomas are mainly hormone-secreting (95%) (Table 26-2). A small portion that occur almost exclusively in men (90%) are nonsecreting. The most common (64%) hormone-secreting adenoma is prolactin secreting, which occurs frequently (85%) in women. Growth hormone and mixed tumors occur about evenly in men and women, whereas adenocorticotropic (ACTH) secreting adenomas occur more often in women (76%).

Prolactin tumors cause amenorrhea and galactorrhea in women and impotence and gynecomastia in men. Growth hormone, mixed tumors, and ACTH tumors cause acromegalic facial features. Bitemporal hemianopsia, an important diagnostic feature in earlier series, is uncommon with the advent of radioimmunoassay measurements of hormones and prompt diagnosis.

Visual field defects occur, chiefly in men, late in the course of pituitary adenomas. The field defect initially affects the superior temporal field and then extends to the inferior temporal quadrant (Fig. 26-2). The defect may be asymmetric, with one eye being blind and temporal field loss in the fellow eye. Optic atrophy lags behind the visual field defect.

Craniopharyngiomas. Craniopharyngiomas originate from secretory vestiges of the Rathke

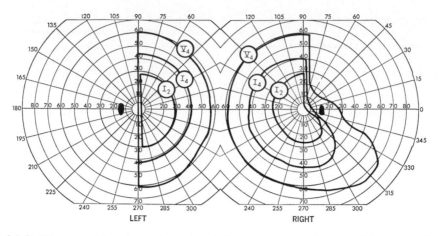

Fig. 26-2. Bitemporal hemianopsia produced by compressive disease of the optic chiasm. The visual field defect is seldom symmetrical in the two eyes and here has affected the decussating axons originating in the nasal retina of the left eye far more severely than the nasal axons originating from the right eye. (From Burde, R.M., Savino, P.J., and Trobe, J.D.: Clinical decisions in neuro-ophthalmology, St. Louis, 1985, The C.V. Mosby Co.)

pouch and are usually suprasellar in position. They are the most common cause of hypopituitarism before puberty and the most common type of tumor involving the pituitary gland in children. They occur most frequently in younger children but occasionally are not apparent until adulthood.

In children, progressive visual loss may not be noted until internal hydrocephalus with papilledema and behavioral changes occur. Obesity, delayed sexual maturation, somnolence, and diabetes insipidus occur. In adolescents, decreased anterior pituitary secretion may cause dystrophia adiposogenitalis (Fröhlich syndrome), cachexia (Simmonds disease), or dwarfism (Lorain disease). In adults, a fluctuating bitemporal hemianopsia that involves the two eyes unequally occurs. An associated hypopituitarism causes impotence or amenorrhea with loss of libido; obesity; fine, silky skin with loss of body hair; and decreased beard growth in males.

Visual field impairment is typically asymmetric with a tendency to initial involvement of the temporal field. Defects tend to be far advanced in one eye before involvement of the fellow eye. Because of the cystic nature of the tumor, the visual fields may fluctuate even without treatment. The viscous, cholesterol-rich suprasellar cysts often calcify, which provides a helpful diagnostic sign on roentgenography.

Frontal lobe tumors. The frontal lobe of the brain is concerned mainly with control of body movements. The cardinal sign of frontal lobe lesions is hemiplegia. Voluntary movements of the eye are initiated in the frontal lobe. Lesions affect conjugate ocular movements (gaze). Changes in psyche caused by lesions include apathy, euphoria, amnesia, and confabulation. Unilateral inability to release voluntarily an object placed in the hand (forced grasping) is of localizing importance. Papilledema is the most common ocular sign.

The Foster Kennedy syndrome consists of optic atrophy on the side of the tumor compression combined with papilledema on the opposite side and anosmia. It occurs rarely with frontal lobe tumors but occurs commonly in tumors of the olfactory groove. It has been described in association with sphenoidal ridge meningiomas, in intracranial aneurysms, and inflammations.

Temporal lobe tumors. Lesions of the temporal lobe induce vertigo, confusion, loss of memory, and often trance-like states. Lesions of the dominant lobe impair motor and sensory functions concerned with speech. Lesions in the area between the frontal, parietal, and temporal lobes (Broca) cause inability to express appropriate words (motor aphasia); posterior lesions cause inability to understand the spoken word. Irritative lesions cause unpleasant odors and tastes (uncinate fits). Visual field defects are usually incongruous and begin in the superior quadrants of the visual field on the side opposite the lesion. Temporal lobe tumors often cause oculomotor nerve palsy.

Parietal lobe tumors. Lesions of the parietal lobe cause astereognosia (faulty recognition of shape and form of objects placed in the hand) and loss of position sense and two-point discrimination on the side of the body opposite the lesion. Lesions in the angular gyrus on the dominant side cause loss of visual recognition of words (alexia) and inability to write (agraphia). Visual field defects are homonymous and the same in extent and intensity (congruous) in each eye. Field defects begin in the inferior quadrants of the visual field on the side opposite the lesion. In parietal lesions, the opticokinetic nystagmus to moving objects is abolished with movement toward the side of the defective field of vision and is normal with movement away from the affected field. In forcible closure of the eyes, patients with parietal lobe lesions may show a deviation of the eyes to the side opposite the lesion.

Lesions of the nondominant parietotemporal lobes cause topographic agnosia in which an individual loses recognition of that which had been familiar so that one may become lost in the community or confused about the position of buttons on one's clothes. There is impairment of ability to construct a diagram, such as the face of a clock (constructional apraxia). There is difficulty in dressing and sometimes failure to recognize faces (prosopagnosia). There may be neglect of the nondominant side so that a right-handed individual leaves the left side of drawings incomplete or neglects food on the left side of the plate.

Occipital lobe tumors. Lesions of the occipital lobe induce a congruous homonymous hemianopsia. If the posterior tip of the occipital lobe is involved, the point of fixation is affected. Flashes of many lights may occur. Bilateral lesions of the occipital lobe cause blindness that may be accompanied by denial of blindness (Anton syndrome). Impairment of the association area may cause inability to recognize people and objects (visual agnosia) or to recognize the relation of objects in space (topographic agnosia).

Infratentorial tumors. Structures derived from the hindbrain include the cerebellum, pons, and medulla oblongata. Ocular lesions involve motor nerves to the eye with supranuclear and infranuclear paralysis and various ocular oscillations.

Cerebellar tumors. Cerebellar tumors cause ataxia, asynergy, dysmetria, and weakness. Ataxia and asynergy are demonstrated by the knee-to-heel test and in testing for diadochokinesis. Dysmetria is demonstrated in the finger-to-finger test. Weakness occurs on the same side. There is a distinct tendency to fall toward the side of the lesion. Acute cerebellar lesions disturb posture, and the patient may be unable to stand or sit up. There is a loss of skeletal muscle tone and coordination.

The earliest ocular sign is jerk nystagmus, which is usually horizontal and accentuated on lateral gaze. Lesions in the vermis cause vertical nystagmus that is accentuated on upward gaze. Papilledema occurs early and may be the initial sign of disease. Other ocular signs are secondary to increased intracranial pressure.

Cerebellopontine angle tumors. Cerebellopontine angle tumors are mainly acoustic neuromas causing cerebellar signs, with lesions of the fifth, sixth, seventh, and eighth cranial nerves. Impairment of hearing occurs initially, followed by cerebellar signs with nystagmus and then cranial nerve involvment. Facial nerve impairment causes a facial tic followed by blepharospasm. Corneal anesthesia indicates trigeminal nerve involvement. Increased intracranial pressure occurs late.

Tumors of the pons and medulla. Tumors of the pons and the medulla are likely to cause disturbance of the abducent nucleus or disturbance of horizontal conjugate gaze. Horizontal jerk nystagmus occurs occasionally, combined with vertical nystagmus. It is usually absent when the eyes are in the primary position and becomes more marked as the eyes are turned toward the side of the lesion. Palsies of the third cranial nerve are uncommon. Corneal anesthesia from trigeminal nerve involvement is common. Increased intracranial pressure does not occur.

Herniation of the hippocampus through the tentorium causes brain-stem compression. The most common signs are decreasing levels of consciousness, dysarthria, and respiratory distress. Mydriasis is the most important ocular sign and, when caused by subdural hematoma, is usually (but not always) on the side of the lesion. Other ocular signs are oculomotor palsy, internuclear ophthalmoplegia, and nystagmus. Blindness occurs if the posterior cerebral arteries are compressed.

Lesions of the midbrain. Lesions in this area may cause predominantly supratentorial or infratenorial symptoms and signs. Compression of the aqueduct of Sylvius may occur initially and cause an internal hydrocephalus and papilledema. Impairment of the supranuclear center for gaze, as in Parinaud syndrome, causes paralysis of conjugate upward movement and mydriasis. Lateral extension to the lateral geniculate body causes an incongruous homonymous hemianopsia. The nuclei of the oculomotor, trochlear, and portions of the trigeminal nerve and medial longitudinal fasciculus are located deep in the midbrain.

CEREBROVASCULAR DISEASE

Sudden intracranial neural death may result from ischemia or hemorrhage. Ischemia is caused by local or general abnormalities that interfere with the supply of blood to the brain. Emboli from the heart are the major local causes. The major general cause is atheromatous occlusion of the internal carotid artery or its branches (Table 26-3). Intracranial hemorrhage, apoplexy, or stroke are caused either by hypertensive cardiovascular disease or rupture of berry aneurysms, acquired fusiform aneurysms, or arteriovenous malformations. The hemorrhage may be limited to the cerebrospinal fluid-filled space between the arachnoid and pia membranes (subarachnoid hemorrhage) or may occur within the brain (intracerebral hemorrhage). Subarachnoid hemorrhage may extend into the substance of the brain and intracerebral hemorrhage may extend into the subarachnoid space, into the ventricles, or both. Only heart disease and cancer cause more deaths in the United States. Stroke is the most common disorder affecting the central nervous system.

The brain is supplied by two internal carotid arteries and two vertebral arteries (Fig. 26-3). The internal carotid artery enters the skull through the foramen lacerum, passes through the cavernous sinus, branches into the ophthal-

Table 26-3. Cerebral vascular disease

I. Occlusive vascular disorders
   A. Thrombotic
      1. Intracranial
      2. Carotid (transient ischemic attacks)
II. Cerebral aneurysms
   A. Infraclinoid
      1. Carotid artery within cavernous sinus
         a. Carotid-cavernous sinus fistula
   B. Supraclinoid
      1. Carotid artery
      2. Middle cerebral artery
      3. Anterior cerebral artery
      4. Basilar artery
III. Subarachnoid hemorrhage
   A. Vascular hypertension
   B. Ruptured supraclinoid aneurysm
   C. Angiomas and arteriovenous malformations
IV. Arteritis
   A. Infectious disease (e.g., syphilis, tuberculosis)
   B. Idopathic
      1. Giant cell arteritis
      2. Wegener arteritis

mic, anterior choroidal, and posterior communicating arteries, and then bifurcates into the anterior and middle cerebral arteries.

The vertebral arteries enter the skull through the foramen magnum, and medial branches immediately join to form the anterior spinal artery; just distal to this, the posterior cerebellar artery branches off. The vertebral arteries supply the medulla oblongata and pons, and then unite to form the basilar artery.

Carotid artery. The internal carotid arterial system or its branches supply the frontal and parietal lobes, part of the temporal lobe, the corpus striatum and the internal capsule. Occlusive disease is associated with contralateral impairment of motor or sensory function of the hand, arm, leg, or lower portion of the face. Ischemia of structures nurtured by the left middle cerebral artery may cause aphasia in right-handed persons. Unconsciousness simulating syncope occurs when an anterior cerebral artery is compromised.

The effects of occlusion of the internal carotid artery proximal to the circle of Willis depend on the adequacy of the collateral circulation. In about 25% of cases of symptomatic stroke, intermittent transient loss of vision occurs in one eye (amaurosis fugax) as a warning symptom. Amaurosis fugax, a type of transient ischemic attack, consists of sudden constriction

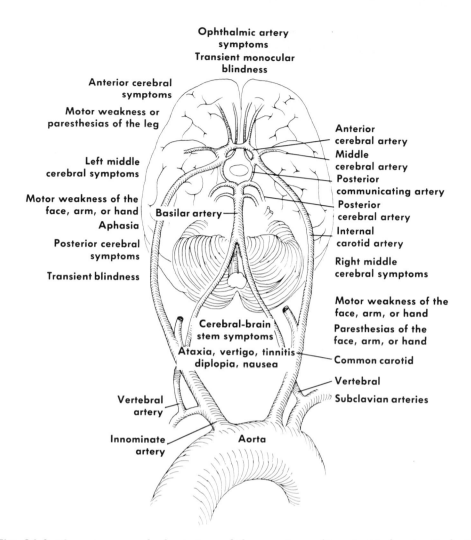

Ophthalmic artery
symptoms
Transient monocular
blindness

Anterior cerebral
symptoms
Motor weakness or
paresthesias of the leg

Left middle
cerebral symptoms

Motor weakness of the
face, arm, or hand
Aphasia

Posterior cerebral
symptoms

Transient blindness

Basilar artery

Anterior
cerebral artery
Middle
cerebral artery
Posterior
communicating artery
Posterior
cerebral artery
Internal
carotid artery

Right middle
cerebral symptoms

Motor weakness of the
face, arm, or hand
Paresthesias of the
face, arm, or hand

Cerebral-brain
stem symptoms
Ataxia, vertigo, tinnitis
diplopia, nausea

Common carotid

Vertebral

Subclavian arteries

Vertebral
artery

Innominate
artery

Aorta

Fig. 26-3. The primary cerebral arteries and the symptoms of transient ischemic attacks in different regions of the brain. Probably less than 20% of individuals have the anatomic configuration illustrated, although it is the most common.

of the visual field of one eye, varying from hemianopsia to loss of light perception. The pupillary light reflex is absent. The retinal arteries are markedly attenuated during an attack. Vision gradually returns within a few minutes. Permanent visual loss does not occur. Amaurosis fugax may also occur in migraine, impending central artery closure, and giant cell arteritis.

Repeated attacks of amaurosis fugax may give an opthalmoscopic picture of cotton-wool patches in one eye, caused by small infarcts secondary to vascular insufficiency. In patients with hypertension, the occluded carotid artery may protect the retinal vasculature from the signs of arteriolar sclerosis or even hemorrhages and papilledema.

Rarely a venous stasis retinopathy develops on the same side as carotid artery insufficiency. Ophthalmoscopically, there are attentuated arteries and veins or, alternatively, dilated and tortuous retinal veins. There may be microaneurysms and flame and blot hemorrhages. New blood vessels may develop on the surface of the optic disk. The intraocular pressure may be high. If the diseased eye is examined without reference to the nearly normal fellow eye, the abnormality might be mistaken for the retinopathy of diabetes, impending central vein occlusion, or pulseless disease.

In both carotid artery and vertebral-basilar system atherosclerosis, there may be showers of emboli from an ulcerating atherosclerotic plaque. Cholesterol emboli appear as bright, yellow-orange plaques near the bifurcation of a retinal arteriole (see Fig. 27-1). With massage on the globe they tumble to the periphery and disappear. Platelet emboli appear as small white bodies. As they course through the arteries, they may cause the sensation of flashing or shimmering vision.

Pulsation in the affected internal carotid artery may be diminished or absent. Palpation through the oropharynx is more reliable than through the neck. Even with complete occlusion of the internal carotid artery, the common and the external carotid artery may be normal to palpation.

Palpation and auscultation over the bifurcation of the carotid artery in the neck may show a thrill and a murmur. A murmur heard with the bell of the ophthalmoscope over the fellow eye indicates augmented blood flow through the patent artery. The bruit of occlusive disease of the vertebral arteries is best heard over the supraclavicular area and is sometimes accentuated by turning the patient's head to the opposite side.

Measurement of the pressure in the ophthalmic arteries with the ophthalmodynamometer has its greatest application in carotid artery insufficiency. The measurement is made by increasing the intraocular pressure until the central retinal artery is seen to pulsate on the optic disk. Most patients with carotid artery occlusive disease that reduces the lumen 90% or more have a 15% to 25% reduction in the systolic pressure of the ophthalmic artery on the side of the occlusive disease. In about one fourth of the patients with proved disease, the pressure is the same or higher on the involved side.

Several noninvasive tests are useful: (1) ultrasound scanning of the carotid arteries using B-mode ultrasound imaging, combined with pulse Doppler analysis of blood flow at each part in the image; and (2) oculoplethysmography to estimate more accurately the pressure within the internal carotid artery than is possible with ophthalmodynamometry.

Compression of the carotid artery may produce syncope suggestive of an insufficiency of the vascular supply of the contralateral anterior cerebral artery. Compression is not recommended and can produce permanent, complete occlusion. In vertebral-basilar artery insufficiency, there may be syncope or convulsive movements.

Cerebral angiography shows the site and extent of the occlusion but carries the risk of permanent complications. It is reserved preferably for distinguishing between carotid occlusive disease, cerebral infarction, and tumor in patients who have symptoms of recent onset, do not have brain infarcts, and are good candidates for surgery if necessary.

Vertebral-basilar system. The vertebral-basilar arterial system supplies the brain stem, cerebellum, occipital lobe, and a portion of the temporal lobe. The vertebral system originates from the two vertebral arteries, which are the first branches of the subclavian arteries. The vertebral arteries traverse the neck in the vertebral canals of the cervical vertebrae and unite within the cranium to form the basilar artery. The basilar artery supplies branches to the brain stem and the cerebellum, and the posterior cerebral artery supplies branches to the occipital lobe. The posterior communicating arteries connect the vertebral-basilar system with the carotid circulation.

Involvement of the cochlear-vestibular system causes vertigo, nausea, and a staggering gait. Auditory system symptoms include partial deafness and unilateral tinnitus. There may be paresthesia, hemiplegia, or hemiparesis. Headache, dysarthria, dysphagia, and hiccoughing occur.

Many patients note ocular symptoms for many months before complete occlusion. There may be blurred vision, diplopia, transient homonymous hemianopsia, and scintillating scotomas. Visual blurring is usually bilateral, and the individual is occasionally momentarily blind.

Complete thrombosis causes a congruous homonymous hemianopsia and motor involvement of the eyes. There may be paresis of conjugate gaze, with a conjugate deviation to one side. Intranuclear ophthalmoplegia may be identical with that seen in multiple sclerosis. Horizontal or rotatory nystagmus is frequent. Horner syndrome is occasionally present.

Recognition of the transient symptoms of

cerebral ischemia, a transient ischemic attack, is important in preventing the development of a cerebral vascular accident. Differential diagnosis includes migraine, epilepsy, carotid sinus syncope, and Ménière syndrome. Diagnostic steps should include auscultation of the neck for bruit, ophthalmoscopy for emboli, comparison of the radial pulses and brachial blood pressure in the two arms, computed tomography, and other noninvasive tests.

Possible causes, such as giant cell arteritis, vascular hypertension, neurosyphilis, systemic lupus erythematosus, polyarteritis nodosa, pulseless disease, and thrombocytopenia from leukemia must be excluded. A sudden decrease in blood pressure or alteration in the heart rhythm or rate may be the cause.

Surgery to correct ischemic attacks is limited to the extracranial portion of the carotid artery system. It may be indicated for patients who have symptoms of recent onset but who do not have brain infarction or widespread atherosclerotic disease. In other patients, anticoagulation may be used. Aspirin, which decreases platelet adhesiveness, is currently popular. Control of vascular hypertension and investigation of its cause are desirable.

Aortic arch syndrome. The aortic arch syndrome is a chronic disorder resulting from obstruction of the subclavian and the carotid arteries. It includes pulseless disease, reversed coarctation of the aorta, and the subclavian steal syndrome. Symptoms are caused by insufficiency of the cerebral blood supply and are similar to those described in carotid and vertebral-basilar insufficiency.

Pulseless disease is a giant cell arteritis of the aorta of unknown origin that occurs mainly in young Japanese women. It causes retinal neovascularization, venous engorgement, microaneurysms, and arterial and venous occlusions. The radial pulse is absent. There may be widespread ischemia of the head and the upper extremities.

Reversed coarctation of the aorta occurs in aortic arch occlusion and is a disorder of collateral circulation in which blood reaches the head, neck, and upper extremities through the intercostal, scapular, axillary, posterior and inferior thyroid, inferior epigastric, and internal mammary arteries.

The subclavian steal syndrome results from stenosis or occlusion of the first portion of the subclavian artery. Blood flows up the contralateral vertebral artery and down the opposite vertebral artery to supply the subclavian artery distal to the occlusion. Cerebral ischemia in the area of distribution of the vertebral-basilar system causes symptoms. A bruit in the subclavicular area and reduction of pulse and blood pressure in the ipsilateral arm suggest the diagnosis.

Brachial-basilar insufficiency occurs in patients with occlusive disease of the proximal segment of the subclavian artery who develop transient ischemic vertebral-basilar symptoms when the arm is exercised. The symptoms result, as in the subclavian steal syndrome, from retrograde blood flow through the ipsilateral vertebral artery.

Arterial aneurysms. Berry aneurysms form most commonly at the anterior portion of the circle of Willis because of a congenital weakness in the wall of the artery. Although the weakness is congenital, the aneurysms do not occur until arterial hypertension accentuates the vessel defect. They are most common at the junction of the internal carotid artery with the posterior communicating artery or middle cerebral artery or with the anterior communicating artery or anterior cerebral artery. Fusiform aneurysms are caused by atherosclerosis that weakens and dilates the basilar artery or the internal carotid artery in the cavernous sinus (infraclinoid).

Symptoms occur suddenly, with severe unilateral headache and pain about the face and eye. Pain in the medial canthal region is common. The pain is caused by meningeal irritation and not by direct involvement of the trigeminal nerve as occurs in infraclinoid aneurysms. Simultaneously with the headache, or within 72 hours, an oculomotor paralysis develops, with blepharoptosis, exotropia, pupillary dilation, and failure of accommodation.

The prognosis for life is poorer with supraclinoid aneurysms than with infraclinoid aneurysms. Death occurs from subarachnoid hemorrhage or from bleeding into the brain. Untreated patients may experience no further episodes, presumably because of intravascular clotting, or may have recurrent attacks. Recovery with regeneration of the oculomotor nerve is seldom complete. A pseudo–von Graefe phenomenon is frequently present, and pupillary abnormalities are observed. There may be loss of pupillary constriction, causing dilation of the pupil with light and constriction with convergence. The pupil may be widely dilated with no reaction to light or convergence.

Aneurysms of the middle and anterior cerebral arteries. Aneurysms of the middle and anterior cerebral arteries are particularly likely to cause defects in the visual fields. Optic atrophy is usually present. The visual field changes are bilateral and tend to be variable. An anterior cerebral artery aneurysm may cause a bitemporal hemianopsia that begins in the inferior temporal quadrant rather than in the superior temporal quadrant, as in early pituitary gland adenoma. With aneurysm of the middle cerebral artery, there may be loss of vision in one eye and a hemianopsia in the fellow eye. Subarachnoid hemorrhage is common.

Basilar artery aneurysms. Congenital berry aneurysms may rarely occur at the anterior end of the basilar artery where it divides into the posterior cerebral arteries or at the posterior end where the vertebral arteries join to form the basilar arteries. The basilar artery is also the most common artery in the body to be affected with atherosclerosis.

The symptoms of basilar-vertebral aneurysms are variable and not characteristic. Dizziness, diplopia, and blurring of vision are the most common symptoms. There may be involvement of motor nerves on the brain stem, occipital headache, deafness, memory impairment, and coma. Diagnosis is often not made until autopsy.

Infraclinoid aneurysms. Dilation of the internal carotid artery within the cavernous sinus occurs most commonly in women during or after the fifth decade of life. The artery gives off no major branches in this location, and atheromatous plaque formation is common. The cavernous sinus contains the motor nerves to the eye and the ophthalmic and maxillary divisions of the trigeminal nerve. An expanding aneurysm thus causes an ophthalmoplegia of all motor nerves and pain and paresthesia in the face. In infraclinoid aneurysms, unlike supraclinoid aneurysms, corneal and facial sensitivity is reduced.

The most conspicuous sign is an insidious, slowly progressive ophthalmoplegia, in which all muscles of the eye are involved. The pupil does not constrict to light but may not be dilated because of interruption of sympathetic nerve fibers on the surface of the artery. Pain is a relatively minor symptom. There is pain or paresthesia of the face, of the side of the head, about the eye, or along the nose on the same side. Corneal anesthesia usually occurs and is usually associated with anesthesia of the face.

The gradual onset is suggestive of tumor, and arteriography is often necessary for exact diagnosis. Large infraclinoid aneurysms are probably reinforced by the walls of the cavernous sinus and do not rupture. Although it is likely that most spontaneous arteriovenous fistulas represent rupture of an aneurysm, usually they are so small before rupture that they do not cause signs of an aneurysm.

If untreated, infraclinoid aneurysms follow one of two patterns. Complete thrombosis of the aneurysm may occur, with resultant spontaneous cure, leaving a residual loss of ocular motility. The artery may expand anteriorly within the cavernous sinus, causing erosion of the optic foramen and the superior orbital fissure, with compression and atrophy of the optic nerve and a proptosis. The development of proptosis is frequently concealed by blepharoptosis. Venous drainage of the orbit is not involved, and there is no chemosis or congestion of bulbar vessels. Posterior expansion may involve the petrous portion of the temporal bone and the acoustic nerve, causing ipsilateral deafness.

The treatment of choice is gradual occlusion of the internal carotid artery, provided arteriography indicates adequate filling of the middle and anterior cerebral arteries on the side of the aneurysm from the contralateral carotid artery and provided there is no untoward effect from digital compression of the common carotid artery for 15 minutes. Patients should be less than 60 years of age, and the operative procedure should be done to relieve severe pain, failing vision, or exophthalmos.

Carotid artery–cavernous sinus fistula. The rupture of an infraclinoid aneurysm shunts blood from the carotid artery into the cavernous sinus, creating an arteriovenous fistula. The arterial blood passes into channels connecting with the cavernous sinus, and congestion of the superior ophthalmic vein draining the orbit causes visual loss, diplopia, headache, and pain.

Carotid-cavernous fistulas are traumatic (75%) or spontaneous. The traumatic fistula follows skull fracture, particularly basilotemporal fracture. A latent period may occur before the onset of symptoms. Spontaneous fistulas occur most commonly in middle-aged women, presumably because of rupture of fusiform aneurysms so small that they did not cause symptoms before rupture. Many may be caused by dural shunts occurring between meningeal branches of the carotid system and dural veins in the region of the cavernous sinus.

The outstanding sign is unilateral or bilateral proptosis (Fig. 26-4), which may pulsate. A bruit synchronous with the pulse is heard by the patient as a rushing, roaring sound. The increased venous pressure with stasis causes chemosis (Fig. 26-5), eyelid swelling, congested conjunctival and retinal veins, and hemorrhages. The abducent nerve may be involved or, less commonly, the third, fourth, or seventh. Visual failure is common from impairment of arterial and venous retinal circulations. Secondary glaucoma, although not obvious, may cause visual loss. Tonography indicates increased arterial pulsation.

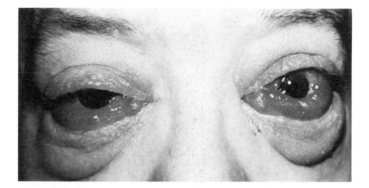

Fig. 26-4. Severe orbital congestion and bilateral proptosis in a spontaneous carotid artery-cavernous sinus fistula in a 57-year-old woman.

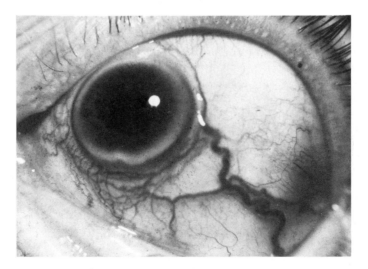

Fig. 26-5. Congested conjunctival vessels in a long-standing carotid artery-cavernous sinus fistula. The dilated blood vessels that surround the corneoscleral limbus are sometimes called "caput medusa."

The ideal treatment is early ligation of the internal carotid artery in the neck combined with simultaneous intracranial clipping of the internal carotid artery and the ophthalmic artery. The anastomoses between the external carotid artery and the ophthalmic artery maintains vision in about 75% of patients in whom the ophthalmic artery is clipped. The recommendations described for infraclinoid aneurysms must be followed. Failure to treat patients promptly who would benefit leads to irreversible changes.

Subarachnoid hemorrhage. The chief causes of spontaneous bleeding into the space between the arachnoid and the pia mater are (1) vascular hypertension, (2) ruptured supraclinoid aneurysms, and (3) angiomas or arteriovenous malformations. Less common causes include blood dyscrasias, necrosis of metastatic or primary brain tumors, and spinal varices.

Subarachnoid hemorrhage is characterized by a sudden, violent head pain of shocking severity followed by photophobia and stiffness of the legs. Unconsciousness persisting for a few hours to days may follow. Later there may be rigidity of the neck and spine. Lumbar puncture, in which only a few drops of fluid should be removed, indicates fresh blood. Bilateral carotid arteriography is indicated to determine whether the circle of Willis is normal and to determine the adequacy of the blood supply from the contralateral side.

The ocular signs are mainly those described for unruptured supraclinoid aneurysms. In addition, there may be sudden loss of vision, papilledema, and exophthalmos. An uncommon but pathognomonic ocular sign is bilateral subhyaloid hemorrhage, at the posterior pole adjacent to the optic disk.

Treatment must be individualized, but modern microsurgical techniques have decreased mortality, although the morbidity is still high. Surgical treatment should be carried out immediately in patients who are conscious or semiconscious, provided the collateral circulation is adequate. Gradual occlusion of the common carotid artery in the neck is moderately effective in subarachnoid hemorrhage caused by ruptured aneurysms of the internal carotid or posterior communicating artery. The treatment of choice is exposure of the aneurysm and either clipping it, coating it with plastic, or in-

ducing intravascular thrombosis with an electric current, animal hair, or wire in the arterial wall.

Sudden severe headache with confusion followed by deep coma with bloody spinal fluid suggests cerebral hemorrhage. Sudden suboccipital headache, stiff neck, nausea, and vomiting are usually caused by subarachnoid hemorrhage from a ruptured saccular aneurysm. Five or more spontaneous subarachnoid hemorrhages suggest a hemangioma rather than a saccular aneurysm. Increasing headache, drowsiness, confusion, and hemiparesis over a period of a few weeks suggest a chronic subdural hematoma. Progressive symptoms over a long period suggest tumor. Hypertensive encephalopathy, tumors, trauma, and syphilis may cause seizures and stupor.

DIABETES MELLITUS NEUROPATHY

Diabetes mellitus in rare instances is complicated by neuropathy involving the cranial motor nerves. There is a severe unilateral headache usually followed by lateral rectus muscle weakness (Chapter 25). More rarely there is weakness of muscles innervated by the oculomotor nerve. The pupil is not impaired in 75% of the instances. Diabetes mellitus neuropathy is usually distinguished from supraclinoid aneurysms by isolated paralysis of the lateral rectus muscle, which rarely is solely affected with an aneurysm. The sparing of the sphincter pupillae muscle aids in the diagnosis of diabetes. Generally, if the pupil is not involved, the cause is a medical disorder that does not require surgery. If the sphincter pupillae muscle is paralyzed, the cause is an aneurysm, tumor, or trauma.

NYSTAGMUS AND OCULAR OSCILLATION

Oscillation of the eyes may be divided into nystagmus, a biphasic involuntary ocular oscillation that always involves slow eye movements, and non-nystagmus, oscillations that are always saccadic or saccadically initiated (fast eye movements: ocular dysmetria, flutter, opsoclonus, myoclonus, and bobbing).

Saccadic eye movements. These fast eye movements involve the interaction of three groups of neurons within the brain stem: burst cells, tonic cells, and pause cells. Burst neurons located within the pontine and mesencephalic-reticular formation initiate a velocity command (saccadic pulse) that generates tonic neurons that move the eye from one position to another (saccadic step). Pause cells within the pons then inhibit the burst neurons so that the eyes are held in the new position.

Abnormalities of ocular movement may involve the burst cells, tonic cells, or pause cells. During head rotation, the vestibulocerebellar complex stabilizes the retinal image so that there is no perception of movement. In ocular dysmetria, the saccade either overshoots or undershoots the target so that a corrective movement is required to bring the eyes on target. The mismatch is caused by an imbalance in the burst cell velocity command innervation and pause cells that inhibit burst cells. It is seen in abnormalities of the vestibulocerebellum, such as Arnold-Chiari malformation.

Ocular flutter consists of spontaneous, conjugate, to-and-fro saccades that interrupt fixation. Patients often demonstrate flutter when recovering from opsoclonus. Opsoclonus (dancing eyes or lightning eye movements) consists of rapid, involuntary, chaotic, repetitive, unpredictable, conjugate eye movements in all directions. The movements prevent fixation and continue during sleep and in darkness. Opsoclonus occurs with cerebellar and brain stem disorders. There is an unexplained association between opsoclonus and occult neoplasms, particularly neuroblastoma. Opsoclonus and ocular flutter are attributed to pause cell dysfunction so that burst neurons are not inhibited after a saccade.

Ocular myoclonus consists of rapid bursts of conjugate saccades often associated with myoclonic jerks of other parts of the body. Myoclonus of the eyes and palate occurs in pseudohypertrophy of the inferior olivary nucleus in the medulla.

Superior oblique muscle myokymia causes a monocular, rapid, fine ocular tremor that may be vertical, torsional, or oblique. There may be an associated monocular oscillopsia. The attacks are recurrent, often precipitated by rotating the eyes into the reading position. The condition may be spontaneous or follow trochlear nerve disorders. Therapy with carbamazepine, a membrane stabilizing drug, may be helpful.

Nystagmus. This is an involuntary, rhythmic, bilateral oscillation of the eyes. It is

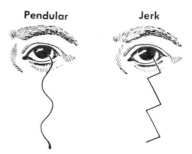

Fig. 26-6. The two general types of nystagmus. The pendular nystagmus has undulating movements of the eyes. The jerk nystagmus shown has a quick phase nasalward and a slow phase templeward. (From Huber, A.: Eye signs and symptoms in brain tumors, ed. 3, St. Louis, 1976, The C.V. Mosby Co.)

usually detected by simple observation of the eyes, but when minimal, it may be observed during ophthalmoscopy, the magnification of the fundus emphasizing the movement. In testing for nystagmus, the ocular movement should be observed in eyes front, right and left, and up and down.

Nystagmus is divided on the basis of its rhythm into pendular and jerk types (Fig. 26-6). The rhythm of pendular nystagmus is regular. In jerk nystagmus, there is a slow movement in one direction, followed by a quick recovery movement in the opposite direction.

Pendular nystagmus. Pendular nystagmus is a to-and-fro oscillation of both eyes that is equal in amplitude and velocity in each direction. Acquired pendular nystagmus in adults reflects vascular or demyelinating disease affecting the brain stem or cerebellum. A head tremor is usual, and there may be a complaint of objects moving (oscillopsia).

Congenital nystagmus is a pendular nystagmus evident at birth or shortly thereafter. There is no consistent lesion causing visual loss, but poor vision increases nystagmus. Congenital nystagmus decreases with convergence and in many cases a direction of gaze angle can be found where nystagmus is minimal (null angle). Treatment with base-out prisms or ocular muscle surgery to place the eyes so that they are in the null position may improve vision. Congenital nystagmus may occur without other ocular defects, but often there are gross opacities of the media, or retinal or optic nerve abnormalities. Albinism (see Chapter 24) is often associated with nystagmus. Nystagmus does not occur in eyes in which the congenital defects cause complete absence of light perception.

Physiologic nystagmus is a high-frequency (50 KHz to 100 KHz), low-amplitude (5 to 30 sec/arc) pendular oscillation that occurs during fixation so that different regions of the foveola will be stimulated.

See-saw nystagmus is a conjugate pendular oscillation in which one eye rises and intorts while the fellow eye falls and extorts. It reflects diencephalic dysfunction and occurs in bitemporal hemianopsia from parasellar lesions, brain-stem lesions, and posttrauma.

Ocular bobbing is generated by fast downward jerks of each eye (sometimes nonconjugate) followed by a slow drift to midposition. It occurs in comatose patients who have extensive pontine destruction, obstructive hydrocephalus, or metabolic encephalopathy.

Spasmus nutans is a rapid nystagmus of small amplitude that occurs in children between 4 months and 2 years of age. There is an associated head nodding and sometimes abnormal head position. It may be bilateral or unilateral and is the most common cause of unilateral nystagmus in children. It has been attributed to poor illumination, but the cause is unknown. It invariably disappears.

Voluntary nystagmus is a pendular nystagmus in individuals who induce rapid ocular oscillations by extreme convergence. It is of no clinical significance.

Jerk nystagmus. Jerk nystagmus is a horizontal oscillation that has a slow component in one direction and a rapid corrective movement (saccadic) in the opposite direction. Reference is made to the direction of the rapid component, although the slow movement reflects the basic disability. Jerk nystagmus in the primary position may indicate vestibular dysfunction, whereas that present in other directions of gaze suggests brain-stem or cerebellar disease or drug ingestion.

Opticokinetic nystagmus is a jerk nystagmus induced by a visual pattern that moves at a constant velocity. There is a slow eye movement in the direction of the moving pattern followed by a fast phase in the opposite direction. Since the subject cannot voluntarily inhibit the eye movements, induction of opticokinetic nystagmus is utilized to measure vision in infants and children. In homonymous hemianopsia caused by parietal lobe lesions, moving the targets from the seeing side to the blind side does not induce an opticokinetic nystagmus.

Clinically, opticokinetic nystagmus is studied by having the subject look at a rotating drum or television screen in which there are moving figures or alternate white and black lines. More simply, a 20-inch strip of alternate 2-inch red and white squares may be used.

Latent nystagmus is a bilateral horizontal jerk nystagmus elicited by covering one eye or making the brightness or clarity of retinal images unequal in the two eyes. The slow component is in the direction of the covered eye, and the rapid component is in the direction of the open eye. With both eyes open, such patients may have normal vision, but when either eye is covered, visual acuity in the open eye is 20/200 or less. There is no treatment. Strabismus is common in this disorder.

Gaze-evoked nystagmus (end-position nystagmus) is seen when the eyes are turned into an extreme position of gaze. It is horizontal or vertical. The slow component is toward the central primary position, and the fast component is toward the extreme position of gaze. It may occur in normal persons who are debilitated or fatigued. It is common after administration of barbiturates or other tranquilizers and may follow use of phenothiazine and anticoagulant drugs. Multiple sclerosis may cause nystagmus in extreme lateral gaze, and nystagmus may be present in brain-stem cerebellar dysfunction.

Vestibular nystagmus. This is a jerk nystagmus that follows asymmetric stimulation of the semicircular canals or their central pathways. There are three semicircular canals in each labyrinth: horizontal, superior, and vertical. The otoliths of the inner ear control body musculature and maintain a conjugate deviation of the eyes with changes in position of the head, so that the eyes tend to maintain a primary position in reference to the environment. The major action of the semicircular canals is evident in torsion of the eyes. The semicircular canals function in acceleration or deceleration of the body, in which the eyes tend to oppose a change of position when the body rotates.

Vestibular nystagmus can be conveniently studied by rotation of the body or by caloric irrigation of the external auditory canal, which sets up convection currents in the semicircular canals. Cold water applied to the tympanic membrane induces a jerk nystagmus in which the fast-phase beats are to the side opposite that to which the cold water was applied.

Vestibular nystagmus occurs in diseases of the end organ, its nuclei, or its central nervous system connections. Peripheral disease may be associated with vertigo, tinnitus, and deafness. The onset is abrupt. The nystagmus is horizontal and tends to decrease in the course of the disease. The common diseases causing peripheral involvement are labyrinthitis and Ménière disease.

Spontaneous vertical nystagmus is virtually always of central origin; spontaneous rotary nystagmus suggests involvement of vestibular nuclei. Nystagmus may occur in multiple sclerosis, encephalitis, vascular disease (particularly occlusion of the posteroinferior cerebellar artery), and cerebellar and cerebellopontine lesions. The latter are likely to produce nystagmus that varies with the position of the head. The fast component is toward the side of the lesion.

DEMYELINATIVE DISEASE

Destruction of the myelin sheath of nerve fibers occurs in a variety of disorders: multiple sclerosis, neuromyelitis optica (Devic disease), subcortical encephalopathy (Schilder disease), and postinfectious disseminated encephalitis. These conditions may all affect vision through involvement of the optic nerve or optic pathways. In addition, they may cause ocular muscle weakness.

Multiple sclerosis. Multiple sclerosis (MS) is a chronic, remittent disease of the white matter of the spinal cord and brain. It is characterized by disseminated areas of demyelination and glial scar formation. It rarely affects individuals younger than 15 years of age. The rate of onset peaks at 30 years of age and rapidly declines thereafter. Onset after 35 years of age occurs occasionally. The prevalence and death rate are relatively high in the northern regions of the United States and Canada and low in the southern United States. The average duration of the disease is 27 years, and in many patients

there are remissions without permanent neurologic residue.

Six criteria are generally accepted for diagnosis: (1) the results of neurologic examination are abnormal; (2) at least two separate parts of the nervous system are involved; (3) fiber tract damage (white matter) predominates; (4) there are at least two separate episodes of worsening, separated by at least 1 month, or alternatively slow stepwise progression over at least 6 months; (5) age of onset between ages 10 and 50 years; and (6) no other condition can explain the disease process.

There may be a mild pleocytosis of the cerebrospinal fluid. The protein content may be slightly increased and the colloidal gold curve abnormal. The gamma globulin of the cerebrospinal fluid shows specific oligoclonal bands in most cases. The mildly abnormal electroencephalogram and demonstration of confluent areas of cerebral demyelination are not specific. The visual-evoked potential is often abnormal in latency or configuration even with no evidence of past or present involvement of the visual system. The auditory-evoked potential may be similarly affected.

Optic neuritis is the initial episode of the disease in 15% of the patients; in another 25% ocular muscle palsy occurs. Of patients hospitalized because of multiple sclerosis, 70% have or have had optic neuritis. The fully developed disease is characterized by the Charcot triad of nystagmus, scanning speech, and optic atrophy. Sheathing of peripheral retinal veins occurs in about 5% of the patients. Diplopia occurs because of an internuclear ophthalmoplegia or because of palsies of individual muscles.

Neuromyelitis optica (Devic). This is a bilateral acute optic neuritis with a transverse spinal cord myelitis. The disease may occur at any age. There are prodromal signs of headache, sore throat, fever, and malaise. The visual loss occurs rapidly, and blindness or near blindness develops within a few days. Paralysis and sensory disturbances caudal to the transverse myelitis occur within a few weeks before or after blindness. Patients may die within a month, or there may be complete remission with recurrences. There is no treatment.

Subcortical encephalopathy. Subcortical encephalopathy (Schilder disease) affects children and adolescents and is characterized by progressive involvement of the brain with loss of vision, spastic paralysis, deafness, mental deterioration, and death in a few months to a year. Papilledema occurs in most of the patients.

Postinfectious encephalitis. Encephalitis may develop after viral infections such as measles, mumps, varicella, and vaccinia. It most commonly follows measles, and the mortality of patients with measles encephalitis is 10%. There may be papilledema, papillitis, or retrobulbar neuritis. Vision recovery is usual.

DYSAUTONOMIA

Familial dysautonomia. Familial dysautonomia or familial autonomic dysfunction (Riley-Day syndrome) is an autosomal recessive neurologic disorder largely confined to Ashkenazic Jews. It is characterized by absence of overflow tears (alacrima), corneal hypesthesia, exotropia, and pupillary constriction after instillation of 0.1% pilocarpine (denervation hypersensitivity). The cause of the disorder is unknown, but there appears to be impaired elaboration or release of neurohumoral transmitter agent, possibly acetylcholine.

Many systemic defects occur: excessive sweating caused by vasomotor instability, skin blotching from eating or excitement, orthostatic hypotension, cyclic vomiting, fixed heart rate with episodes of tachycardia, and episodic fever. There is a striking indifference to pain, but proprioception and vibration sense are normal. There may be self-mutilation or mutilation from trauma. The patients are unsteady, uncoordinated, and unable to perform fine repetitive movements or ride a bicycle. Response to touch stimuli is excessive (dysesthesia). Deep tendon reflexes are absent or hypoactive. Emotions are labile, and patients are often sullen and uncommunicative; breathholding is common in infancy. Few patients survive to adulthood, and most succumb to pneumonia, cardiovascular collapse, and intercurrent illness after a progressively downhill course during childhood.

The fungiform papillae of the tongue, the site of most of the taste buds, are absent. Disturbed swallowing causes drooling, feeding problems, and sometimes aspiration pneumonia. Intradermal injection of $1:1,000$ histamine causes a wheal but not the usual flare.

The initial finding may be the absence of tears in a crying infant who has a feeding problem. By 2 years of age, the child drools constantly, is undernourished, and walks on his toes with a stumbling gait. High fever of unexplained origin is common and sometimes is accompanied by convulsions.

In about half the patients, deficient lacrimation is associated with chronic, indolent, corneal ulcers that cause little or no pain because of the reduced corneal sensation. Artificial tears and intermarginal eyelid adhesions may be required. The Schirmer test indicates reduced tear formation. Myopia occurs in about 80% of the patients, and about one third of these have more than 1.5 diopters difference in the refractive error in the two eyes (anisometropia). Exotropia occurs in about two thirds of the patients, but it is not clear whether this is secondary to decreased vision resulting from keratitis or myopia or is caused by a central defect.

Ocular differential diagnosis includes congenital absence of the lacrimal gland and anhidrotic hereditary ectodermal dysplasia, in each of which the corneal sensitivity is normal. Keratoconjunctivitis sicca occurs in later years and, in addition to punctate or filamentary keratitis, has a stringy, mucoid discharge not present in autonomic dysfunction. Vitamin A deficiency with keratomalacia presents feeding problems, decreased tearing, and corneal ulcers, but the conjunctiva is affected initially and loses its luster, with dry spots appearing in it in contrast to the glistening, normal-appearing conjunctiva in autonomic dysfunction. Neuroparalytic keratitis is usually unilateral, follows trigeminal nerve injury, and has no associated systemic findings.

Subacute sclerosing panencephalitis. This is a slowly progressive disease of children and young adults caused by a persistent measles-virus infection. The serum and cerebrospinal fluid lack antibodies to the M protein of the measles virus although there are high titers to other measles-virus proteins. It usually develops before 11 years of age in previously well children who had measles before 2 years of age. Mental deterioration is followed by intractable myoclonic seizures. A focal retinitis of the central retina leads to atrophy of the retinal pigment epithelium and sensory retina. Cortical blindness, papilledema, and optic atrophy may occur with associated cranial nerve lesions. Death occurs within 1 year of onset.

HEADACHE

Headaches may be divided into those that originate from intracranial sources and those that originate from extracranial sources (Table 26-4). Iridocyclitis, high intraocular pressure, impending zoster ophthalmicus, and temporal arteritis cause orbital pain. Retrobulbar neuritis is associated with pain behind the eye aggravated by ocular movements. The ocular muscle palsy of diabetic neuropathy begins with severe retrobulbar pain. Refractive errors are commonly thought to cause discomfort and pain in the head, but usually the cause is vascular, neurologic, or psychogenic.

Migraine. This is a familial symptom complex of transient (usually), paroxysmal, neurologic dysfunction that often but not exclusively, occurs with headache. Common migraine (sick headache) is initiated by depression, diarrhea, or constipation and is followed by headache that is unilateral and throbbing at the beginning but eventually involves the whole head. Nausea and vomiting may be followed by relief or more often by intensified head pain.

Classic migraine is similar to common migraine except that it is preceded by an aura that is often visual with scintillating scotomas of bright lights or rhythmically flashing zigzag lines (Fig. 26-7). Classic migraine may occur with multiple attacks over a few days. Some individuals, often middle-aged, have only the visual aura of migraine without headache or other symptoms. Spontaneous remission is the usual course.

Complicated migraine (Table 26-5) is associated with motor, sensory, and visual signs, and individuals may develop permanent hemianopsias, speech difficulties, and hemiplegia. Ophthalmoplegic migraine is associated with transient or permanent ocular muscle paralysis with exotropia, blepharoptosis, and pupillary dilation.

In migraine of the anterior visual pathway, there may be ischemic papillitis, vitreous hemorrhage, serous chorioretinopathy, and optic

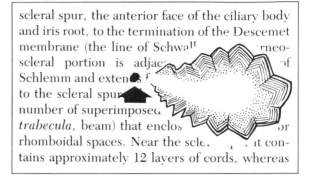

Fig. 26-7. The scintillating scotoma of migraine. The arrow points to the fixation point. The scotoma expands and contracts and always involves both eyes.

atrophy. Typically a young adult with migraine develops permanent visual loss.

Ergotamine preparations are the chief therapy. Methysergide and propranolol are used in prophylaxis.

Benign intracranial hypertension. In this chronic condition, obese young women with a history of menstrual irregularity, often with amenorrhea, develop bilateral papilledema and headache. The headache is often worse upon awakening and is aggravated by coughing and straining. The papilledema may be associated with dimming or blurring of vision, sometimes often during a day. Visual symptoms may be minimal despite severe papilledema. The disorder may persist for years without serious sequelae.

Papilledema also develops with vascular hypertension, chronic emphysema, chronic fibrosing meningeal disease, Addison disease, corticosteroid withdrawal, vitamin A overdosage, and hypothyroidism.

Recurrent nocturnal orbital (cluster) headaches. These are characterized by constant, unilateral orbital localization, occurrence in men between 20 and 50 years of age, and onset within 2 to 3 hours of falling asleep. There is lacrimation, sometimes flush and edema of the cheek, and sometimes Horner syndrome. The nostril is blocked, followed by rhinorrhea. The attack disappears within several hours. The attacks recur nightly for days or weeks (hence, cluster) and then disappear for years.

Some pains behind the eye, nose, or upper jaw associated with a blocked nostril are de-

Table 26-4. Some causes of headache

Intracranial sources
  Traction and displacement
    Venous sinuses and tributaries
    Middle meningeal arteries
    Intracranial arteries at base of brain and their
      major branches
    Pain-sensitive cranial nerves
    Trigeminal neuralgia
  Dilation and distention
    Intracranial arteries
    Increased or low intracranial pressure
  Cranial nerve neuralgias
    Tic douloureaux (V)
    Glossopharyngeal neuralgia (IX)
  Intracranial inflammation
    Meningitis
    Subarachnoid hemorrhage
    Arteritis
    Phlebitis
    Raeder syndrome
    Altitude
Extracranial sources
  Vascular headache
    Migraine
      Classical
      Common
      Complicated
        Cerebral
        Ophthalmoplegic
        Retinal
        Basilar artery
    Cluster headache
    Posttrauma
    Vascular hypertension
    Fever
  Occipitofrontal muscular contracture
  Sinus
  Aural
  Dental
  Extracranial arteritis
  Ocular
  Greater occipital neuralgia
  Preherpetic and herpetic neuralgia
  Temporomandibular joint pain

Table 26-5. Migraine accompaniments

Visual problems
  Scintillations with or without fortification
  Blurring
  Blindness
  Hemianopsia
  Transient monocular blindness
  Diplopia
  Oculosympathetic palsy
  Mydriasis
Paresthesias
Dysarthria
Hemiplegia
Confusion, stupor
Cyclic vomiting
Deafness
Recurrence of old stroke deficit
Chorea
Car sickness

From Burde, R.M.: Discussion of Cohen, R.G., Harbison, J.W., Blair, C.J., and Ochs, A.L.: Clinical significance of transient visual phenomena in the elderly, Ophthalmology **91:**436, 1984.

BIBLIOGRAPHY
General

Anderson, D.R.: Testing the field of vision, St. Louis, 1981, The C.V. Mosby Co.

Bosley, T.M., Rosenquist, A.C., Kushner, M., Burke, A., Stein, A., Dann, R., Cobbs, W., Savino, P.J., Schatz, N.J., Alavi, A., and Reivich, M.: Ischemic lesions of the occipital cortex and optic radiations: positron emission tomography, Neurology **35:**470, 1985.

Burde, R.M., Savino, P.J., and Trobe, J.D.: Clinical decisions in neuro-ophthalmology, St. Louis, 1985, The C.V. Mosby Co.

Cogan, D.G.: Neurology of the visual system, Springfield, Ill., 1980, Charles C Thomas, Publisher.

Ebers, G.C.: Optic neuritis and multiple sclerosis, Arch. Neurol. **42:**702, 1985.

Glaser, J.S.: Neuro-ophthalmology, New York, 1978, Harper & Row, Publishers.

Harrington, D.O.: The visual fields, ed. 5, St. Louis, 1981, The C.V. Mosby Co.

Lessel, S., and van Dalen, J.T.W., editors: Neuro-ophthalmology, vol. 3, Amsterdam, 1984, Elsevier Science Publishers B.V.

Rowland, L.P., editor: Merritt's textbook of neurology, ed. 7, Philadelphia, 1984, Lea & Febiger.

Toole, J.F.: Cerebrovascular disorders, ed. 3, New York, 1984, Raven Press.

Walsh, T.J., editor: Neuro-ophthalmology: clinical signs and symptoms, ed. 2, Philadelphia, 1985, Lea & Febiger.

scribed as neuralgia affecting specific nerves: sphenopalatine (Sluder), petrosal, vidian, and ciliary (Charlin). They probably are instances of cluster headache or variants thereof.

Paratrigeminal syndrome (of Raeder). This consists of severe daily unilateral headaches with Horner syndrome without anhydrosis and often with lacrimation and conjunctival injection. Men are commonly affected (7:1). The average age of onset is 46 years. The attacks last 1 or 2 months and rarely recur.

Wiederholt, W.C., editor: Neurology for non-neurologists, New York, 1982, Academic Press.

Ocular muscles

Cogan, D.G.: Neurology of the ocular muscles, ed. 2, Springfield, Ill., 1978, Charles C Thomas, Publisher.

von Noorden, G.K., Tredici, T.D., and Ruttum, M.: Pseudointernuclear ophthalmoplegia after surgical paresis of the medial rectus muscle, Am. J. Ophthalmol. **98**:602, 1984.

Vascular disease

Kearns, T.P.: Differential diagnosis of central retinal vein obstruction, Ophthalmology **90**:475, 1983.

Tomsak, R.L.: Ischemic optic neuropathy associated with retinal embolism, Am. J. Ophthalmol. **99**:490, 1985.

Nystagmus

Carl, J.R., Optican, L.M., Chu, F.C., and Zee, D.S.: Head shaking and vestibulo-ocular reflex in congenital nystagmus, Invest. Ophthalmol. Vis. Sci. **26**:1043, 1985.

Lee, J.P.: Superior oblique myokymia, Arch. Ophthalmol. **102**:1178, 1984.

Safran, A.B., and Berney, J.: Synchronism of inverse ocular bobbing and blinking, Am. J. Ophthalmol. **95**:401, 1983.

Simon, J.W., Kandel, G.L., Krohel, G.B., and Nelsen, P.T.: Albinotic characteristics in congenital nystagmus, Am. J. Ophthalmol. **97**:320, 1984.

Tumors

Anderson, D., Faber, P., Marcovitz, S., Hardy, J., and Lorenzetti, D.: Pituitary tumors and the ophthalmologist, Ophthalmology **90**:1265, 1983.

Grossman, A., and Besser, G.M.: Prolactinomas, Br. Med. J. **290**:182, 1985.

Randall, R.V., Scheithauer, B.W., Laws, E.R., Jr., Abboud, C.F., Ebersold, M.J., and Kao, P.C.: Pituitary adenomas associated with hyperprolactinemia: a clinical and immunohistochemical study of 97 patients operated on transsphenoidally, Mayo Clin. Proc. **60**:753, 1985.

Tolis, G., Stefanis, C., Mountokalakis, T., and Labire, F., editors: Prolactin and prolactinomas, New York, 1983, Raven Press.

Headache

Cohen, G.R., Harbison, J.W., Blair, C.J., and Ochs, A.L.: Clinical significance of transient visual phenomena in the elderly, Ophthalmology **91**:436, 1984.

27

CARDIOVASCULAR DISORDERS

The ocular fundus is the only region where small arteries, arterioles, and their accompanying veins may be directly observed in vivo. These blood vessels are subject to the same systemic disorders as similar-sized vessels elsewhere in the body but also may be affected by local ocular diseases such as glaucoma or retinitis pigmentosa, which have no systemic counterpart. The vascular pressure within the eye must exceed the intraocular pressure to prevent collapse of the vessels. This is thus a highly specialized vascular bed, and changes in retinal vessels are extrapolated to similar changes in the cardiac, cerebral, or renal blood vessels with caution.

A number of cardiovascular disorders of the eye have been discussed: the increased incidence of myocardial infarction before 50 years of age in men who smoke and have corneal arcus, amaurosis fugax in occlusive disease of the carotid artery, occlusive disease of the central retinal artery and vein and their branches, giant-cell vasculitis, and cerebral hemorrhage and ischemia.

This chapter is mainly directed to discussion of age-related retinal vascular changes, arteriosclerosis of the central retinal artery, and arteriolar sclerosis of accelerated vascular hypertension that affects branches of the central retinal artery. Particulars concerning the ophthalmoscopic examination are discussed elsewhere (Chapters 6 and 16).

AGING (INVOLUTIONAL SCLEROSIS)

Abnormalities of the retinal blood vessels are common in elderly persons and occasionally occur in younger individuals who do not have and have not had vascular hypertension. The outstanding ophthalmoscopic characteristic of involutional sclerosis is localized involvement of medium-sized retinal arterioles in which much of the vasculature looks normal. The light reflex from the convex surface of arterioles is of diminished intensity and more diffuse than normal. A slight reduction in the caliber of arterioles may occur. Associated with the vascular changes are degenerative changes of the retinal pigment epithelium, such as drusen and depigmentation.

The involutional changes occur with aging but do not necessarily parallel any aging processes elsewhere in the body. Their cause is not known, but in all probability they are the consequence of loss of elasticity and arteriolar fibrosis.

ARTERIOSCLEROSIS

Arteriosclerosis is a nonspecific, broadly inclusive term that describes all processes in which thickening of the arterial wall has occurred. The three conditions generally included in the term are Mönckeberg medial sclerosis, atherosclerosis, and diffuse arteriolar sclerosis. Mönckeberg medial sclerosis affects medium-sized arteries, particularly in the extremities; there is never ocular involvement. Atherosclerosis affects large and medium-sized arteries; the central retinal artery and its

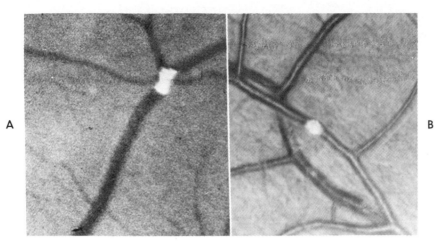

Fig. 27-1. **A,** Cholesterol embolus at bifurcation of a branch of a retinal artery in a 57-year-old woman with an atheroma of the common carotid artery. **B,** Fibrin embolus in the inferior temporal artery of the left eye of a 23-year-old man with mitral regurgitation after rheumatic heart disease. Four months later, the embolus was no longer present. There were no symptoms.

branches immediately adjacent to the optic disk may be involved. Diffuse arteriolar sclerosis involves all arterioles in the body in a similar manner. It occurs solely as a result of vascular hypertension. The retinal arteries beyond the first bifurcation are arterioles.

Retinal vein obstruction causes changes in adjacent arterioles identical with those in arteriolar sclerosis. The adjacent vein obstruction and the focal arteriolar sclerosis indicate the cause.

Atherosclerosis

Atherosclerosis is characterized by focal necrosis and thickening of the arterial intima, combined with intimal and subintimal lipid deposition. There are hyperplastic and degenerative changes in the wall of the artery, particularly of the internal elastic lamina. The disease affects arteries of all diameters, but it has a predilection for the aorta and its major branches. The condition is minimal in puberty, but thereafter its extent and severity increase with advancing age. Atheromas are asymptomatic unless blood supply to a region is reduced or emboli are released that occlude distant vessels. The lesions may be multiple, but atheromas in one vessel do not indicate atheromas in another. Their cause is unknown, but they are associated with vascular hypertension,

turbulence eddies within blood vessels, hyperlipoproteinemia, and heredity.

Atherosclerosis of retinal vessels. Atherosclerosis involves the central retinal artery either within the optic nerve or in its branches immediately adjacent to the optic disk.

An atheroma of the central retinal artery within the optic nerve reduces its lumen and draws the retinal arterioles toward the disk. As the bifurcations of arterioles are drawn onto the optic disk, more blood vessels cross the disk margins, the retinal vessels become straighter, and the bifurcations occur at more acute angles.

Atheromas in papillary branches of the central artery near the optic disk cause subtle changes. Localized indentations in the wall of the central retinal artery reduce the caliber of the lumen as the result of projection of an atheromatous plaque into the lumen. Fibrosis causes a whitish opacification in the wall of the involved blood vessel.

Ocular atherosclerosis may obstruct the central retinal artery, compress the adjacent central retinal vein, and cause venous obstruction.

A cholesterol embolus dislodged from an atheromatous plaque in the carotid artery appears as a glistening, crystalline body within a retinal artery, often at a vessel bifurcation (Fig. 27-1, *A*). The embolus may cause an amaurosis fugax or retinal ischemia. The presence of such an embolus should lead to a full study of the patient's vascular status.

A fibrin embolus originates from a damaged heart valve or other cardiac lesion. It is dull white to yellowish-white with ill-defined margins and is less likely to be lodged at a vessel bifurcation (Fig. 27-1, *B*) than a cholesterol embolus.

Platelet emboli are minute white accumulations. As they course through the arteries, they cause flashing or shimmering vision.

Arteries and veins are bound together in a common adventitial sheath at the lamina cribrosa and at arteriovenous crossings within the eye. Atheromatous plaque formation in the artery may compress the vein, causing venous closure at the lamina cribrosa (central retinal vein occlusion) or obstruction at one of the crossings (branch vein occlusion). Glaucoma increases the possibility of central retinal vein occlusion, since the increased intraocular pressure favors stagnation of blood and thrombus formation.

Retinopathy of carotid occlusive disease

Low perfusion pressure in the retinal arterioles may lead to a slowing of blood flow in the retinal veins. The condition is also called venous stasis retinopathy, chronic ischemic retinopathy, and ischemic oculopathy or ophthalmopathy.

The ophthalmoscopic picture resembles a central vein occlusion, but the optic disk is likely to be free of congestion and hemorrhages. The hemorrhages, microaneurysms, and edema are likely to be located in the midperiphery, often the superior temporal quadrant. Visual acuity fluctuates, and blurring of vision may be noted upon entering a less well-lighted area from a brighter area. This impaired dark adaptation likely reflects impaired choroidal circulation with decreased nutrition of the retinal pigment epithelium. Amaurosis fugax with variation in vision may occur, as well as other transient ischemic attacks. Ophthalmodynamometry indicates pressure in the central retinal artery to be at least 50% less than that of the opposite side. The intraocular pressure is lower unless a secondary glaucoma has developed. Treatment must be directed to the occluded carotid artery, often an endarterectomy.

Arteriolar sclerosis

Arteriolar sclerosis is the result of prolonged severe vascular hypertension with resultant thickening of the walls and narrowing of the lumen of arterioles. In contrast to the spotty, plaquelike involvement of atherosclerosis, the arteriolar sclerosis is generalized and affects all arterioles throughout the body to a similar degree. One of two changes occurs in arteriolar sclerosis.

1. Replacement fibrosis develops in slowly increasing, moderately severe hypertension, associated chiefly with an increase of the systolic blood pressure in the range of 170 to 200 mm Hg, and diastolic pressure usually less than 100 mm Hg. There is increased collagen and elastic tissue in all layers of the blood vessel, loss of cells, and lipid and hyaline deposition beneath the endothelium.

2. Hyperplastic thickening and fibrinoid necrosis occur as acute, severe reactions to a sudden marked increase in the blood pressure in which the systolic blood pressure exceeds 200 mm Hg and the diastolic blood pressure exceeds 120 mm Hg. Hyperplastic thickening and fibrinoid necrosis occur in vessels containing muscle fibers. Vessels that have been the site of involutionary sclerosis or previous replacement fibrosis are not affected. These changes appear to protect the arterioles from the effects of severe hypertension, and they may explain the infrequency of hyperplastic thickening and fibrinoid necrosis in patients with involutional sclerosis.

Replacement fibrosis and fibrinoid necrosis cause two main groups of ophthalmoscopic changes (Table 27-1). If ophthalmoscopy in a patient with severe hypertension indicates no arteriolar sclerosis, the hypertension either is not severe or is of recent onset. If the changes of replacement fibrosis are present, the disease is of long duration and has affected arterioles throughout the body similarly. If the ophthalmoscopic changes are those of hyperplastic thickening and fibrinoid necrosis, the hypertension is severe, is likely of recent onset, and may be associated with renal insufficiency, encephalopathy, and impairment of cardiac function.

Retinal vascular changes. Healthy retinal blood vessels are transparent tubes through which blood inside is visible. The oxygenated blood in arteries is brighter red than that in

Table 27-1. Ophthalmoscopic signs of arteriolar sclerosis

Replacement fibrosis: long-duration, moderately severe hypertension	Fibrinoid necrosis: recent-onset, severe hypertension
Attenuation of arterioles	Severe focal attenuation of arterioles
Arteriovenous crossing changes	Edema of retina
Concealment	Cotton-wool patches
Depression or elevation	Hemorrhage
Deviation	Papilledema
Stenosis	Ophthalmoscopic changes of replacement fibrosis may precede above
Changes in vascular light reflex	signs or remain after condition is corrected
Irregularities of caliber	
Widening	
Copper-wire arteries	
Silver-wire arteries	
Sheathing	
Tortuosity	
Hard yellow exudates	
Hemorrhage	
Microaneurysms	

veins. With ophthalmoscopy, a light streak is reflected from the convex wall of arteries, presumably from the medial coat. With replacement fibrosis, the blood vessel wall becomes less transparent and the thickening of the medial coat is indicated by variation in the light reflex. To avoid confusing congenital anomalies that resemble sclerotic changes, attention is directed to blood vessels after they have traversed 1 disk diameter on the surface of the retina.

The difficulty of interpretation of retinal vascular changes is emphasized in the critical study by Salus of the accuracy of his own ophthalmoscopy, a field in which he was preeminent. In a careful experiment, he found that his diagnosis of hypertensive cardiovascular disease was correct in only 50% of patients with arteriosclerosis. In young adults who did not have arteriosclerosis and whose facial features and figures were covered except for their eyes, he incorrectly diagnosed arteriosclerosis in more than 50%.

Attenuation of arterioles. Attenuation of the arterioles is the most consistent sign of hypertension but is the most difficult to evaluate. Both generalized and focal constriction may be observed, but only the generalized attenuation seems to result from arteriolar spasm. Generalized attenuation is best appreciated by observing arterioles beyond their second bifurcation. They appear as thin red threads that disappear from view at the equator. The ophthalmoscopic change can be seen in accelerated arterial hypertension in young persons who have not developed replacement fibrosis.

Errors in diagnosis may occur either because arteries are concealed by retinal edema or the retinal veins are dilated, causing the arteries to appear narrower. Many believe that the ratio of arterial diameter to venous diameter is of no value and that attention should be directed to the diameter of arterioles.

Arteriovenous crossing changes. Abnormalities affecting all arteriovenous crossings are observed solely in arteriolar sclerosis and differentiate it from the occasional crossing change seen in involutional sclerosis. Replacement fibrosis of a retinal arteriole produces a variety of changes at the point at which it crosses over or under a vein. The arteriovenous crossing changes in arteriolar sclerosis include the following:

1. *Concealment.* The underlying vein is concealed because of loss of transparency of the wall of the retinal arteriole, which is caused by replacement fibrosis of its wall. The venous blood column appears to terminate abruptly on either side of the crossing. Alternatively, there may be a tapering type of concealment, with the vein fading on either side of the crossing. The concealment appears to cause a narrowing of the vein, commonly described as "nicking" (Fig. 27-2). The venous lumen is not narrowed.

2. *Depression or elevation.* A vein may be deflected deep into the retina or may hump abruptly over the artery (Fig. 27-3). The thick-

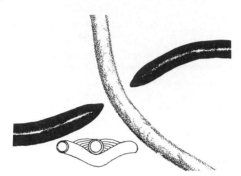

Fig. 27-2. Tapering concealment of the vein appearing as "nicking."

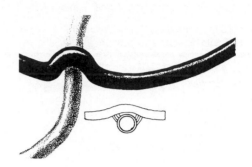

Fig. 27-3. Elevation of the vein over the artery.

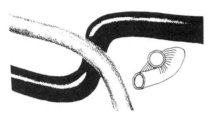

Fig. 27-4. Deviation of the vein out of its path.

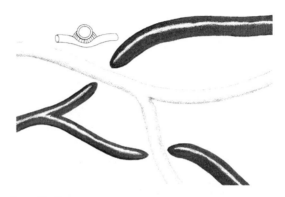

Fig. 27-5. Compression of the vein at the arteriovenous crossing, causing stenosis of the distal vein.

ened wall of the arterioles causes displacement of the vein.

3. *Deviation.* Displacement of a vein at the point of crossing is characterized by an abrupt turn in the course of the vein just as it reaches the artery (Fig. 27-4). At a similar distance beyond the artery it again assumes the same direction as before the crossing. This gives the vein an S-shape bend.

4. *Stenosis.* Because of compression or constriction at the arteriovenous crossing, the vein distal to the crossing becomes dilated and swollen (Fig. 27-5). The crossing is concealed, and thereafter the vein has a normal diameter.

Changes in light reflex. In the early days of ophthalmoscopy, much attention was directed to light reflected from the surface of blood vessels.

The major changes in light reflex are as follows.

1. *Widening of light reflex.* Light is reflected from the medial wall of arterioles. The earliest sign of arteriolar sclerosis is widening of the light reflex, which becomes broader and softer with less distinct borders. In time, there is variation in width of the light reflex.

2. *Copper-wire arteries.* As the reflex broadens, it eventually occupies most of the width of the blood vessel. Early ophthalmoscopists used reflected light having less intensity than that provided by the modern direct ophthalmoscope and described the burnished, metallic reflections as copper-wire arteries.

3. *Silver-wire arteries.* As replacement fibrosis continues, the vessel wall obscures the blood column, and the arteriole appears as a whitish tube containing a red fluid. This is not the white, threadlike appearance of the artery that follows occlusion of the central retinal artery.

4. *Sheathing.* Sheathing may occur as a result either of arteriolar sclerosis or of an atheromatous plaque involving an artery adjacent to the optic disk. Normally arterioles near the disk are sheathed with glial tissue. In arteriolar sclerosis, white parallel lines appear at arterio-

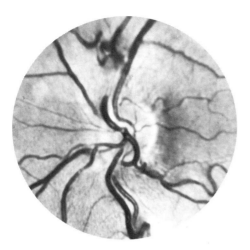

Fig. 27-6. Congenital tortuosity of retinal veins in a 27-year-old man with normal vision.

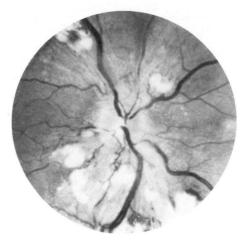

Fig. 27-7. A 39-year-old woman with fibrinoid necrosis. Her blood pressure is 250/160. Visual acuity is 20/25 in each eye. The optic disk margins are slightly blurred superiorly. The arterioles are extremely attenuated. There are numerous cotton-wool patches.

venous crossings and encase the arteriole, giving the appearance of a white, fibrous-looking cord. Sheathing also occurs in arterioles after a vasculitis subsides, and the arteries appear as white cords long after an arterial occlusion.

5. *Tortuosity.* In fibrous replacement, the arterioles increase in length and diameter, resulting in increased tortuosity. This may also be a congenital condition (Fig. 27-6), and its development in hypertension can only be evaluated by seeing the change develop.

Cotton-wool patches. Cotton-wool patches occur in fibrinoid necrosis when the diastolic blood pressure exceeds 120 mm Hg. They are located in the nerve fiber layer of the retina at the posterior pole, number usually less than 10, and are about one third of the disk diameter in size (Fig. 27-7). They may reflect impaired axoplasmic transport. Cotton-wool patches occur in many conditions (see Chapter 16), but the occurrence of even a solitary patch can indicate an accelerated hypertension.

Hard deposits. Hard deposits (chronic edema residues or hard yellow exudates) are focal accumulations of free fat and fat-laden macrophages in the outer plexiform layer of the retina or between the sensory retina and retinal pigment epithelium. They often circle an area of intraretinal microvascular abnormalities or occur diffusely in generalized retinal vascular leakage. These exudates are observed mainly at the posterior pole, vary in number from a few to 50 or more, and are scattered throughout the outer plexiform layer of the retina. In severe hypertension they may be concentrated around the fovea centralis (Henle layer), creating a star-shaped figure.

Hemorrhages. Hemorrhages in arteriolar sclerosis are located in the nerve fiber layer and are splinter- or flame-shaped.

Papilledema. The occurrence of cotton-wool patches of the retina indicates that hypertension has entered an accelerated phase (malignant). Shortly after their appearance, papilledema occurs, and patients complain of headache, blurred vision, and dizziness. About one half of patients have uremia. The diastolic blood pressure is above 110 mm Hg and sometimes as high as 170 mm Hg. There is fibrinoid necrosis of arterioles throughout the body.

Hypertensive encephalopathy occurs in accelerated hypertension with fibrinoid necrosis of the cerebral arterioles. Papilledema with retinopathy may or may not be present. The high arterial pressure impairs consciousness and gradually leads to coma.

Choroidal changes. The vasculature of the choroid is obscured by the retinal pigment epithelium and cannot be seen distinctly with the ophthalmoscope. Vascular changes of the choroid, however, are similar to those elsewhere in the body and the eye. Atherosclerosis of choroidal vessels is common, but the rich anastomoses minimize ischemia. Severe hypertension may cause fibrinoid necrosis of the choroidal arterioles. The retinal pigment epithelium becomes necrotic, and there may be atrophy of the sensory retina along with the formation of bright yellow spots (Elschnig) and lines three to four times the diameter of a retinal artery (Siegrist). The lesions cause a bilateral, multilobular, exudative, bullous retinal separation that commonly occupies the lower half of the fundus. The detachment disappears when the hypertension is corrected.

GRADING OF ARTERIAL HYPERTENSION

Ophthalmoscopic examination of the fundus in arterial hypertension is done to exclude papilledema and cotton-wool patches. These may be present with nearly normal blood pressure if cardiac decompensation has complicated accelerated hypertension.

Grading of the ocular changes of hypertension has caused confusion because the replacement fibrosis of arterial hypertension and that of involutional sclerosis (aging) cause similar changes. Grading is important in indicating vascular disease in a young individual, but controlled studies indicate that skilled ophthalmoscopists often disagree as to whether or not minor changes are present.

Keith-Wagner-Barker grouping. This 1938 classification is traditional and widely cited. It relates only to vascular hypertension and the arteriolar sclerosis caused by hypertension. It is not intended for classification of the involutional sclerosis of aging or atherosclerosis. Since hypertension causes generalized, diffuse changes, one should not use the classification for focal changes or for changes secondary to retinal inflammation that causes venous stasis. Both eyes should have similar changes; involvement of only one eye suggests impaired internal carotid circulation on the side of the normal eye. Glaucoma tends to minimize the ophthalmoscopic changes of vascular hypertension.

Group I. The light reflex from arterioles is brightened, and there is an increased luster with a burnished copper-wire or polished silver-wire appearance. There is moderate arteriolar attenuation often combined with focal constriction. No marked changes are seen in arteriovenous crossings, although there may be widening with increased translucency of the ar-

teriole, making the underlying vein nearly invisible. Patients in this group have an essential benign hypertension with adequate cardiac and renal function; the heart size and the electrocardiogram are usually normal. The majority of cases of hypertension fall into this group. The vascular changes of the fundi are virtually identical with those occurring in aging sclerosis without hypertension. With adequate treatment of the hypertensive disease, the ophthalmoscopic changes will probably not progress.

Group II. The light reflex has a definite burnished copper-wire or polished silver-wire luster. Arteriovenous crossing changes may be marked and include all the various abnormalities. The arterioles are about half the size of normal, and there are areas of localized constriction. Hard deposits as well as minute linear hemorrhages may develop late in the course of the disease. These patients have a more sustained hypertension with higher diastolic pressure than those in Group I. Their cardiac and renal functions tend to be normal, but cardiomegaly may develop, along with corresponding changes in the electrocardiogram. Angina pectoris and proteinuria may also be present.

Group III. Marked attenuation of the arterioles occurs. The retina appears wet and edematous. One or more cotton-wool patches and hemorrhages are present. The significant change is the cotton-wool patch. These patients have an accelerated hypertension and a diastolic blood pressure of more than 120 mm Hg. Depending on the cause of hypertension, there may be cardiac symptoms, changes in the electrocardiogram, and renal changes of proteinuria and insufficiency.

Group IV. The patients in Group IV have all the ophthalmoscopic signs of those in Group III, in addition to papilledema. The degree of papilledema may vary from blurring of the optic disk margins to complete obliteration of the optic disk structure. Cardiac and renal functions may be seriously impaired. Papilledema and cotton-wool patches may disappear shortly before death.

Systemic abnormalities such as eclampsia and pheochromocytoma cause hypertensive retinopathy of Groups III and IV in previously normal fundi. When alleviated, the ophthalmoscopic appearance of the fundus may be restored to normal. If the hypertension has caused fibrinoid necrosis, and is then corrected, the fundus will resemble that seen in Group II. The authors of this classification did not describe the hard deposits that may occur in Group II. An error is introduced if such deposits, rather than cotton-wool patches, are the basis for classifying the fundus disease as Group III.

GLOMERULONEPHRITIS, ECLAMPSIA, AND PHEOCHROMOCYTOMA

The retinal manifestation of glomerulonephritis is entirely related to the vascular hypertension produced. The fundi show advanced arteriolar sclerosis. Superimposed on these changes is the development of cotton-wool patches and retinal hemorrhages. The combination suggests a severe hypertensive vascular disease that has been present for a long period.

In eclampsia, the hypertensive vascular changes occur in a fundus that has not previously been the site of vascular change. The rapid onset of a severe hypertension causes a generalized arteriolar spasm. Cotton-wool patches occur together with much retinal edema, giving the retina a wet, edematous, "shot silk" appearance. The hemodynamic disturbances may be so severe that a bilateral retinal detachment occurs without holes in the retina. Once the hypertension is corrected, the fundi rapidly return to normal.

Pheochromocytoma and unilateral renal disease cause hypertension with the fundus changes of severe hypertension without antecedent vascular disease. Usually the hypertension develops more slowly than that seen in eclampsia, and the retina is less edematous. If the condition is corrected early in the course of hypertension, the fundus returns to normal. If the condition persists for some time before correction of the hypertension, the hemorrhages and deposits disappear, but the arteriolar constriction and variation in caliber tend to persist.

RENAL TRANSPLANTATION

About one third of patients receiving a kidney transplant develop some type of ocular complication. Many have had severe hypertension for many years before the transplant, and their retinal blood vessels have severe changes of arteriolar sclerosis. Except when the donor kidney is obtained from an identical twin, nearly all patients develop signs of rejection and require prolonged therapy with immunosuppressive drugs. After successful transplantation, there is a period of severe hypertension, and in many patients the preexisting arteriolar sclerosis limits the capacity of the vasculature of the eyes to respond to another episode of hypertension. Posterior subcapsular cataracts, seldom reducing visual acuity below 20/40, develop in about one fourth of the patients. The incidence parallels the high corticosteroid dosage. Corticosteroid-induced glaucoma may occur, but less frequently than when corticosteroids are instilled topically. Cytomegalic virus inclusion disease, fungal retinitis, herpes keratitis, and opportunistic ocular infections with organisms usually considered nonpathogenic are seen. Cancers develop in 4% to 6% of renal transplant patients. Malignant skin neoplasms with squamous cell carcinoma are the most common type. The eyelids and ocular adnexa may be involved. Early excision rather than observation is indicated.

BIBLIOGRAPHY

Anderson, W.B.: Examination of the retina. In Hurst, J.W., editor: The heart, ed. 6, New York, 1986, McGraw-Hill Book Co.

Arruga, J., and Sanders, M.D.: Ophthalmologic findings in 70 patients with evidence of retinal embolism, Ophthalmology 89:1336, 1982.

Braunwald, E., editor: Heart disease: a textbook of cardiovascular medicine, vol. 1, ed. 2, Philadelphia, 1984, W.B. Saunders Co.

Cogan, D.G.: Major problems in internal medicine, vol. 3, ophthalmic manifestations of systemic vascular disease, Philadelphia, 1974, W.B. Saunders Co.

Hayreh, S.S., Servais, G.E., and Virdi, P.S.: Fundus lesions in malignant hypertension: IV. Focal intraretinal periarteriolar transudates, Ophthalmology 93:60, 1986.

Hayreh, S.S., Servais, G.E., Virdi, P.S., Marcus, M.L., Rojas, P., and Woolson, R.F.: Fundus lesions in malignant hypertension: III. Arterial blood pressure, biochemical, and fundus changes, Ophthalmology 93:45, 1986.

Michaelson, I.C.: Textbook of the fundus of the eye, ed. 3, Baltimore, 1980, The Williams & Wilkins Co.

Nover, A.: The ocular fundus, ed. 4, translated by F. Blodi, Philadelphia, 1980, Lea & Febiger.

Raitta, C., and Kaitila, I.: The ophthalmological findings in autosomal recessive severe juvenile arteriosclerosis, Acta Ophthalmol. 63:175, 1985.

28

HEMATOLOGIC AND
HEMATOPOIETIC DISORDERS

Diseases of the blood and blood-forming organs can be divided into disorders affecting primarily the erythrocytes, leukocytes, or platelets. Abnormalities in their number, shape, survival time, metabolism, cell membranes, or special function may lead to marked ocular changes. Sometimes ocular signs or symptoms, or both, lead to the appropriate diagnostic tests, as in some hemoglobinopathies and macroglobulinemias. In other instances, the ocular changes are only incidental to the blood disease. This topic is so encompassing that reference will be made here mainly to those diseases in which there are more or less specific ocular changes.

HEMOGLOBINOPATHIES

Hemoglobin consists of a protein molecule, globin, bound to four molecules of heme, an iron and protoporphyrin compound. The globin is composed of two pairs of amino acid chains that differ in the sequence and composition of their constituent amino acids. Four normal amino acid chains occur in humans: alpha, beta, gamma, and delta. Separate pairs of allelic genes control their structure.

Normal adult hemoglobin consists mainly (97%) of hemoglobin A (Hb A), which has a pair of alpha amino acid chains and a pair of beta amino acid chains. Normal adults also have a minor amount of hemoglobin (3%) composed of a pair of alpha chains and a pair of

delta chains (Hb A_2). Fetal hemoglobin (Hb F), which is normally formed in trace amounts after birth, contains a pair of alpha chains and a pair of gamma chains.

An alteration in the sequence of amino acids in the amino acid chains may cause changes in the shape, oxygen affinity, electrophoretic mobility, pliability, solubility, and life span of the hemoglobin molecule. Most variations of clinical importance (Table 28-1) involve the beta chain. The variants are tabulated according to the position in the amino acid chain in which the amino acid substitution has occurred. Thus, sickle hemoglobin (Hb S) is designated $\alpha_2\beta_2^{6 \ glu \ \to \ val}$ indicating that valine has been substituted for glutamic acid in the sixth position of the beta chain. Hb C has a structure of $\alpha_2\beta_2^{6 \ glu \ \to \ lysine}$.

SICKLE CELL SYNDROMES

Sickle cell anemia or homozygous HbS disease occurs when each parent provides a gene for hemoglobin S. From 70% to 98% of the individual's hemoglobin is hemoglobin S and the remainder is hemoglobin F. Deoxygenated hemoglobin polymerizes to form a gel and subsequently a crystal. This results in an elongated, distorted erythrocyte, the sickle cell. The cell passes through capillaries with difficulty and is responsible for sluggish blood flow, tissue hypoxia, and infarction. Patients with sickle cell anemia experience symptoms caused by hemo-

Table 28-1. Hemoglobinopathies of major ophthalmic interest

Sickle cell anemia: SS disease ($\alpha_2\beta_2^{6\ glu \rightarrow val}$ and $\alpha_2\beta_2^{6\ glu \rightarrow val}$)
  Each parent provides Hb S
Sickle cell trait: SA disease ($\alpha_2\beta_2^{6\ glu \rightarrow val}$ and $\alpha_2\beta_2$)
  One parent provides Hb S and one parent provides normal Hb A
Sickle cell disease: SC disease ($\alpha_2\beta_2^{6\ glu \rightarrow val}$ and $\alpha_2\beta_2^{6\ glu \rightarrow lysine}$)
  One parent provides Hb S and one parent provides Hb C
Hemoglobin C trait: AC disease ($\alpha_2\beta_2$ and $\alpha_2\beta_2^{6\ glu \rightarrow lysine}$)
  One parent provides normal Hb A and one parent provides Hb C
Sickle cell β-thalassemia: S-β-thalassemia ($\alpha_2\beta_2^{6\ glu \rightarrow val}$ and $\alpha_2\delta_2$)
  One parent provides Hb S and one parent provides β-thalassemia

lytic anemia and microvascular thrombi. Vascular thrombi result in strokes, retinal infarcts, atrophy of the spleen (with resultant susceptibility to bacterial infection), aseptic necrosis of bones, inability to concentrate urine, priapism, and placental insufficiency with spontaneous abortion. Episodic painful crises are caused by bone and organ infarction.

In sickle cell trait, Hb SA disease, one parent provides the gene for sickle cell hemoglobin (Hb S) and the other provides a gene for normal hemoglobin (Hb A). In sickle cell disease, Hb SC disease, one parent provides the gene for sickle cell hemoglobin and the other for hemoglobin C. The resultant Hb SC is the origin of the most severe retinopathy caused by sickle cell syndrome.

The ocular lesions are caused by conjunctival or retinal arteriole thrombi. The conjunctival changes have no symptoms. They consist of multiple, short, comma-shaped, or distorted isolated capillary segments that do not seem to be connected to the vascular network. Conjunctival changes are most marked in Hb SS anemia, mild in Hb SC disease, and rare in Hb SA trait.

The retinal changes are similar to those caused by other diseases that result in occlusion of the arterioles of the peripheral retina. Initially there is capillary occlusion, and the retina peripheral to the occlusion appears white because of edema. This is followed by narrowing of the peripheral arterioles and tortuosity of the veins. An occluded arteriole ends abruptly, and the retina beyond appears avascular (Fig. 28-1) Salmon-patch hemorrhages in the peripheral retina are followed by retinoschisis as blood absorbs. The retinoschisis is lined with iridescent hemosiderin-filled macrophages (iridescent deposits). Retinal pigment epithelium proliferation at the equator with areas of chorioretinal atrophy having black stellate borders causes black sunburst lesions.

The zone between the ischemic and normal retina is the site of arteriolar-venular anastomosis that is followed by neovascularization on the surface of the retina. The new blood vessels initially lie flat on the retina and have a sea-fan configuration. These new blood vessels continue to grow and, with collapse of the vitreous, are drawn into the vitreous cavity, and subsequently rupture with vitreous hemorrhage.

Of all sickle cell syndromes, patients with Hb SC disease are most vulnerable to retinal complications. Generally, retinal infarction is uncommon in Hb SS anemia and Hb SA trait.

White persons of Mediterranean ancestry or black persons who develop hemolytic anemia, angioid streaks, peripheral retinal neovascularization, or recurrent vitreous hemorrhages should have hemoglobin electrophoresis. Correction of rhegmatogenous retinal separation in patients with hemoglobinopathies is difficult, since encircling bands may cause anterior segment ischemia. Subsequent sickling with anterior ciliary artery occlusion may cause anterior segment necrosis. The risk may be minimized by preoperative exchange transfusion. Tractional retinal detachment and persistent vitreous hemorrhage are managed by vitrectomy.

Photocoagulation of newly formed blood vessels by means of a xenon arc (Fig. 28-1, C) or argon laser photocoagulator may minimize bleeding into the vitreous.

THALASSEMIA SYNDROMES

The thalassemia ("the sea") syndromes are hereditary abnormalities in which the rate of normal hemoglobin synthesis is impaired and in which the number of alpha or beta chains may be insufficient. The major group occurs because of a deficiency in the rate of synthesis of beta chains (beta-thalassemia) and substitu-

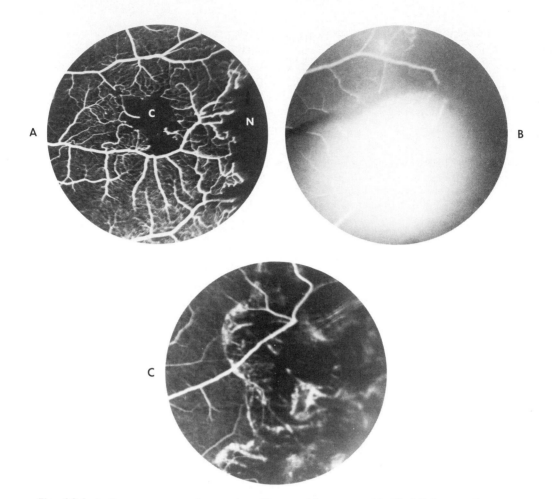

Fig. 28-1. A, Late venous angiogram in a 23-year-old woman with Hb SC disease. Because of arteriolar occlusion there is a central area *(C)* of failure of capillary filling with fluorescein. There is distal occlusion in the periphery and early neovascularization adjacent to this area *(N).* **B,** In the extreme periphery new blood vessels leak fluorescein. **C,** The new blood vessels have been destroyed by xenon photocoagulation of the retina.

tion of delta chains. A deficiency of alpha chains (alpha-thalassemia) is more difficult to recognize and less clinically severe.

Hemolytic anemia and excessive deposition of iron in spleen, liver, and kidneys dominate the systemic aspects of the condition. The onset is in infancy, and the children have flat hypoplastic facies with prominent epicanthal folds. There may be neovascularization of the peripheral retina as in sickle cell disease. The thalassemia syndromes may be combined with sickle cell hemoglobinopathies.

POLYCYTHEMIA

Polycythemia is a myeloproliferative disorder in which the red blood cell count, hemoglobin, and hematocrit exceed the normal. It occurs as absolute and relative types.

Absolute polycythemia (Rubra vera) is caused by an increase in the red blood cell mass. There is decreased erythropoietin and generalized increased hematopoiesis causing a panmyelosis. Relative polycythemia is caused by a decrease in plasma volume. There is excessive release of erythropoietin, a high normal red blood cell mass, and a low normal plasma volume. Relative polycythemia occurs most commonly in obese, hypertensive men who smoke, and the resulting blood hyperviscosity is a factor in some retinal vascular occlusive disease. Relative polycythemia also occurs in dehydration; in response to low oxygen tension in mountain dwellers; in patients with obstructive pulmonary disease, hypernephromas, kidney cysts, cerebellar hemangiomas, and uterine myomas; and in cyanotic types of congenital heart disease.

In absolute polycythemia, the increased red blood cell mass increases the volume and decreases the velocity of the blood. There is venous engorgement, skin cyanosis, headache, tinnitus, and nasal and gastric bleeding. The spleen and liver are enlarged. The conjunctival and retinal veins are dilated. The fundus is dusky red (cyanosis retinae) with the appearance of an impending vein occlusion. The ocular abnormalities may disappear with phlebotomy. Retinal vein occlusion, papilledema, retinal neovascularization, and retinal arteriolar spasm may occur.

LEUKOCYTE ABNORMALITIES

Leukocytes (and erythrocytes) develop from a common precursor stem cell that becomes committed to the production of macrophages, granulocytes (neutrophils, eosinophils, and basophils), lymphocytes, or monocytes.

Neutrophilic (polymorphonuclear) leukocytes function in phagocytosis and destruction of microorganisms by mobilization, adherence, chemotaxis, phagocytosis, cytolysis, digestion, and extracellular release. Leukocyte mobilization (leukocytosis) and adherence to the endothelial wall in the affected area are direct effects of microbial invasion. Many factors affect chemotaxis: low molecular weight compounds of bacteria, complement-derived factors released by bacteria and damaged tissues, agents from lymphocytes and macrophages, and other products.

Eosinophilic leukocytes function as part of the immunologic system and congregate around certain antigens, especially reactions involving immunoglobulin E. The eosinophil modulates IgE-mediated allergic reactions in which histamine is released from mast and basophilic cells.

Basophilic leukocyte and mast cells are the cellular mediator of immediate hypersensitivity reactions. Their cell membranes contain receptors for IgE, which when bound to an antigen cause the cells to release histamine, eosinophilic chemotactic factors, and other mediators of the immediate hypersensitivity reaction.

Stem cells from bone marrow may mature to B lymphocytes or T lymphocytes. B lymphocytes mature under control of "bursal equivalent" cells (gut-associated lymphoid tissue: Peyer patches, appendix, and others), whereas T lymphocytes mature under control of the thymus gland.

B lymphocytes bind macrophage-processed antigens in a process aided by the helper T cell (some simple antigens elicit an antibody response without helper T cells). After activation, B lymphocytes are transformed to lymphoblasts and plasma cells and subsequently produce immunoglobulins, usually an antibody of a single class: IgG (four subclasses), IgA (two subclasses), IgD, IgE, and IgM. Suppressor T cells activated by interleukin-2 suppress the immune response, probably by acting on helper T cells (see chapter on infectious diseases).

T lymphocytes are associated with cell-mediated immune reactions against targets such as transplants, infectious agents, and tumors. Macrophages bind antigen and become highly immunogenic for T lymphocytes. Sensitized T lymphocytes in turn regulate the differentiation of B lymphocytes into immunoglobulin-producing plasma cells by stimulation (helper) and suppression (suppressor). Stimulation of activated T lymphocytes by an antigen not only regulates B lymphocytes but produces a variety of lymphokines that activate macrophages and participate in cell-mediated immunity and lymphocyte transformation. Mediators include migration inhibitor factor that prevents macrophages from leaving an inflammatory site together with macrophage aggregation factor that brings macrophages to the site, and macrophage activity factor that increases the biologic activity of macrophages. Other mediators include interferon, lymphotoxin, chemotactin, skin reactive factor, and transfer factor. Cytotoxic T lymphocytes specifically attach to and destroy target cells such as tumor cells. K or killer T lymphocytes act in conjunction with antibody to attack target cells (antibody-mediated lympholysis). Target specificity occurs only through the specific antibody with which it functions.

PLASMA CELL DYSCRASIAS

Plasma cell dyscrasias are disorders resulting from a proliferation of a clone of B lymphocyte-derived cells that synthesize an excessive amount of a specific immunoglobulin. Those with ocular features include multiple myeloma, macroglobulinemia, and primary amyloidosis.

Multiple myeloma. This is a malignant neoplasm of plasma cells involving mainly bone and bone marrow. The malignant plasma cell clone elaborates an excess of a single immunoglobulin (M protein). Most patients (55%) have an excess of IgG; about 25% have IgA. In both of these groups of patients and the remainder, the two light chains of the immunoglobulin molecule are not linked to the two heavy chains. The light chains appear in the urine (Bence-Jones protein) and may accumulate in the serum. The peak age for occurrence of multiple myeloma is 50 to 70 years; it is slightly more common in men than women, and is particularly common in blacks.

Patients have chronic bone pain, pathologic fractures, recurrent infection, and renal failure. Osteolytic bone lesions are characteristic. Bone marrow aspiration and biopsy, serum and urine electrophoresis of protein, and complete skeletal x-ray survey are required.

The ocular signs may be divided into two main groups: (1) those resulting from the neoplasm itself, such as orbital tumor, compression of cranial nerves within the orbit or head, and papilledema; and (2) those secondary to blood hyperviscosity, such as retinal hemorrhage and vascular occlusion. Cysts of the pars plana that are filled with protein, possibly a myeloma globulin, are found in about one third of the eyes removed at autopsy from patients with multiple myeloma.

Diffuse uveal accumulation of leukocytes may occur. Sludging and dilation of conjunctival blood vessels occur in cryoglobulinemia, and the signs may be accentuated by irrigating the conjunctiva with cold water. Treatment consists of cytotoxic agents, ambulation, and adequate hydration.

Waldenström macroglobulinemia. This is a generalized abnormality of plasma cells that synthesize and secrete IgM. The onset of the disease in the fifth or sixth decade is characterized by severe anemia, lymphadenopathy, splenomegaly, and hepatomegaly. The IgM globulins and cryoglobulins increase the blood viscosity, which may cause vascular occlusions involving almost any system.

The blood hyperviscosity produces a spectacular fundus appearance of dilated veins, hemorrhages, cotton-wool patches, and exudative retinal detachment. Treatment is by means of cytotoxic agents. When increased blood viscosity causes severe ocular or systemic signs, plasmaphoresis may bring about prompt improvement.

Crystalline inclusions of the cornea and conjunctiva occur in both multiple myeloma and Waldenström macroglobulinemia. The crystals are intracytoplasmic, light kappa chains of immunoglobulins. They may appear as early as 5 years before the onset of the overt disease.

Leukemia. The leukemias are a neoplastic disorder of hematopoietic tissue characterized by abnormal proliferation of leukocytes, leukocyte precursor cells, or both. They may be classified as acute or chronic according to the maturity of cells in the peripheral blood or bone marrow and according to cell type involved: granulocytic or lymphocytic. The greatest incidence is before 5 years and after 50 years of age.

Clinically, leukocytes infiltrate bone marrow, liver, spleen, and lymph nodes. Subperiosteal infiltration causes bone pain, and pathologic fractures may occur. Infiltration into the brain may cause ophthalmoplegia, deafness, or Ménière syndrome. Leukemic meningitis is common in treated cases, presumably because the chemical antileukemic agents do not cross the blood-brain barrier, so that leukemic cells proliferate in the meninges. Internal hydrocephalus may occur, causing headache, nausea, increased cerebrospinal fluid pressure, and papilledema.

The ocular changes in leukemia are caused by infiltration, hemorrhage, or both into the conjunctiva, sclera, retina, and choroid. Acute leukemia is more likely to cause ocular signs than chronic leukemia, but in both types changes usually are reversible with remission. There is no clinical difference in ocular changes in lymphocytic leukemia and in myelocytic leukemia.

Leukemic retinopathy occurs in both acute and chronic forms of leukemia, but is more common in a relapse of an acute type. The main ophthalmoscopic signs are (1) dilated, tortuous retinal veins of irregular caliber that may be sausage-shaped; (2) sheathing of retinal ves-

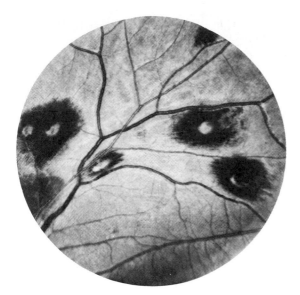

Fig. 28-2. Retinal hemorrhages in a 19-year-old man with acute myelogenous leukemia. The white spots at the center of the hemorrhage are leukocytes.

sels as a result of leukocytic perivascular infiltration; (3) pallor of the blood column caused by anemia or high leukocyte concentration; (4) round or flame-shaped intraretinal hemorrhages, which commonly have a central white area of leukemic cells (Fig. 28-2); (5) a subhyaloid hemorrhage, which rarely occurs and may break into the vitreous; and (6) hard yellow-white deposits (exudates) and occasionally cotton-wool patches. Peripheral retinal microaneurysms demonstrated with fluorescein angiography may occur in chronic forms of leukemia. The choroid is often packed with leukemic cells, but visual symptoms are usually absent.

The conjunctiva is subtly and frequently involved in acute leukemia. There is a slight thickening of conjunctiva near the corneoscleral limbus from leukemic infiltrates. Infiltrates in the sclera are found on histologic study but do not cause clinical signs.

Hemorrhage usually occurs when the platelet count is less than 20,000/mm^3. It may involve the mucous membranes, skin, kidney, conjunctiva, orbit, and retina. The retinal hemorrhage may be a large preretinal collection of blood with a meniscus. Subarachnoid hemorrhage may cause death.

Leukemic infiltration compresses the lacri-mal drainage system and predisposes to infection (dacryocystitis). Intracranial infiltration may cause papilledema and cranial nerve palsies. Optic nerve infiltration reduces vision and causes an afferent pupillary defect.

Myeloid sarcoma (granulocytic sarcoma or chloroma) is a tumor manifestation of granulocytic leukemia that develops preferentially in the periosteum of the skull. It occurs mainly in children, and boys are more frequently affected than girls. Proptosis attributable to orbital involvement may be severe. Histologic stains for esterase activity aid in the diagnosis when the tumor precedes overt leukemia. The differential diagnosis of a rapidly progressing orbital tumor in a child includes rhabdomyosarcoma, Burkitt lymphoma, metastatic neuroblastoma, and myeloid sarcoma, provided retinoblastoma is excluded by ophthalmoscopy.

Lymphocytic neoplasms. Malignant lymphoma of the orbit and lacrimal glands develops painlessly and rapidly in middle-aged adults. Most develop from monoclonal B lymphocytes and have immunoglobulins other than IgG on the cell surface membranes. Histologic study is necessary for diagnosis. In 25% of the patients, the disease is limited to the orbit, whereas the other 75% have systemic lymphoma.

Evaluation for systemic lymphoma should include a chest x-ray, complete blood cell count, serum protein electrophoresis, bone marrow biopsy, liver and bone scans, lymphangiography, and computed tomography for retroperitoneal lymphoma. The orbit should be treated with radiotherapy and the systemic lymphoma with chemotherapy. If the lymphoma is limited to the lacrimal gland or orbit, only radiation is indicated.

The ocular changes include the following: (1) eyelid involvement, with painless, progressive infiltration; (2) a characteristic subconjunctival tumor, frequently with smooth surfaces in the lower cul-de-sac; and (3) orbital or lacrimal gland enlargement, with proptosis causing diplopia, ocular compression, and the like.

Treatment is individualized as to site of involvement and symptoms and includes surgery, irradiation, chemotherapy, and corticosteroids. Commonly the ocular manifestations can be resolved with a dosage of radiation too low to cause cataract.

The signs and symptoms of reactive lymphoid hyperplasia are similar to those of malignant lymphoma, and histologic differentiation is necessary. About 20% of patients with reactive lymphoid hyperplasia subsequently develop systemic lymphomas. Reactive lymphoid hyperplasia of the uvea may cause signs of uveitis.

Intraocular reticulum cell sarcoma (histiocyte type of lymphoma) causes signs of uveitis in middle-aged men who may have microgliomatosis of the brain.

SYSTEMIC HEMORRHAGE

Ischemic optic nerve atrophy may follow severe spontaneous gastrointestinal hemorrhage. Loss of vision occurs either immediately or several days later. The retinal arteries and the veins are attentuated, the fundus is pale, and the optic disk may be edematous. Cotton-wool patches may occur. There may be permanent, complete blindness, or vision may improve to normal. More often the vision remains at the 20/200 level, and optic atrophy is evident. Acute blood loss may also cause visual defects from cortical ischemia without ocular fundus changes.

Chronic or acute anemia may cause a transient loss of vision in one or both eyes. The symptoms strongly suggest occlusive disease involving the carotid-basilar system. Hypoxia secondary to hemorrhage may aggravate the visual defects of glaucoma.

AMYLOIDOSIS

Many different disease processes result in the extracellular deposition of an inert protein: B-pleated sheet (amyloid). Amyloid deposition occurs in association with plasma cell dyscrasias as a reaction to recurrent acute and chronic suppurative or granulomatous infections (tuberculosis), chronic inflammations (rheumatoid arthritis), tumors of nonlymphoreticular origin (Hodgkin disease), or renal and bladder adenocarcinoma. It occurs as a hereditary disease in generalized neuropathic and nonneuropathic forms and in a localized form in lattice dystrophy of the cornea.

In systemic amyloidosis the material is present in the conjunctiva, in the eyelids, in the uveal tract, and in the retina and vitreous body. The protein is apparently secreted into the vitreous cavity without causing retinal abnormalities. Early prominent perivascular sheathing may be observed in the retina. Amyloid in the vitreous humor may originate from the walls of the retinal blood vessels. Ophthalmoscopically, the vitreous opacities look like veils of glasswool. Rarely, patients with hereditary systemic amyloidosis have orbital amyloidosis with deposition in the ciliary ganglion that may cause pupillary abnormalities. Additionally, external ophthalmoplegia, diplopia, and optic neuropathy have been reported in isolated cases. Conjunctival biopsy material may indicate the accumulation of amyloid.

Lattice dystrophy of the cornea, an autosomal dominant abnormality, is a type of localized amyloidosis. A similar lattice dystrophy has also been seen in patients with hereditary amyloidosis. The lesions appear as centrally located, raised, gelatinous masses that resemble the hereditary lattice degeneration.

A protein related to the light-chain of immunoglobulins (L) is the major component of deposits associated with plasma cell dysproteinemias. A protein (protein AA) unrelated to immunoglobulins is the major component of deposits occurring with reactive amyloidosis. The protein in lattice dystrophy of the cornea is protein AA.

Diagnosis is based on demonstration of β-fibrils in a tissue specimen stained with congo red and examined by polarization microscopy. Systemic amyloidosis is almost invariably fatal. In reactive amyloidosis, recovery depends on control of the underlying disorder. Vitrectomy improves vision in amyloidosis causing opacification of the vitreous humor. Keratoplasty improves vision in a patient with lattice corneal dystrophy.

JUVENILE OCULAR XANTHOGRANULOMA

This is an ocular complication of what is usually considered to be a disease solely of the skin. Inconspicuous, small, yellow-orange plaques on the head and trunk develop during the first 3 years of life. They disappear without treatment. If removed for histologic study, the scar may be infiltrated with a similar plaque.

Tumors of the iris, ciliary body, or both are the most common ocular involvement. Episodes of spontaneous bleeding cause hyphema and secondary glaucoma. Glaucoma and enlargement of the globe may occur without hyphema. The iris and the ciliary body are infiltrated with histiocytes, which become fused to form giant (Teuton) cells. The ocular disease is responsive to small doses of radiation.

Other causes of hyphema, such as retinoblastoma, leukemia, injury, and persistent primary vitreous, should be excluded. The occurence of typical skin lesions should distinguish secondary glaucoma from congential glaucoma caused by either a malformation of the chamber angle or neurofibromatosis of Recklinghausen.

BIBLIOGRAPHY
General

Smolin, G., and O'Connor, G.R.: Ocular immunology, Philadelphia, 1981, Lea & Febiger.

Leukocyte abnormalities

Rosenthal, A.R.: Ocular manifestations of leukemia, Ophthalmology **90**:899, 1983.

Amyloidosis

Doft, B.H., Rubinow, A., and Cohen, A.S.: Immunocytochemical demonstration of prealbumin in the vitreous in heredofamilial amyloidosis, Am. J. Ophthalmol. **97**:296, 1984.

Gorevic, P.D., Rodrigues, M.M., Krachmer, J.H., Green, C., Fujihara, S., and Glenner, G.G.: Lack of evidence for protein AA reactivity in amyloid deposits of lattice corneal dystrophy and amyloid corneal degeneration, Am. J. Ophthalmol. **98**:216, 1984.

Rubinow, A., and Cohen, A.S.: Immunocytochemical demonstration of prealbumin in the vitreous in heredofamilial amyloidosis, Am. J. Ophthalmol. **97**:296, 1984.

29

DISORDERS OF CONNECTIVE TISSUE AND JOINTS

Connective tissue provides the structural and supportive elements of the body including the eye. It consists of the following elements: (1) the fibrous proteins, collagen and elastin; (2) proteoglycans, in which proteins are imbedded; and (3) cellular elements.

Collagen is the major structural protein of the body. Its molecules each consist of three polypeptide chains coiled around each other in a triple helix. Each collagen fibril, under electron microscopy, shows characteristic cross-striations, which are repeated at intervals of 60 to 70 nm. Collagen contains a high content of glycine (35%) and alanine (11%), and the distinctive amino acids (21%) proline and 4-hydroxyproline. Eight genetically distinct types of collagen are known; all are present in the cornea. Types IV and V are present in basement membrane, and thus in Descemet membrane, but not in the sclera.

Elastin consists of molecules of two proteins: elastic and elastic fiber microfibrillary protein. They are rich in glycine and alanine but, rather than proline, contain lysine. Elastic properties are due to the amino acid desmosine, a lysine derivative that joins protein so that they can be stretched reversibly in all directions. Elastin forms the middle layer of Bruch membrane and is abundant in the sclera, conjunctiva, and blood vessels. It is absent in the cornea.

The proteoglycans are molecules of protein and polysaccharides in which the polysaccha-ride constitutes most of the weight (the protein predominates in glycoproteins). They constitute an intercellular cement that fills the space between tissues and cells and that also occurs in synovial fluid. Hyaluronic acid, a glycosaminoglycan (an acid mucopolysaccharide), gives the vitreous humor its characteristic viscosity.

The cellular elements of connective tissue are derived from mesenchyme and include: (1) fibroblasts, which are responsible for the elaboration of collagen, elastin, and proteoglycans; (2) macrophages, which function as phagocytes; (3) mast cells, which are rich in histamine and serotonin and are involved in the formation of heparin and possibly of hyaluronic acid (both proteoglycans); (4) B lymphocytes, which produce immunoglobulins; and (5) T lymphocytes with many immune functions.

Connective tissue disorders (Table 29-1) include hereditary defects (see Chapter 24), disorders of abnormal collagen biosynthesis, and a heterozygous group of inflammations of connective tissue sometimes associated with the deposition of a fibrinoid material (an acellular, eosinophilic, proteinaceous deposit, with staining characteristics of fibrin) along connective tissue fibers and within vessel walls.

Marfan syndrome. This is a relatively common autosomal dominant disorder of connective tissue. The major clinical manifestations include ectopia lentis, aortic dilation, dissecting aortic aneurysm, and multiple skeletal de-

Table 29-1. Connective tissue disorders

I. Hereditary disorders
   A. Marfan syndrome
   B. Pseudoxanthoma elasticum
   C. Cutis laxa
   D. Ehlers-Danlos syndrome
      1. Type I: gravis, autosomal dominant.
      2. Type II: mitis, autosomal dominant
      3. Type III: benign hypermobile, autosomal dominant
      4. Type IV: ecchymotic, autosomal dominant or recessive (arterial type)
      5. Type V: X-chromosome-linked recessive
      6. Type VI: autosomal recessive ocular fragility
      7. Type VII: autosomal recessive
         a. Arthrochalasis
         b. Multiplex congenita
      8. Type VIII: Autosomal dominant peridontitis
      9. Type IX: autosomal recessive mental retardation
   E. Osteogenesis imperfecta
   F. Stickler syndrome
II. Acquired disorders
   A. Seropositive conditions
      1. Sjögren syndrome
      2. Polyarthritis
         a. Rheumatoid arthritis
         b. Juvenile rheumatoid arthritis
      3. Systemic lupus erythematosus
      4. Scleroderma (progressive systemic sclerosis)
      5. Psoriatic arthritis
      6. Polymyositis and dermatomyositis
      7. Mixed connective tissue diseases
   B. Seronegative conditions
      1. Polyarthritis of unknown etiology
         a. Ankylosing spondylitis
         b. Reiter syndrome
      2. Necrotizing angiitis
         a. Periarteritis nodosa
         b. Hypersensitivity angiitis
         c. Giant cell arteritis
         d. Wegener granulomatosis
         e. Takayasu disease
         f. Cogan syndrome
      3. Other conditions
         a. Ulcerative colitis
         b. Crohn disease
         c. Behçet syndrome
         d. Erythema nodosum
         e. Relapsing polychondritis
         f. Sarcoidosis
         g. Amyloidosis

fects, particularly excessive length of long bones. The pubis-to-sole measurement is characteristically in excess of the pubis-to-vertex measurement, and the arm span is in excess of the height. The more distal bones tend to demonstrate excessive length (arachnodactyly: spider fingers). There is a weakness of the joint capsule, causing flatfoot, hyperextensibility of the joints, recurrent dislocation of the hip, and kyphoscoliosis. Pigeon breast (pectus excavatum) may occur. Frequently the patient has a long, narrow face, a highly arched palate, and prognathism. Degeneration of the medial coat of the aorta is the usual cause of death.

Subluxation of the lens (ectopia lentis) is the major ocular change. Both lenses subluxate early in life, possibly in utero. The lenses are displaced upward and the inferior zonule is attenuated or fragmented. The zonular fibers superiorly appear shortened and taut. Ectopia lentis may be suspected only because of the abnormal mobility of the iris (iridodonesis), which lacks the support of the lens. The lens may be smaller than normal and may be spherical. In some patients, ectopia lentis may be the only sign of the Marfan syndrome.

Patients tend to be myopic and to develop peripheral retinal degeneration (lattice) that can cause holes and retinal detachment. The retinal degeneration is apparently related to an elastin defect and not to the myopia. Heterochromia iridis, translucence of the iris, keratoconus, megalocornea, and blue scleras may be present. In general, surgical removal of the subluxated lens is not indicated. Complications are common, and surgery should be deferred unless necessitated by secondary glaucoma caused by lens dislocation.

The major differential diagnosis includes other causes of ectopia lentis, particularly cystathione β-synthase deficiency (homocystinuria), Stickler syndrome, or Weill-Marchesani syndrome.

Pseudoxanthoma elasticum. This is either an autosomal recessive or dominant abnormality characterized by changes in the skin, cardiovascular system, and eyes. The basic defect is presumably in elastin, and widespread systemic changes occur secondary to degeneration of the medial wall of arteries. The skin of the face, neck, axillary folds, inguinal folds, and cubital and periumbilical areas becomes lax, grooved, redundant, relatively inelastic, and resembles coarse-grained Moroccan leather. Involvement of the small arteries may cause hemorrhages in the gastrointestinal tract, brain, kidney, uterus, bladder, and nose. A severe hypertension that aggravates the hemorrhagic tendency commonly occurs.

The characteristic ocular change is angioid streaks, a bizarre network of pigmented lines affecting particularly the posterior pole of the retina and often associated with subretinal neovascularization and focal chorioretinal atrophy. They are the result of degeneration of the elastic layer of Bruch membrane. A subretinal neovascular network extending beneath the fovea centralis results in a fibrovascular proliferation that destroys the fovea centralis.

Ehlers-Danlos syndrome. This is a heterogeneous group of hereditary defects of collagen biosynthesis (see Table 29-1). There is hyperextensibility of the joints, fragile skin, easy bruising, and poor wound healing. Poor synthesis of fetal membranes often causes premature birth. Minor trauma often causes gaping lacerations that must be repaired with adhesive bridges, since the friable skin will not hold sutures. Arterial rupture with death may follow relatively minor accidents. Systemic abnormalities include arterial aneurysms, diaphragmatic hernia, and congenital defects of the heart, the respiratory and gastrointestinal tracts, and the genitalia.

The skin of the eyelids is often involved. Epicanthal folds may be present. The eyelids are easily everted. Esotropia is common, as are blue scleras and microcorneas. Glaucoma has been recorded. Myopia is common. Additionally, there may be keratoconus, ectopia lentis, proliferative retinopathy, hemorrhages into the retina, and traction detachment of the retina.

In the ocular type there is a deficiency of lysyl hydrolase, which catalyzes the hydroxylation of lysine to hydroxylysine, resulting in weakening of collagen cross-linking. Microcornea or megalocornea, extreme thinning of the cornea, corneal rupture caused by slight trauma, ectopia lentis, cataract, and retinal separation occur. Every patient with blue scleras should be warned against contact sports, because the thinning of their corneas (fragilitas oculi) predisposes the eye to rupture.

Osteogenesis imperfecta (brittle bones, blue scleras, and premature deafness). This is a defect of type I collagen (the only collagen of adult bone). Some 80% of the patients have mild bone disease and autosomal dominant inheritance. Fractures occur mainly in childhood, deformity is minimal, and eventual stature is nearly normal. Blue scleras are prominent. There is early onset of deafness, joints are hypermobile, tendons may rupture, and aortic valves are thin and sometimes incompetent. In a rare, dominantly inherited type (IV), the scleras are of normal appearance, but the bone disease is considerably more severe. Infants with a grossly abnormal skeleton die at or near birth (type II), while the rare survivor joins children with a progressively severe deformity (type III).

The scleras in patients with osteogenesis imperfecta type I are vividly blue. The color, described as robin's egg blue, slate blue, and Wedgwood blue, is apparently caused by thinning of the sclera so that the choroid is seen beneath. Often the corneoscleral limbus is white, resulting in a Saturn ring. Corneal arcus is common. The eyes are frequently hyperopic, and there may be keratoconus, megalocornea, and maculas of the cornea.

Treatment is symptomatic.

Sjögren syndrome. This is a chronic connective tissue disorder that predominantly affects women (90%). It is manifested by keratoconjunctivitis sicca (dry eyes), xerostomia (dry mouth), and rheumatoid arthritis or other connective tissue disease. HLA-B8 is more common in patients with Sjögren syndrome (53%) than in a control population. There is dryness of the eyes, nose, mouth, pharynx, tracheobronchial tree, vagina, stomach, and skin. Small lymphocytes, plasma cells, and reticulum cells infiltrate salivary glands and, occasionally, lacrimal glands, which causes enlargement. Histologic and immunologic abnormalities suggest involvement of both T cell and B cell immunologic mechanisms.

The disorder predominantly affects middle-aged women but may have its onset at extremes of 5 and 72 years of age. It is found in 10% to 15% of patients with rheumatoid arthritis. The syndrome may include dry skin, pancreatitis, interstitial nephritis, hepatobiliary disease, thyroid abnormalities, and lymphoma. Excessive proliferation and abnormal distribution of lymphoid and plasma cells may impair function of major organs.

Keratoconjunctivitis sicca (L. *siccus*, dry) causes burning or smarting of the eyes, sometimes associated with severe photophobia. The symptoms are aggravated by a dry, hot environment. Occasionally filamentary keratitis occurs, in which minute strands of corneal epithelium extend from the corneal surface. Thick, tenacious secretion may gather on the inner corner of the eyelids. Punctate lesions of the conjunctival and corneal epithelium stain with rose bengal or fluorescein. Conjunctival and episcleral vasculitis originating from hypersensitivity (Type III: immune complexes with complement) may cause necrosis of the sclera with perforation of the adjacent cornea. The Schirmer test indicates less than a 5 mm wetting of the filter paper strip. The enzyme lysozyme (muramidase) is decreased in tears. Dryness of the mouth (xerostomia) causes burning pain and paresthesia of the mouth and tongue and atrophy of the lip and oral mucous membrane. Patients are unable to swallow a tablet of medication without drinking water.

The laboratory signs indicate a widespread abnormality of immunologic mechanisms. Plasma cells synthesize large amounts of IgG and IgM, including rheumatoid factor. There are often autoantibodies directed against thyroglobulin, smooth muscle, salivary ducts, and mitochondria. The erythrocyte sedimentation rate is increased. Antinuclear antibodies are common.

Treatment is often unsatisfactory. The dry eye is treated with artificial tears and by avoiding conditions that favor the rapid evaporation of tears, such as hot, dry rooms. Artificial tears may be instilled as often as every 30 to 60 minutes. Closure of the lacrimal puncta to conserve the remaining tears is not often effective and is used only in severe cases.

In some patients malignant lymphomas develop. In severe progressive disease, treatment by means of immune suppression seems useful.

Rheumatoid arthritis. This is a chronic, progressive systemic disease of unknown cause that has a familial tendency and onset between 25 and 50 years of age. Women are affected more commonly (75%) than men. The histocompatibility antigen HLA-DRw4 is found in 70% compared to 28% in the controls. The onset is insidious, with pain and swelling in one or more joints that may become chronic and involve all joints, causing contraction and deformity. There may be systemic disturbances such as lymphadenopathy, splenomegaly, fever, tachycardia, leukocytosis, and increased erythrocyte sedimentation rate. Subcutaneous rheumatoid nodules occur at sites of pressure over bones. They vary in size from 2 or 3 mm to 3 cm in diameter. They contain a central necrotic area surrounded by a zone of monocytic cells enveloped in lymphocytes and monocytes.

Iritis may precede or follow the acute disease but usually accompanies it. Most iritis is mild, may involve either eye, and may be recurrent. The severity of attacks varies. The iritis usually responds quickly to systemic and local corticosteroids. In some patients the inflammation is extremely severe and is unresponsive to therapy, with progression to secondary glaucoma and cataract formation. About 4% of the patients with rheumatoid arthritis develop iritis.

Rheumatoid nodules in the sclera cause scleromalacia perforans (Fig. 29-1), in which the sclera appears to melt away. Additionally, rheumatoid nodules in the sclera may cause a massive granuloma (brawny scleritis or annular scleritis), in which there is massive scar formation, or necroscleritis nodosa, limited to small areas of the anterior sclera.

Juvenile rheumatoid arthritis. This is a chronic inflammation of the joints that occurs before the age of 16 years. It may occur as a systemic illness with fever, rash, and spleen, liver, and heart involvement. Polyarticular juvenile rheumatoid arthritis occurs at about 2 years of age, mainly in girls, and affects mainly the small joints of the hands and feet. Pauciarticular arthritis affects mainly girls with onset at about 5 years of age. Commonly, the knees or ankles are affected, often only one joint.

Iridocyclitis most commonly occurs in patients with pauciarticular involvement, particularly boys with HLA-B27. The iridocyclitis is bilateral and resistant to treatment. Secondary cataract may develop. A band-shaped keratopathy develops (90%), with a deposition of calcium in the Bowman zone of the cornea. It usually accompanies the iridocyclitis. Posterior inflammation is uncommon, but bilateral exudative retinal detachment may occur. Band keratopathy also occurs in degenerated eyes, after excessive vitamin D intake, and in hypercalcemia.

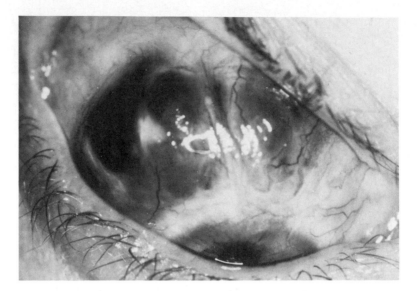

Fig. 29-1. Scleromalacia perforans in a 39-year-old woman with rheumatoid arthritis. The condition has remained unchanged for the past 10 years.

Ankylosing spondylitis (Marie-Strümpell disease). This is a chronic and often progressive inflammatory disease of the lumbosacral and cervical spine often combined with a synovitis of the hips and shoulders. It has a variable course and commonly causes back pain in white men during the third decade of life. Acute anterior uveitis occurs in 20% to 30% of the patients. The diagnosis is often suggested when a young man with recurrent iritis has difficulty in adjusting himself to the chin-rest of a biomicroscope. Histocompatibility typing indicates that 90% to 95% of patients with ankylosing spondylitis have HLA-B27 antigen, as contrasted with 7% in the normal white population. Individuals with Reiter syndrome and acute anterior uveitis also have HLA-B27 antigens but less often than those with ankylosing spondylitis.

Giant cell arteritis. Giant cell arteritis (temporal arteritis, cranial arteritis) is a chronic, disseminated, inflammatory disease of segments of large and medium-sized arteries that occurs mainly in elderly individuals. Possibly it is an autoimmune hypersensitivity to the elastic tissue of arteries. It is probably a part of the same disease process as polymyalgia rheumatica, which occurs without arteritis.

Headache at the onset is severe, boring, and may be intractable to treatment. The temporal arteries, when affected, become prominent and tender. There is often erythema of the overlying skin. Pain on chewing is a common complaint. The erythrocyte sedimentation rate is increased; fever may be present.

One to 4 weeks after the onset of the headache, sudden loss of vision may be caused by inflammation of the central retinal artery or of the short posterior ciliary arteries that supply the optic nerve. There may be occlusion of branches of retinal arteries, retinal hemorrhage, exudates, and occasionally ocular pain. Often both eyes are affected, the second eye from 1 to 21 days after the first.

Palsies of extraocular muscles, especially of the lateral recti muscles, may occur. Loss of vision may occur in some patients without obvious evidence of temporal artery involvement, but biopsy of the temporal artery may indicate the typical histiocytes, epithelioid cells, and multinucleated giant cells in intima and media adjacent to a highly fragmented or absent elastic lamina. Some patients appear curiously unconcerned about the devastating loss of vision.

The diagnosis of giant cell arteritis should be considered in all cases of sudden loss of vision, ocular vascular occlusion, and unexplained ophthalmoplegia in elderly individuals. If ocular symptoms are associated with an increased erythrocyte sedimentation rate, temporal artery biopsy is indicated. Serum alkaline phosphatase and C-reactive protein are increased.

Once vision is lost it seldom improves, but remarkable recovery has been reported. Corticosteroids should be administered before visual loss has occurred in the fellow eye.

Systemic lupus erythematosus. This is a generalized disorder that may involve nearly any system and may be associated with severe constitutional signs. Young women are affected predominantly. The disease appears to result from an initial development of antibodies to many cellular components of the body: nuclear antigens (DNA), cytoplasmic antigens (RNA, ribosomes), clotting factors, and antigens on red and white blood cell surfaces. These antibodies form antigen-antibody-complement complexes (type III hypersensitivity) in the vascular and glomerular basement membranes with resultant damage.

Fever, a facial rash with a "butterfly" distribution, and arthralgia may occur. Glomerulonephritis, pericarditis, myocardial and endocardial lesions, or pleurisy may develop. Mental changes and convulsions may occur. There may be diplopia, nystagmus, and decreased vision. Leukopenia is common. Lupus erythematosus may simulate almost any disease, and the diagnosis may be overlooked because of failure to associate successive involvement of different systems with the same disorder.

External involvement of the eye is mainly erythema and puffiness of the eyelids. Keratoconjunctivitis sicca may occur. The most common ocular sign is cotton-wool patches of the posterior pole. Successive crops of lesions appear and fade during the acute phase of the disease and disappear with remission. Changes other than cotton-wool patches have also been described: optic neuritis (autoimmune), secondary optic atrophy, papilledema, retinal vasculitis, superficial and deep retinal hemorrhages, and arterial or venous occlusion. Chloroquine is widely used in therapy and may itself cause retinal damage.

Dermatomyositis. This is an acute or chronic disease of middle life characterized by dermatitis and diffuse muscle inflammation and degeneration. In patients over 50 years of age, it may be associated with a neoplasm (20%). In childhood, a periorbital edema associated with a lilac-colored erythema of the eyelids (heliotrope rash) is frequent. Cotton-wool patches are the most common ocular finding. Ophthal-

moplegia, nystagmus, and episcleritis have been described.

Periarteritis nodosa. This is a necrotizing angiitis that causes a variety of symptoms depending on the blood vessels involved. Men are affected most frequently (75%), usually between 20 and 50 years of age. Signs of fever, weight loss, and arthralgia occur. Symptoms include abdominal pain, renal disease often causing a vascular hypertension when healed, peripheral neuritis, myocardial infarction, pulmonary infiltration, and asthma, Leukocytosis is present, often with marked eosinophilia, and the sedimentation rate is increased. The disease is often fatal, but remissions and recovery occur. Symptomatic relief follows administration of corticosteroids.

Inflammation of cerebral vessels may cause subarachnoid hemorrhage, headache, vertigo, and convulsions. There may be involvement of motor nerves of the eye or decreased vision caused by angiitis of the optic tract blood vessels or radiation.

Angiitis of ciliary vessels causes conjunctival injection, chemosis, and scleral necrosis. Involvement of the pericorneal arcade may be followed by corneal necrosis beginning at the corneoscleral limbus. Periarteritis of the choroidal vessels has been found histologically with choroidal function not impaired. Ophthalmologic findings are common. Hypertensive retinopathy with papilledema, cotton-wool patches, and vasospasm may follow renal disease and not seem different from any other accelerated (malignant) hypertension. Cotton-wool patches may develop as a sign of vasculitis. They are unrelated to hypertension, as in the other collagen diseases.

Miscellaneous connective tissue disorders. A variety of conditions with prominent ocular signs may be classified in the group of connective tissue disorders. Reiter syndrome (urethritis, conjunctivitis, uveitis) and Behçet syndrome (aphthous ulcers, uveitis) are discussed in the section on uveitis. Cogan syndrome, in which there is interstitial keratitis, deafness, and vestibular signs, is described in the chapter on diseases of the cornea. The several aortic arch inflammations that may be variants of polyarteritis are described in Chapter 26. A variety of localized ocular disorders reflect connective tissue abnormalities but are seldom classed as such: pterygia, pingueculas, corneal dystrophies, and keratoconus.

MUSCLE DISORDERS

Myotonic dystrophy. This is an autosomal dominant disorder characterized by muscle weakness and atrophy, testicular or ovarian atrophy, mental deterioration, and widespread ocular abnormalities. Muscles do not relax normally after voluntary constriction and there may be inability to release after shaking hands. Frontal baldness, atrophy of the facial muscles, enophthalmos, and blepharoptosis combine to produce a long, dull, expressionless face.

Bilateral cataract is the most common ocular sign. The opacities are located in a narrow zone just beneath the lens capsule. They consist of minute, brilliantly colored, scintillating specks (iridescent dust) or snowball-shaped opacities. They result from whorls of plasma membrane of the lens fibers. The intraocular pressure may be low and there is atrophy of the ciliary muscles and vacuolization of the nonpigmented ciliary epithelium. The pupils are miotic and constrict poorly to light. Blepharoconjunctivitis, blepharoptosis, and myotonia of the extraocular muscles occur. There is peripheral retinal pigmentation, retinal arteriolar attenuation, reduced amplitude of the scotopic electroretinogram, and impaired dark adaptation.

Myasthenia gravis. This is a chronic autoimmune disorder of skeletal neuromuscular junctions, characterized by easy fatigability and weakness of voluntary muscle. In normal muscle contraction the neurotransmitter acetylcholine interacts with nicotinic acetylcholine receptors located in the postsynaptic membrane of the motor end plate (see Chapter 3). In myasthenia gravis there is a decrease in both the number of receptors and the sensitivity of the postsynaptic membrane to acetylcholine as the result of an autoimmune hypersensitivity directed against the acetylcholine (nicotinic) receptors. Antibodies in the patient's serum against acetylcholine receptors are diagnostic of myasthenia gravis. The antibody titers, however, do not correlate with the severity of the disease. Women are affected in 65% of the cases when onset occurs before 35 years of age; thereafter there is no sex predilection. Weakness is often exacerbated in the premenstrual period in young women.

Initial symptoms include blepharoptosis, double vision (from extraocular muscle weakness), or blurred vision in about one half of the patients. The remainder develop systemic signs of the disease. Diagnostic ocular signs or symptoms do not occur in the remaining patients, although there may be weakness of the orbicularis oculi muscle in nearly all. In patients with otherwise marked ocular muscle weakness there may be a twitching of the upper eyelid, which strongly suggests myasthenia gravis. It is elicited by asking the patient to change gaze from downward to straight ahead. There also may be rapid movement of the eyes of 3° to 4°, described as quiver, lightning twitches, or oscillations.

The diagnosis is based on the history of fluctuations in strength, single fiber nerve stimulation and electromyography, increased antiacetylcholine-receptor antibody titers, and positive response to edrophonium (Tensilon). (Atropine sulfate, 0.4 mg, should be available to counteract cholinergic toxicity.) Two to ten milliliters of edrophonium are administered intravenously. If myasthenia gravis is present, relief of blepharoptosis, improvement of speech, and generalized muscle strengthening will occur within 30 to 60 seconds and persist 2 to 3 minutes, although the effect of the drug may be unusually short. The extraocular muscles tend to be resistant to cholinergic effects, and ophthalmoplegia may not be grossly responsive, although diplopia may decrease slightly, intraocular pressure may increase, and electromyography of an affected ocular muscle may show increased activity. Diplopia testing is more accurate than the patient's response to awareness of double vision. Intramuscular neostigmine (after premedication with atropine) may provide a more effective test agent in ocular myasthenia gravis.

Hyperthyroidism occurs in 3% to 8% of patients with myasthenia gravis and must be excluded. A syndrome resembling myasthenia occurs in association with oat cell carcinoma of the lung. Topical beta blockers in the treatment of glaucoma may aggravate the symptoms and signs of myasthenia gravis as may treatment with penicillamine.

Systemic anticholoinesterase therapy with neostigmine or pyridostigmine is classic. Blepharoptosis responds well, but extraocular muscle paresis (and diplopia) may be resistant. Corticosteroids, azathioprine, cyclophosphamide, and plasmapheresis may be used. Thymectomy should probably be reserved for seriously ill patients. Intensive respiratory care and support is required for severe systemic exacerbations.

SKIN

Erythema multiforme (Stevens-Johnson syndrome). This is an acute perivascular inflammatory systemic disease that varies in severity from mild skin and mucous membrane lesions to a severe, sometimes fatal systemic disorder. Ophthalmologists describe the disease with conjunctival involvement as Stevens-Johnson syndrome. The disease affects all ages. The cause is not known, but the condition is associated with systemic and ocular herpes simplex infections, toxic reactions to systemic and ocular drugs, mycoplasma infection, and neoplasms. Topical sulfacetamide sodium, topical anesthetics, systemic sulfonamides, acetazolamide, phenytoin (Dilantin), and antibiotics have all been implicated as sensitizing agents.

The onset is variable, with mild to severe constitutional symptoms of fever, malaise, myalgia, and arthralgia and the symptoms of an upper respiratory tract infection. Bullous erosions of skin and mucous membrane develop 1 to 14 days later, often with malaise (Fig. 29-2). The skin lesions develop symmetrically and in crops and vary considerably in appearance. Vesicles and bullae may develop on preexisting macular papules or wheals. A pale white center may be surrounded by shades of erythema, called iris, target, or bull's-eye lesion. Ulcerations and scaling take place with healing, leaving pigmented and depigmented areas. The mouth, pharynx, vagina, and rectum may have erosions and ulcerations. These heal, leaving scarred areas that suggest the diagnosis long after the disease has cleared.

The skin of the eyelids may be involved. A conjunctivitis develops, varying in severity from catarrhal to pseudomembranous. There may be marked swelling of the eyelids. An acute iritis may occur. In severe cases, the cornea may perforate (see Fig. 29-2). The active inflammation may persist for weeks. Treatment during the acute phase is mainly supportive.

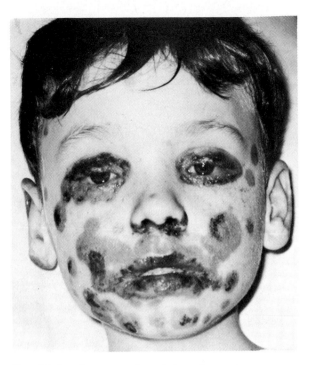

Fig. 29-2. Ulceration of eyelids and mouth in erythema multiforme.

With healing there are often adhesions between the tarsal and the bulbar conjunctivas (symblepharon). Trichiasis is common. The most marked symptom is decreased mucus of the tears as the result of destruction of goblet cells. Scarring and occlusion of the orifices of the accessory and major lacrimal glands reduce the aqueous component of tears. Additionally, the eyes are dry, uncomfortable, and injected. Corneal vascularization occurs easily. Treatment is by means of soft contact lenses, artificial tear substitutes, and all-trans vitamin A ointment.

BIBLIOGRAPHY
General

Foster, C.T., and Yee, M.: Corncoscleral manifestations of Graves' disease, the acquired connective tissue disorders, and systemic vasculitis, Int. Ophthalmol. Clin. **23**:131, 1983.

Malinow, K.L., Molina, R., Gordon, B., Selnes, O.A., Provost, T.T., and Alexander, E.L.: Neuropsychiatric dysfunction in primary Sjögren's syndrome, Ann. Intern. Med. **103**:344, 1985.

Pinals, R.S., Masi, A.T., and Larsen, R.A.: Preliminary criteria for clinical remission in rheumatoid arthritis, Arthritis Rheum. **24**:1308, 1981.

Roidman, C.M., Lavi, S., Moore, A.T., Morin, D.J., Stein, L.D., and Gelfand, E.R.: Tenosynovitis of the superior oblique muscle (Brown syndrome) associated with juvenile rheumatoid arthritis, J. Pediatr. **106**:17, 1985.

Osteogenesis imperfecta

Kaiser-Kupfer, M.I., Podgor, M., McCain, L., Kupfer, C., and Shapiro, J.R.: Correlation of ocular rigidity and blue sclerae in osteogenesis imperfecta, Trans. Ophthalmol. Soc. U.K. **104**:191, 1985.

Smith, R.: Osteogenesis imperfecta 1984, Br. Med. J. **289**:394, 1984.

Giant cell arteritis

Monteiro, M.L.R., Coppeto, J.R., and Greco, P.: Giant cell arteritis of the posterior cerebral circulation presenting with ataxia and ophthalmoplegia, Arch. Ophthalmol. **102**:407, 1984.

Myasthenia gravis

Grob, D., editor: Myasthenia gravis: pathophysiology and management, Ann. N.Y. Acad. Sci. **33**:1981.

Miller, N.R., Morris, J.E., and Maguire, M.: Combined use of neostigmine and ocular motility measurements in the diagnosis of myasthenia gravis, Arch. Ophthalmol. **100**:761, 1982.

Oosterhuis, H.J.G.H.: Myasthenia gravis, Clinical Neurology and Neurosurgery Monographs, vol. 5, New York, 1984, Churchill Livingstone.

Erythema multiforme

Edmond, B.J., Huff, J.C., and Weston, W.L.: Erythema multiforme, Pediatr. Clin. North Am. **30**:631, 1983.

Genvert, G.I., Cohen, E.J., Donnenfeld, E.D., and Blecher, M.H.: Erythema multiforme after use of topical sulfacetamide, Am. J. Ophthalmol. **99**:465, 1985.

Wright, P., and Collin, J.R.O.: The ocular complications of erythema multiforme (Stevens Johnson syndrome) and their management, Trans. Ophthalmol. Soc. U.K. **103**:338, 1983.

Lupus erythematosus

Donzis, P.B., Insler, M.S., Buntin, D.M., and Gately, L.E.: Discoid lupus erythematosus involving the eyelids, Am. J. Ophthalmol. **98**:32, 1984.

APPENDICES

A
GLOSSARY

aberration Difference in focus or magnification as a result of difference in refraction of different wavelengths composing white light.

ablepharon Absence of the eyelids.

abnormal (anomalous) retinal correspondence Condition in which corresponding points on the two retinas do not have the same relative direction in space.

  disharmonious Angle of abnormality is less than the angle of strabismus.

  harmonious Angle of abnormality is the same as the angle of strabismus.

accommodation Process by which the refractive power of the lens is increased through contraction of the ciliary muscle (N III), causing an increased thickness and curvature of the lens.

  amplitude The difference in refraction of the eye at rest and when fully accommodated.

accommodative esotropia Inward deviation of the eyes characteristically more marked for near than far and increased by ciliary muscle contraction in accommodation.

achromatopsia Color vision deficiency.

  atypical Incomplete achromatopsia with normal visual acuity and no nystagmus.

  typical Severe congential deficiency in color vision with reduced vision and nystagmus.

acoria Absence of pupil.

after-cataract Opacity of posterior capsule after extracapsular lens extraction. Secondary cataract.

after-image Persistence of visual response after stimulus stops.

agnosia (visual) Inability to recognize objects by sight while retaining the ability to recognize by touch; a sign of lesions of the angular gyrus of the parieto-occipital fissure.

agraphia (optic) Loss of ability to copy.

albinism Inherited deficiency or absence of melanin in skin, hair, and eyes, or eyes only, caused by an abnormality in melanin synthesis.

  ocular Hereditary absence of melanin in eye transmitted as X chromosome-linked abnormality.

  tyrosinase negative Albinism with an absence of tyrosinase.

  tyrosinase positive Albinism with normal tyrosinase that does not enter pigment cells.

alternating cross-eyes Deviation of the eyes in which either eye may be used for fixation while the other deviates.

amaurosis Blindness.

  fugax Transient blindness, often monocular.

  of Leber Autosomal recessive rod-cone abiotrophy with severely reduced vision.

amblyopia Unilateral decreased visual acuity often caused by deprivation of form vision during visual maturation.

  ex anopsia Functional, refractive, sensory, strabismic, or stimulus deprivation amblyopia now preferred.

  functional Cortical inhibition as in refractive or strabismic amblyopia.

  refractive Results from a refractive error, particularly a marked difference in refraction of the two eyes (anisometropia).

  relative Associated with sensory amblyopia on which is superimposed an inhibition as in strabismic amblyopia.

  sensory Caused by organic disease such as optic atrophy, central retinal degeneration, or cataract.

  strabismic Associated with crossing of the eyes that occurs before the establishment of normal visual acuity in each eye; there appears to be active inhibition of perception of the retinal image transmitted by one eye.

amblyoscope A reflecting stereoscope used to evaluate binocular function.

ametropia Optical condition in which, with eyes at rest, the retina is not in conjugate focus with light rays from distant objects (see hyperopia, myopia, astigmatism, presbyopia).

angiography, fluorescein, ocular Photographic visualization of the passage of fluorescein through the intraocular vessels after intravenous injection.

angioid streaks Degeneration of the elastic layer of lamina basalis (Bruch membrane) causing pigmented striations of the ocular fundus; associated with a variety of systemic diseases such as pseudoxanthoma elasticum, sickle cell disease, and osteitis deformans (Paget disease) and a variety of generalized diseases affecting the elastic lamina of blood vessels.

angioscopy Ophthalmoscopic visualization of passage of fluorescein through the intraocular vessels after intravenous injection.

angle of anomaly (abnormality) In strabismus, the degree an eye deviates from parallelism.

angle-closure glaucoma See closed-angle glaucoma.

angstrom (Å) Unit of wavelength equal to 10^{-10} meter (nanometer now preferred [10^{-9} meter]).

aniridia Almost total absence of iris.

aniseikonia Optical condition in which the retinal images in the two eyes are of different sizes.

anisocoria Condition in which the pupils of the two eyes are of unequal size.

anisometropia Condition in which the refractive errors in the two eyes are different.

ankyloblepharon Condition in which the margins of the eyelids are fused together.

anomalous retinal correspondence *See* abnormal retinal correspondence.

anomalous trichromatism Defect of color vision in which there appears to be a deficiency of one of the cone pigments

anophthalmia Absence of the eye.

aphakia Absence of the crystalline lens of the eye.

aqueous flare Tyndall beam observed with a biomicroscope when excessive protein is present in the anterior aqueous humor.

aqueous humor Fluid that fills the posterior and anterior chambers.

arcuate scotoma Area of blindness in the field of vision of characteristic arc shape; caused by interruption of a nerve fiber bundle in the retina; most often seen in glaucoma.

arcus cornealis Deposition of lipid in the peripheral cornea mainly in the aged (arcus senilis; gerontoxon) and rarely in youth (arcus juvenilis; embryotoxon).

argyria Discoloration of the skin or mucous membranes produced by prolonged administration of silver salts with deposition of metallic silver in tissue.

asteroid hyalosis Fixed opacities composed of a calcium lipid complex that occur in an otherwise normal vitreous humor; there are no symptoms.

asthenopia Ill-defined ocular discomfort attributed to use of the eyes.

astigmatism Optical condition in which the refractive power is not uniform in all meridians; when regular, there are two main meridians of refractive power; when irregular, there are a number of meridians of different power.

avulsion of caruncle Term usually applied to a laceration involving inner one sixth (lacrimal portion) of lower eyelid with rupture of the inferior canaliculus.

band keratopathy Deposition of calcium in the cornea most marked in the horizontal meridian; occurs in degenerating eyes, hypercalcemia, hypophosphatemia, and juvenile arthritis (of Still).

bedewing of cornea Subepithelial corneal edema, often associated with sudden prolonged increase in intraocular pressure or wearing of contact lenses for an excessively long period (Sattler veil).

Bell palsy Peripheral paralysis of the facial nerve (N VII).

Bell phenomenon Upward and outward rotation of the eyes that occurs in sleep or with forcible closure of the eyelids.

Bergmeister papilla Small mass of glial cells that surrounds the fetal hyaloid artery in the center of the optic disk; occasionally it persists and obliterates the physiologic cup of the optic disk.

biomicroscope Microscope for examining the eye; consists essentially of a dissecting microscope combined with a light source that projects a rectangular light beam that can be changed in size and focus (a slit lamp).

Bitot spot Highly refractile mass with silver-gray hue and foamy surface that appears on the bulbar conjunctiva in vitamin A deficiency.

black out Amaurosis fugax.

blenorrhea Discharge from mucous surfaces.
   adult Gonorrheal conjunctivitis.
   inclusion Chlamydial conjunctivitis.
   neonatorum ophthalmia neonatorum.

blepharadenitis Inflammation of marginal glands of eyelid: meibomian, Moll, and Zeis.

blepharitis Inflammation of the margin of the eyelids; occurs in squamous (seborrheic) and ulcerative forms.

blepharochalasis Relaxation of the skin of the eyelid caused by atrophy of the elastic tissue; the upper eyelid is commonly involved, and a fold of tissue hangs over the eyelid margin.

blepharoclonus Exaggerated reflex blinking.

blepharophimosis Decreased size of the palpebral fissure, often associated with excessive distance between the inner canthi (telecanthus) and drooping of the upper eyelid (blepharoptosis).

blepharoplasty Plastic correction of the eyelid abnormality.

blepharoptosis Drooping of the upper eyelid caused by paralysis of the oculomotor nerve (N III) or the sympathetic nerves or by excessive weight of the upper eyelids.

blepharospasm Tonic spasm of the orbicularis oculi muscle.

blepharostat Instrument for holding eyelids apart in eye surgery.

blind spot (of Mariotte) Area of blindness in the visual field marking the site of the optic disk in the eye where there are no photoreceptors.

blindness Loss of sense of sight; defined by Internal Revenue Service as reduction of best corrected visual acuity to 20/200 or less in better eye or restriction of the visual field to 20° or less; defined by Social Security Agency as reduction of visual acuity in best corrected eye to 5/200 or less; in industry, reduction of the best corrected visual acuity to less than 20/200.

    color *See* achromatopsia, protanopia, tritanopia, deuteranomaly, protanomaly.

    cortical Caused by a lesion in the cortical visual center.

    night Inadequate dark adaptation so that vision is markedly reduced in reduced illumination.

    snow Inability to open the eyes to see; secondary to ultraviolet keratitis.

blood-aqueous and -retina barrier Limitation of diffusion of lipid-insoluble substances by tight junctions of iris vasculature, pigmented epithelium of ciliary body, retinal pigment epithelium, and retinal vasculature.

blowout fracture of orbit Fracture of the roof of the maxillary sinus with prolapse of the intraorbital contents into the antrum; there is enophthalmos, blepharoptosis, inability to turn the eye upward, and usually infraorbital anesthesia.

blue sclera Abnormality in which the sclera is thin and has a blue appearance caused by the underlying pigmented choroid.

bobbing Disordered ocular movements in comatose patients with lower pontine lesions; intermittent rapid downward movement of eyes with slow return to primary position.

Bowman zone Anterior condensation of the corneal stroma.

break up time, tears Time in seconds for dry spot to form on corneal epithelium in absence of blinking.

Bruch membrane Tissue between the choriocapillaris and the retinal pigment epithelium.

Brushfield spots Transient whitish areas in the iris at birth that occur in Down syndrome and in many normal children.

buckling operation For retinal detachment with scleral indentation.

buphthalmos Enlargement of the eye usually occurring as a result of congenital glaucoma.

Busacca floccule Accumulation of macrophages on surface of iris, lens, and anterior chamber angle in anterior uveitis.

campimeter Alternative term for perimeter.

canal of Cloquet Central area of vitreous humor that transmits hyaloid vascular system in embryonic life.

canaliculitis Inflammation of a lacrimal canaliculus, often caused by fungus infection.

candela Unit of luminous intensity; one candela is defined as the luminous intensity of ⅟₆₀ of a square centimeter of projected area of a blackbody radiator operating at the temperature of solidification of platinum.

candle power Luminous intensity as expressed in candelas.

canthotomy Cantholysis, surgical division of the canthus.

canthus Angle at either end of palpebral fissure.

capillary-free zone Region of foveola; area adjacent to retinal arterioles.

caput medusae Dilated ciliary blood vessels girdling the corneoscleral limbus in rubeosis iridis.

cardinal points Three pairs of points of an optical system (principal, nodal, and focal) that determine its refractive characteristics.

cardinal positions of gaze Eyes right, eyes right and up, eyes right and down, eyes left, eyes left and up, eyes left and down.

carotid-cavernous fistula Rupture of a carotid aneurysm into the cavernous sinus (infraseller) that causes an increased venous pressure in the sinus; also occurs with dural shunt.

caruncle, lacrimal Red, modified skin at inner angle of palpebral fissure.

cataract Opacity of the crystalline lens

    after Opacity of the lens capsule after cataract extraction.

    complicated Opacity that follows intraocular inflammation

    hypermature Opacity in which lens cortex is liquefied and nucleus gravitates within capsule (Morgagnian).

    immature Opacity in which transparent lens fibers remain.

    intumescent Swollen and mature.

    mature Opacity in which all lens fibers are opaque.

central serous choroidopathy Detachment of sensory retina from retinal pigment epithelium in macular region, induced by a defect in pigment epithelium that permits serous fluid to enter subretinal space.

centrocecal scotoma Area of blindness in a field of vision involving both the fixation point and the blind spot (cecum); characterizes toxic amblyopias.

cerclage Operation for retinal detachment in which a band encircles sclera posterior to insertions of recti muscles.

chalazion Chronic lipogranuloma of a meibomian gland. Internal stye.

chalcosis Deposition of copper in tissues.

Charcot triad Nystagmus, intention tremor, and scanning speech, all of which occur as a late sign in demyelinating disease, particularly multiple sclerosis.

chemosis Edema of the bulbar conjunctiva.

cherry-red spot Ophthalmoscopic appearance of the fovea centralis (which contains only the outer layers of the retina adjacent to the choroid) when surrounded by either edematous or lipid-filled inner layers of the retina, as occurs in occlusion of the central retinal artery, and lysosomal enzyme deficiency.

chlorolabe Pigment of retinal cone that absorbs maximally middle wavelengths of light.

chloroma Granulocytic sarcoma; localized accumulation of myelocytes in leukemia.

chorioretinitis Inflammation of choroid and retina.

choristoma Tumor of a tissue not normally belonging in an area.

choroideremia X chromosome-linked abnormality characterized by atrophy of the choriocapillaris and degeneration of the retinal pigment epithelium.

choroiditis Inflammation of the choroid.

chromatic aberration Imperfection of an image produced by variations in the refractivity of the various wavelengths of white light.

chrysiasis Deposition of gold in connective tissue including sclera and cornea.

C.I.E. observer Hypothetical observer having color vision sensitivity recommended in 1931 by Commission Internationale de l'Eclairage (C.I.E.).

circinate retinopathy Circular or oval figure, often incomplete, of hard retinal deposits (edema residues) in macular area that surrounds a region of abnormal vascular permeability of retinal vasculature.

closed-angle glaucoma Ocular abnormality in which the intraocular pressure increases, often quickly, because the anterior aqueous humor is mechanically prevented from reaching the trabecular meshwork.

Coats white ring Oval or round 0.5-mm deposition of lipid in superficial layer of cornea.

collarette Junction of ciliary and pupillary zones of iris.

collyrium Eyewash.

coloboma Absence of some ocular tissue resulting from defective closure of fetal fissure.

color That aspect of the appearance of light and objects that may be specified as to hue, brightness, and saturation. The portion of the electromagnetic spectrum between 370 and 760 nm specified as to wavelength, luminosity, and saturation.

  complementary Pairs of light of different wavelengths that produce white light when combined.

  opponent Pairs of color that share color channels in retina (red-green, blue-yellow).

  primary The three colors of the retinal cone pigments (red, green, blue) that may be combined to match any hue; spectral colors.

  saturated A color containing a minimum amount of whiteness.

commotio retinae Traumatic lesion of the posterior pole with edema and hemorrhage following contusion of the anterior ocular segment.

congruous field defects Visual field defects that are exactly the same in extent and intensity in both eyes; characterizes lesions in the optic radiation and occipital cortex.

conical cornea Keratoconus.

conjugate ocular movements Similar ocular movements of both eyes, such as eyes right, eyes left, eyes up, eyes down (version).

conjunctival follicles Lymphatic hypertrophy in response to conjunctival inflammation.

conjunctivitis Inflammation of the conjunctiva.

conjunctivorhinostomy Surgical procedure to provide a passageway from conjunctival sac to the nasal cavity.

conoid of Sturm In optics, the pattern of rays formed by a spherocylinder.

consensual light reflex Constriction of the pupil in the fellow eye when the retina is stimulated by light.

conus of optic disk Condition in which the choroid and retinal pigment epithelium do not extend to the optic disk, allowing the sclera to be observed ophthalmoscopically at its margin.

convergence Simultaneous adduction of both eyes to fix a nearby object (vergence).

corectopia Displacement of pupil from its normal position.

corneal erosion Loss of corneal epithelium that may follow minor injury or may occur as a corneal dystrophy.

corresponding points Areas on the two retinas that have the same directional value in space.

cotton-wool patch Retinal microinfarct with impaired axonal transport that results in a white area with poorly defined margins in the nerve fiber layer of retina. Histologically, a cytoid body composed of intracellular organelles.

couching An ancient surgical procedure of dislocating the lens out of the visual axis.

cover-uncover test Alternate covering and uncovering of one eye to distinguish between a phoria and a tropia.

craniosynostosis Premature fusion of cranial bone sutures.

Credé prophylaxis Instillation of 1% silver nitrate in the eyes of a newborn infant to prevent gonococcal conjunctivitis.

cross-cylinder Spherocylinder lens used in refraction, composed of a cylinder of twice the strength and the opposite sign of the sphere.

cryopexy Use of a freezing probe in retinal detachment operation.

cryotherapy Procedure carried out with a freezing probe.

cryptophthalmia Congenital absence of eyelids so that skin covers the eyes.

cup/disk ratio Ratio of horizontal or vertical diameter of physiologic cup of optic disk to diameter of optic disk.

cupping Increase in diameter and depth of the physiologic optic cup that occurs in glaucoma.

cyanolabe Pigment of retinal cone that maximally absorbs short wavelengths of light.

cyanosis retinae Obsolete term for vascular dilation in blood hyperviscosity syndromes, particularly polycythemia.

cyclectomy Excision of a portion of the ciliary body.

cyclitis Inflammation of the ciliary body.

cyclocryotherapy Destruction of a portion of ciliary body by freezing to reduce the quantity of aqueous humor produced in glaucoma.

cyclodialysis Surgical procedure for glaucoma to establish a communication between the anterior chamber and the suprachoroidal space.

cyclodiathermy Destruction of a portion of the ciliary body by heat to reduce the quantity of aqueous humor produced in glaucoma.

cycloplegia Paralysis of accommodation.

cylinder In optics, a lens with no refracting power in one meridian and maximal refracting power in the meridian at right angles to this.

cystoid macular degeneration Edema of the central retina caused by abnormal permeability of capillary bed surrounding fovea centralis.

cytoid body Accumulation of cell organelles in neuron.

dacryoadenitis Inflammation of the lacrimal gland, often chronic and caused by a granulomatous disease; acute dacryoadenitis occurs with mumps and infectious mononucleosis.

dacryocystitis Inflammation of the lacrimal sac that usually results from interference with lacrimal drainage.

dacryocystography Roentgenographic study of lacrimal system after injection of radiopaque compound in lacrimal drainage system.

dacryocystorhinostomy Surgical procedure in which the mucous membrane of the lacrimal sac is anastomosed with the mucous membrane that lines the middle meatus of the nose to establish lacrimal drainage.

dacryolith Concretion in lacrimal system.

dacryosintography Graphic recording of passage of a radioactive isotope through lacrimal drainage system.

dacryostenosis Atresia of the lacrimal duct.

dark adaptation Biochemical and neurologic process by which the eye becomes more sensitive to light.

dellen Shallow excavations of peripheral corneal epithelium caused by localized deficiency of precorneal tear film.

dendritic keratitis Inflammation of the corneal epithelium by *Herpesvirus hominis*.

denervation supersensitivity Increased sensitivity to neural effector substance that follows postganglionic interruption of the nerve supply of organs innervated by the autonomic nervous system.

deorsumversion Simultaneous movement of eyes downward from primary position.

descemetocele Herniation of the basement membrane of the corneal endothelium through corneal stroma.

deturgescence Mechanism by which corneal stroma remains relatively dehydrated.

deuteranomaly Form of anomalous trichromatism in which there appears to be a deficiency of middle wave length sensitive cones so that there is poor green-purple and red-purple discrimination, green insensitivity, and normal luminosity function.

deuteranopia Form of dichromatism in which there are only two cone pigments present and there is complete insensitivity to middle wavelength (green).

deviation

  conjugate The simultaneous rotation of the eyes in the same direction.

  primary The abnormality in ocular parallelism in paralysis of an ocular muscle when the nonparalyzed eye is used for fixation.

  secondary The abnormality in ocular parallelism in paralysis of an ocular muscle when the paralyzed eye is used for fixation.

  skew A hypertropia in which the eyes move equally in opposite directions.

dextroversion Simultaneous movement of eyes to right from primary position.

dialysis of retina Separation at the ora serrata of the sensory retina from the retinal pigment epithelium.

diaphanoscopy Transillumination of a body cavity; used in ophthalmology to demonstrate the diminution of pigment in the iris (pigmentary dispersion syndrome) in the female carriers of ocular albinism or to diagnose intraocular tumors.

dichromatism The abnormality of color vision in which only two of the three retinal cone pigments are present (in protanopia, long-wave sensitive [red] cones are absent; in deuteranopia, middle-wave sensitive [green] cones are absent; and in tritanopia, short-wave sensitive [blue] cones are absent). Also called dichromatopsia, dyschromatopsia, parachromatism, parachromatopsia.

diopter Unit of measurement of refraction power of lenses equal to the reciprocal of the focal length of the lens expressed in meters; with prisms, the image displacement in centimeters at 1 meter.

diplopia Double vision; simultaneous perception of a single object as two objects.

  crossed Double vision in which the image from the right eye is observed to the left of the image from the left eye; associated with conditions in which the eyes turn outward.

diplopia—cont'd

monocular Diplopia as a result of opacities in the visual axis.

uncrossed Condition in which the image of the right eye is to the right of the image from the left eye; observed in conditions in which the visual axes of the eye are directed toward each other, as in esotropia.

disciform degeneration of central retina Secondary type of central retinal degeneration caused by a subretinal neovascular membrane.

disciform keratitis Stromal type of corneal inflammation, roughly circular, often seen as secondary stromal involvement in a herpes simplex keratitis.

disinsertion of retina Retinal dialysis at the ora serrata in which the sensory retina is separated from the retinal pigment epithelium.

dislocation of lens Condition in which the crystalline lens is completely unsupported by the zonular fibers so that the lens is free, either in the vitreous humor or in the anterior chamber.

disparity, retinal The slight difference in retinal images that arises because of the lateral separation of the two eyes that stimulates stereoscopic vision.

distichiasis Supernumerary row of eyelashes.

districhiasis Two hairs share a single hair follicle.

divergence Outward rotation of eyes from primary position.

drusen Hyaline excrescences of the retinal pigment epithelium or acellular laminated bodies of the optic nerve.

dry eye Keratoconjunctivitis sicca.

ductions Ocular rotations of one eye only.

dyscoria Abnormality in the shape of the pupil.

dyslexia Psychologic abnormality in which, despite adequate intelligence, motivation, and instruction, and in the absence of a physical handicap, emotional disturbance, or cultural deprivation, an individual fails to master printed and written language.

dysmetria Disturbance of power to control range movement in muscular action; in ophthalmology, overshoot or undershoot of eyes on attempted fixation.

dystrophy Noninflammatory developmental, nutritional, or metabolic abnormality.

eccentric fixation Visual abnormality in which a retinal area other than the fovea centralis is used for visual fixation.

ecchymosis Extravasation of blood beneath the skin.

echography Use of ultrasound as diagnostic aid.

ectasia of sclera Localized bulging of the sclera lined with uveal tissue; staphyloma.

ectopia Displacement or malposition, especially congenital.

ectropion Turning outward of the margin of the eyelid occurring in spastic, cicatricial, and paralytic forms.

eikonometer Instrument used to measure aniseikonia, a difference in image size of each eye.

electromagnetic spectrum Range of radiant energy that has a variable frequency and a constant velocity (energy-Planck's constant × frequency).

electro-oculogram (EOG) Ratio of standing potential between retina and cornea in light and dark adaptation.

electroretinogram (ERG) Action potential that follows stimulation of the retina.

ELISA Acronym for *enzyme-linked immunosorbent assay test*. Specific antigens available for variety of organisms.

Elschnig pearls Proliferated anterior capsule epithelium after extracapsular cataract extraction.

embryotoxon

anterior Arcus cornealis.

posterior Proliferation of peripheral corneal endothelium at Schwalbe ring.

emmetropia Refractive condition in which no refractive error is present with accommodation at rest.

endogenous uveitis Inflammation of the uveal tract from causes within the body in contrast to that introduced from outside the body, as in injuries (exogenous).

endophthalmitis Purulent inflammation of the intraocular contents.

enophthalmos Recession of the eye within the orbit.

entropion Inward turning of the eyelid, observed in cicatricial, spastic, and paralytic forms.

enucleation Removal of the eye.

epiblepharon Supernumerary fold of skin along lower eyelid margin that turns eyelashes against the globe.

epicanthus Crescentic fold of skin of lower eyelid extending upward at inner canthus.

epidemic keratoconjunctivitis Inflammation of the cornea and conjunctiva caused by adenovirus type 8 or 19.

epiphora Tearing in which faulty drainage of tears permits their overflow.

episcleritis Localized inflammation of the superficial tissues of the sclera.

epithelial downgrowth Epithelization of the interior of the eye that may follow faulty wound healing of the anterior segment.

esodeviation Inward deviation of the eye.

esophoria Latent inward deviation of the eyes in which, with binocular vision suspended, an eye deviates inward.

esotropia Manifest inward deviation that occurs with both eyes open.

evisceration In ophthalmology, the surgical procedure in which the intraocular contents are removed, retaining the cornea (sometimes) and the sclera.

excyclodeviation Deviation of upper pole of vertical axis of eye toward the temple (plus cyclodeviation).

exodeviation Turning outward of the eyes.

exophoria Latent outward deviation of the eyes in which, with binocular vision suspended, an eye deviates outward.

exophthalmometer Instrument to measure protrusion of eye.

exophthalmos Abnormal protrusion of both eyes.

  endocrine Associated with abnormalities of the thyroid gland.

  ophthalmoplegic Inability to move the eye because of exophthalmos.

  pulsating Associated with a carotid-cavernous fistula.

exotropia Outward deviation of the eyes.

extorsion Temporal rotation of 12 o'clock corneal meridian.

eye

  cat's Yellow pupillary reflection in retinoblastoma and intraocular granulomas.

  dominant Preferred eye for monocular fixation.

  exciting Initially injured eye in sympathetic ophthalmia; the fellow eye is the sympathizing eye.

  fixating In strabismus, the eye directed to the object of regard.

  reduced, schematic Simplified eye used in optics.

  squinting Deviating eye in strabismus.

faden suture Placed between muscle and posterior sclera to limit ocular muscle overaction.

Farnsworth-Munsell color test 84 colored chips arranged in order of increasing hue.

far-point Remotest point where object is clearly seen without accommodation.

Fasanella-Servat procedure Resection of levator palpebrae superioris muscle through the conjunctival surface.

field of vision Area simultaneously visible to an eye without movement.

filtering operation One designed to establish a fistula between the anterior chamber and subconjunctival space.

fixation Coordinated accommodation and ocular movements that maintain the image of objects on the retina.

floater Object seen in the field of vision that originates in the vitreous humor; the most common floaters are muscae volitantes, minute residues of the hyaloid vasculature seen in bright, uniform illumination.

fluorescein angiography Serial photography of ocular fundus after intravenous administration of fluorescein solution.

fluorescence Reradiation of energy with increase of wavelength by an absorbing substance.

flux Short form for radiant flux, or luminous flux, according to context.

focus Point of convergence of light rays; starting point of disease.

fogging Method to determine refractive error in which accommodation is relaxed by means of convex spheres that make the patient artificially myopic.

foot-candle Unit of illuminance equal to one lumen incident per square foot.

foot-lambert Unit of luminance.

fornix In ophthalmology, the reflection of the conjunctiva from the eyelid to the eye.

fovea centralis Rod-free area of the retina that contains the foveola.

foveola Capillary-free area of the sensory retina.

Frost sutures Temporary marginal sutures used in blepharoptosis surgery.

Fuchs black spot Area of proliferation of the retinal pigment layer in the foveal area in degenerative myopia.

Fuchs dystrophy Corneal abnormality in which there is initially a degeneration of the endothelium followed sometimes by epithelial and stromal edema and scarring.

funduscope Many organs have a fundus; a more precise term for the instrument used in ophthalmoscopy is *ophthalmoscope.*

fusion Reflex; the stimulus to unify similar images that fall upon retinal areas that have the same directional value in space.

  fusion with amplitude Blending of the similar images from the two foveas into a single perception (Grade 2).

  simultaneous central retinal perception (normal correspondence) Ability of the brain to receive and comprehend images from the fovea centralis of each eye simultaneously.

  stereopsis Blending of slightly dissimilar images from the two eyes with the perception of depth.

fusion-free Position of the eyes when binocular vision is suspended.

gerontoxon Corneal arcus.

glare Sensation produced by brightness within the visual field that is sufficiently greater than the luminance to which the eyes are adapted to cause annoyance, discomfort, or loss in visual performance and visibility.

glaucoma An ocular disease in which increased intraocular pressure causes atrophy and excavation of the optic nerve, producing characteristic field defects.

goblet cells Mucin-secreting cells in the conjunctiva.

gonioscope Optical instrument for studying the angle of the anterior chamber of the eye.

goniosynechiae Adhesions between the iris and cornea at the anterior chamber angle.

goniotomy Operation for congenital glaucoma in which the trabecular meshwork in the region of the canal of Schlemm is incised.

hallucinations Perception without external stimulus that may occur in every field of sensation; formed visual hallucinations are composed of scenes, and unformed hallucinations are composed of sparks, lights, and the like; formed hallucinations characterize temporal lobe disturbances, and unformed hallucinations characterize occipital lobe disorders.

hamartoma Localized tumor composed of an abnormal proportion of a single tissue element of tissues normally present in the areas.

haploscope Type of stereoscope used to measure ocular functions.

Hassall-Henle bodies Hyaline deposits of Descemet membrane that occur with aging.

hemianopsia Loss of vision in one half of the visual field in one or both eyes.

> **congruous** Hemianopsia in which the hemianopsia of each eye is completely symmetrical in extent and intensity.

> **homonymous** Blindness in corresponding parts (right or left) of the visual field of each eye.

hemeralopia Defective vision in bright light.

Henle layer Outer plexiform layer of the retina in the region surrounding the foveola.

Herbert pits Characteristic defect at corneoscleral limbus after healing of follicle in trachoma.

Hering's law of equal innervation Impulse to each muscle involved in turning the eyes in the same direction is equal in duration and intensity.

heterochromia of iris Condition in which the irises of the two eyes are different colors.

heterophoria Condition in which there is a latent tendency of the eyes to deviate that is prevented by fusion.

heteroptropia Condition in which the eyes deviate; strabismus.

hippus Spasmodic rhythmic dilation and contraction of the pupil, independent of stimulation with light.

"histo" spot Area of atrophic choroid and retina in presumed ocular histoplasmosis.

Hollenhorst plaque Cholesterol embolus in retinal artery from atheromatous plaque in carotid artery.

homonymous In ophthalmology, having the same side of the field of vision; thus, a right homonymous hemianopsia is right half-blindness and results from a defect involving the nasal fibers of the right eye that decussate and the noncrossing fibers of the left eye; the lesion is on the left side, posterior to the optic chiasm.

hordeolum Acute inflammation caused by infection of one of the sebaceous glands of Zeis; a sty; the term "internal hordeolum" is sometimes applied to a chalazion.

horopter Plane in space that localizes the visual direction of corresponding retinal points.

Hruby lens Concave lens to neutralize corneal refractive power and permit study of retina with biomicroscope.

Hudson-Stähli line Pigmented iron line of the cornea.

humor, aqueous The watery fluid that fills the anterior and posterior chambers of the eye. It is secreted by the ciliary processes and passes through the posterior chamber and the pupil into the anterior chamber, where it passes through the trabecular meshwork and is reabsorbed into the venous system at the iridocorneal angle by way of the sinus venosus sclerae (canal of Schlemm).

humor, vitreous The fluid component of the corpus vitreum.

hyalitis Inflammation of the corpus vitreum. Vitreitis.

hyalosis Degenerative changes in the corpus vitreum.

> **asteriod** Benson disease: numerous small spherical bodies ("snowball" opacities) in the corpus vitreum visible ophthalmoscopically; an age change, usually unilateral, and not affecting vision.

hydrops of cornea Corneal edema usually caused by failure of deturgescence mechanism.

hydrops of iris Vacuolization of the iris pigment layer when these cells are filled with glycogen in diabetes mellitus.

hyperopia Refractive state of the eye in which rays of light cannot be brought to focus on the retina except by interposition of a convex lens or by accommodation.

> **absolute** Cannot be neutralized completely by accommodation so that there is indistinct vision both for near and for distance.

> **axial** Caused by abnormal shortness of the anteroposterior diameter of the eye.

> **latent** Portion of total hypermetropia that cannot be overcome, or the difference between the manifest and total hypermetropia.

> **manifest** Amount of hypermetropia indicated by the strongest convex lens a patient will accept while retaining normal visual acuity.

> **total** Entire hypermetropia, both latent and manifest.

hyperphoria Tendency for the eyes to deviate vertically that is prevented by binocular vision.

hypertelorism Excessive width between two organs; in ocular hypertelorism there is increased distance between the eyes (telecanthus) that is often associated with mental deficiency and exotropia.

hypertropia Deviation of the eyes in which one eye is higher than the other.

hyphema Blood in the anterior chamber.

hypopyon Pus in the anterior chamber.

illuminance Luminous flux incident per unit area of a surface.

illusion, optical A false interpretation of the color, form, size, or movement, of a visual sensation.

image Visual impression of an object formed by a lens or mirror.

> **false** In diplopia, the image in the deviating eye.

> **Purkinje-Sanson** The images reflected from anterior and posterior surfaces of the cornea and the lens.

> **real** In optics, the inverted image formed by actual rays of light from an object.

> **true** In diplopia, the image received by the nondeviating eye.

> **virtual** In optics, the erect image formed by projection of divergent rays from an optical system.

image jump Abrupt shift in field of view as direction of gaze moves across segment line of bifocal lens.

inclusion body Irregular-shaped particles in cytoplasm and nuclei of cells containing virus particles.

incongruous field defects Visual field defects that are dissimilar in the two eyes; occur in lesions involving that portion of the visual pathways anterior to the lateral geniculate body.

incyclodeviation Deviation of upper pole of vertical axis of eye toward the nose (negative cyclodeviation).

infrared radiation Portion of the electromagnetic spectrum that has a wavelength of more than 700 nm and less than 10,000 nm.

interstitial keratitis Inflammation of the corneal stroma with neovascularization, often complicating congenital syphilis.

intorsion Nasal rotation of 12 o'clock corneal meridian.

intrascleral nerve loop (of Axenfeld) Condition in which a long ciliary nerve loops in the anterior sclera; causes a minute dark spot of uveal tissue on the sclera.

iridectomy Excision of a part of the iris.

> **peripheral** Removal of a portion of the peripheral iris.
>
> **sector** Removal of an entire sector, extending usually from the pupillary margin to the root of the iris.

iridencleisis Surgical procedure to correct glaucoma in which an incision is made at the corneoscleral limbus and the iris is incarcerated in the wound to create a filtering wick between the anterior chamber and subconjunctival space.

iridescent vision Halos around lights, particularly in corneal edema.

iridocycletomy Surgical excision of a portion of the iris and ciliary body.

iridocyclitis Inflammation of the iris and ciliary body.

iridodialysis Separation of the base of the iris from the ciliary body; the main cause is blunt trauma to the eye.

iridodonesis Tremulousness of the iris; occurs following loss of support after lens removal.

iridoplegia Paralysis of the sphincter pupillae muscle of the iris.

iridoschisis Separation of the mesodermal layer of the iris from the ectodermal layer.

iridotomy Opening in iris by cutting or photocoagulation.

Iris bombé Condition in which the pupillary border is adherent to the lens so that aqueous humor accumulates in the posterior chamber.

iris coloboma Defect of the iris that occurs either as a congenital abnormality or after iridectomy.

iritis Inflammation of the iris.

irradiance Density of radiant flux incident on a surface.

Ishihara color plates Devices for screening for color discrimination using forms composed of different colored dots.

isopter Curve of equal sensitivity in the visual field.

jaw-winking (Marcus Gunn) Abnormality in which movements of the face cause retraction of upper eyelid, often associated with blepharoptosis.

joule Ten million ergs.

K reading Corneal curvature as measured with keratometer.

kappa angle Angle between a line through the center of the pupil and the visual axis; when the visual axis is nasal to the center of the pupil (common), the angle is positive; when the visual axis is temporal, the angle is negative.

Kayser-Fleischer ring Golden deposit of copper in the periphery of Descemet membrane observed in hepatolenticular degeneration (Wilson disease).

keratectomy Excision of a portion of the cornea.

keratic precipitates Clumps of leukocytes adhering to the corneal endothelium in uveal tract inflammation; customarily divided into mutton-fat (macrophages and epitheloid cells) and punctate (lymphocytes and plasma cells).

keratitis Inflammation of the cornea.

keratocele Anterior herniation of Descemet membrane through the cornea; descemetocele.

keratocentesis Aqueous humor paracentesis.

keratoconjunctivitis Simultaneous inflammation of the cornea and conjunctiva.

keratoconus Conical protrusion of the cornea.

keratoglobus Enlargement of the cornea.

keratomalacia Softening of the cornea, often occurring in severe vitamin A deficiency.

keratome Knife with a triangular blade used for corneal incision.

keratometer Instrument for measuring the radius of curvature of the cornea.

keratomileusis Surgical procedure that reshapes the cornea to modify refractive error.

keratomycosis Keratitis caused by fungus infection.

keratopathy Noninflammatory disorder of the cornea.

keratoplasty Transplantation of a portion of the cornea.

> **lamellar** Replacement of superficial layers.
>
> **partial** Replacement of a portion of the cornea.
>
> **penetrating** Replacement of entire thickness of the cornea; may be partial or total.
>
> **tectonic** To reconstruct tissue.
>
> **total** Replacement of entire cornea.

keratotomy Incision of the cornea.

> **radial (refractive)** Radial incisions through peripheral cornea to reduce curvature of optical portion of the cornea and reduce myopia.

Koeppe nodule Accumulation of epithelioid cells at the pupillary margin in granulomatous uveitis.

Krükenberg spindle Accumulation of pigment on the corneal endothelium in the shape of a vertical spindle that occurs in pigmentary glaucoma.

lacrimation Secretion of tears.

lagophthalmos Condition in which the globe is not entirely covered with the eyelids closed.

lambert Unit of luminance.

laser Acronym for *light amplification by stimulated emission of radiation;* the laser produces a nearly monochromatic and coherent beam of radiation.

lens Glass or other transparent material used optically to modify the path of light.

    achromatic A compound lens made of two or more lenses having different indices of refraction, so correlated as to minimize chromatic aberration.

    bandage Contact lens used in management of corneal disease.

    biconcave Both surfaces concave.

    biconvex Both surfaces convex.

    bifocal Spectacles that contain two foci, usually arranged with the focus for distance above and a small segment for near below; such lenses are used in the correction of presbyopia and to relieve excessive accommodation in accommodative strabismus of children.

    colored Selectively absorb or reflect certain wavelengths of light.

    concave Causes divergence of incident light rays.

    contact Worn beneath the eyelids.

    crystalline Transparent biconvex tissue located behind the pupil and in front of the vitreous.

    cylindrical Lens that is a section of a cylinder and used to correct astigmatism.

    decentered Lens in which the ocular visual line does not pass through its center.

    meniscus Lens that has one concave and one convex surface.

    omnifocal Spectacles that contain both near and distance portions with gradual increase in reading power.

    prism Transparent solid with two converging sides; separates white light into its spectral components and bends rays of light toward its base; used to measure or to correct ocular muscle imbalance.

    safety Lens resistant to shattering made either of plastic or by means of case-hardening, coating, or lamination.

    spherical Concave or convex.

    toric Meniscus lens with a cylinder on one surface.

lensectomy Removal of lens by small incision through pars plana (orbicularis ciliaris) of ciliary body.

lensometer Instrument for determining the refractive power of a lens.

lensopathy Condition in which tear proteins are deposited on a contact lens.

lenticonus Rare abnormality of the lens characterized by a conical prominence on the anterior or posterior lens surface.

lentiglobus Excessive curvature of crystalline lens.

leukocoria Whitish pupillary reflex caused by intraocular mass.

leukoma Opacity of the cornea; a less marked opacity is a macula, and the least type of opacity is a nebula.

    adherent Corneal opacity to which the iris is adherent.

levoversion Rotation of eyes to the left.

light That portion of the electromagnetic spectrum that stimulates the retina and causes a visual sensation.

lightning streaks (Moore) Flashes of light, usually within the temporal field, with movements of eyes occurring after detachment of vitreous humor and caused by impingement of separated vitreous on the retina or by vitreous traction.

Lisch nodules Bilateral hamartomatous nodules of the iris, possibly pathognomic neurofibromatosis.

Listing plane Transverse vertical plane perpendicular to the anterior posterior axis of the eye that contains the center of rotation of the eye.

lumen and related terms Refer to the action of radiant energy upon the photopic vision of a standard observer.

lumen Unit of luminous flux equal to the flux in a unit of solid angle (one steradian) from a uniform point source of one candela.

luminance Luminous flux per unit of solid angle emitted per unit of projected area.

luminosity Ratio of lumens per watt of any kind of radiant energy.

luminous emittance Density of luminous flux emitted from a surface.

luminous flux Rate of flow of radiant energy.

lux Unit of illuminance equal to one lumen per square meter.

lysozyme (muramidase) Antibacterial enzyme found in tears, leukocytes, egg albumin, and plants; mainly destructive of nonpathogenic gram-positive bacteria.

macula corneae Minute corneal opacity.

macula lutea Yellow spot; the ill-defined retinal area surrounding the fovea centralis.

mandibulofacial dysostosis Hereditary hypoplasia of zygoma and mandible.

medulloepithelioma Embryonal tumor of nonpigmented layer of ciliary epithelium.

megalocornea Cornea with a diameter of 12 mm or more.

melanocytoma Nevus with giant melanosomes on the surface of the optic disk.

mesopic Intermediate illumination between daylight (photopic) and twilight (scotopic).

metamorphopsia Condition in which objects appear distorted, usually caused by foveal disturbance.

microaneurysms Capillary outpouching in the retina in diabetes mellitus, pulseless disease, hypertension.

microcornea Cornea with a diameter of less than 9 mm.

microphakia Anomaly in which the crystalline lens is abnormally small.

microphthalmia Condition in which the eyeball is abnormally small.

micropsia Disturbance of visual perception in which objects appear smaller than their true size.

microtropia Strabismus of less than 4°.

millimicron Unit of wavelength equal to 10^{-9} meter; nanometer now preferred.

miosis Condition in which the pupil is constricted.

miotic Pertaining to or characterized by constriction of the pupil.

Mittendorf dot Opacity of the posterior lens capsule marking the site of hyaloid artery attachment.

monochromatism Achromatopsia.

Mooren ulcer Chronic, peripheral necrotic keratitis in the aged.

Morgagnian cataract Hypermature cataract in which the cortex is liquefied, permitting the lens nucleus to float within the capsule.

movement

    cardinal ocular Eye rotations to the right and left, upward to the right and left, and downward to the right and left; the diagnostic positions of gaze.

    cog-wheel ocular Loose, jerky ocular rotations replacing smooth following movements.

    conjugate movement of the eye Rotation of the two eyes in the same direction. See also version.

    disjugate movement of the eyes Rotation of the two eyes in opposite directions, as in convergence or divergence.

    fixational ocular Rotation of the eyes during voluntary fixation on an object; tremors, flicks, and drifts occur.

    fusional A reflex movement that tends to move the visual axes to the object of fixation so that stereoscopic vision is possible.

    lightning eye Ocular myoclonus.

    paradoxical movement of eyelids Spontaneous, involuntary elevation or lowering of the eyelids, associated with movement of extraocular muscles or muscles of mastication (external pterygoid muscles).

    perverted ocular A condition in which attempts to move eyes affected by partial ophthalmoplegia initiate a movement in another direction.

    rapid eye movements (REM) Symmetrical, quick, scanning rotations occurring in clusters for 5 to 60 minutes during sleep; associated with dreaming.

    saccadic (1) A quick rotation of the eyes from one fixation point to another as in reading; (2) the rapid correction movement of a jerky nystagmus, as in labyrinthine and optokinetic nystagmus.

mural cells Pericytes in retinal capillary walls.

muscae volitantes Remnants of the fetal hyaloid system that appear as opacities in the vitreous humor (floaters).

mydriasis Dilation of the pupil.

myectomy Excision of a portion of a muscle.

myoclonus, ocular Lightning eye movements; rapid bursts of small ocular saccadic movements that usually follow gaze toward the paretic or ataxic side of the body.

myokymia Persistent quavering of a muscle.

myopia Optical condition in which parallel rays of light come to focus in front of the retina.

    axial Caused by abnormal length of anteroposterior diameter of the eye.

    degenerative Associated with conus of optic disk and retinal abnormalities.

    refractive Caused by increased index of refraction of the lens, as in nuclear sclerosis.

myopic crescent Term applied to a conus of the optic disk in myopia.

myotomy Disinsertion of a muscle.

Nagel anomaloscope Device for mixing two colors to match a third; used for analysis of color perception.

nanometer (nm) Unit of wavelength equal to 10^{-9} (one one-billionth) meter; formerly called millimicron (mμm).

nanophthalmos Microphthalmos.

near point Nearest point an eye can distinctly perceive an object.

    convergence Nearest point eyes can converge on an object without double vision.

near reflex Convergence, accommodation, and miosis on viewing a nearby object.

nebula of cornea A faint translucent corneal opacity.

neuroglia Supporting structure of neural tube composed of astroglia (macroglia), oligodendroglia, and microglia.

neuropathy, ischemic optic Inflammation of optic nerve; arteritic, arteriosclerotic; nonarteritic vascular inflammation.

neuroretinitis Inflammation of the optic nerve and retina.

neurotrophic keratitis Keratitis occurring because of anesthesia of the cornea.

nodal points Locations in an optical system toward and from which are directed corresponding incident and transmitted rays that make equal angles with the optic axis.

nyctalopia Night blindness.

nystagmus Ocular ataxia; rhythmic oscillation of the eyeballs, either pendular or jerky.

    after-nystagmus Occurring after the abrupt cessation of rotation in the opposite direction of the rotatory nystagmus.

    amaurotic Ocular nystagmus.

    ataxic A unilateral nystagmus with impairment of horizontal conjugate movement, most commonly caused by multiple sclerosis.

    caloric Jerky nystagmus induced by labyrinthine stimulation with hot or cold water in the ear.

nystagmus—cont'd

central Reflex from stimulation originating in the central nervous system.

cervical originating from a lesion of the proprioceptive mechanism of the neck.

compressive A jerky nystagmus resulting from unilateral changes of pressure in semicircular canals.

congenital (1) Present at birth, caused by lesions sustained in utero or at the time of birth; (2) inherited, usually X chromosome-linked, without associated neurologic lesions and nonprogressive; (3) the nystagmus associated with albinism, achromatopsia, or hypoplasia of the macula.

conjugate A nystagmus in which the two eyes move simultaneously in the same direction.

deviational End-position nystagmus.

dissociated Dysjunctive, incongruent nystagmus, or irregular nystagmus; a nystagmus in which the movements of the two eyes are dissimilar in direction, amplitude, and periodicity.

down-beat A vertical nystagmus with a rapid component downward, occurring in lesions of the lower part of the brain stem or cerebellum.

dysjunctive Dissociated nystagmus.

end-position Deviational nystagmus; a jerky, physiologic nystagmus occurring normally on attempts to fixate a point at the limits of the field of fixation.

fixation A nystagmus aggravated or induced by ocular fixation, occurring as opticokinetic nystagmus, or resulting from midbrain lesions.

galvanic Involving galvanic stimulation of the labyrinth.

gaze A nystagmus occurring in partial gaze paralysis when an attempt is made to look in the direction of the palsy.

incongruent Dissociated nystagmus.

irregular Dissociated nystagmus.

jerk Nystagmus in which there is a slow drift of the eyes in one direction, followed by a rapid recovery movement; it usually results from labyrinthine or neurologic lesions or stimuli.

labyrinthine Vestibular nystagmus.

latent Jerk nystagmus evoked by covering one eye.

micronystagmus Of minimal amplitude.

miner's Nystagmus described in coal miners and related to reduced illumination and other factors.

ocular Amaurotic nystagmus; pendular nystagmus in severely reduced vision.

opticokinetic; optokinetic Railroad nystagmus; nystagmus induced by looking at moving visual stimuli.

pendular A nystagmus that, in most positions of gaze, has oscillations equal in speed and amplitude, usually originates from reduced vision.

positional Occurring only when the head is in a particular position.

rotational Jerk nystagmus arising from stimulation of the labyrinth by rotation of the head around any axis and induced by change of motion.

rotatory A movement of the eyes around the visual axis.

seesaw A nystagmus in which one eye rotates upward as the other rotates downward, often combined with a torsional rotation.

strabismic Nystagmus associated with esotropia.

up-beat A vertical jerk nystagmus with a rapid component upward, occurring with brain-stem lesions.

vertical An up-and-down oscillation of the eyes.

vestibular Labyrinthine nystagmus; nystagmus resulting from physiological stimuli to the labyrinth that may be rotatory, caloric, compressive, or galvanic, or caused by labyrinthal lesions.

ocular deviation

primary Ocular deviation seen in paralysis of an ocular muscle when the nonparalyzed eye is used for fixation.

secondary Ocular deviation seen in paralysis of an ocular muscle when the paralyzed eye is used for fixation.

supranuclear Binocular paralysis of the volitional ocular movements that occur because of abnormalities in the frontal or occipital cortex.

ocular flutter Involuntary, intermittent, to-and-fro movements of eye occurring in cerebellar disease.

ocular hypotony Diminished ocular pressure.

ocularist One skilled in design, fabrication, and fitting of artificial eyes and the making of prostheses associated with the appearance or function of the eyes.

oculist Ophthalmologist.

open-angle glaucoma Condition of increased intraocular pressure in which the aqueous humor has access to the trabecular meshwork.

operculum, ocular The attached flap of a retinal tear.

ophthalmia Conjunctivitis.

ophthalmodynamometer Instrument for measuring blood pressure in the ophthalmic artery through observation of collapse of the central retinal artery.

ophthalmologist A specialist in diseases and surgery of the eye.

ophthalmoplegia Paralysis of the ocular muscles.

externa Paralysis of the external ocular muscles.

interna Paralysis of the muscles of the iris and the ciliary body.

total Combination of both internal and external paralysis.

ophthalmoscope Instrument for examining the interior of the eye.

direct Provides an upright image of about 15 diameters magnification.

indirect Convex lens is held in front of the eye and an inverted image is observed; provides a magnification of about four times, but allows examination of a more peripheral portion of the fundus than direct ophthalmoscopy.

opsin The protein of the light-sensitive pigment of retinal rods and cones.

opsoclonus Irregular jerks of the eyes in all directions in cerebellar disease.

optic atrophy Atrophy of the optic nerve.

optical filter Device or material that changes the distribution of incident radiation flux.

optometrist A professional concerned with examination and correction of vision problems and eye disorders.

optotypes Test symbols of graduated size for measuring visual acuity.

orbital emphysema Air in the orbit; generally follows traumatic rupture of a nasal sinus, particularly the lamina papyracea of the ethmoid bone.

orbital exenteration Removal of all of the orbital tissues, including the eye and its nervous, vascular, and muscular connections.

orbitonometer Instrument for measuring resistance to compression of orbital contents.

orthokeratology A method of molding the cornea with contact lenses to improve unaided vision.

orthophoria Tendency for the eyes to be parallel; normal ocular muscle balance.

orthoptics Technique of providing correct and efficient visual responses, usually by the form of visual training; these measures include the treatment of functional amblyopia, management of convergence insufficiency, and diagnosis of muscle imbalance and strabismus.

oscillopsia Oscillatory vision in which objects seem to move back and forth, and symptom of multiple sclerosis.

palsy Paralysis.

pannus Subepithelial fibrovascular tissue in the cornea.

   corneal A fibrovascular pannus affecting the superior portion of the cornea mainly, a frequent complication of trachoma. Three forms occur: *crassus* (thick), in which there are many blood vessels and the opacity is very dense; *siccus* (dry), pannus with dry, glossy surface; and *tenuis* (thin), in which there are few blood vessels and the opacity is slight.

panophthalmitis Purulent inflammation of all parts of the eye.

pantoscopic Adapted to both near and far vision; bifocal lenses.

Panum area Spatial area surrounding the horopter in which objects are viewed with stereopsis; outside this area, diplopia occurs.

papilla Small nipplelike eminence.

   Bergmeister Small mass of glial tissue on the surface of the disk.

   lacrimal Small conical eminence on the upper and lower eyelid at the inner canthus pierced by the lacrimal punctum; particularly evident in the elderly.

optic Misnomer in that the optic disk does not project into the eye.

papilledema Passive edema of the optic disk.

papillitis Inflammation of the optic nerve at the level of the optic disk.

paracentesis Puncture of cavity for removal of fluid; anterior chamber keratocentesis.

parallax Apparent displacement of an object resulting from a change in observer's position.

paresis Partial paralysis.

pars planitis Inflammation of ciliary body or peripheral retina often associated with foveal edema.

perception Conscious mental registry of a sensory stimulus.

perimeter Device to measure peripheral visual field.

perimetry Measurement of the field of vision.

   stasis Perimetry in which the test object and its location remain constant as illumination increases.

   kinetic Perimetry in which the location of the test object moves and its intensity remains constant.

persistent hyperplastic vitreous Abnormality caused by failure of the hyaloid system to regress.

phacoanaphylaxis Uveitis induced by hypersensitivity to lens protein.

phacoemulsification Fragmentation of the lens with ultrasound combined with aspiration.

phakomatoses Group of hereditary diseases characterized by the presence of spots, tumors, and cysts in various parts of the body; types recognized as associated with ocular findings are tuberous sclerosis, Lindau-von Hippel disease, Recklinghausen disease, Bourneville disease, and Louis-Bar syndrome (*see also* syndrome).

phlyctenule Cell-mediated hypersensitivity with localized lymphocytic infiltration of the conjunctiva.

phoria Tendency for deviation of eyes when fusion is suspended.

phosphene Sensation of light produced by electrical or mechanical stimulation of the visual system.

photocoagulation Use of laser or xenon arc energy to coagulate tissue.

photon A quantum of light (Troland).

photopsia Subjective sensation of lights induced by mechanical or electrical stimulation of retina.

phthisis bulbi Degenerative shrinkage and disorganization of the eye.

pinguecula Small yellowish-white subconjunctival elevation composed of elastic tissue located between the corneoscleral limbus and the canthus.

pits Incomplete coloboma of the optic disk, sometimes associated with central serous choroidopathy.

Placido disk Device composed of concentric black and white lines that are reflected onto the anterior surface of the cornea to detect astigmatism.

pleoptics Method of reestablishing foveal fixation.

poliosis Premature graying of hair; in ophthalmology, of eyelashes.

polycoria Condition of multiple pupils; true polycoria if surrounded with sphincter muscle.

precorneal tear film Layer of tears covering the anterior surface of the cornea.

presbyopia Refractive condition in which there is a diminished power of accommodation because of impaired elasticity of the crystallin lens, as occurs with aging.

prism Lens with converging sides that splits light into constituent colors and deflects light rays toward its base.

proptosis Forward displacement of any organ, specifically, protrusion of the eyeball(s).

prosthesis Artificial substitute for body part.

protanomaly form of anomalous trichromatism for which, in a red-green mixture, more than the normal amount of red is required than for a normal observer.

protanopia Form of dichromatism in which red and bluish-green are confused and relative luminosity of red is much lower than for a normal observer.

pseudoglioma Any intraocular opacity liable to be mistaken for retinoblastoma.

pseudoisochromatic plate Ishihara color plates.

pseudopapilledema Blurring of optic disk margins in hyperopia.

pseudostrabismus Appearance of crossed eyes caused by epicanthal folds or a visual axis not centered in the pupil.

pseudotumor Nonneoplastic progressive cellular proliferation.

pterygium Abnormality originating in the cornea in which a triangular patch of conjunctiva extends into the cornea; apex of the patch points toward the pupil.

pupil Aperture in the iris of the eye for the passage of light.

    Adie Abnormality in the reaction of the pupil to light and associated with hypotonic deep reflexes.

    Argyll Robertson Pupil that does not constrict to light but constricts to convergence; pupils are small, unequal in size, and irregular; seen mainly in tabes dorsalis.

    cat's eye Pupil with a white reflex when light is directed into it; most commonly associated with retinoblastoma.

    Marcus Gunn Unilateral afferent nerve pupillary defect.

pupillary membrane Anomaly of the iris, usually minor, in which the fetal pupillary membrane fails to atrophy; often a persistent strand extends between the iris collarette and the anterior lens capsule; a fibrovascular occlusion after surgery.

Purkinje image Reflected image from surface of cornea and anterior and posterior surfaces of crystalline lens.

Purkinje phenomenon If intensity of illumination is reduced in fields of equal brightness, green becomes brighter than other colors.

Purkinje shift Luminosity curve of dark-adapted individual peaks at 500 nm, whereas the luminosity curve of light-adapted individual peaks at 550 nm; indicates two types of retinal photoreceptors.

quadrantanopia Loss of one quadrant of the visual field; homonymous inferior considered pathognomonic parietal lobe involvement; homonymous superior vascular lesion of temporal loop of the visual radiation.

radiance and related terms Refer to physical aspects of energy.

radiant absorptance Ratio of absorbed radiant flux to incident flux.

radiant emittance Radiant flux emitted per unit area of a source.

radiant energy Energy being transferred, unaccompanied by transfer of matter.

radiant flux Rate of transfer of radiant energy.

radiant intensity Flux radiated per unit of solid angle.

radiant power Alternative term for radiant flux.

radiant reflectance Ratio of reflected radiant flux to incident flux.

red eye Lay term applied to any condition with dilation of conjunctival or ciliary blood vessels.

reflex Involuntary, invariable, adaptive response to a stimulus.

    accommodative Constriction of the pupils when the eyes converge for near vision; an associated reaction and not a reflex.

    auditory Brief closure of the eyelids resulting from a sudden sound.

    conjunctival (eyelid) Closure of the eyelids induced by touching the conjunctiva (also called corneal reflex).

    consensual light (crossed) Constriction of the pupil when the opposite retina is stimulated with light.

    direct light Contraction of the sphincter pupillae muscle induced by stimulation of the retina with light (also called pupillary reflex).

    eye compression (oculocardiac) Decrease of cardiac rate caused by pressure on the eye.

    fixation Direction of the eye so that an image remains on the fovea centralis of each eye.

    foveolar Bright dot of light originating from the foveola when an ophthalmoscope light is directed on the region of the fovea centralis.

    lacrimal Secretion of tears induced by irritation of the cornea and conjunctiva.

    red Red glow of light seen to emerge from the pupil when the interior of the eye is illuminated.

refraction Deviation of rays of light when passing from one transparent medium into another of a different density.

retinal detachment Separation of the sensory retina from the retinal pigment epithelium.

    combined Including choroid and retina.

    rhegmatogenous With hole formation.

    secondary Resulting from tumor.

    retinal hole Opening in the continuity of the sensory retina so that there is a communication between the vitreous cavity and the potential space between the sensory retina and the retinal pigment epithelium.

Appendices **567**

retinitis Inflammation of the retina.

retinoblastoma Malignant retinal tumor of infancy.

retinopathy Noninflammatory degenerations of the retina.

retinopexy Surgical procedure to correct retinal detachment by means of diathermy.

retinoschisis Retinal abnormality in which the sensory retina splits at the level of the inner plexiform layer.

retinoscopy Objective method of determining the refraction of the eye by observing the movements of the reflection of light from the eye (skiascopy).

retrobulbar neuritis Inflammation of the optic nerve occurring without involvement of the optic disk.

retrolental fibroplasia Retinopathy of prematurity; a condition of cicatricial neovascularization of the retina that occurs predominantly in infants who weigh less than 1,500 g at birth.

rhegmatogenous With hole formation.

rhodopsin Light-sensitive photopigment of rods.

rubeosis iridis Neovascularization of the iris.

saccadic movements Ocular rotation in ductions and versions.

salmon patch Central area of intense vascularization that occurs in interstitial keratitis as the result of the confluence of all blood vessels at the center of the cornea; also retinal hemorrhage in sickle cell disease.

Sattler veil Subepithelial corneal edema that occurs after prolonged wearing of a contact lens.

scintillating scotoma Unformed visual hallucination with flashing, bursting lights occurring in occipital lobe disorders, particularly migraine.

scleritis Inflammation of the sclera.

scleromalacia perforans Degenerative condition of the sclera in which localized rheumatoid nodules cause necrosis.

sclerosing keratitis Inflammation in which the cornea becomes white and opaque, resembling the sclera.

scotoma Area of blindness in the field of vision.

scotopic adaptation. Adaptation to low levels of luminance at which only rod vision is operative.

Seidel test Dilution of fluorescein on surface of eye caused by aqueous humor leaking through fistula.

siderosis Chronic inflammation of the eye caused by a retained iron foreign body within the eye.

skiascopy Retinoscopy.

slit lamp Biomicroscope.

Snell laws of refraction (1) The incident ray, the normal to the surface at the point of incident, and the refracted ray lie in one plane. (2) The sine of the angle of refraction bears a constant relation to the angle of incidence and the value of the ratio depends on the nature of the two media and the nature of the incident light.

Snellen letter Letter so constructed that at a given distance from the eye it subtends an angle of 5 minutes, with each portion of the letter subtending an angle of 1 minute.

specular microscopy Visualization of human corneal endothelium in reflected light.

spherical aberration Unequal refraction of light rays that pass through the center and periphery of the lens.

squamous blepharitis Seborrheic inflammation of the eyelid margins.

squint Cross-eyes (strabismus).

staphyloma Ectasia of the wall of the eye line with the uveal tract.

stereoscope An instrument providing two horizontally separated images of the same object to provide a single image with an appearance of depth.

Stiles-Crawford effect Light passing through the center of the pupil of the eye is more effective in evoking the sensation of brightness than the same amount of light passing through an equal area near the edge of the pupil.

strabismus Condition in which the eyes are not simultaneously directed to the same object.

    concomitant Deviation of the eye in which there is no ocular muscle paralysis and the degree of crossing is the same in all directions of gaze.

    nonconcomitant Deviation of the eyes from parallelism in which a muscle is paretic or paralytic.

sty Purulent inflammation of a gland of Zeis; hordeolum.

subconjunctival hemorrhage Bleeding beneath the conjunctiva, often occurring spontaneously.

subhyaloid hemorrhage Hemorrhage between the sensory retina and the vitreous body; a meniscus level is often present.

subluxation of lens Condition of the lens when a portion of the supporting zonule is absent and the lens lacks support in one or more quadrants.

suppression Physiologic mental process whereby the retinal image transmitted by one eye is ignored.

sursumversion Upward rotation of the eyes.

symblepharon Adhesion between the palpebral and bulbar conjunctivas.

sympathetic ophthalmia Granulomatous uveitis caused by perforating wound of the uvea followed by similar uveitis of the fellow eye; the eye secondarily affected is called the sympathizing eye, and the injured eye is called the exciting or activating eye.

synchysis Fluid condition of the vitreous body.

syndrome Group of symptoms and signs that occur together; disease or definite morbid process having a characteristic sequence of symptoms; may affect the whole body or any of its parts.

    A and V Cross-eyes in which the eyes are closer together in looking up than down (A) or closer looking down than up (V).

    Adie *See* pupil.

    Anton Form of anosognosia in which the patient denies his blindness; usually accompanied by confabulation, with the patient claiming to see objects in the blind field.

    Axenfeld anomaly Posterior corneal arcus, glaucoma (and hypertelorism).

syndrome—cont'd

Bassen-Kornzweig Progressive ataxic neuropathy associated with retinal pigmentary degeneration and a crenated appearance of erythrocytes (A-beta-lipoproteinemia).

Batten-Mayou Neuronal ceroid lipofuscinosis.

Behçet Aphthous ulcers (canker sores) of mouth and genitalia combined with uveitis, iritis, and hypopyon.

Benedikt Hemianesthesia and involuntary movements of a choreiform nature in the extremities on the side opposite the lesion in the medial lemniscus and region of the red nucleus.

Berlin disease Perimacular retinal edema following trauma (commotio retinae).

Best disease Autosomal dominant vitelliruptive central retinal degeneration characterized by a central retinal lesion with an ophthalmoscopic appearance of an egg fried "sunny side up" and associated in this stage with good vision; when egg is "scrambled," vision deteriorates.

Biedl-Bardet Autosomal recessive disorder of the pituitary gland characterized by girdle-type obesity, hypogenitalism, mental retardation, polydactyly, and pigmentary retinal degeneration.

Bielschowsky-Lutz-Cogan Internuclear ophthalmoplegia with medial rectus muscle paralysis for versions, intact convergence, and nystagmus of abducted eye.

Bourneville disease Mental deficiency, tuberous sclerosis, and adenoma sebaceum; glaucoma and conjunctival and retinal tumors may occur.

Bowen disease Intraepithelial epithelioma; when the eye is affected, it commonly involves the conjunctiva at the corneoscleral limbus in chronically irritated eyes.

Brown Contracture of superior oblique muscle with apparent paralysis of ipsilateral inferior oblique muscle.

cavernous sinus Thrombosis of the cavernous sinus with third, fourth, and sixth carnial nerve palsy, edema of the face and eyelids, and infection.

cerebellopontine angle tumor Ataxia, tinnitus, deafness, ipsilateral paralysis of the sixth and seventh cranial nerve, involvement of the fifth cranial nerve, vertigo, and nystagmus.

Chandler Iris atrophy, dystrophy of corneal endothelium, and secondary glaucoma.

Chédiak-Higashi disease Recessive albinism with leukocytic inclusions.

chiasmal Optic atrophy and bitemporal hemianopsia.

Coats disease Chronic progressive retinal abnormality characterized by retinal deposits and malformation of retinal blood vessels.

Cogan (1)Nonsyphilitic interstitial keratitis with associated nerve deafness. (2) Oculomotor apraxia with absence of voluntary ocular movements with full random movements. Fixation by jerky head movements with overshooting.

Cogan-Reese Iris nevi, iris atrophy, dystrophy of corneal endothelium.

Collins (Franceschetti) Mandibulofacial dysostosis.

crocodile tears Spontaneous lacrimation that occurs with the normal salivation of eating; follows facial nerve paralysis and is caused by aberrant regenerating nerve fibers so that some destined for the salivary glands go to the lacrimal gland.

Crouzon disease Craniofacial dysostosis with eyes widely separated.

Devic disease Subacute encephalomyopathy with severe demyelination of optic nerves.

Down Mental retardation with retarded growth, flat hypoplastic face, muscle hypotonia, and other abnormalities.

Doyne Autosomal dominant drusen of retinal pigment epithelium.

Duane retraction Narrowing of the palpebral fissure on the side on which the lateral rectus muscle is paralyzed when the patient looks toward the opposite side.

Eales disease Retinal phlebitis characterized by inflammation, occlusion, neovascularization, and recurrent retinal hemorrhages, occurring particularly in young men.

Ehlers-Danlos Widespread systemic disorder with overextensibility of joints, hyperelasticity of the skin, fragility of the skin, and pseudotumors following trauma; there may be epicanthal folds, esotropia, blue sclera, glaucoma, ectopic lenses, proliferating retinopathy, and acanthocytosis.

Fabry X chromosome-linked sphinogolipidosis with deficiency of α-galactosidase.

Foster Kennedy *See* syndrome, Kennedy.

Foville Paralysis of the limbs on one side of the body and of the face on the opposite side together with loss of power to rotate the eyes to that side.

Franceschetti (Collins) Mandibulofacial dysostosis.

François Dysephaly, microphthalmia, and cataract.

Fuchs Unilateral heterochromia, inflammation of the iris and ciliary body, and secondary cataract.

Gaucher disease Familial disorder characterized by splenomegaly, skin pigmentation, and pigmented pingueculas.

Goldenhar Mandibulofacial dysostosis with epibulbar dermoids and vertebral anomalies.

Gradenigo Palsy of the lateral rectus muscle (N VI) and severe unilateral headache in suppurative disease of the middle ear.

Graves disease Hyperthyroidism, goiter, and exophthalmos (Basedow, Parry).

Grönblad-Strandberg Angioid streaks of the fundus and pseudoxanthoma elasticum of the skin.

Gunn (Robert Marcus Gunn) (1) Unilateral blepharoptosis with marked opening of the eye during chewing. (2) Unilateral afferent pupillary defect.

Hallerman-Streiff Mandibulofacial dysostosis with microphthalmia and congenital cataract (François).

Hand-Schüller-Christian disease Insidious and progressive abnormality in children characterized by exophthalmos, diabetes insipidus, and softened areas in the bones, particularly in femurs and in bones of the skull, shoulder, and pelvic girdle.

Harada Vogt-Koyanagi syndrome combined with retinal detachment.

Heerfordt disease Uveitis, fever, and parotid gland swelling; now recognized as a manifestation of sarcoidosis.

hepatolenticular degeneration (Wilson) Abnormality of copper metabolism associated with progressive degeneration of the liver and lentate nucleus, mental retardation, and a brownish ring (Kayser-Fleischer) composed of copper at the periphery of the cornea.

Horner Sympathetic nerve paralysis with miosis, blepharoptosis, and anhydrosis of the face.

Hunter X chromosome-linked form of mucopolysaccharidosis (type MPS II) in which the corneas remain clear until the third decade.

Hurler (gargoylism) Autosomal recessive mucopolysaccharidosis (type MPS I H) characterized by dwarfism with short, kyphotic spinal column; short fingers; depression of bridge of the nose; heavy, ugly facies; stiffness of joint; cloudiness of the cornea; retinal degeneration; hepatosplenomegaly; and mental retardation.

Hutchinson (1) Interstitial keratitis, deafness, and notched, narrow-edged permanent incisors in congenital syphilis. (2) Neuroblastoma with orbital metastasis.

Irvine-Gass Cystoid central retinal edema with corneal-vitreous adhesions after cataract extraction.

Jensen disease Chorioretinitis adjacent to the optic disk (juxtapapillary).

Kearns-Sayre Ophthalmoplegia, pigmentary degeneration of retina, and cardiac conduction defect.

Kennedy (Foster Kennedy) Ipsilateral optic atrophy and contralateral papilledema in frontal lobe tumors, aneurysms, or abscesses.

Kimmelstiel-Wilson Hypertension, retinopathy, and intercapillary glomerulosclerosis in diabetes mellitus.

Kufs disease Late juvenile form of cerebromacular degeneration.

Leber Autosomal recessive congenital retinal degeneration.

Leber disease Retrobulbar neuritis and optic atrophy occurring at about 20 years of age in men.

Letterer-Siwe disease Nonfamilial reticuloendotheliosis of early childhood.

Lignac-Fanconi Cystinosis with renal rickets (Abderhalden–de Toni–Debré).

Lindau disease Angioma of the central nervous system, particularly in the cerebellum, and associated Lindau–von Hippel disease with angioma of the cerebellum, retina, pancreas, and kidney.

Louis-Bar Cerebellar ataxia with oculocutaneous telangiectasia.

Lowe Oculocerebrorenal X chromosome-linked glaucoma, cataract, growth and mental retardation, and aminoaciduria.

Marcus Gunn *See* syndrome, Gunn.

Marfan Spider fingers and toes (arachnodactyly), ectopia lentis, cardiovascular defects, and widespread defects of elastic tissue.

Marinesco-Sjögren Autosomal recessive stationary cerebellar ataxia, mental retardation, cataract, and oligophrenia.

Maroteaux-Lamy Mucopolysaccharidosis type MPS III.

Mikulicz Chronic lymphocytic infiltration and enlargement of the lacrimal and salivary glands (Sjögren).

milk-alkali Hypercalcemia induced by peptic ulcer management with milk and calcium carbonate.

Millard-Gubler Paralysis of sixth and seventh cranial nerves and contralateral hemiplegia of extremities.

Möbius (1)Migraine headache with recurrent oculomotor paralysis (ophthamoplegic migraine). (2) Bilateral lateral rectus and facial nerve paralysis.

morning glory Unilateral enlarged optic disk with funnel-shaped excavation and elevated peripapillary tissue annulus.

Morquio-Brailsford Mucopolysaccharidosis type MPS IV.

Neimann-Pick disease Heredofamilial lipid disorder mainly caused by sphingomyelinase deficiency.

Oguchi disease Autosomal recessive night blindness found almost exclusively in Japanese.

orbital apex Oculomotor paresis and neuralgia resulting from involvement of structures at the apex of the orbit by a tumor, often a neoplasm of the nasopharynx.

osteogenesis imperfecta (van der Hoeve) Bone fragility, blue sclera, and deafness.

Ota nevus Pigmented nevus of the eyelids, nose, and zygomatic and frontal regions.

Paget disease Bone thickening and thinning, sometimes with angioid streaks.

paratrigeminal (Raeder) Rare abnormality caused by a lesion of the semilunar ganglion and related sympathetic fibers from the carotid plexus; characterized by trigeminal neuralgia; often followed by sensory loss on the affected side of the face, weakness and atrophy of the muscles of mastication, miosis, and blepharoptosis.

Parinaud (1) Necrotic lesion of conjunctiva associated with palpable preauricular lymph nodes. (2) Paralysis of conjugate in upward gaze, usually associated with lesions at the level of the superior colliculi.

Peter anomaly Adherent corneal leukoma with absence of Descemet membrane and endothelium.

syndrome—cont'd

Posner-Schlossman Glaucomacyclitic crisis; recurrent cyclitis with glaucoma.

Purtscher disease Traumatic angiopathy of the retina.

Raeder *See* syndrome, paratrigeminal.

Recklinghausen disease Autosomal dominant neurofibromatosis.

Refsum disease (heredopathia atactica polyneuritiformis) Autosomal recessive pigmentary degeneration of the retina with polyneuritis, deafness, and cerebellar signs with excretion of phytanic acid.

Reiter disease Disease of males marked by initial diarrhea and followed by urethritis, conjunctivitis, and migratory polyarthritis.

Rieger Autosomal dominant mesodermal dysgenesis of the cornea and iris; corneal opacities, hypoplastic iris, iridotrabecular adhesions, and posterior corneal arcus occur.

Riley-Day (familial autonomic dysfunction) Reduced or absent tears, postural hypotension, excessive sweating, corneal anesthesia, exotropia, and absence of taste buds.

Rollet Orbital apex syndrome with involvement of the second, third, fourth, fifth, sixth, and sympathetic nerves.

Roth spot Retinal hemorrhage with white center in subacute bacterial endocarditis.

Rothmund (-Thomson; Bloch-Stauffer) Autosomal recessive congenital cataract with skin telangiectasis and pigmentation.

Sanfilippo Mucopolysaccaridosis type MPS III.

Scheie Mucopolysaccharidosis type MPS I S.

Sjögren Keratoconjunctivitis sicca, xerostomia, enlargement of the parotid gland, and polyarthritis.

Stargardt disease Fundus flavimaculatus with atrophic central retinal degeneration.

Stevens-Johnson Form of erythema multiforme characterized by constitutional symtoms and marked inflammation and later by scarring of the conjunctiva and oral mucosa.

Stilling-Duane-Türk Abnormality of ocular musculature innervation with absence of abduction combined with retraction of the globe and blepharoptosis on adduction.

Sturge-Weber-Dimitri disease Nervus flammeus (port wine), often associated with glaucoma.

Tay-Sachs disease Infantile amaurotic familial idiocy; a sphingolipidosis.

Usher Autosomal recessive pigmentary degeneration of the retina with nerve deafness.

vitreoretinal, familial, exudative Autosomal dominant peripheral pigmentary retinopathy, vascular abnormalities, choroidal atrophy, and vitreous opacities.

Vogt-Koyanagi Bilateral uveitis, poliosis, vitiligo, alopecia, and dysacousia.

Waardenburg-Klein Autosomal dominant hypertrophy of the root of the nose, heterochromia iridis, white forelock, and deafness.

Weill-Marchesani Short fingers and toes, compact body, glaucoma, and spherophakia.

Wilson Autosomal recessive deficiency of ceruloplasmin with cirrhosis of the liver, lenticular degeneration, and visible deposition of copper in the periphery of Descement membrane (Kayser-Fleischer ring).

synechiae Adhesions between the iris and adjacent structures.

anterior Adhesions between the iris and the cornea.

peripheral anterior Occurs with unrelieved attacks of angle-closure glaucoma; may occur following injury or surgery when the anterior chamber does not form.

posterior Adhesions between the iris and the lens as occur commonly in uveitis.

syneresis Concentration of particles of the dispersed phase of a gel with separation of the dispersed phase and shrinkage of the gel.

talbot Unit of light equal to one lumen-second

tangent screen Instrument used for the study of the field of vision within 30° of the fixation point; testing is carried out 1 or 2 m from the eye; called tangent because it would be tangent to the arc of a perimeter.

tapetoretinopathy Hereditary degeneration of the retinal pigment epithelium and sensory retina.

tarsorrhaphy Operation in which the eyelids are sutured together, as in lagophthalmos.

telecanthus Increased distance between medial canthi.

temporal arteritis Giant cell arteritis.

tension, ocular Resistance of coats of eye to deformation.

Terrien marginal degeneration Bilateral stromal degeneration of the cornea with gutter formation followed by ectasia.

Thygesson superficial punctate keratitis Bilateral, coarse, multiple, transient epithelial opacities of cornea.

tonography Test to determine the volume of fluid forced from the eye by a constant pressure during a constant period.

tonometer Instrument for measuring ocular tension.

torsion Rotation of eye about its anteroposterior axis.

trabeculectomy A filtering operation for glaucoma by creation of a fistula between the anterior chamber of the eye and the subconjunctival space, through a subscleral excision of a portion of the trabecular meshwork.

trachoma Cicatrizing conjunctivitis caused by *Chlamydia trachomatis*.

TRIC agents Acronym for *trachoma* and *inclusion conjunctivitis*, members of the psitacosis–lymphogranuloma venereum–trachoma *(Chlamydia)* group of microorganisms.

trichiasis Condition in which there are ingrown eyelashes.

tritanopia Form of dichromatism in which there are only two cone pigments present and there is a complete insensitivity to blue.

tropia Strabismus.

Uthoff sign Weakness with warming of the body in multiple sclerosis.

uveitis Inflammation of the uveal tract.

vergence Binocular disjunctive rotations of the eyes as in convergence and divergence.

vernal conjunctivitis Anaphylactic hypersensitivity (Type I) of the conjunctiva characterized by giant papillary hypertrophy of the conjunctiva.

version Binocular conjugate movements of the eyes.

VISC Acronym for *v*itreous *i*nfusion *s*uction *c*utter used in vitreous surgery.

vision

  binocular Faculty of using both eyes synchronously, with diplopia.

  color Ability to distinguish subjectively a large variety of wavelengths of light in the visible spectrum.

  iridescent Perception of colored halos around light; occurs because of corneal edema particularly in glaucoma.

  mesopic Vision in illumination between photopic and scotopic ranges.

  photopic Vision in bright illumination.

  scotopic Vision in dim illumination or vision following the biochemical or neurologic changes occurring in dark adaptation.

  stereoscopic Vision in which objects are perceived in three dimensions.

visual angle Angle that an object or detail subtends at the point of observation; usually measured in minutes of arc.

visual axis Straight line connecting an object seen with the foveola.

visual field Locus of objects or points in space that can be perceived when the head and eyes are kept fixed; the field may be monocular or binocular.

visual line Line that connects a point in space with the fovea centralis.

visuscope Ophthalmoscope that projects a pattern that the patient fixates for diagnosis of eccentric fixation.

vitelliform degeneration Autosomal dominant retinal degeneration (Best).

vitrectomy Surgical removal of the vitreous.

closed Through pars plana incision.

open Through corneoscleral limbal incision.

Vossius lenticular ring Pigment on anterior lens capsule after contusion of eye.

xanthelasma Flat, sharply circumscribed deposits of lipid in the eyelids, sometimes associated with hypercholesterolemia.

xerophthalmia Dryness of conjunctiva and cornea in vitamin A deficiency.

xerosis Abnormal dryness.

yellow spot Term applied to macula lutea.

yoke muscles Muscles of the eys that function in rotations in the same direction.

zonulolysis Dissolution of the zonule by α-chymotrypsin in intracapsular cataract extraction.

B

A NOTE ON GENERAL REFERENCES

The *American Journal of Ophthalmology*, the *Archives of Ophthalmology*, the *British Journal of Ophthalmology*, and *Ophthalmology* provide current discussion of many clinical conditions. The *Transactions of the American Ophthalmological Society* and the *Transactions of the Ophthalmological Societies of the United Kingdom* are clinically oriented. *Investigative Ophthalmology and Visual Science* and *Experimental Eye Research* contain more basic studies.

The normal eye and the diseased eye are richly described in many monographs, textbooks, and multivolume works. Duane's looseleaf *Clinical Ophthalmology* (five volumes), Duke-Elder's *System of Ophthalmology* (fifteen volumes), Harley's *Pediatric Ophthalmology* (two volumes), and Miller's revision of *Walsh and Hoyt's Clinical Neuro-Ophthalmology* (two volumes) are comprehensive. Duane and Jaeger's looseleaf *Biomedical Foundations of Ophthalmology* (three volumes) and Davson's *Physiology of the Eye* (six volumes) provide extensive basic material. Spencer's *Pathology of the Eye* (three volumes), Yanoff and Fine's *Ocular Pathology*, and Garner and Klintworth's *Pathobiology of Ocular Disease* (two volumes) are standard sources.

Reviews are published in the *Survey of Ophthalmology* and in *International Ophthalmology Clinics*. The theses of candidates for membership in the American Ophthalmological Society often provide comprehensive reviews. The annual publications of the meetings of the New Orleans Academy of Ophthalmology and the Bascom Palmer Eye Institute contain surveys of general ophthalmology topics and reports of neuro-ophthalmology topics.

Abstracts of ophthalmic reports are available in the *American Journal of Ophthalmology*, *Excerpta Medica*, and *Ophthalmic Literature*. Indexes of the *American Journal of Ophthalmology* appeared in 1953, 1963, 1973, 1978, and 1983, and another is scheduled for 1988. The *Year Book of Ophthalmology* abstracts recent literature and provides comments. The *Medical Letter on Drugs and Therapeutics* provides current authoritative commentary. The Medline system, of course, is unexcelled as a key to both refereed and nonrefereed medical publications.

C

CENTRAL VISUAL ACUITY: DISTANCE, SNELLEN

Feet	Meters	Reduced	Percent loss of central vision
20/16	6/5	1.2	0
20/20	6/6	1.0	0
20/25	6/7.5	0.8	5
20/30	6/9	0.66	9
20/40	6/12	0.5	15
20/50	6/15	0.4	25
20/60	6/18	0.33	35
20/80	6/24	0.25	40
20/100	6/30	0.2	50
20/200	6/60	0.1	80
20/300	6/90	0.066	85
20/400	6/120	0.05	90
20/800	6/240	0.025	95

Conversion factors to obtain SI Units		Conversion Factor to Give cd m^{-2}
Unit	Geometry	Multiply Column Units By
Candela per meter squared (nit or meter-candle)	$1\ cd\ m^{-2}$	1
Lambert	$(1/\pi)\ cd\ cm^{-2}$	3183
Millilambert	$10^{-3}\ (1/\pi)\ cd\ cm^{-2}$	3.183
Stilb	$1\ cd\ cm^{-2}$	10,000
Apostilb	$(1/\pi)\ cd\ m^{-2}$	0.3183
Footlambert	$(1/\pi)\ cd\ ft^{-2}$	3.4258

D

COMMON OPHTHALMIC ABBREVIATIONS

+	Convex lens	I	Luminous intensity
−	Concave lenx	ICCE	Intracapsular cataract extraction
Δ	Prism diopters	IOL	Intraocular lens
A	Ocular tension by Goldmann applanation tonometer; initial negative deflection of electroretinogram; accommodation	IOP	Intraocular pressure
		J-1	Jaeger test type number 1
		K	In optics, coefficient of scleral rigidity
AC	Anterior chamber	K	Refractive power of cornea
AC/A	Accommodative convergence/accommodation ratio	KP	Keratitic precipitates
		LE	Left eye
Acc	Accommodation	LP/DT	Light-peak/dark-trough ratio
ARC	Abnormal retinal correspondence; anomalous retinal correspondence	LPerc	Light perception
		LProj	Light projection
Ax	Axis of cylindrical lens	NLP	No light perception
B	Large positive defection of electroretinogram; base of prism	NPA	Near point accommodation
		NPC	Near point convergence
C	Coefficient of facility of outflow in tonography; cylinder	OD	Oculus dexter: right eye
		OS	Oculus sinister: left eye
cc	Cum correction (with lenses)	OU	Oculi uterque: both eyes
CF	Counting fingers	PC	Posterior chamber
cyl	Cylindrical lens	PD	Interpupillary distance; prism diopters
D	Diopter; dextro: right	P_o	Intraocular pressure
DA	Dark adaptation	RE	Right eye
dd	Disk diameters (1.5 mm)	S	Spherical lens; sinister: left
E	Esophoria for distance	SC	Sine correction (without lenses)
E′	Esophoria for near	TT	Tactile tension of eye
ECCE	Extracapsular cataract extraction	VA	Visual acuity (without correction)
EOG	Electro-oculography	VA_{cc}	Visual acuity with correction
EOM	Extraocular muscles; extraocular movements	VA_{ph}	Visual acuity with pinhole
		VA_{sc}	Visual acuity without correction
ERG	Electroretinography	VEP	Visual-evoked potential
ET	Esotropia for distance	X	Exophoria distance
ET′	Esotropia for near	X′	Exophoria near
FC	Finger counting	XT	Exotropia distance
HM	Hand movements	XT′	Exotropia near
HT	Hypertropia	YAG	Acronym for yttrium-aluminum-garnet

E

CASE STUDIES

CASE ONE

A 49-year-old woman who wears a biofocal correction to correct a moderately severe myopia (-6.00 diopters) and presbyopia states that one week ago there was a sudden shower of floaters in the left eye. Initially these caused no difficulty, but during the past 24 hours she has noticed that her left nasal field is restricted. She feels that her nose has suddenly become extremely large.

Examination

- *Visual acuity, with correction:* R.E., 20/20, 4 pt. L.E., 20/20, 4 pt.
- *External eye:* Normal. Pupils react normally to light.
- *Confrontation field:* Indicates a field defect in the left nasal visual field.
- *Ophthalmoscopy:* Through the dilated pupil the optic disk is normal. The temporal retina appears grayish and with small folds. The arteries and veins have the same color.

Diagnosis

- Left retinal detachment.

Treatment

- Surgical repair.

Comment

The initial shower of particles were erythrocytes freed in the vitreous humor as traction by a vitreous attachment opened in the retina. Fluid gradually collected beneath the sensory retina, causing a rhegmatogenous (with hole)

retinal detachment. The fovea centralis is still attached, so central vision is not affected.

The differential diagnosis involves a solid retinal detachment resulting from a malignant melanoma of the choroid that would likely not be preceded by a vitreous traction. It would appear brownish and likely have a much longer history of visual difficulty. A branch arterial or venous obstruction of a temporal artery or vein would diminish vision in the nasal visual field. These are unlikely in an individual who does not have vascular hypertension or valvular heart disease, or does not use oral contraceptives.

CASE TWO

A 21-year-old college student awakens suddenly with severe pain in each eye. The pain is so severe that his roommate must lead him into the emergency room.

Examination

- *Visual acuity:* Cannot open eyes to measure.
- *External:* Eyes squeezed closed; externally normal, much tearing.
- *Corneas:* Rapid glimpse, seem clear.
- *Local anesthetic instilled:* Pain relieved; visual acuity: R.E., 20/25, L.E., 20/25. Mild conjunctival injection.
- *Sterile fluorescein:* Punctate staining of cornea.
- *Further history:* Uses sunlamp intermittently.

Diagnosis

- Ultraviolet keratitis.

Treatment

- Patch both eyes until comfortable. Sulfacetamide drops may be used prophylactically. Usually the eyes are comfortable within 24 hours.

Comment

Ultraviolet burns are cumulative on the external eye as on the skin. Unwise exposure can cause keratitis.

CASE THREE

A 42-year-old man wears contact lenses for cosmetic reasons. He developed a red painful left eye 24 hours earlier.

Examination

- *Visual acuity with correction:* R.E., 20/30, 4 pt. L.E., 20/30, 4 pt.
- *External:* R.E., normal. L.E., slight ciliary injection.
- *Sterile fluorescein:* Small, sharply demarcated staining area, central cornea.
- *Pupils:* React normally to light.
- *Tension:* Not done.
- *Ocular movements:* Normal.

Diagnosis

- Keratitis, left eye; possibly secondary contact lens trauma.

Treatment

- Discontinue contact lens wear, left eye. Patch eye (remove patch if more comfortable with eye open). Instill topical 10% sulfacetamide drops every 2 hours.

Comment

A common occurrence, usually entirely amenable to treatment. Exception: Forty-eight hours later the eye is more painful. The staining area has increased in size, it has a white infiltrate, and the eye is violently red. An ophthalmic emergency. Get help. Gram stain of ulcer exudate and culture. Treatment every hour based initially on Gram stain and the results of a culture.

CASE FOUR

A 38-year-old office worker complained that since morning, when he walked to work, he had discomfort and watering in his right eye.

Examination

- *Visual acuity:* R.E., 20/20. L.E., 20/20.
- *External:* R.E., conjunctival injection and tearing. L.E., normal.
- *Pupils:* Reactive.
- *Ocular movements:* Normal.
- *Fluorescein:* No corneal staining.
- *Topical anesthetic:* Complete relief.

Diagnosis

- Foreign body in right eye.

Treatment

- Upper eyelid everted and cinder found on tarsal plate. Wiped off with moist cotton-tipped applicator.

Comment

This is a common ocular emergency. Remember to have the cotton-tipped applicator ready when eyelid is everted, since the foreign body may migrate and be difficult to locate if the eyelid is released.

CASE FIVE

A healthy 66-year-old man, with a history of glaucoma well controlled with medication, complained of visual decrease caused by pupillary constriction from the pilocarpine medication.

Examination

- *Visual acuity:* R.E., 20/30. L.E., 20/30.
- *External:* Conjunctiva, cornea, extraocular movements, normal. Pupils, pinpoint; cannot see reaction to light.
- *Ophthalmoscopy:* Cannot see details through miotic pupils.
- *Tension:* Seems soft.

Treatment

- Timolol 0.50% twice daily was substituted for pilocarpine.

Course

- *Four days later:* Occasional diplopia at end of the day.

Examination

- *Visual acuity:* R.E., 20/20. L.E., 20/20.
- *External:* Pupils do not react.
- *Ophthalmoscopy:* Optic disk normal.
- *Ocular movements:* Normal.

Course

- *Two months later:* Constant diplopia; drooping of eyelids; frequent deep inspiration.

Examination

- As before, possibly ocular movements less full. Testing with edrophonium chloride momentarily improved the blepharoptosis. The acetylcholine receptor antibody level was 4.0 nmol (normal range, 0.00 to 1.0 nmol).

Diagnosis

- Myasthenia gravis aggravated by timolol administration.

Comment

Timolol is a rare cause of extraocular motility problems, precipitation of myasthenia gravis, and aggravation of pulmonary insufficiency. All unexpected complaints of patients receiving timolol should be investigated.

Coppeo, J.R.: Timolol-associated myasthenia gravis, Am. J. Ophthalmol. **98:**244, 1984.

CASE SIX

A 74-year-old man complained of irritated and burning eyes for several months. Treatment at home with topical sulfisoxazole (Gantrisin) resulted in slight improvement in the symptoms.

Examination

- *Visual acuity:* Pinhole, R.E., 20/40. L.E., 20/30.
- *External:* Scurf and sleeving of eyelashes; thickening of eyelid margins. Cornea clear; moderate conjunctival injection. Pupils react to light.
- *Ocular movements:* Full.
- *Tactile tension:* Soft eyes.
- *Ophthalmoscopy:* Normal.
- *Fluorescein staining:* Diffuse punctate staining of the cornea.

Culture

- Cultures of the conjunctiva grew *Staphylococcus epidermidis* resistant to penicillin, methicillin, and ampicillin and sensitive to cephalosporins, gentamicin, chloramphenicol, erythromycin, and clindamycin.

Diagnosis

- *Staphylococcus epidermidis* blepharitis.

Treatment

- Topical gentamicin 0.3% instilled four times daily. Eyelid cleansing with cotton-tipped applicators moistened with baby shampoo twice daily and warm soaks twice daily. Ten days later the eyelid symptoms were markedly improved.

Comment

Chronic blepharitis may cause persistent ocular irritation. Usually, mechanical cleaning of the eyelid margins is required in addition to effective local antibacterial treatment.

Kahn, J.A., Hoover, D., and Ide, C.H.: Methicillin-resistant *Staphylococcus epidermidis* blepharitis, Am. J. Ophthalmol. **98:**562, 1984.

CASE SEVEN

A 61-year-old woman mentioned that, after watching television in the evening, she had a dull, ocular discomfort and slight blurring of vision. She fell asleep promptly and woke without discomfort. She did not have symptoms when she watched television during the day.

Examination

- *Visual acuity:* R.E., 20/20. L.E., 20/20.
- *External:* Conjunctiva and cornea normal; pupils round and react promptly to light; possibly anterior chamber is shallow.
- *Ocular movements:* Normal.
- *Tactile tension:* Eyes soft.
- *Ophthalmoscopy:* Normal.

Treatment

- Suggest ophthalmic consultation. Possible closed-angle glaucoma.

Consultant's report

When the patient rested for 45 minutes with her head and hands on a table in front of her, the pressure in each eye increased from 18 to 29 mm Hg. Gonioscopy indicated that the anterior chamber angle was closed. You concur in the recommendation for an argon laser iridotomy to relieve a closed-angle mechanism.

After the iridotomy in each eye, the patient reported that headaches no longer occurred in the evening after watching television.

Comment

The pupillary dilation that occurs in semidarkness may cause closed-angle glaucoma with ocular discomfort. The patient might also see halos around lights, caused by corneal edema. The corneal edema also reduces vision. With sleep, the pupils become constricted and the attack is relieved. The head forward in the prone position is an excellent test for closed-angle glaucoma, as is a 45-minute stay in a dark room. A combination of the two is additionally effective (be certain the patient does not sleep and cause pupillary constriction). Halos around lights occur with minor forms of cataract (usually this is combined with multiple images at the source of light).

CASE EIGHT

A 65-year-old construction foreman complained of a nodule of the left lower eyelid that had been present for 3 months. There were no other complaints related to the eyes.

Examination

- *Visual acuity, corrected:* R.E., 20/20, 4 pt. L.E., 20/20, 4 pt.
- *External:* 9 mm nodular mass with central ulceration orbital portion left lower eyelid.
- *Tension Schiøtz:* R.E., 17 mm Hg. L.E., 18 mm Hg.
- *Pupils:* Round, equal, react to light.
- *Ocular movements:* Normal.
- *Ophthalmoscopy:* Normal.

Diagnosis

- Tumor left lower eyelid.

Treatment

- Wide excision.

Histologic diagnosis

- Adenoid squamous cell carcinoma.

Comment

Clinically, adenoid squamous cell carcinoma has no distinctive features and may resemble keratocanthoma, basal cell carcinoma, and squamous cell carcinoma. The tumor occurs mainly in white, fair-skinned, elderly men who have outdoor activities and occupations. The diagnosis must be established by microscopic examination. The differential diagnosis involves solar keratosis as well as basal cell and squamous cell carcinoma. Local excision usually suffices for treatment.

Caya, J.G., Hidayat, A.A., and Weiner, J.M.: A clinicopathologic study of 21 cases of adenoid squamous cell carcinoma of the eyelid and periorbital region, Am. J. Ophthalmol. **99**:291, 1985.

CASE NINE

A 67-year-old man was operated on 5 years previously for open-angle glaucoma. Ocular pressures had been well controlled thereafter with timolol 0.5% twice daily. Three days before he was seen the right eye became swollen and teared. The next day vision decreased and the eye was painful.

Examination

- *Visual acuity:* R.E., light perception, no projection. L.E., corrected to 20/20, 4 pt.
- *External:* R.E., Eyelids: swollen red, mucous on eyelashes. Cornea: edematous and cloudy. Filtering bleb pus-filled. Severe conjunctival and ciliary injection.
- *Tension:* Not done.
- *Pupils:* R.E., seen with difficulty; questionable reaction to light. L.E., normal reaction to light; no consensual reaction. R.E., stimulation.
- *Ophthalmoscopy:* R.E., faint red light reflex; no details. L.E., normal.

Diagnosis

- Right endophthalmitis.

Treatment

- Patient was hospitalized and vitreous and aqueous humor removed for culture. Gentamicin, clindamycin, and dexamethasone were used intravitreally. The patient received intravenous gentamicin and clindamycin orally. Topical gentamicin and cefazolin eyedrops were also started.

Comment

Thin-walled cystic blebs after filtering surgery for glaucoma may provide an entry for pathogenic organisms. Other factors that may contribute to the development of endophthalmitis are contact lenses, hypotony, and trauma to the bleb. Early diagnosis and treatment are essential if the eye is to be saved. High doses of antibiotics and corticosteroids should be administered simultaneously by systemic, intravitrealy, and subconjunctival routes. Intravitreal cultures should be obtained before therapy as they are much more adequate in identifying the causative organism than either aqueous or conjunctival cultures.

Lobue, T.D., Deutsch, T.A., and Stein, R.M.: *Moraxella nonliquefaciens* endophthalmitis after trabeculectomy, Am. J. Ophthalmol. **99**:343, 1985.

CASE TEN

Saturday evening a 25-year-old man in previous good health complains of a sudden onset of double vision. This disappeared when he developed a bilateral blepharoptosis, more marked on the right side. Additionally, he has difficulty in swallowing, generalized weakness, and increasing difficulty in speaking.

Examination

- *Visual acuity with correction:* R.E., 20/20, no J. L.E., 20/20, no J.
- *External:* R.E. and L.E. blepharoptosis and ophthalmoplegia. Pupils dilated and do not react to light. No convergence.
- *Ophthalmoscopy:* Normal.
- *Confrontation visual fields:* Normal.
- *Physical examination:* Temperature, pulse, blood pressure, normal. Questionable weakness of extremities. Two hours later a descending symmetrical motor paralysis was evident.

Diagnosis

Botulism is characterized by an onset with diplopia, dry mouth, blurred vision, dysphagia, or dysphonia. There may be other cranial nerve dysfunction, extremity weakness, or respiratory failure. Onset with ocular signs is predictive of respiratory failure.

Treatment

If food was recently ingested, remove unabsorbed toxin from gastrointestinal tract, using ipecac (30 to 45 ml) as an emetic and magnesium sulfate as a cathartic. Administer antitoxin. Hospitalize in intensive care unit with arrangements for mechanical respirator and tracheotomy, if necessary.

Before antitoxin administration, obtain 30 ml of blood in a vacutainer tube. Culture bowel contents.

Comment

Sudden onset of diplopia, bilateral ocular muscle weakness, pupillary signs, and blepharoptosis would originate only with a bilateral brain-stem lesion that would have additional CNS signs, probably including coma. The signs of a cerebrovascular accident would be unilateral. Myasthenia gravis would not have such a sudden widespread onset. Atropine poisoning has a rapid onset, facial flushing, and fever. Mushroom poisoning causes severe abdominal pain, violent vomiting, diarrhea, and coma. Guillain-Barré syndrome has an ascending paralysis, and cranial nerve signs are late.

Donadio, J.A., Gangaros, E.J., and Faich, G.A.: Diagnosis and treatment of botulism, J. Infect. Dis. **124**:108, 1971.
MacDonald, K.L., Spengler, R.F., Hatheway, C.L., Hargrett, N.T., and Cohen, M.L.: Type A botulism from sauteed onions, J.A.M.A. **253**:1275, 1985.

CASE ELEVEN

A 67-year-old professor noted flashing lights in the periphery of vision several times each month. The lights are present in both eyes and with the eyes open or closed. At the onset the lights are so slight as to be almost unnoticeable, but then they become brighter, larger, and interfere with reading. They disappear over a period of 15 to 20 minutes. They are unrelated to his activities and are not followed by headache or any other ocular or neurologic disturbance.

Examination

- *Visual acuity with correction:* R.E., 20/20. L.E., 20/20.
- *External:* Ocular movements, normal. External eyes, normal. Pupils react promptly to light.
- *Ophthalmoscopy:* Normal.
- *Ocular tension:* Normal.

Diagnosis

- Visual hallucination.

Treatment

- Reassurance.

Comment

This is probably a mild, transient ischemic attack or migraine without headache. The attacks appear to be without significance.

CASE TWELVE

A 46-year-old woman noticed the sudden appearance of a translucent object in her field of vision. She described it as being comma-shaped and as she turns her eye to fix on it, it darts away. It is best noticed against the blue sky.

Examination

- *Visual acuity:* R.E. 20/20. L.E., 20/20.
- *External:* Conjunctiva and cornea, normal. Ocular movements, normal. Pupils react promptly to light.
- *Ophthalmoscopy:* Normal.
- *Ocular tension:* Normal.
- *Mydriacyl instilled for pupillary dilation:* A small, translucent floater is seen in the vitreous.

Diagnosis

- Detachment of the vitreous.

Treatment

- Reassurance. Although the floater will not disappear, it impinges less on the consciousness with passing time.

Comment

Vitreous detachment is a common phenomenon that probably results from dehydration of the vitreous. It tends to be bilateral within 6 months.

CASE THIRTEEN

A 72-year-old woman is told by a companion that her right eye is brilliantly red. Inspection indicates a bright red dot on the temporal side. There are no symptoms.

Examination

- *Visual acuity:* R.E., 20/20. L.E., 20/20.
- *External:* A bright red dot, measuring approximately 6 mm in diameter, is present beneath the conjunctiva of the right eye. It looks like a drop of blood. Results of examination are otherwise normal.

Diagnosis

- Subconjunctival hemorrhage.

Treatment

- There is no treatment. The blood absorbs spontaneously.

Comment

A subconjunctival hemorrhage is caused by the same process as a black-and-blue spot elsewhere in the body. Generally it is of no significance and the patient should be reassured.

CASE FOURTEEN

A routine examination of a 3-month-old infant indicates the right eye to be strongly deviated inward. The mother states that the eyes have never been straight and that the right eye has always turned inward.

Examination

- *Vision:* The child appears bright and alert and seems to see adequately with the left eye. Vision cannot be measured in the right eye.
- *External:* The eyes appear normal. The pupils react. One cannot be certain that lateral rotation of the right eye is full.
- *Ophthalmoscopy:* Difficult, but there appears to be a red reflex in each eye.

Diagnosis

- Right esotropia.

Treatment

- The child requires ophthalmic examination with pupillary dilation to exclude intraocular disorders. In the event that the eyes are normal except for the strabismus, corrective surgery will likely be recommended at age about 6 months. Usually bilateral medial rectus muscle recessions are carried out. If the squint is severe, a right lateral rectus muscle resection will be added.

Thereafter the child will be treated by occlusion of the left eye, if necessary, to prevent the development of strabismic amblyopia or to correct it if it is already present.

CASE FIFTEEN

A 36-year-old obese man was seen because of fatigue and loss of weight. Physical examination is essentially normal, but laboratory studies establish a type II diabetes. Despite adequate weight reduction and dietary modification, he requires insulin.

Examination

- *Visual acuity:* R.E., 20/20. L.E., 20/20.
- *External:* Normal.
- *Ophthalmoscopy:* Normal.

Ophthalmic diagnosis:

- Normal eyes.

Comment

Many ophthalmologists believe that annual examination is desirable to observe the earliest signs of development of diabetic retinopathy. Many believe that routine fluorescein angiography of each eye is desirable. Visual acuity should be maintained at the best level possible and, if retinopathy develops, photocoagulation may be necessary.

CASE SIXTEEN

A preschool examination in a 5-year-old girl indicated a healthy child.

Ocular examination

- *Visual acuity:* R.E., 20/20. L.E., 20/80.
- *External:* Conjunctiva and cornea are clear. Pupils react normally to light.
- *Ophthalmoscopy;* The disks appear normal.

Diagnosis

- Reduced vision, left eye.

Treatment

- Complete ocular examination is required, using a cycloplegic. Amblyopia appears likely. If the eyes appear grossly normal, it is possible that on cover test a microtropia is present (no correctional movement when a 5-diopter prism is placed in front of ei-

ther eye). Treatment consists of optical correction, if necessary, combined with patching of the right eye to force use of the left eye.

Comment

Ideally, every child should have vision tested after about the age of 3 years. Amblyopia becomes more difficult to correct with increasing years and may be impossible to correct after the seventh year.

CASE SEVENTEEN

A 44-year-old woman mentioned in passing that she is unable to read the telephone book in a telephone booth and she seems to require increasingly bright lights to read. She has never worn glasses and has no other complaints related to her eyes.

Examination

- *Visual acuity:* R.E., 20/20, Jaeger 4 pt. L.E., 20/20, 4 pt.
- *External:* Normal. Pupils react normally to light.
- *Ophthalmoscopy:* No abnormality.

Diagnosis

- Hyperopia and presbyopia.

Treatment

- Correction of refractive error.

Comment

Difficulty in reading, the need for bright illumination to read, and a receding region of comfortable reading all suggest hyperopia combined with presbyopia. This is common after age 40; the age of onset is often directly related to the severity of the hyperopia. Symptoms occur somewhat later in life in individuals with myopia. Often they compensate by reading without correction.

CASE EIGHTEEN

A 28-year-old man complained of chronically red eyes. He has used a variety of eyedrops and has been examined twice by ophthalmologists without effective medication being prescribed. He was treated at age 22 for gonorrhea but has been in otherwise good health.

Examination

- *Visual acuity:* R.E., 20/20. L.E., 20/20.
- *External:* Diffuse conjunctival injection of each eye. Eversion of the lower eyelids indicates small, translucent, tapioca-like swellings along the lower tarsal plate. Corneas are clear. Pupils react promptly to light.
- *Ophthalmoscopy:* Fundus appears normal.

Diagnosis

- A chronic inflammation of the conjunctiva is strongly suggestive of a chlamydial infection. The urethra should be studied for *Chlamydia trachomatis.*

Treatment

- Treatment consists of systemic and ocular instillation of tetracycline ointment. Treatment may be necessary for several weeks. Repeated reinfection is possible, and sexual contacts must also be vigorously treated.

Comment

Chronic inflammation of the conjunctiva should be distinguished from inflammation of the eyelid margins. Consistent conjunctival inflammation with follicles of the conjunctiva of the lower eyelid is strongly suggestive of inclusion conjunctivitis. Trachoma involves the upper eyelid initially and is a curiosity in the United States. Other chronic inflammations are vernal conjunctivitis (seasonal, severe itching) and herpes simplex (intermittent, corneal).

CASE NINETEEN

A mother complained that the right eye of an 8-week-old infant has begun to tear. Examination indicates a healthy child with no apparent ocular abnormality. The mother is reassured, but 6 weeks later returns, stating that there is an intermittent discharge from the right eye.

Examination

- *External:* Pressure over the right medial canthus causes regurgitation of pus.

Diagnosis

- Infantile dacryocystitis.

Treatment

- Instillation of a mild ophthalmic drop or ointment, such as erythromycin, will minimize infection. Daily massage of the lacrimal sac will prevent accumulation of pus. Usually opening is spontaneous before the sixth month. If not, I prefer to open the sac by probing at this time. Many ophthalmologists prefer to defer it a year or even later.

Comment

The lacrimal system is not canalized until shortly after birth, and lacrimal secretion does not begin until after birth. Usually the lacrimal system opens spontaneously, but, if occluded, a dacryocystitis may occur.

CASE TWENTY

A 9-year-old girl in fifth grade complained of her eyes being stuck together in the morning. There are not other ocular complaints.

Examination

- *Visual acuity:* R.E., 20/20. L.E., 20/20.
- *External:* Mild conjunctival injection of each eye. The eyelashes are slightly agglutinated. There is no preauricular adenopathy. The corneas are clear. The pupils react normally.

Diagnosis

- Conjunctivitis.

Treatment

- The cause is probably infectious. Be careful of instruments, towels, and one's own hands and those of office staff. Warn the parents of contamination. Instruct the child to use separate washcloths and towels and not to touch siblings. Do not allow the child to attend school until eyes clear. Instill an ophthalmic antibiotic, such as gentamicin or neosporin, every 2 hours. Instill an ophthalmic antibiotic at bedtime to prevent the eyelids from being stuck together.

Comment

The absence of preauricular adenopathy tends to eliminate the diagnosis of adenovirus inflammation.

INDEX